D0566271

APHASIOLOGY

APHASIOLOGY

DISORDERS AND CLINICAL PRACTICE

G. ALBYN DAVIS

University of Massachusetts, Amherst

ALLYN AND BACON

Boston London Toronto Sydney Tokyo Singapore

Executive Editor: Stephen D. Dragin
Vice President, Editor in Chief: Paul A. Smith
Editorial Assistant: Bridget McSweeney
Marketing Manager: Brad Parkins
Editorial Production Service: Bernadine Richey Publishing Services
Manufacturing Buyer: David Repetto
Cover Administrator: Jennifer Hart
Electronic Composition: Omegatype Typography, Inc.

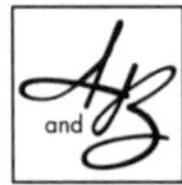

Copyright © 2000 by Allyn & Bacon
A Pearson Education Company
160 Gould Street
Needham Heights, MA 02494

All rights reserved. No part of the material protected by this copyright notice may be reproduced or utilized in any form or by any means, electronic or mechanical, including photocopying, recording, or by any information storage and retrieval system, without written permission from the copyright holder.

Internet: www.abacon.com

Library of Congress Cataloging-in-Publication Data

Davis, G. Albyn (George Albyn), 1946–
Aphasiology : disorders and clinical practice / G. Albyn Davis.
p. ; cm.
Includes bibliographical references and index.
ISBN 0-205-29834-6 (hardcover)
1. Aphasia. 2. Language disorders. I. Title.
[DNLM: 1. Aphasia. WL 340.5 D261a 1999]
RC425 .D379 1999
616.85'52—dc21

99-044519

Printed in the United States of America

10 9 8 7 6 5 4 04 03

To Dr. Audrey Holland

Contents

Preface

Aphasiology: Disorders and Clinical Practice began as a comprehensive overhaul of *A Survey of Adult Aphasia and Related Language Disorders* published in 1993. Everything was rewritten, and the new book took on a life of its own.

Some of the modifications are organizational. The previous two chapters on assessment were reduced to one, which was moved forward for early clinical emphasis. Now, many supplemental tests are introduced as extensions of research in other chapters. Background on cognition and psycholinguistics is integrated into presentation of disorders. Information about pragmatics is combined into single chapters on disabilities and treatment. A richer presentation of closed head injury has its own chapter. In general, literature review has been sacrificed for an attempt to be instructive about basic concepts. Reporting every study is replaced by illustrating with key examples.

This book retains *Survey*'s attempt to present a comprehensive and balanced knowledge base of experimental and clinical information. *Aphasiology*'s psycholinguistic orientation should not be considered to be a peculiar, idiosyncratic approach. Rather, it is an attempt to show how aphasiology has become like other communicative disorders that are aligned with appropriate communication sciences. For example, developmental language disorders are understood with respect to cognitive development and language acquisition. Similarly, acquired language disorders in adults are being studied with paradigms used in the study of normal language use.

Aphasiology addresses the health care environment, namely, managed care. Texts and college courses are often criticized for lacking practical training. Sometimes this criticism is fair, other times it is shortsighted. The criticism is fair when universities provide relatively little coursework for the medical setting relative to coursework for the school setting and when teaching is not supported by clinical experience. College preparation for working with aphasic clients is quite varied, and universities have experienced pressure from practicum supervisors in medical settings for students and graduates to be "battle-ready" when entering a pre-certification training experience. It is as if our texts and colleges should be providing practicum for practicum.

However, this text is written with the assumption that fundamental knowledge can be useful, especially in the sense that basic research predicts the future of diagnostic and treatment practices. College is the time to explore these possibilities. Also, no text can replace good supervision of practical experience.

About three months before the final copyediting of the manuscript, my mother suffered a subcortical stroke. She did almost no walking or talking for a couple of months. The situation challenged my capacity to respect the difference between personal and professional involvement, and it has given me unique insight into each. My mom's physical and occupational therapists have been a terrific team. However, her first speech-language pathologist avoided dialogue with them and me, and she informed my family that I would be of little use because I am "an academic." These experiences inspired a few revisions regarding the practice of speech-language pathology in the "real world." Most importantly, my mother has been getting better. She has been on her feet, and she has started talking a little.

I want to gratefully acknowledge the patience and understanding of my family and my colleagues and students at the University of Massachusetts, Amherst. Our department chair, Dr. Harry Seymour, was especially kind. Steve Dragin at Allyn and Bacon put up with me in the transition between books and gave me plenty of room to try this one. Bernadine Richey was special. I want to thank Lynn Serper for inspiring the story that weaves throughout the book. Cynthia Paulk, a doctoral student, helped with proofreading. Substantial assistance was also provided by Pat Piekara and Juliet Hossack. Dr. Jennifer Horner Catt gave me advice and information about the real world that went right into the book. I would like to thank Dr. Catt and Harry Seymour for their helpful reviews of the text. Betsy Elias, "the whip," combed all the chapters, kept me alive, and saw to it that I finished.

Chapter 1

INTRODUCTION TO ACQUIRED LANGUAGE DISORDERS

Not long ago, Professor Martin Exeter was home practicing an important lecture when he suddenly stopped, stared at his wife Jackie, and dropped to the floor. An ambulance rushed him to the hospital. He did not recognize Jackie at first, was not quite sure where he was, and could not talk. She tried to get him to write, but he had to hold the pen with his left hand and just threw it at his feet. "I can't…talk" was all he could say. He looked frightened, and she was scared to death. The doctor told her that her husband probably had suffered a stroke, and a couple days later she remembered the doctor also mentioned something called "aphasia." She thought she knew what a stroke was, but she had never heard of aphasia before.

The doctor also told Jackie of someone at the hospital who was trained to help people with aphasia. This has not been a common situation for very long. In 1925 in the United States, the field of speech-language pathology was established mainly to provide "speech correction" in public schools. However, the great wars left many young adults to struggle with longlasting language disorders. Neurologists, psychologists, and speech pathologists created rehabilitation programs in military hospitals throughout the world. Therapies were quickly borrowed from speech correction, classroom teaching, and psychotherapy. Since then, veterans have been living longer, and pathologies of aging have challenged the health care system. In addition, aphasia is now understood to be a unique communicative disorder.

This introductory chapter has two main goals. One is to help the reader acquire a good idea of what aphasia is. A device used for this purpose is to revise a traditional definition of aphasia. The other goal is to help the reader acquire a foundation of thought that underlies the study of aphasia. **Clinical aphasiology** is an evolving discipline that includes (a) research intended to help us identify and explain aphasia and (b) rehabilitation intended to help patients and their families tackle their challenges.

Throughout this text, we shall occasionally check in on Martin Exeter and his family. We shall look into his recovery, language therapy, and adjustments to a new life. Toward the end of the first day after his stroke, Jackie was asking lots of questions: "When can he come home? How soon will he walk again? How soon will he get his speech back? Marty talks for a living."

DEFINING APHASIA

The physician's first task is to preserve a patient's life (see Chapter 2). Once survival is assured, the doctor starts considering a plan for discharge from acute care. This plan includes rehabilitation. When there is paralysis, a patient is referred to a physical therapist. When a patient is likely to have communication problems, the patient is referred to a speech-language pathologist. A written request for services is conveyed on a *consultation* or *referral* form. The form includes a provisional diagnosis, the patient's location in the hospital, and perhaps some medical history. The clinician's first responsibilities are to evaluate oral motor function and communicative capacity (see Chapter 3). The clinician also determines whether or not the patient has aphasia.

At the Mayo Clinic nearly 20 years ago, Frederic Darley pointed out the fundamental diagnostic features of aphasia in a relatively long definition that reads as follows:

> *Impairment, as a result of brain damage, of the capacity for interpretation and formulation of language symbols; multimodality loss or reduction in efficiency of the ability to decode and encode conventional meaningful linguistic elements (morphemes and larger syntactic units); disproportionate to impairment of other intellective functions; not attributable to dementia, confusion, sensory loss, or motor dysfunction; and manifested in reduced availability of vocabulary, reduced efficiency in application of syntactic rules, reduced auditory attention span, and impaired efficiency in input and output channel selection (Darley, 1982, p. 42).*

This expansive definition includes the cause of aphasia, some linguistic elaboration, and some indication of what is *not* aphasia. We need much of this information to make a diagnosis, but we do not need all of it to define aphasia. Let us think about what is tricky about defining aphasia later. For now, we shall focus on the key distinguishing elements that Darley noted, namely:

- multimodality deficit in the communicative modalities of speaking, writing, listening, and reading
- language is more impaired than "other intellective" or mental functions

Multimodality Deficit

When someone's name is on the tips of our tongues, it is also on the tips of our fingers. Finding words is the most common problem with aphasia, and it is manifested through writing as well as speech. The same patient also has problems comprehending when reading as well as listening. Moreover, the modalities are not impaired equally, and there is a typical pattern of comparative deficit. Aphasic people nearly always comprehend better than they talk or write, and reading-writing skills are usually more impaired than auditory-speech skills (Basso, Taborelli, and Vignolo, 1978; Duffy and Ulrich, 1976; Schuell and Jenkins, 1961; Smith, 1971). When language skills in each modality are measured, the results look like the graph in Figure 1.1.

How does a clinical aphasiologist measure language skill in each modality? Martin Exeter was evaluated for possible aphasia with a test structured like the one shown in Table 1.1. The clinician administers tasks involving language at different levels of difficulty. The patient deals with words in some tasks, sentences in others, and paragraph-length material in the most difficult tasks. A common result is that the fewest errors are made at the word level and the most errors are made at the paragraph level. The measure in Figure 1.1 is the percentage of correct responses in each modality. No matter what the severity of aphasia is, a patient usually displays the pattern in Figure 1.1.

Jackie did not need a test to tell her that her husband had difficulty talking, but the test was informative with respect to subtle pockets of expressive ability displayed in a controlled situation. The test was particularly informative regarding level of comprehension, which is difficult to ascertain when a patient is not talking much in conversation. The clinician also uses the test to

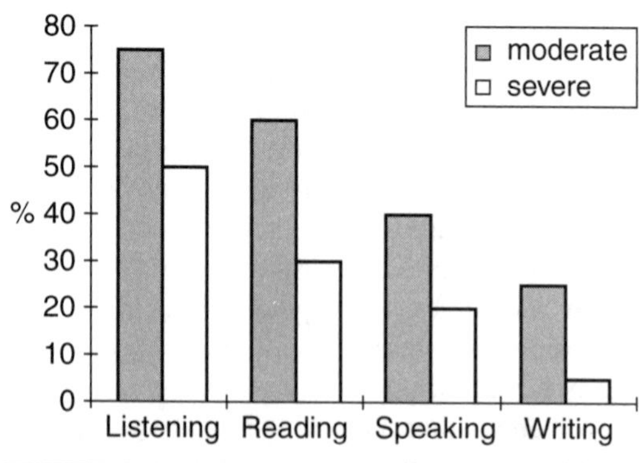

FIGURE 1.1 General pattern of aphasia at two severity levels, when comparing performance among the language modalities.

TABLE 1.1 A model of assessment for aphasia consisting of tasks at different levels of language in each modality. The level of multiple sentences is represented by discourse (spoken) and text (written).

	COMPREHENSION		PRODUCTION	
LEVEL	*Listening*	*Reading*	*Speaking*	*Writing*
Word	Listen to a word, then point to an object	Read a word, then point to an object	Name objects	Write names of objects
Sentence	Follow simple command	Follow simple instruction	Describe simple actions	Describe action
Discourse/Text	Listen to a story, answer questions about it	Read a paragraph, then answer questions	Describe a complex picture	Write a letter

confirm diagnosis of aphasia as opposed to impairment of a specific sensory or motor channel. Let us review some of the modality-specific disorders that were not part of Martin's aphasia.

Martin's doctor did not find sensory problems in the initial evaluation. Aphasia per se does not include **sensory disorders** involving channels for transmitting information to the brain, such as hearing, sight, or touch. When someone has only aphasia, he or she hears speech and sees print as well as before the stroke. Nevertheless, once Martin started going to a speech-language clinic, he received a hearing test anyway. When someone with aphasia does have a severe hearing loss, the graph in Figure 1.1 is likely to look quite different. The listening score may be well below the reading score, an exception to the aphasic pattern.

Another general category of modality-specific disorders is somewhat enigmatic. **Agnosia** is the impairment of the ability to recognize a stimulus even though sensory transmission is intact. With *visual agnosia,* an object can be seen but it is unfamiliar. With *auditory agnosia,* a person hears a common sound, such as a hissing teapot, but does not turn off the stove because of failure to recognize what the sound is. *Tactile agnosia,* also called astereognosis, is the inability to recognize an object by touch even though the patient senses pain, texture, and temperature. Although agnosias are not inherent features of aphasia, they still present the following challenges for clinical diagnosis:

- whether one patient has aphasia *or* an agnosia (or sensory deficit)
- whether one patient has aphasia *and* an agnosia (or sensory deficit)

In either case, the multimodality test pattern again would differ from the one shown in Figure 1.1. The affected input modality would be distinctly depressed relative to the other input modality.

An aphasic individual often speaks easily. Aphasia does not include muscle weakness or other neuromuscular abnormalities such as rigidity or uncontrollable movement. One type of motor speech disorder is the **dysarthrias** which are impairments of the ability to execute movement with the muscles used for speaking. With dysarthria, speech may be slowed or slurred; and the patient may also have difficulty chewing and swallowing food (i.e., dysphagia). Dysarthria accounted for 46 percent of around 3,400 cases of neurogenic communicative disorders evaluated at the Mayo Clinic between 1987 and 1990 (Duffy,

1995). Aphasia accounted for 27 percent. Duffy indicated that aphasia may constitute a larger proportion of the caseload in a long-term rehabilitation setting.

Another motor disorder is called **apraxia of speech** (AOS), which is a little like the agnosias because of intact peripheral transmission. AOS is an impaired programming of movement for the purpose of speaking *without* neuromuscular deficit. Someone with this disorder is quite likely to have no difficulty chewing and swallowing.

Like the diagnostic challenges for sensory deficits, one person can have aphasia, another person can have a motor speech disorder, and someone else can have aphasia *and* a motor speech disorder. Although a referring neurologist examines a patient for these problems, it is the job of a speech-language pathologist to make a definitive diagnosis. Many aphasic patients also have apraxia of speech. When dysarthria accompanies aphasia, it is usually fairly mild; and a swallowing problem, if there is one, does not last long.

As a multimodality disorder, aphasia is not simply the sum of separate auditory, visual, speaking, and writing disorders. The damage causing aphasia is in one location in the brain, not four locations. Aphasia is often called a **central disorder,** suggesting that language functions are somewhat independent of each of the transmissive or peripheral functions of the nervous system (Table 1.2). Centralized functions have been identified historically with linguistic components, because word-meaning relationships are the same whether we are listening or reading. We do not learn one grammar for talking and another one for writing. Wepman suggested that aphasia occurs "in the arousal of a meaningful state, in the semantic process of word selection, or in the syntactic processes" (Wepman, Jones, Bock, and Van Pelt, 1960, p. 328).

Language Disorder

When Jackie first met the speech-language pathologist, she remarked that "Marty doesn't talk but his mind is OK." This is what Darley (1982) meant when he wrote that aphasic language impairment is "disproportionate to impairment of other intellective functions." Both statements characterize a pattern of impaired and retained mental faculties across the range of everyday things people do such as dressing, cooking, and driving as well as reading, writing, and conversing. With aphasia, many of the so-called nonverbal skills may be downright preserved. A day or two after a stroke, people with aphasia are not forgetting who everyone is; or, when able to move about, they are not getting lost in the maze of hospital corridors. They just have trouble with names for people, places, and things. When these skills are measured in a clinic, the pattern of results is roughly low marks for linguistic tasks and high marks for nonverbal tasks such as drawing a flower or putting a puzzle together.

Brain damage can cause other patterns of difficulty and success. Let us go back to where Darley wrote that the language problems of aphasia are "not attributable to dementia, confusion…" and so on. Let us consider **confusion.** Robert Wertz (1985) wrote about the "language of confusion" in which discourse can be twisted by disorientation, inability to sustain attention, failures of recollection, and extreme impatience and irritation. A patient may be said to be incoherent.

TABLE 1.2 Differentiation of aphasia from modality-specific communicative impairments, similar to Wepman and Van Pelt's (1955) historic construct.

	INPUT TRANSMISSION		CENTRAL PROCESSES	OUTPUT TRANSMISSION	
Function	sensation	recognition	language	programming	execution
Dysfunction	hearing loss	agnosia	aphasia	apraxia	dysarthria

Many of these problems are associated with the intellective functions of attention and memory.

In particular, we may be familiar with theatrical portrayals of *amnesia,* which is a problem with remembering people, places, and events (see Chapter 9). Distinguishing amnesia from aphasia may help in making a diagnostic distinction that can be subtle for the layperson. Brain damage has shown that retrieving a memory of a person or event is different from retrieving their names. That is, an amnesic person may be unable to recognize a friend or remember a birthday party, whereas an aphasic person recognizes the friend and remembers the party but has difficulty retrieving the words "Marsha" or "birthday party." An aphasic person often expresses frustration when saying, "I know what I want to say but I cannot think of the words." The scientific approach to this distinction is introduced in Chapter 4.

Dementias are somewhat similar to confusion because of their involvement of varied intellectual skills, but the two terms are commonly associated with (but not necessarily tied to) different causes. Confusion is associated with traumatic brain injury. Irreversible dementias are associated with insidious onset and relentessly progressive deterioration over months or years (although progression is not necessary for a diagnosis of dementia). Alzheimer's disease is one well-known progressive neuropathology. Patients with confusion or dementia tend to have substantially reduced performance on clinical tests beyond the tests for language. The pattern of deficit is often uneven with some retained strengths as well as multiple deficiencies.

Besides language skills, visuospatial or musical skills can be uniquely impaired by stroke. These functions contribute to artistic expression as well as orientation to everyday sights and sounds (Gardner, 1974). A music lover may no longer tolerate listening to the radio due to a problem with recognizing melodies called *amusia.* The general pattern of performance is the opposite of the pattern with aphasia, namely, deficits of nonverbal functions with verbal functions relatively spared. For a long time, physicians did not refer persons with **nonverbal dysfunctions** to speech-language pathologists, because these patients exhibit impressive word-finding and grammatical abilities. Nevertheless, communicating with some of these individuals can be disconcerting. For example, they do not get the punch line of jokes, or they randomly stray from the point of a conversation. Researchers have been studying the question of whether nonverbal dysfunctions or a more elusive dysfunction leads to this occasionally bizarre language use.

In addition to comparing speech and language abilities, the initial evaluation is structured broadly around a comparison between verbal and nonverbal abilities. However, the speech-language pathologist's training is still mainly for dealing with speech and language disorders. The clinical aphasiologist may rely on information from a **clinical neuropsychologist** who conducts a comprehensive evaluation of attention, perception, memory, and reasoning. Many of these specialists, who were trained as clinical psychologists, employ familiar IQ tests that balance examination of certain verbal and nonverbal skills.

Propositional Use of Language

Jackie was amazed when the speech-language pathologist got Martin to count to 10. The clinician had to prod him a little, but counting came out so much easier than any talking Martin had been attempting. Fluent counting illustrates one fundamental feature of aphasia that is absent from Darley's definition. Aphasic people tend to retain so-called *subpropositional* forms which "come 'ready made' or preformulated for the speaker" (Eisenson, 1984, p. 6). These speaking acts include counting to 10, singing a song, or producing routine greetings like "How are you?" or "I'm fine." Also, usually silent patients may curse uncharacteristically when frustrated. Jackie did not know enough about aphasia to be relieved that Martin was not hurling profanities across the room.

Aphasic impairment concentrates on the *propositional* language that we use for normal conversation. Eisenson defined it as "a creative formulation of words with specific and appropriate regard to the situation." Propositional deficit distinguishes aphasia from dysarthria. That is, dysarthrias diminish all levels of verbal expression, whereas aphasia is manifested mainly in the propositional mode of language formulation. Fluent counting or reciting a daily prayer is proof that an aphasic person's neuromuscular mechanism for speaking is intact.

Acquired Disorder

The term "aphasia" is also applied to language-specific disorders in childhood, and this double usage can lead to some confusion. Consumers of speech-language services may wonder if the adult and child verisons are the same disorder, which may lead to the same expectations for recovery and rehabilitation. "Aphasia in adults" is said to be an acquired disorder because its onset occurs after a substantial or completed period of normal language development. **Developmental language disorders** of childhood are diagnosed at an early age, and the cause often appears to have germinated prior to birth. One major classification of developmental delay in childhood is broadly consistent with Darley's definition but is not called aphasia. This disorder is known as specific language impairment (SLI), an often used but highly debatable classification (e.g., Aram, Morris, and Hall, 1993).

There is a crucial overlap between the broad categories of acquired and developmental disorder such that we should not identify them strictly with adulthood and childhood, respectively. Young children who were normal at birth can acquire aphasia, sometimes by stroke. The term aphasia is used with these children who have been studied extensively by Dorothy Aram in Cleveland and Boston (Aram, 1991). Also, when developmentally delayed children start to go to school, they may be diagnosed as having a learning disability; and they may carry the learning disability with them into adolescence and adulthood (Wiig and Secord, 1994). The key distinction is not the age at which aphasia is diagnosed. It is whether the developmental process is compromised.

DESCRIBING APHASIA

The grist for our clinical mill is a patient's behavior. It is what we can observe for evaluation and manipulate for rehabilitation. Different types of behavior arise because of the effects of brain damage. For his best-selling book about "the man who mistook his wife for a hat and other clinical tales," Oliver Sacks (1985) organized chapters around two kinds of abnormality, namely, *loss* of function (e.g., not talking enough) and *excess* of function (e.g., talking too much). Also, some behaviors are the effect of the damage, and other behaviors are the product of intact brain tissue. A broad classification of symptoms is indicated with the following:

- negative symptoms (indicative of impaired processing)
- positive symptoms (indicative of processes remaining intact)
- symptoms of omission (units of language that are missing)
- symptoms of commission (language that was not normally present before the brain injury)

A linguistic sensitivity enhances our precision in looking for symptoms of omission and commission in expressive language. We analyze utterances with respect to units at the sound-level, word-level, and sentence-level.

Word-Finding

Martin Exeter got to the point of saying things like, "I know what I want to say, I just can't think of the words." All of us experience having a word on the tip of our tongue; but, for someone with aphasia, saying any word at any time can be like reaching for a distant fruit on a tree. **Anomia** (also, *dysnomia*) is a broad term for the problem of finding words, and it is the most consistent feature of aphasia. A patient may be just unusually slow coming up with intended words. Upon being unable to find a word, some patients talk around it saying, "I wear it right here, and I tell time with it. Mine goes tick, tick." This positive symptom is called **circumlocution,** which tells us that a patient has found a concept without the word for it.

Another possibility is that an aphasic person says "clock" when thinking about a watch. Word substitution errors are a symptom of commission and are called **paraphasias.** Paraphasias are produced unintentionally, and patients may be surprised upon hearing these mistakes. Paraphasias differ according to the linguistic relationship between the intended word and the error. Without a circumlocution or clear context, the patient's target can be difficult to identify during conversation. Types of paraphasia are revealed best when a clinician already knows the targeted word. Therefore, we ask patients to name objects, repeat words, or read words aloud.

Paraphasias are divided into two broad categories (Table 1.3). A real word is substituted for another, called lexical errors; or a nonword is produced, called sublexical errors (Dell, Schwartz, Martin, Saffran, and Gagnon, 1997). The assumption underlying the notion of sublexical errors is that the correct word has been accessed but its sound has been transformed. Formal and phonemic paraphasias are usually produced in fluent utterances and, thus, are not the same as sound substitutions occurring in motor speech disorders: "the distorted pronunciation of patients with poor articulation does not come under this heading" (Goodglass and Kaplan, 1983, p. 8).

The basis for identifying neologisms varies and their origin is debatable (*see* Chapter 5). We may be properly ambivalent about whether one particular error is phonemic or neologistic, and some investigators speak of target-related versus unrelated neologisms. Someone might say "spork" for spoon and fork, an error that Eisenson (1973) called a neologism but one that Lecours and Vanier-Clement (1976) would have called a "phonemic telescopage." The ambiguities are perplexing, but clinicians rarely rely on a single instance for diagnosing the type of paraphasia dominating a patient's expression. A tendency to produce one type of error during controlled testing may lead to a decision about the ambiguous ones that occur in conversation.

Sentence Production

Aphasic people tend to differ according to two styles of spontaneous verbal production. Right after his stroke, Martin Exeter's utterances were similar to **nonfluent aphasia,** in which patients produce fewer words than normal. Although Martin's words tended to be accurate, getting each word or phrase out was hard work. Jackie felt like she was waiting forever for the next word to come. His remarks about not being able to talk were islands of fluency amidst exhausting struggle. A listener has to be patient, which is something Jackie had to learn.

Labored nonfluent aphasias often contain a problem with grammar. The behavior is a symptom of omission called **agrammatism,** in which

TABLE 1.3 Classification of errors for naming *cat,* according to Dell and others (1997).

LEVELS	PARAPHASIAS	DEFINITION	ERROR
lexical	semantic	word related to target in meaning (not sound)	dog
	formal	word related to target in sound (not meaning)	mat
	mixed	word with sound and meaning relationship	rat
	unrelated	word with no apparent relationship to target	log
sublexical	phonemic	nonword obviously related in sound	lat
	neologistic	nonword with a remote relationship to target	soth

certain types of linguistic units tend to drop out of utterances. When asked to tell what happened before coming to the hospital, a patient might say one of the following:

- "Bathroom...shave."
- "Sleeping...get up...bathroom...fall down... um...wife...um...ambulance."
- "I was standing mirror...shave...the...uh... fall on floor...and I did, too...I could not talk."

Knowing the situation, these fragments make sense. They represent different degrees of grammatical deficit. The omitted units are what linguists call *grammatical morphemes,* including inflectional word endings such as *-ing* and closed-class or function words (e.g., *the, is, on*). The agrammatic patient produces mainly open-class or content words or what has been called "telegramese" (Gardner, 1974). In severe agrammatism, just one or two nouns are produced. It should be noted that the words in the examples are not necessarily simple to pronounce, which is indicative of language disorder rather than a mechanical speech disorder.

The other general style is called **fluent aphasia,** in which patients talk with an easy flow of complete sentences. The main problem is with selection of words. Patients either have trouble finding a word they want to use, or they make many word-finding errors. With mild forms of fluent aphasia, patients communicate fairly well. They have problems finding common words from time to time. When a word does not come to them, they often resort to vague wording or circumlocution. In the following example, an auto mechanic explains how to drive a car:

> *When you get into the car, close your door. Put your feet on those two things on the floor. So, all I have to do is pull...I have to put my...You just put your thing which I know of which I cannot say right now, but I can make a picture of it...you put it in...on your...inside the thing that turns the car on. You put your foot on the thing that makes the stuff come on. It's called the, uh...*

Another type of fluent production makes little sense, and this is called **jargon.** Talking has the sound of normal statements and questions, but it is peppered with paraphasias that transform utterances into pervasive nonsense. A listener is likely to be amazed and sometimes a bit amused at what is depicted informally as word salad or jibberish. It is nearly the opposite of agrammatism (Table 1.4). Two kinds of jargon are recognized based on the type of paraphasias dominating utterances. Mostly semantic paraphasias is called *semantic jargon,* sounding like a confused version of the speaker's language. When neologisms dominate, *neologistic jargon* sounds like a strange language invented by the patient. Semantic jargon is thought to be a less severe deficit because, at least, it contains mostly real words.

In his popular book about brain dysfunction, Howard Gardner (1974) reported asking a patient to talk about what brought him to the hospital. The following reply is mainly semantic jargon with one neologism tossed in:

> *"Oh sure, go ahead, any old think you want. If I could I would. Oh, I'm taking the word the wrong*

TABLE 1.4 Traditional contrasting features of agrammatism and jargon.

	AGRAMMATISM	JARGON
Utterance length	Reduced	Normal or increased
Content words	On target	Paraphasic substitutions
Grammatical morphemes	Omissions or errors	Occasional substitutions
Initiation and flow	Hesitant	Smooth
Prosody	Reduced	Seemingly normal

way to say, all of the barbers here whenever they stop you it's going around and around, if you know what I mean, that is tying and tying for repucer, repuceration, well, we were trying the best that we could while another time it was with the beds over there the same thing..." (p. 68).

Martin was talking more by the end of the first week after his stroke. This progress is called "spontaneous recovery" (see Chapter 10). Moreover, the experts were starting to have a hard time deciding whether his language was nonfluent or fluent. Longer phrases were appearing, but with some of the same struggle. Grammatical morphemes were not always missing.

Recurring or Stereotypic Utterance

Some people with severe aphasia are unable to say anything except some repeated involuntary and seemingly subpropositional utterances. These **stereotypic utterances** occur at the onset of aphasia and tend to persist for months "without apparent modification of their structure" (Alajouanine, 1956). They may appear in any attempt to respond, as if they were the only language forms available. A patient may produce a recurrent syllable called iterative stereotype (e.g., "dee, dee, dee") or a jargonized or neologistic stereotype. A neologistic version was heard by Hughlings Jackson, a nineteenth-century neurologist, during a boyhood seaside holiday:

> *...he lodged at a house where the landlady—as he discovered to his wonderment and awe—could say nothing but "watty." This unlikely disyllable was articulated with such a range of cadence that it could express a variety of emotions. Her laugh was merry and ringing, and when anything amused her she would say: "Watty, watty, watty" (Critchley, 1960, p. 8).*

When stereotypy consists of dictionary words, a common example is the use of "yes" and "no" (often incorrectly) as the only verbalization. Another example is a phrase such as "down the hatch." Ask the patient how he is doing, and he will say, "Down the hatch."

EXPLAINING APHASIA

Why does one aphasic person speak in fragmented sentences, whereas another speaks in fluent jargon? The explanation of these behaviors lies hidden inside a patient's head. Figure 1.2 represents the internal processes of propositional speaking as "encoding" an idea or message into sounds and the process of listening as "decoding" the message from sounds. These notions are certainly vague. They will not help us to understand why one patient does one thing, and another does something else. There are two types of explanation of human behavior, and they originate in an ancient philosophical conundrum called the "mind-body problem."

The Mind-Body Problem

Aphasiologists differ in their orientation to the internal processes of communication. Many focus on the concrete wiring of the brain, speaking of *neural* processes that encode and decode messages. Others are more "psychological," which is to say that they speak of *mental* processes that encode and decode messages. To be psychological is to speak of ideas or memories instead of cerebral convolutions or neurons. Aphasiology was born with a neurological orientation over a hundred years ago, whereas a truly scientific approach to the mind has been emerging only since the early 1970s. The brain and the mind are not usually treated as alternative versions of the truth. The brain is the physical mechanism responsible for mentalistic things like memory and comprehension.

For centuries philosophers have been contemplating the nature of the mind, arguing over whether it exists or where it lives (Campbell, 1970). In medieval times, the clergy was the government. Laws were based on such beliefs as the earth is the center of the universe, and material and spiritual worlds cannot cohabitate. Anatomic dissection was frowned upon in medical schools, and dissecting sex organs and the brain was forbidden. Drawings by Leonardo da Vinci provide

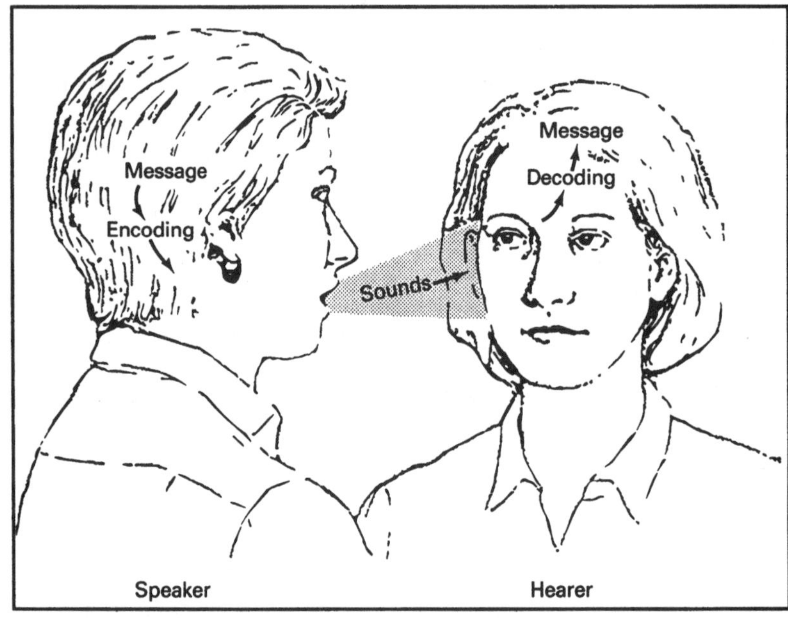

FIGURE 1.2 A simplified indication of psychological or "mental" mechanisms of communication.

Reprinted by permission from Akmajian, A., Demers, R. A., & Harnish, R. M., *Linguistics: An introduction to language and communication* (Second Edition). Cambridge, Ma: MIT Press, 1984, p. 393.

evidence of a belief that the mind or soul inhabits little spaces inside the brain. During the 1600s or "the age of reason," Rene Descartes was one of the first to speculate that memory and thought are managed in a material part of the brain. This was about as upsetting as Copernicus having the nerve to claim that the sun is the center of the universe.

Now, experimental psychologists speak of the mind as cognition. **Cognition** is "the collection of mental processes and activities used in perceiving, remembering, thinking, and understanding" (Ashcraft, 1994, p. 12). Cognitive science was born when these processes could be measured in the fractions of a second in which they occur. Just as archaeologists build models of Pompeii based on tiny fragments of its remains, cognitive scientists construct the most likely "functional architecture" of the mind from bits and pieces of behavior (e.g., Anderson, 1983).

While most psychologists believe that cognition represents the jobs performed by the brain, they approach their work as if "the mind can be studied independently from the brain" (Johnson-Laird, 1983). Cognitive psychologists, "by and large, simply seem not to worry about the mind-brain problem" (Flanagan, 1984). Johnson-Laird (1983) added: "Once you know the way in which a computer program works, your understanding of it is in no way improved by learning about the particular machine on which it runs" (p. 9). Many psychologists have been reluctant to shackle models of cognition with neurological speculations (Mehler, Morton, and Jusczyk, 1984). At one time texts on cognitive psychology contained almost nothing about the brain (e.g., Ashcraft, 1989; Solso, 1988), but the 1990s have seen inclusions of at least a chapter on brain studies (e.g., Anderson, 1990; Ashcraft, 1994; Solso, 1991).

The ensuing instruction is managed by attending to neurological and cognitive orientations as independent entities. This separation is not entirely artificial. A neuroscientist learns important things from studying pathologic brain tissue under a miscroscope without any knowledge of the patient's cognitive or communicative dysfunction. A speech-language pathologist can evaluate a patient's language abilities without attending to what went on in the patient's brain.

Neurological Explanation

The importance of neurological explanation was advanced by Brookshire (1997) from the start of his text, where he wrote that "features and severity of neurogenic communication disorders depend on location and magnitude of the damage ...clinicians who wish to understand these communication disorders must have a rudimentary understanding of the human nervous system and what can go wrong with it" (p. 1). The nervous system is divided into central and peripheral components. The peripheral modalities are wired for transmissive input to and transmissive output from the central nervous system. The brain is the principal integrating device in the central nervous system.

Distribution of faculties in the brain was contemplated when even the appearance of materialistic explanation of the human spirit was rejected by church-guided authorities. Early in the 1800s, Franz Gall traveled to a tolerant Paris to escape the Austrian Kaiser's wrath, because Gall was relating traits such as pugnacity and love of wine to areas of the brain. People with a quarrelsome disposition were assumed to have large pugnacity cortex. Based on a "science" called phrenology, Gall would detect wine lovers or those with strong "alimentariness" by feeling bumps on their skulls. Physicians, however, were looking forward to serious proof that human faculties could be localized in cerebral matter.

Reported in 1861, Paul Broca performed an autopsy on a patient with a dissociated speech disorder and discovered a lesion in a frontal region of left cerebral cortex (Broca, 1960). Broca's discovery was enthusiastically received by the medical community. In 1874, Carl Wernicke wrote of someone with a severe comprehension deficit and a lesion in left temporal cortex (Wernicke, 1977). Medical journals filled with descriptions of specific disorders linked to sites of damaged brain. Physicians were convinced that these relationships indicated sites of normal functions.

Aphasiologists are most familiar with the topographical view of the brain or **cerebrum** depicted in the upper left of Figure 1.3. The brain has two halves or **hemispheres,** and we see the left cerebral hemisphere in the figure. Also, we see the gross geography of the cerebral **cortex,** which is formed by a 2 to 2½ square foot sheet folded into wormy convolutions so that it can fit within the skull. The cortex is actually a layered sheet that is less than two typewriter spaces thick, consisting of 30 billion delicately networked neurons (Calvin and Ojemann, 1980). The thin spaces between convolutions provide important boundaries for regions of the cortex. The central sulcus, for example, divides each half of the brain into what are known as anterior and posterior regions.

Figure 1.3 also illustrates that the Russian neuropsychologist A. R. Luria (1970a) divided the central nervous system (CNS) into three functional levels. The first level has something to do with general awareness and distribution of sensory input. It includes deep cerebral nuclei (e.g., thalamus) and the reticular formation running through the brainstem. The **reticular activating system** (RAS) distributes nerve impluses to all areas of the cortex. The second level is the posterior cortex which perceives, recognizes, and integrates sensory information. The third level is the anterior cortex which generates volitional response.

Returning to the upper left of the figure, four main **lobes** provide a frame of reference for identifying more specific locations of the cerebral cortex. The frontal lobe coincides with the anterior cortex, and a part of this region serves motor functions. Posterior cortex receives auditory input in

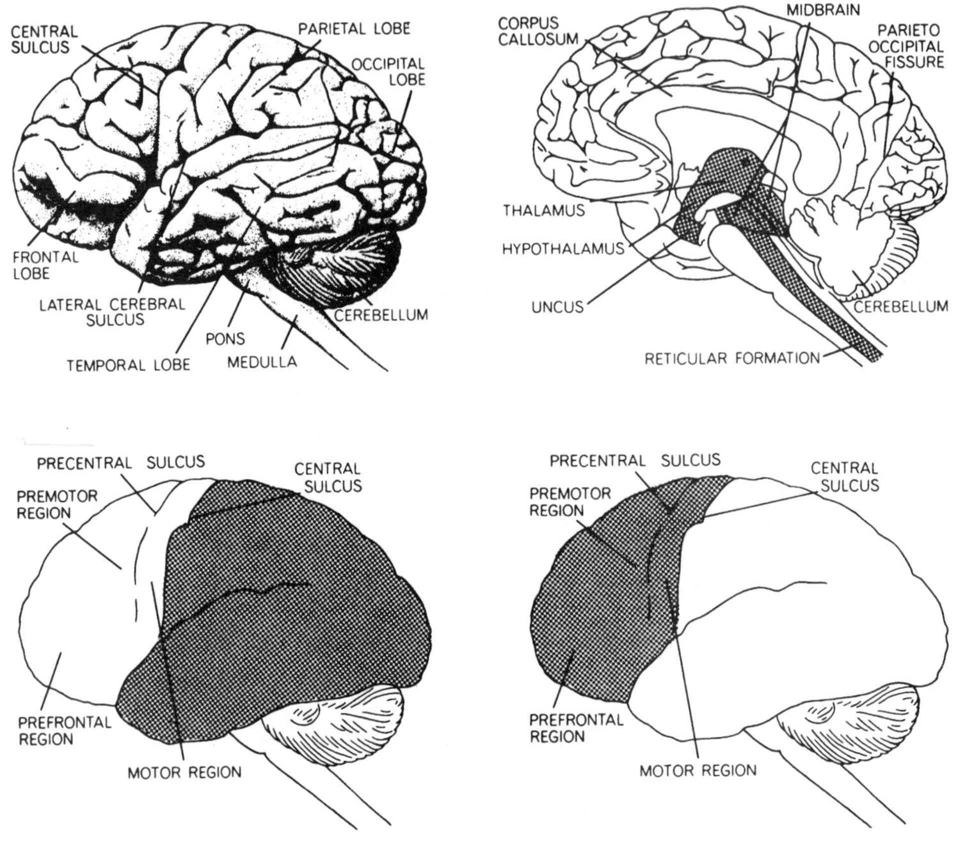

FIGURE 1.3 Gross anatomy of the brain is depicted in the upper left (lateral view) and upper right (medial view). The shaded regions represent Luria's three functional levels or "blocks": reticular formation, posterior cortex, and anterior cortex.

Reprinted by permission of Lorelle Raboni from Luria, A. R., The functional organization of the brain. Scientific American, 222(3), 66–78, 1970. Copyright © 1970 by Scientific American, Inc. All rights reserved.

the temporal lobe, visual input in the occipital lobe, and tactile input in the parietal lobe. To summarize simply, posterior cortex receives a stimulus, and anterior cortex makes a response.

Now, let us turn to the vocabulary of pathology. Damaged tissue is called a *lesion.* Aphasia is thought to be most clearly caused by a lesion in the cerebral cortex. A few neuropathologies can destroy a small part of the brain, and such localized damage is called a **focal lesion.** Focal lesions are a typical result of disrupted blood flow or *stroke.* However, stroke is not the only cause of focal lesions. A region of the cortex can gradually shrink (called atrophy) for mysterious reasons. Small parts of the brain can be scraped during life-saving surgery. Surgeons are quite serious about avoiding the areas for speech and language. A person may also accumulate multiple lesions by suffering several little strokes through the years, called a **multifocal lesion** pattern. Finally, damage spread evenly throughout the brain is referred to as being "diffuse."

We learned a great deal about the effects of focal lesions from extensive studies of soldiers who fought in the world wars decades ago. From his studies, Luria (1970b) characterized *traumatic brain injury* (TBI) as "a cleanly punched out defect in a cerebrum." Yet, contemporary life can inflict damage that is more varied or complex depending on whether the damage was caused by modern firearms, motor vehicle accidents, or other forms of violence. To put it simply for now, TBI can be multifocal and diffuse.

The anterior and posterior regions of the cortex serve the same peripheral sensory and motor functions in each hemisphere. However, the left and right hemispheres have different intellectual functions. When one hemisphere is damaged, its functional specialty is impaired and the other hemisphere's expertise is relatively preserved. For most people, the left hemisphere is specialized for language functions, and the right hemisphere is specialized for fundamental nonverbal functions. Within the left hemisphere, lesions in an anterior region produce nonfluent aphasia, and posteriorly located lesions produce fluent aphasias. When taking a neurological perspective, some researchers speak materially of anterior aphasia and posterior aphasia.

The objective of neurological diagnosis is to figure out what has happened to the brain. Bruce Porch (1986) once argued that aphasia tests should reveal "the relative efficiency of various 'brain circuits'" (p. 295). However, our knowledge of the brain does not allow us to take him too literally, because we do not know, for example, how brain circuits comprehend sentences. It is still hard to tell in neurological terms why someone just names objects slowly or why someone produces more neologisms than semantic paraphasias or why someone else omits certain kinds of grammatical morphemes. To understand fully why a particular lesion causes aphasias, we need a better understanding of the functional significance of fairly specific parts of the brain and how they work together.

Cognitive Explanation

A mechanism for encoding and decoding messages could also be represented with respect to ideas and words stored in our heads. Encoding would start with an idea that would be connected to a word. Decoding starts with a word that is connected to an idea. This is the start of characterizing a "cognitive chain" of events.

There are two fundamental features of cognition. One is our relatively stable storage of information, or our fund of **knowledge.** It includes knowledge of the world and knowledge of the language we speak. Frequent reference to "architecture" is indicative of the use of spatial metaphors to characterize knowledge. Our mental vocabulary is said to have form and structure. The other feature of cognition is **process,** or the fleeting activity of the mind. A cognitive process is not just a complicated act of problem-solving. It is also a "mental response" to a stimulus. Connecting a word to an idea is a type of mental process. Processes are temporal. In principal, their duration can be measured.

A fundamental question in cognitive sciences applies to both knowledge and process. How is information in our heads represented? What form does it take? The form of information in our heads differs from the form of a stimulus. This inner form is called a **mental representation.** Information is represented either in permanent storage or in a transient state. A theory of the neural representation of a new memory can appeal to concrete tissues and chemicals. Characterizing a memory in functional terms, however, is more problematic. Again, scientists use analogies or metaphors. For example, a mental image may be like a photograph. Characteristics of the brain are invoked to depict the mind, such as talking about knowledge as being stored like a "network" or talking about a representation as being "activated."

All cognitive functions are carried on the shoulders of **memory.** Ashcraft (1989) wrote that cognition is "the coordinated operation of active mental processes within a multicomponent memory system" (p. 39). All sorts of notions about memory exist. The basic nature of memory is that it is the retention of information in the mind beyond the life of an external stimulus. Thus, a stimulus is represented and retained. A memory can last just a small fraction of a second. The ability to hold information in our heads is fundamental to the mind's (or brain's) ability to perform various functions, including simple ones like perception and recognition.

Let us take a moment to become familiar with the overall organization of the memory system. Figure 1.4 is a traditional model. This information management system is much like a library. A library system stores books, acquires new ones, and has procedures for efficient access to books on the shelves. In the mind, knowledge is shelved in **long-term memory** (LTM). The store of books in a library is organized so that we do not wander around all day looking for a particular book. Cognitive scientists test theories of lexical organization by determining which theory predicts the speed of finding words. In this way, structure has an influence on process.

Also like a library, LTM contains different types of information. Knowledge may have a verbal format like novels and a photographic format like picture books. The following types of knowledge representation were given to us by Tulving (1972) and Anderson (1983):

- **episodic memory** for individually experienced events (also, *autobiographical memory*)
- **semantic memory** for common knowledge of the world
- **procedural memory** for knowledge of skills like swinging a golf club
- **lexical memory** for words and information about words

Aphasia provides evidence for the notion that words and world knowledge are kept in different stores. That is, an aphasic person knows what he or she wants to convey but just cannot access the words. In general, the validity of memory stores is supported by many case studies showing that neu-

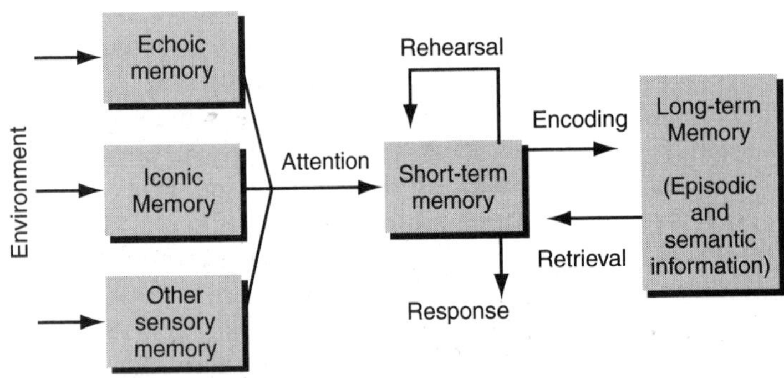

FIGURE 1.4 Three levels of memory have implications for language function. Processing for comprehension and production takes place within the capacity and time constraints of short-term memory, also called "working memory." The knowledge-base for communication is housed in long-term memory. (Reprinted by permission from Smith, A. D., and Fullerton, A. M., Age differences in episodic semantic memory: Implications for language and cognition. In D. S. Beasley and G. A. Davis, (Eds.), *Aging: Communication Processes and Disorders.* New York: Grune & Stratton, 1981)

ropathologies can impair access to one type of memory but not others (Schacter, 1996).

Now, let us turn to cognitive processing. Our processing system has a limited capacity for doing work. That is, the mind can do only so much at one time. The short-term memory in Figure 1.4 is now called **working memory** (WM), which is the "work space" for any cognitive activity. It constrains our capacity for keeping information active and for processing information, just as computers have a limited capacity for the number of programs that can run at the same time. Asking someone to do two things at once is one way of assessing WM capacity. In addition to being informed by the external environment, WM is informed by the **activation** of information in long-term storage.

Short-term memory (STM) is now considered to be one component of working memory. The memory span test of STM tells us the amount of a stimulus that can be represented in working memory.

Diagrams of the memory system show the relationships of working memory to external stimuli and the long-term store of knowledge (Figure 1.4). These relationships are expressed as directions of the flow of information in the cognitive system. Processes are said to be **bottom-up** (or *data-driven*) to the extent that they are influenced by the environment. For example, the complexity of a linguistic stimulus can influence comprehension processes. Processing is also **top-down** (or *concept-driven*) to the extent that it is directed by what we already know. That is, we fill in blanks or "read between the lines" as we comprehend. Partial theories of a language function or dysfunction emphasize either bottom-up or top-down processing, whereas a comprehensive explanation incorporates both directions.

Are we aware of information activated in working memory? We are aware of some information, but "intellective" activity is more than our conscious thoughts. Cognitive processing occurs at both subconscious and conscious levels of awareness. Subconscious processing is said to be automatic. Scientists use so-called *fast tasks* and millisecond timers to measure automatic activity, such as comprehending a common word. **Automatic processing** has the following characteristics:

- it is subconscious or beneath our awareness
- it is obligatory (i.e., mandatory)
- it takes up little or no room in working memory

In the presence of a stimulus, the brain does not just sit there waiting for our conscious commands. It responds or activates on its own. Fundamental decoding and encoding for communication is automatic and obligatory. When we hear an utterance, comprehension happens whether we want it to or not.

Clinical aphasiologists are most experienced with assessment and treatment of **controlled processing,** which has the following features:

- it can be conscious or in our awareness
- it can be intentional and, therefore, optional
- it is effortful and takes up room in working memory

Also known as strategic processing, controlled processing is studied with *slow tasks* that allow enough time for decision-making or planning to occur. Unlike automatic processes, strategic processes clog the system. When a patient scans picture-choices in a typical comprehension task, there is time for all sorts of controlled processing to occur, and a pointing response is the result of both automatic and controlled processing. Language processes become particularly effortful in "metalinguistic" tasks, such as sorting words into categories or editing a manuscript (see Table 9.7 for similar terminology).

This introduction to the fundamental characteristics of information processing should leave the impression that language functions operate within a cognitive framework. For example, both comprehension and production are accomplished with bottom-up and top-down informational flow through working memory. Language processing is constrained by the capacity of working memory and draws from knowledge stored in long-term memory.

The constructs of cognition coincide with common explanations of aphasia. For example, Martin Exeter would explain that he knows what he wants to say but cannot find the words. Focusing on language, Schuell's (1969) clinical experience led her to believe that "the language storage system is at least relatively intact." Most aphasiologists consider aphasia to be an impairment of processing rather than an erasure of linguistic knowledge. In this way, cognitive constructs help us to put into words what we think aphasia is. They provide a framework for "locating" a disorder in the human information processing system.

Implications for Basic Terminology

Hopefully this temporary separation of neurological and cognitive domains helps to put some basic concepts in their proper place. Problems with terminology are reflected in a mixing of neurological and functional terms. For example, this book refers to "aphasia" for some chapter titles and to traumatic brain injury and the right hemisphere for other titles. Thus, some titles refer to the brain, whereas most others refer to dysfunction. Another mixing problem is a growing list of aphasias such as optic aphasia, subcortical aphasias, and so on. "Subcortical" refers to a part of the brain, and "optic" refers to a functional modality. Table 1.5 shows a logical alignment of terms. For example, "stroke" refers to something that happens to the brain. "Aphasia" is a dysfunction caused by stroke and, therefore, is logically parallel to other dysfunctions like amnesia.

TABLE 1.5 Basic terminology and classification of function, neuropathology, and dysfunction.

FUNCTION	NEUROPATHOLOGY (CAUSE)	DYSFUNCTION (EFFECT)
language	stroke	aphasia
music	stroke	amusia
memory	traumatic brain injury	amnesia
general intellect	late stage Alzheimer's disease	dementia

The faulty parallelism of chapter titles is indicative of a difficulty in coming up with a single classification of dysfunctions that are unique to head trauma or right hemisphere stroke. We often say they are not language disorders. Clinical professionals refer to these dysfunctions collectively as cognitive disorders, perhaps, to put a positive spin on "nonverbal disorders." Then, cognitive disorders are often distinguished from language disorders, despite the fact that language disorders are impairments of a part of the cognitive system. Attention and memory have been considered to be cognitive, whereas linguistic skills have been thought to be something else. As Rosenbek (1982) put it, "most traditional aphasiologists would like to separate cognition and language and leave cognitive deficit out of the definition of when aphasia is aphasia" (p. 364).

Re-Defining Aphasia

It is possible that what we thought 25 years ago or so may need some minor adjustments. After all, the cognitive science of language functioning did not get underway until around 1970, and clinical practice has yet to incorporate the fast tasks that measure automatic obligatory processes. In order to modernize a bit, a reconsideration of Darley's definition of aphasia may be worthwhile.

To help with re-definition, we should recognize that clinical diagnosis is a process of using behavioral clues to diagnose a disorder that exists in someone's brain or mind. Neurologists use clinical evaluation to make an initial guess about what literally happened to the brain. A stroke can cause sudden changes in language comprehension and word-finding, both of which happen in the brain. Clinical evaluation of behavior is employed to support a diagnosis of aphasia or something else, and it has been suggested here that aphasic disorder is specified in terms of the jobs performed by the brain (i.e., cognition).

So, let us consider another definition: *Aphasia is a selective impairment of the cognitive system specialized for comprehending and formu-*

lating language, leaving other cognitive capacities relatively intact. This definition differs from Darley's in the following ways:

- brevity, because specifying basic language functions should be discriminating enough, and details about language should be part of what we learn as we delve into the subject further;
- omission of any reference to etiology, simply because a logical sorting of concepts suggests that the cause of a dysfunction does not comprise the dysfunction;
- re-wording in cognitive terms for the idea that aphasia is impairment of the language processing system.

Subtracting reference to brain damage places a burden on specifying dysfunction as the basis for defining and, thus, diagnosing aphasia. By speaking of aphasia as a cognitive impairment, it does not necessarily become something that is different from what Darley thought. The new wording is problematic only if we continue to believe that language is one thing and cognition is something else. By putting aphasia squarely in the domain of cognition, this text points to cognitive science as the fundamental framework for the study of dysfunction, with neuroscience being the fundamental framework for studying the causes of aphasia.

Of course, neither Martin or Jackie Exeter were interested in our problems with terminology. They did want a correct diagnosis of Martin's communicative difficulties, however. A diagnosis of "aphasia" leads to recommending a particular plan of rehabilitation that is conducted at great cost with respect to time and energy as well as money. In this sense, our understanding of what aphasia is becomes important for clinical practice.

TREATING APHASIA

The treatment of aphasia is conducted within a medical environment or, more broadly, according to guidelines established for health care services in a variety of environments. This section introduces some general concepts that define the health care environment, and these concepts provide a framework for discussions of clinical practice throughout this text. Because the practice of clinical aphasiology is so integrated with the health care system and occurs along with the treatment of other neurogenic communicative disorders, some clinicians now include this practice in the category of *medical speech pathology* (Golper, 1992; Miller and Groher, 1990).

The World Health Organization recommended that medical conditions be evaluated and treated with respect to three levels, namely, the impairment, disability, and handicap (Table 1.6). In clinical aphasiology, rehabilitation has historically emphasized evaluation and treatment of the language impairment. Attention to disability and handicap increases the likelihood of caring for the "whole patient." The overall objectives of post-stroke rehabilitation are to **maximize functional independence** and **improve quality of life.** More specific goals pertain to minimizing the impairment and the disabilities caused by the impairment.

The structure of health care delivery is based largely on how it is paid for. In theory, payment

TABLE 1.6 World Health Organization's levels for medical conditions (see Frattali, et al., 1995).

LEVEL	GENERAL DEFINITION	APHASIA
impairment	the disordered system	language disorder
disability	functional consequences of the *impairment*	communicative difficulties
handicap	social consequences of the *disability*	loss of employment, isolation or dependency

could be provided by the "first party" (patient) or by the "second party" (service provider). Because the expense is too great for either party, health care is usually supported by **third-party payers** who cover the cost on behalf of patients. A third-party payer can be public (i.e., the government) or private (i.e., insurance). In many countries, the third-party is the government exclusively which leads to some variation in rehabilitation programs that can be offered around the world.

For a moment, let us concern ourselves with health care in the United States. Between World War II and the mid-1970s, physicians and speech-language pathologists provided services without much interference. During this period, most of our major clinical tests and many treatment strategies were developed in government-supported Veterans Administration Hospitals. In the 1980s, health care costs skyrocketed along with double-digit inflation. **Managed care** became the collective term for new approaches to the delivery of health care in a way that would improve quality as well as contain costs (see Chapter 11).

There has been a highly publicized concern over an apparent shift from a service-provider-driven system to a payment-provider-driven system in which health care decisions are made by insurance companies. The National Committee for Quality Assurance (NCQA) is a private non-profit organization that monitors managed care. NCQA began accrediting managed care organizations in 1991. The organization provides information to help consumers distinguish among plans. Each plan receives a score based on physician credentials, members rights and responsibilities, preventive health services, appropriateness of services, and adequacy of medical records.

One fundamental distinction has implications for reimbursement plans. An **inpatient** is someone who "resides" in the facility providing service, whereas an **outpatient** is someone who comes to the facility during the day for services. Other general categories of care pertain to time following onset of disease (Table 1.7). A stroke patient receives *acute care* upon admission to a hospital. Hospital stays are as brief as medically reasonable, because inpatient treatment is more expensive than outpatient treatment. *Subacute care* is a new category established by the managed care industry to focus on rehabilitation as soon as possible. It is thought to be a bridge between acute hospitalization and independence at home. *Chronic care* is provided for long-term residual impairments such as aphasia. Substantial rehabilitation used to be provided in many acute care hospitals. Now, stroke survivors leave the acute setting as soon as possible and receive therapies at home or at a rehabilitation center.

The health care system has several mechanisms for providing "quality assurance" or the more current concept of **quality improvement** (Frattali, 1994). Quality is evaluated with respect to standards developed by each health care profession. One standard is the **care path,** which is a hierarchy of steps or protocols for rehabilitation of each disorder (Cornett, 1994). Care paths guide decisions about diagnostic and treatment services for each patient, and each decision is documented

TABLE 1.7 General categories of health care and typical settings in the United States.

CATEGORY	DEFINITION	SETTING
Acute	immediate and short-term (e.g., stroke unit)	acute care hospital
Subacute or Postacute	transition between acute hospitalization and independence at home	rehabilitation hospital (inpatient or outpatient)
Chronic	persistent diseases or conditions; living with permanent residual impairment	rehabilitation center (outpatient) home health care nursing home

in a patient's records. This documentation is one basis on which a **utilization review** can evaluate the appropriateness of services at a health care facility.

Standards of care are constructed at different levels. The hospital has *critical paths* for different diagnoses, and each department has its own guideline. A hospital has a critical path for stroke with hemiplegia. Speech-language evaluation should be on this path. When it is not on the critical path, speech-language pathologists should advocate for its inclusion. The following "care path," without a decision hierachy, outlines most basic stages in speech-language services for someone with aphasia:

- receive referral or consult from a physician
- review medical chart
- evaluate patient at bedside
- report results of evaluation to physician (in medical chart)
- administer standardized language evaluation in clinic
- report results of evaluation and recommendation for treatment
- document treatment goals and plan
- administer treatment
- document progress relative to goals

SUMMARY AND CONCLUSIONS

This chapter had two principal goals. One was to help the reader acquire a general idea of what aphasia is. Aphasia is an acquired disruption of the cognitive system responsible for language comprehension and production. Stroke is a neuropathology that can cause a distinctly isolated language disorder, leaving other cognitive functions relatively intact. Many patients with aphasia have other problems such as a motor speech disorder or attentional difficulties. In some aphasias, finding nouns is harder than producing sentences. The reverse can also happen, namely, producing sentences is harder than retrieving nouns. Such observations lead to decisions about targeting language rehabilitation.

The other goal of this chapter was to help the reader acquire a foundation of thought that underlies clinical decision-making as well as the study of aphasia. The main point is that post-stroke behavior is symptomatic of an internal dysfunction. This dysfunction may be characterized in cognitive as well as neurological terms. Taking this distinction literally is intended to minimize the fuzzy reference to the mind as the brain (and the brain as the mind) that occurs in public discourse. Moreover, someone may claim that a behavioral therapy "rewires the brain." Yet, there may be no evidence that the brain has been physically rewired, and the claim is supported instead with mushy cognitive theorizing that seems to pass as reference to the brain. Our clarity about what is the brain and what is cognition ought to contribute to public confidence in rehabilitation fields.

The clinical distinction between cognition and language coincides with a division of labor in which an aphasiologist speaks of assessing language disorders and a clinical neuropsychologist speaks of assessing cognitive disorders. Debates over boundaries may arise when a clinical neuropsychologist learns that language is a cognitive function or when an aphasiologist begins thinking of aphasia as a "cognitive-communicative disorder." It is unclear how clinical professionals will deal with the scientific notion that cognition is common ground and that divisions pertain to more specific functions such as attention and language.

Meanwhile, we know that Martin Exeter suffered a stroke while practicing an important lecture. He had been invited to speak about psycholinguistics at a conference on aphasia in Brussels. He was going to take Jackie with him, and it would have been their first trip to Europe. After the conference they were going to see London, Paris, and Rome. Martin wanted to sip espresso at a Left Bank cafe like Hemingway, and Jackie wanted to reminisce about her high school Latin teacher while walking through the Roman Forum. However, paralysis and aphasia seemed to have destroyed these dreams; but Martin and Jackie learned that a lot is possible with rehabilitation. We shall see.

Chapter 2

CAUSES OF APHASIA

The ambulance arrived at Martin Exeter's home a few minutes after he collapsed. In another 20 minutes, he was in the emergency room of the hospital. He was conscious but could not move his right side. The doctor had been informed of what had happened, and, upon preliminary evaluation, he suspected that a stroke was a strong possibility. His main objectives were to preserve life and stabilize the patient's vital functions. Martin was hooked up for electrocardiogram monitoring and blood pressure readings. The doctor asked him questions. Do you know your name? Do you know where you are? Martin nodded inconsistently and could not speak.

Meanwhile, Jackie Exeter had been separated from her husband. She paced around the waiting area as the ER team decided whether to admit Martin to the hospital. After about 15 minutes and while she was starting to fill out admission forms, the doctor appeared and told her of his preliminary diagnosis. Martin would be taken to the Stroke Unit for specialized "intensive care." He asked about Martin's primary care physician at the university health center, who in managed care is called the "gatekeeper physician." Jackie recalled that their insurance plan allowed 48 hours to contact the gatekeeper in case of emergencies, and the ER physician said that he would take care of it the next day.

STROKE

A stroke (or cerebrovascular accident) disrupts blood flow to the brain. Brookshire (1997) noted that some professionals have disdain for the acronym "CVA." Neverthless, stroke is the third most common cause of death over age 45 in the United States. The National Stroke Association reported that the number of strokes has been increasing from 550,000 per year twenty years ago to 730,000 estimated in the mid-1990s (www.stroke.org). Surveys indicated that 20 to 33 percent of stroke survivors have aphasia shortly after their stroke, and 10 to 18 percent have aphasia months later (Wade, Hewer, David, and Enderby, 1986). The National Stroke Association also reported a Gallup survey stating that 40 percent of the American public does not know that a stroke occurs in the brain.

To understand what happens in the brain, we should have some knowledge of the cerebral circulatory system. Like other tissue in the body, neurons thrive on the process of **metabolism** or the exchange of nutrients and waste products between the circulatory system and neurons. Arteries transport nutrients in the bloodstream, including oxygen and glucose, from the heart to the brain. The brain's large appetite is indicated by its use of 15 to 20 percent of the body's blood while taking up only two percent of body weight (Metter, 1986). The nutrients pass through the capillary membrane at the end of arteries, cross a space, and then pass through the neural membrane. The nerve cell transforms the nutrients into waste products that are carried away through veins. The effectiveness of medications depends on the permeability of the capillary membrane which is impermeable to many substances (i.e., *blood-brain barrier*).

Two mechanisms can disrupt metabolism. One is an **ischemic stroke** (or ischemia) which is a blockage or occlusion of an arterial vessel. The occlusion keeps blood from getting to an area of the brain. The other general type of stroke is a **hemorrhage,** which is a bursting artery causing blood to accumulate around nearby brain tissue. Ischemic stroke is much more common than hemorrhage. Different patterns of deficit are related to site of occlusion or hemorrhage in the circulatory system.

The blood supply to the brain has three structural levels: arteries in the neck that transport blood from the heart to the base of the brain, interconnecting arteries in the base of the brain, and cerebral arteries on the surface of the cortex. In the neck, the left and right common carotid arteries course upward and divide near the larynx. The left and right **internal carotid arteries** proceed to the interconnecting arteries at the base of the brain. Behind the carotid arteries, the left and right *vertebral arteries* are held in place along the vertebral column. The vertebral arteries join to become the *basilar artery* at the level of the medulla in the brainstem. Branches of the basilar artery supply the brainstem and cerebellum.

Three cerebral arteries supply the cortical surface for each hemisphere, and their locations are sketched in Figure 2.1 in relation to key speech and language areas of the left hemisphere. The main vessel of the **middle cerebral artery (MCA)** runs along the Sylvian fissure and branches to most of the lateral cortical convexity. Figure 2.1a shows the left hemisphere's middle cerebral artery (or **LMCA**) supplying key language areas including Broca's area, Wernicke's area, and the ideational speech area. It is continuous with the internal carotid artery and, thus, can suffer effects of occlusion in the carotid. The *anterior cerebral artery* (ACA) is distributed mostly throughout medial frontal and parietal regions (Figure 2.1b). The *posterior cerebral artery* (PCA) covers the medial surface of the occipital lobe and the base of the temporal lobe. In Figure 2.1a, it can be seen reaching around the posterior portion of the occipital region.

The cerebral arteries originate in the *communicating arteries* at the base of the brain, which collectively form the *Circle of Willis.* This polygon of small arteries is one **collateral system** in which some compensation may occur for occlusion in a carotid artery below. For example, the anterior communicating artery allows for collateral flow between the left and right anterior cerebral arteries. If flow in the left ACA is reduced by left carotid occlusion, the right carotid can be an alternative source through the communicating artery. This possibility is often prohibited in persons with communicating arteries narrowed by vascular disease.

Also in the lateral view (Figure 2.1a), we see areas in which the cerebral arteries approach each other, almost touching. These are called **watershed areas** or zones. For example, end-branches of the MCA and ACA meet anteriorly in the frontal lobe. An occlusion in one artery may not cause damage to neural tissue in a watershed area if collateral circulation from the other artery is effective.

ISCHEMIC STROKE

As indicated earlier, an ischemic stroke is an occlusion of an artery that keeps the bloodstream from reaching areas of the brain. The most common cause of occlusion is *atherosclerosis,* which is a proliferation of cells (i.e., blood platelets) along arterial walls and an accumulation of fatty substances (i.e., lipid) within associated connective tissue. Another factor that could lead to ischemic stroke is high cholesterol or too much fat in the blood (Shimberg, 1990). Atherosclerosis is an untreatable risk factor, whereas high cholesterol is a treatable risk factor.

Types of Ischemic Stroke

Two types of ischemic stroke produce similar clinical characteristics but result from different processes. Most strokes are a **thrombosis** which occurs from accumulation of atherosclerotic platelets and fatty plaque on the vessel wall at the site of occlusion. Thrombus formation may take minutes or weeks to clog an artery. Dysfunction arises suddenly and increases in severity over minutes, hours, or even days during the final

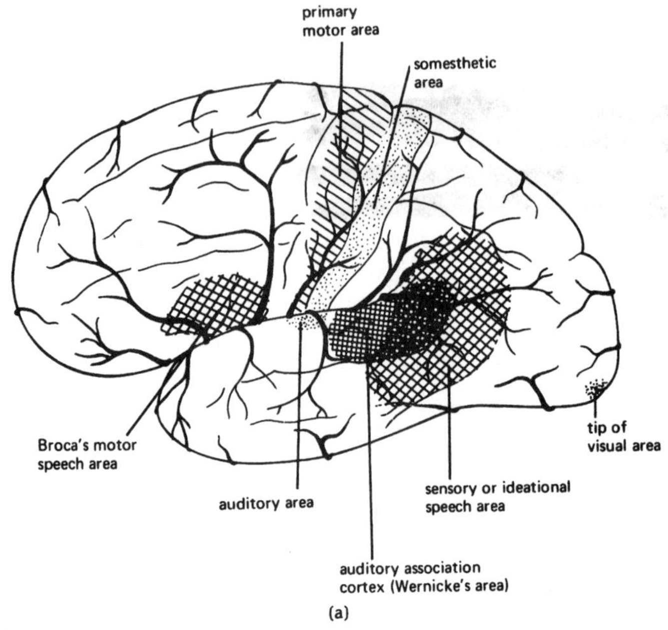

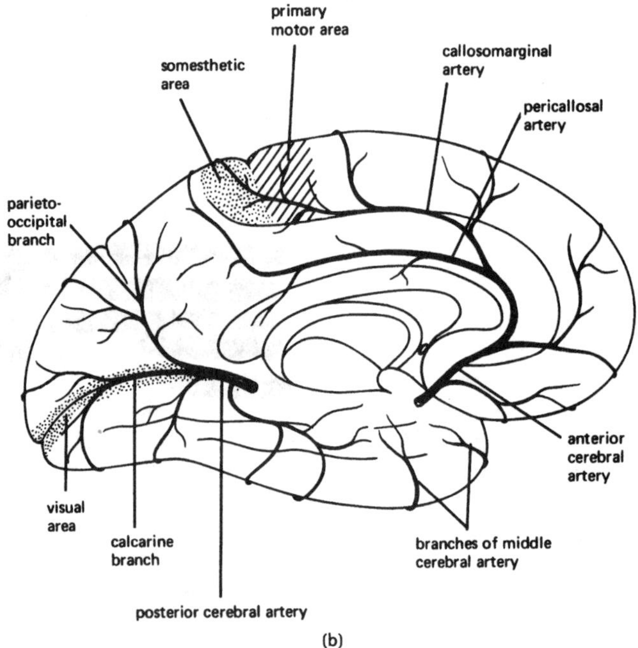

FIGURE 2.1 Distribution of the three cerebral arteries to the (a) lateral and (b) medial surfaces of the brain are shown relative to functional areas for speech and language (also see Figure 3.1). The lateral view primarily depicts the middle cerebral artery.

Reprinted by permission from Barr, M. L., *The human nervous system*. Hagerstown, Md.: Harper & Row, 1974.

stages of accumulation. This *stroke-in-evolution* (or "progressing stroke") may proceed in a stepwise fashion, and maximum deficit is referred to as *completed stroke.* There is higher incidence of thrombosis among people with diabetes mellitus and hypertension (or high blood pressure) than in the general population.

A frequent signal of impending thrombosis is the *transient ischemic attack* (TIA), or "little stroke." TIAs are temporary disruptions of blood flow. They produce transient neurological signs indicating that platelet formation is underway, generally in the internal carotid artery. The neurological signs include blurring of vision, numbness or weakness on one side, speech difficulty, imbalance or unsteadiness of gait, or a combination of these. The event frequently lasts a few minutes and usually less than an hour. However, it is defined as completed within 24 hours. There is about 20 percent chance of suffering a stroke during the first year after TIAs begin and a 30 to 60 percent chance in five years (Metter, 1986).

Whereas the sites of origin and occlusion are the same in thrombosis, these sites differ with an **embolism.** Platelets and fatty plaque break off a vessel wall and then travel until they become stuck in a smaller cerebral artery. The heart is the most common source of embolic material, and medical history is likely to include cardiac disease. Embolism may also be a secondary effect of trauma. Clinical onset is quicker or more abrupt than thrombosis. Time to maximum deficit takes only seconds or minutes. Thus, stroke-in-evolution is less frequent. There are usually no warnings. Often physicians are unable to determine whether an ischemia is thrombotic or embolic, so that they may refer to "thromboembolic CVA" in a medical report.

When metabolism is prohibited for about two minutes, the result is death (or necrosis) of neural tissue. The necrotic tissue is called an **infarction.** A physician may report that a patient has suffered a "thromboembolic infarct." Over time the damaged tissue softens and liquifies. This waste is removed by a process called gliosis because of the assistance from star-shaped astroglial cells (astrocytes) that hold neurons in place. Gliosis leaves a cavity on the surface of cortex that looks like a crater on the moon.

Technically, ischemia refers to the occlusion in an artery, whereas infarction is the resultant necrosis of brain tissue. However, in medical reports, we may see the terms used interchangeably when identifying type of stroke.

Acute Phase

The doctor informed Jackie Exeter that Martin has weakness on only one side of his body and intact sensory functions. The doctor added, "It is hard to know the extent of damage until some pictures can be taken of Martin's brain and he gets past his confusion. This bewilderment is common and temporary in most cases." Stroke is unlike more familiar medical conditions with specific treatments and recuperation periods. It took a few days to know more about what happened in Martin's head, and it took a few days more to have some idea about the more lasting outcome.

Caution about prognosis is prompted by **diaschisis,** which is a temporary suspension of functions that depend on structures remote from an infarct. Upon infarction or other injury to the brain, a swelling of surrounding tissue develops due to accumulation of water called **edema.** It takes two or three days to peak and one or two more weeks to subside. Sometimes edema extends throughout the brain. In addition, a reduction of blood flow extends to both hemispheres following a single occlusion. Flow to the uninfarcted side improves dramatically within two or three weeks after onset. Edema and reduced blood flow are likely to cause temporary generalized deficits for most patients.

In a hospital's Stroke Unit, a physician's main concern is the patient's survival. The patient is confined to bed with feet slightly elevated to avoid rapid lowering of blood pressure during stroke-in-evolution. Patients with low levels of consciousness are nourished with intravenous fluids. Within two or three days after a completed stroke, physical exercises may be started a few times per day to prevent muscle contractures. Self-care activities are started for psychological and physical well-being.

Several medications are indicated for treating stroke in the acute period (Table 2.1). Some are for preventing additional strokes, and others are for treating the physiologic effects of a stroke. Some drugs have been used for a long time, and many are still being investigated. *Anticoagulants* (also "anti-thrombotic") improve blood flow and prevent clotting. *Antiplatelets* are "clot dissolving." Thrombosis can be delayed or avoided with anticoagulants prescribed judiciously. In the 1990s, a great deal of publicity was given to medications, such as Nimodipine and Nadroparin, that may minimize damage when administered within the first six hours after an episode.

Chronic Phase

Five days after admission to the Stroke Unit, Martin was transferred to the Rehabilitation Unit in the same facility for subacute care. Patients in smaller acute care hospitals may be discharged to a freestanding rehabilitation center or even to home. For Martin, diaschisis had not completely subsided. It generally takes two or three weeks before edema has largely cleared and the pattern of dysfunction attributable to the infarct emerges.

Because neural tissue in the cortex does not regenerate, infarction presents a permanent neurological condition. Speech-language pathologists often delay full examination two or three weeks after onset, until medical stability is established and the specific disorder is manifested. In Martin's situation, he was examined briefly at bedside while in the Stroke Unit, and the clinician explained his aphasia to Jackie. Once in the Rehab Unit, he was immediately evaluated by the rehabilitation team for overall functional status as an initial baseline before therapy began (see Chapter 7).

For a long time, we thought that chronic dysfunction is caused soley by the size and location of infarction. However, studies of cerebral metabolism support a more complex picture of pathophysiology because of **remote effects** some distance from infarction. For years beyond the period of diaschisis, a patient may still have a reduction of blood flow. Such reduction of blood flow is called *hypoperfusion* (a term mainly associated with inadequate cardiac function).

This diminished blood flow reduces metabolism (called *hypometabolism*) and potentially causes an ischemic *penumbra* or insufficient operation of structurally intact regions of cortex. The research shows that, with an infarct in left language areas, hypometabolism occurs in adjacent and distant cortex of the same hemisphere and in some subcortical regions (Metter and Hanson, 1994). Around 57 percent of aphasic subjects showed hypometabolism in the left prefrontal region, anterior to Broca's area (see Figure 1.3); but only 22 percent had structural damage in that re-

TABLE 2.1 Medications used in stroke prevention and acute stroke therapy.

MAIN USE	PROCESS	DRUG	COMMENT
stroke prevention	anticoagulant	Enoxaparin	
		Nadroparin	low molecular weight heparin
		Warfarin	
	antiplatelet	Aspirin	
		Clopidigrel	may be more effective than aspirin
acute stroke therapy	anticoagulant	Heparin	prevention
	antiplatelet	Abciximab	prevention
	neuroprotective	Nimodipine	calcium antagonist or channel blocker
		Ebselen	free radical scavenger

gion. In general, a chronic symptom pattern may be attributed to tissue damage and these remote effects. Metter and Hanson concluded that frontal remote effects may also be indicative of the brain's attempt to adjust to infarction in language areas.

HEMORRHAGE

"Dr. K. begins to talk, I hear almost nothing after the words 'brain hemorrhage'...My mouth hangs open, and my respiration comes in percussive bursts, like a cap gun. Each breath pokes the fingertip of this new danger into my ribs, and hurts. My eyes work the shadows, I can't meet Dr. K.'s gaze...I imagine a navy-blue baseball jacket with a gold team patch, the one I wore as a clumsy teen to make me feel pride. This isn't like me to be so sick..." (Fishman, 1988, pp. 65–66).

While in a hotel lobby in Nicaragua, journalist Steve Fishman's vision suddenly became fuzzy and undulating, and then an arcing pain pounded in his head with each heartbeat. He wrote a book about his experiences, including neurological evaluations and neurosurgery. A hemorrhage is a bursting artery causing blood to flood the brain's surface or invade brain tissue. The accumulation, called a **hematoma,** is a rapidly expanding mass that displaces and compresses adjacent structures. Common initial symptoms of this sudden "space-occupying lesion" include excruciating headache, nausea, and vomiting. A hemorrhage can be caused by naturally weakened vessel walls or by tearing of arteries during traumatic brain injury.

Hemorrhages are classified with respect to location. Mostly occurring in patients with high blood pressure, an **intracerebral hemorrhage** invades deep regions of the thalamus, internal capsule, and lenticular nuclei or basal ganglia (Figure 2.2). About half of these cases lose consciousness in minutes to hours after rupture, which may be precipitated by a sudden increase of blood pressure during physical activity or emotional stress. Branches of the Circle of Willis and basilar artery are most susceptible. Medication reduces edema and blood pressure, and surgical evacuation of the hematoma is possible from some areas.

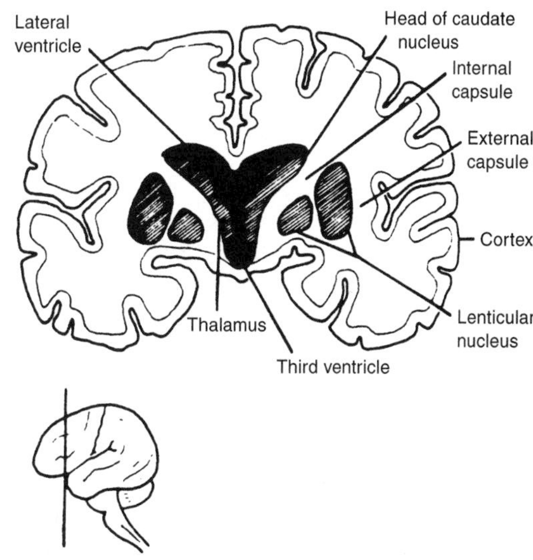

FIGURE 2.2 Frontal (coronal) section of the cerebrum shows location of the layer of cortex and certain interior structures.

From Willard R. Zemlin, *SPEECH AND HEARING SCIENCE: Anatomy and Physiology,* © 1968, pp. 466, 469. Reprinted by permission of Prentice-Hall, Inc., Englewood Cliffs, N.J.

Subarachnoid hemorrhage occurs in the pia-arachnoid space surrounding the brain and can be caused by a ruptured aneurysm near the Circle of Willis. An *aneurysm* is a dilated blood vessel from the size of a pea to an orange, stretching and weakening the vessel wall (Chusid, 1979). Rupture of an aneurysm may be provoked by sudden physical exertion but can be prevented by surgery when the dilation is accessible. Procedures include "trapping" the reservoir by applying clips on both sides, clipping the neck of the bulge, or packing muscle around the aneurysm. Plastics may be sprayed on the dilation and surrounding vessels.

Arterial walls are also weakened in the condition of *arteriovenous malformation* (AVM), in which the capillary network between arteries and veins is absent. Vessels are twisted and tangled. It may occupy a tiny area or an entire hemisphere. Presumably a congenital condition, presence of

AVM may not be signaled until hemorrhage or seizures occur in adulthood. Bleeding occurs in the subarachnoid space. A hemorrhaging AVM is usually less damaging than a bursting aneurysm.

TUMOR

A tumor (or neoplasm) is an abnormal mass of tissue caused by an increased rate in the reproduction of cells. A neoplasm is a space-occupying lesion that presses against adjacent tissue and obstructs circulation. *Benign* tumors do not spread to other parts of the body and are not recurrent. However, in the brain they can grow large enough to be dangerous. *Malignant* or cancerous tumors expand uncontrollably and are resistent to treatment. They may spread to other parts of the body via the bloodstream (called metastasis).

Medical Diagnosis

Early symptoms of malignant neoplasms usually are quite general reductions of function. Like hemorrhage, space-occupying pressure causes headache, nausea, and vomiting. Sensory impairments and dulled mental function may occur; and, if the tumor is allowed to enlarge, impairment may evolve to stupor and coma. Specific dysfunctions depend on location and may include loss of vision or hearing when there is pressure on the optic or acoustic cranial nerves.

To determine whether a tumor is benign or malignant, a pathologist performs a *biopsy* in which tissue or cells are removed from the body with a needle for examination under a microscope. Cells of a benign tumor are very much like their tissue origin. Cells of a malignant tumor are less recognizable. For areas that are difficult to reach, a "guided" biopsy can be performed with the aid of neuroimaging techniques such as CT or ultrasound scanning that help the physician follow progress of the needle (discussed later in this chapter). Another advance is the use of very fine needles, called stereotactic biopsy.

A study was done to determine if CT-guided stereotactic biopsy in the left hemisphere causes deterioration of language functions. Language was assessed with standard aphasia tests before and after a biopsy sample was obtained. Results showed that the particular biopsy procedure carries a nine percent risk of impairing language functions if the patient is not aphasic preoperatively. If the patient is aphasic preoperatively, there is a high risk of aggravating the aphasia (Thomson, Taylor, Fraser, and Whittle, 1997).

Classification

Neoplasms are named according to their tissue origin. A common source is supportive cells throughout the central nervous system called glial cells. For example, an **astrocytoma** originates in the housekeeping astroglia mentioned earlier with respect to infarction. Several grades of malignancy can be determined based on rate of cell growth, differentiation of cell types, and number of abnormal cells.

Astrocytoma grades 3–4 (also, *glioblastoma multiforme* or malignant glioma) is the most common primary brain tumor in adults. It is a rapidly growing mass likely to infiltrate both hemispheres through the commissures. George Gershwin, composer of "Porgy and Bess," suffered the earliest signs of a temporal lobe glioblastoma multiforme while conducting the Los Angeles Philharmonic Orchestra at age 38. Preferred treatment is surgery which consists of craniotomy (i.e., opening the skull) followed by resection of tissue. Surgeons may report "gross total removal of the tumor," but it usually recurs in months (Weiss, 1982). Survival averages about one year. Gershwin died two days after his surgery (Rolak, 1993).

Astrocytoma grades 1–2 (low-grade astrocytoma) is much less common but has a more favorable prognosis. It expands slowly, and symptoms may appear years before the tumor is discovered. Complete removal is seldom accomplished, but repeated surgery can be beneficial when the neoplasm is accessible. Prognosis after surgery has been reported variably at three to six years.

Meningioma is a benign tumor arising from the arachnoid tissue covering the brain. After glioblastoma, it is the second most common primary brain tumor in adulthood. Unlike other tumors, it occurs more frequently in women than men. Fifty percent occur over the lateral surfaces, and 40 percent occur at the base of the brain. They grow slowly and usually do not invade the cortex. Complete removal is often possible, with prolonged survival being a frequent outcome of surgery. Recurrence is possible in a small proportion of cases.

OTHER NEUROPATHOLOGIES

Some debate has swirled around whether other neuropathologies, especially progressive ones, cause aphasia. The traditional position in speech-langauge pathology is reflected in Rosenbek and others' (1989) declaration that "aphasia in adults does not creep, it erupts" (p. 53). This is based on the pronounced language-specificity of aphasia subsequent to erupting strokes and a traditional association of progressive diseases with diffuse damage and "generalized intellectual impairment" (e.g., Wertz, 1985). However, with some intense study of progressive diseases, a significant revelation is that damage can be more localized than we once thought. A fairly specific impairment may emerge from progressive disease. This type of discovery is one reason for not including causation in the definition of aphasia.

Dementing Diseases

Dementia is a category of heterogeneous disorders, and the term often gives the misleading impression that patients have sweeping cognitive dysfunctions. **Alzheimer's disease** is the most frequent cause of dementia in adulthood. It is one of several progressive and irreversible neuropathologies with a gradual onset and relentless deterioration. One characterisic change is a presence of *neurofibrillary tangles* which are unusual triangular and looped fibers in nerve cell bodies. A microscope also picks up granular deposits and remains of degenerated nerve fibers called *neuritic plaques.* These phenomena cause a gradual disruption of patterns of neural connection.

Alzheimer's disease has a fairly consistent pattern of pathology. Fibrillary tangles are pronounced in the *inferior temporal lobe* and accumulate in the *parieto-temporal juncture.* Studies of cerebral blood flow and metabolism reveal bilateral reduction in parietal and posterior temporal lobes. There can be more hypoperfusion in one hemisphere than the other hemisphere in early stages (Gray and Cummings, 1994). This concentration of pathology results in fairly specific impairments, especially of memory and language in the early stage. Some patients appear to have aphasia, despite some debate a few years ago over whether a language-specific disorder can be observed with Alzheimer's disease (Au, Albert, and Obler, 1988; Swindell, Boller, and Holland, 1988).

Early identification of Alzheimer's disease is difficult and precarious. Diagnosis is termed "probable dementia of Alzheimer's type" (or DAT) according to criteria developed at the National Institutes of Health in Washington, D.C. (McKhann, Drachman, Folstein, Katzman, Price, and Stadlan, 1984). It is identified clinically when there are two or more declining functions such as language (e.g., misnaming), memory (e.g., forgetting appointments), orientation (e.g., getting lost in familiar settings), and judgment (e.g., not wearing a coat in freezing weather). Diagnosis can also be a process of elimination, and DAT is considered in the absence of depression, multiple infarcts, alcoholism, malnutrition, or other conditions that produce similar symptoms. "The confirmation of the diagnostic hypothesis is a matter of histologic study of the post-mortem brain specimen" (Damasio, Van Hoesen, and Hyman, 1990, p. 91).

The course of Alzheimer's disease is a continuum of changes encompassing six-to-twelve years. Table 2.2 summarizes three stages. The individual in *Stage I* conducts household chores carelessly but can follow well-established routines. Conversation contains word-finding errors. The next stage places an increasing burden on family members, and a spouse becomes a parenting caregiver. In this *Stage II* memory impairments are more obvious and disruptive. Shoes are put on before socks. There is frequent pacing and

TABLE 2.2 Stages in the Progression of Dementia of Alzheimer's Type (DAT).

	OTHER TERMS	INTELLIGENCE	PERSONALITY	LANGUAGE
Stage I	Early Mild	Forgetful Disoriented Careless	Apathetic Anxious Irritable	Usually comprehends Vague words in talk Naming may be impaired Word fluency impaired Good repetition
Stage II	Middle Moderate	Recent events forgotten Math skills reduced	Restless	Comprehension reduced Paraphasias, jargon Irrelevant talk Naming becomes wordy Poor self-monitoring
Stage III	Late Severe	Recent events fade fast Remote memory impaired Family not recognized Incontinence		Becomes unresponsive Becomes mute

staring into space. In terminal *Stage III* sensory and neuromotor disabilities appear. The individual sits motionless in a corner and becomes totally dependent on others for tasks of daily living. When discussing someone with DAT, clinicians often identify if they are referring to an "early stage" or "late stage" condition.

Dementing diseases may be classified as progressive or nonprogressive (Table 2.3). A cortical-subcortical distinction is another basis of classification. For example, location of pathology in Alzheimer's disease and Pick's disease has been thought to be concentrated in cerebral cortex, whereas pathology in Parkinson's disease and Huntington's disease is below the level of cortex. However, white matter pathology has been found with Alzheimer's disease, and frontal lobe hypometabolism has been detected in some subcortical pathologies (Stuss and Levine, 1996). Because patterns of cognitive impairment differ between cortical and subcortical pathologies, the distinction is still considered by many to be clinically useful (Darvesh and Freedman, 1996).

One category of denegerative disease receiving more attention in the literature is **frontal lobe degenerations** (FLD). *Pick's disease* is the most well-known FLD. Neuroimaging techniques demonstrate hypoperfusion and hypometabolism in frontal lobes as well as atrophy of frontal convolutions (Gray and Cummings, 1994). It may also involve the temporal lobe. Pick's disease causes changes in organizational skills, language, and personality. Kertesz and Munoz (1997) suggested that it may be the second most common degenerative dementia. They also suggested that aphasia is a common early manifestation, an example of what is known as primary progressive aphasia.

Focal Cortical Atrophy

Primary progressive aphasia (PPA) or "aphasia without dementia" is an isolated language deterioration with relative preservation of other cognitive abilities. Mesulam's (1982) report of six cases led to widespread recognition of the syndrome.

TABLE 2.3 Summary of dementing diseases or conditions (e.g., Ross, Cummings, and Benson, 1990).

	DIAGNOSIS	SITE OF DAMAGE	DISEASE PROCESS
Progressive	Alzheimer's disease	bilateral parietal and temporal lobes (including hippocampus)	accumulation of neuritic plaques and neurofibrillary tangles
	Pick's disease	frontal lobe degeneration; more temporal lobe atrophy than in Alzheimer's disease	absence of plaques and tangles; neuronal loss; presence of "Pick's bodies"
	Parkinson's disease	"subcortical dementia" substantia nigra in the brain stem	cell loss reducing production of the neurotransmitter dopamine
	Huntington's disease	"subcortical dementia" caudate nucleus of the basal ganglia	inherited atrophy of the caudate
Nonprogressive	multiple infarcts	any location	accumulated small ischemic strokes; also called stroke-related dementia (SRD)
	herpes simplex viral encephalitis (HSVE)	medial temporal areas extending into orbitofrontal regions; usually bilateral	infection causing acute necrosis, edema and hemorrhage; sometimes evolves to coma in 2–3 days

Westbury and Bub (1997) reviewed 119 cases appearing in the literature since Mesulam's report. The reviewers found the case studies to be unsystematic, relying on a wide variety of neuropsychological instruments. "These limitations have made it difficult to place the published reports into a coherent theoretical structure" (p. 381).

PPA usually starts as a difficulty with a particular language function, and then it spreads to other language functions. The most common early deficit is misnaming. By the third year after initial appearance of symptoms, cases are quite heterogeneous. About 45 percent have a severe naming deficit, 30 percent still have a mild deficit, and most of the rest have no naming deficit. Many have no comprehension deficit in the first two years. Reading deficits are rarely seen before the fourth or fifth year. Thus, the classic multimodality deficit does not necessarily factor into diagnosis of aphasia in early stages.

Some investigators suggest that isolated language deficit may last at least two years, before dementia begins to develop. Kertesz and Munoz (1997) noted that the aphasia may be nonfluent leading to mutism (i.e., frontal lobe degeneration) or it may be fluent (i.e., temporal lobe degeneration). Some researchers in Great Britain considered PPA to be nonfluent (e.g., Croot, Patterson, and Hodges, 1998). They used the term "semantic dementia" for a fluent aphasia caused by predominantly left anterior temporal degeneration (see Chapter 6).

These specific deficits are possible because progressive pathologies can be localized to a region the size of an infarction. The pathologies may be referred to as **non-Alzheimer lobar degeneration.** Damage can be bilateral but with one side more impaired than the other. Pick's disease is considered to be a focal cortical degeneration (Black, 1996). In neuroimaging, degeneration shows up as *atrophy* or shrinkage of a portion of the brain. Interior spaces or ventricles are enlarged because of the decreased mass of adjacent brain matter. Atrophy is also viewed as enlarged sulci or spaces between cerebral convolutions.

With PPA, damage is concentrated in the perisylvian region of the left hemisphere. The existence of focal progressive neuropathologies suggests that aphasia and other specific cognitive disorders may indeed creep occasionally.

CLINICAL NEUROLOGICAL EXAMINATION

A *neurologist* is the specialist responsible for evaluation and treatment of persons with brain damage. He or she is able to examine the basic status of sensory, motor, and cognitive systems in about thirty minutes. In addition to determining if deficits are caused by neurological dysfunction, the physician wants to know the nature and site of damage. Radiological tests confirm and elaborate preliminary diagnosis based on clinical examination. With the accuracy and availability of brain imaging technology, the neurologist no longer has to rely on clinical examination to localize lesion. This specialist relates clinical findings to radiological findings and orders referrals to rehabilitative specialists so that impairments can be evaluated more thoroughly.

Clinical examination begins the instant the physician first sees a patient. Alertness indicates the status of the reticular activating system in the brain stem (see Figure 1.3). The doctor presses a stethoscope lightly to each temple to listen for unusual rushing sounds in the cerebral bloodstream called *bruits.* This examination is called *auscultation.* An initial interview yields clues about cognition, including language. The doctor may carry a brief screening test such as the *Mini-Mental State Examination* (Folstein, Folstein, and McHugh, 1975).

Systematic examination begins with motor and sensory systems to assess the peripheral and central nervous systems. Simple reflexes are tapped from head to toe, with hypoactivity indicating peripheral damage and hyperactivity indicating central damage. Balance and coordination are indicative of cerebellar function. Loss of sensation on one side is called *hemianesthesia,* and paralysis on one side is called *hemiplegia.* Left and right sides are compared with the normal side being a standard for estimating severity of unilateral impairment in the aphasic individual. Motor and/or sensory impairment of one side signify damage to the contralateral cerebral hemisphere, and deficits of specific body parts reflect damage to particular locations along pre- and postcentral gyri.

Visual deficits are particularly informative regarding the site of neuropathology. The visual system is not a directly contralateral connection between the eyes and the occipital lobes. Instead, contralaterality exists between *fields of vision* and the cerebral hemispheres. When we look straight ahead, we see objects to the left and right of the center. Moreover, we can see to the left and right of center with each eye. The right occipital lobe receives what we see in the left visual field (LVF), and the left occipital lobe receives vision in the right field (RVF). The left and right optic nerves make these connections by crossing only partially at the base of the brain. Neurology books have a diagram that displays this crossing point, called the optic chiasm.

Specific visual deficits are indicative of location of a tumor or other pathology, especially relative to the optic chiasm. Damage between the optic chiasm and one eye produces blindness of that eye, but a patient can still see each field with the other eye. Because of the unique structure of the optic tracts (i.e., partial crossing), damage between the optic chiasm and the left occipital lobe causes blindness for the RVF, which is a problem for each eye. The loss of a field of vision is called *homonomous hemianopia.* A "right field cut" can occur with aphasia, because the optic nerve radiates through the parietal and temporal lobes on its way to the occipital lobe. The speech-language pathologist should ask a patient to look straight ahead and then should present objects to the left or right in order to determine if visual field matters in responding to visual stimuli.

CLINICAL BRAIN IMAGING

Scientists are inventing increasingly safe, efficient, and accurate means of viewing the living brain. Some newer or more expensive procedures are currently used to observe normal brain function for basic research and are not routine clinical procedures. There are two general types. One is spatial or *structural neuroimaging* which produces a static picture of brain anatomy. The other is temporal or *functional neuroimaging* which is sensitive to neural activity that may be associated with cognitive processes. Researchers are discovering pathologies with these procedures, such as focal cortical atrophies, that had been only hypothesized or even denied a couple decades ago.

Procedures in either category can be *invasive* in that a foreign substance (e.g., "contrast medium") is injected in the body so that structures can seen more clearly, or they can be *noninvasive* in that no substance is introduced. Because injecting any foreign substance into the circulatory system increases risks in a procedure, research is partly devoted to decreasing or eliminating the invasiveness of imaging procedures.

Structural Neuroimaging

Cerebral **angiography,** or **arteriography,** is an X-ray procedure for observing arteries in the head and neck. As an invasive approach, an iodinated opaque fluid is injected usually in a carotid artery so that the cerebral arteries can be seen on X-ray film. With ischemia, vessels cannot be seen beyond the point of an occlusion. Tumors or other space occupying lesions are inferred from distortion of the arterial pattern. *Digital-subtraction angiography* is a recent development based on computer computation that improves image quality and reduces the amount of contrast medium injected in the blood stream.

Computerized tomography (CT scan) permits detailed imaging of cerebral structures through computerized reconstruction. Scanners have undergone stages or generations of development, and a fourth-generation scanner is sketched in Figure 2.3. CT scan uses narrow beams of X-rays on a scanner that rotates around the head. Intensity of the x-rays is detected and sent to a computer which transforms the data into absorption coefficients indicative of tissue densities. Results are displayed as tiny blocks of tissue, which is a

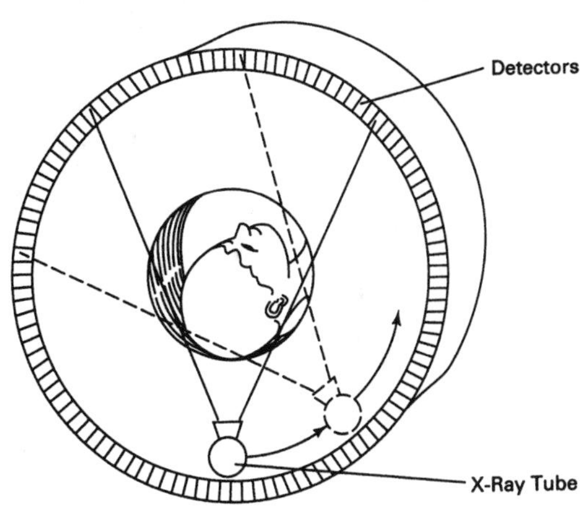

FIGURE 2.3 Schematic representative of a fourth generation CT scanner. An X-ray tube revolves around the body while emitting a beam wide enough to encompass the width of a patient. Stationary detectors measure the activity penetrating the body.

Reprinted by permission from Patronas, N. J., Deveikis, J. P., & Schellinger, D., The use of computer tomography in studying the brain. In H. G. Mueller & V. C. Geoffrey (Eds.), *Communication disorders in aging: Assessment and management.* Washington, D.C.: Gallaudet University Press, 1987, p. 110.

"reconstruction" of structures in a particular plane of the cerebrum.

Images of several planes are obtained in about 30 minutes. Figure 2.4 shows locations of infarction as they might be found in a horizontal plane: anterior to the central sulcus (including the insula), deep in lenticular nuclei, medial (including posterior insula), and posterior invading the occipital lobe. Simple anterior-posterior classification may put the medial infarction in the posterior category.

An advantage of the CT scan lies in power of resolution of a lesion and detection of longstanding CVAs. Pathology is indicated by alterations in the normally expected densities of brain structures. Infarct is shown as decreased tissue density, and hemorrhage is shown as increased density. Identifying an infarction can be improved with injection of a contrast material. CT scan is particularly good at distinguishing between infarct and intracerebral hemorrhage. Methods for calculating lesion size and tissue density were detailed in CT studies of aphasia (Naeser, Hayward, Laughlin, and Zatz, 1981). The main concern with this procedure is its exposure of radiation to the patient.

A much sharper image without radiation exposure is achieved with **magnetic resonance imaging** (MRI). This noninvasive procedure capitalizes on areas of high water density. It is based

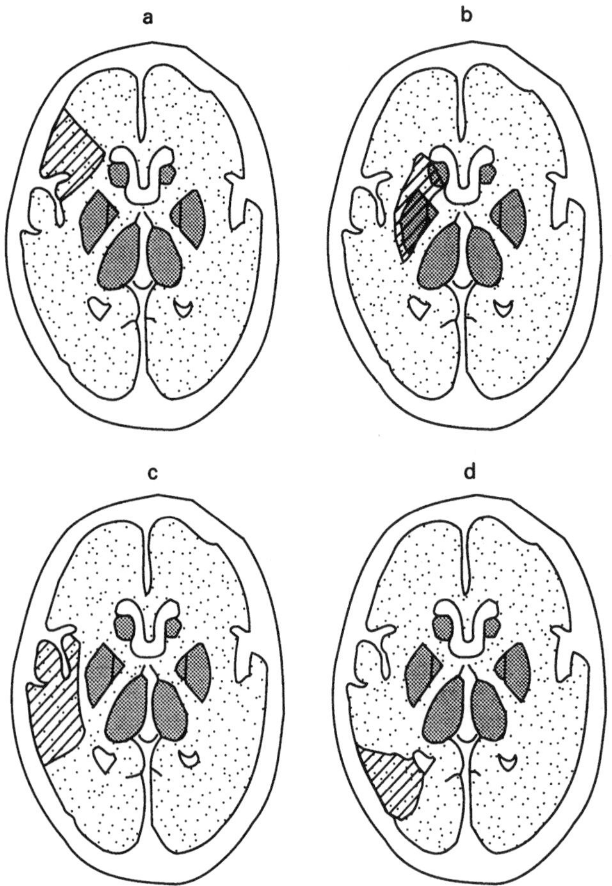

FIGURE 2.4 Four areas of infarction within the territory of the middle cerebral artery: (a) anterior, (b) deep, (c) medial, and (d) posterior. (Reprinted by permission from Habib, M., Ali-Cherif, A., Poncet, M., & Salamon, G., Age-related changes in aphasia type and stroke location. Brain and Language, 31, 1987, p. 247. Academic Press, publisher.)

on the "spin" of molecules within the nucleus of an atom. First, the body is placed in an area surrounded by a large electromagnet (meaning that persons with metallic implants cannot be assessed). The magnet manipulates the spin of hydrogen molecules with the magnetic field and radio waves. Then, a computer creates a picture of the brain from the electromagnetic signals generated by this manipulation.

MRIs produce clear images of bone and soft tissue, and they contrast gray and white matter in the brain. They are superior to CT scans in their sensitivity to subtle neuropathologies and their early detection of diseases involving physiological changes. Because the procedure is noninvasive, it may be used repeatedly on the same patient and, therefore, is well suited for longitudinal studies. Brookshire (1997) noted that "MRI scans take a long time, and the patient must remain motionless in a noisy, confining space, sometimes leading to claustrophobia and blurring the MRI image because of patient movement" (p. 67).

Another noninvasive procedure is the application of **ultrasound scanning,** which has been commonly employed in obstetrics for obtaining pictures of a fetus about 16 to 18 weeks into the pregnancy. For obtaining pictures of the brain, inaudible high frequency sound waves are transmitted into the head, and reflected echoes are detected and analyzed with a computer. Ultrasound is used to scan the brain of a newborn child for diagnosing hemorrhage or tumors. As indicated earlier, it is being used to guide stereotactic biopsy.

Functional Neuroimaging

Two aspects of neurophysiology are measured in functional neuroimaging. One is the electrical activity of neurons, called electrophysiological neuroimaging. The other approach, called metabolic neuroimaging, is a little less direct and measures blood flow and metabolism. Because of their experimental use, Martin Exeter did not receive any of these procedures.

Perhaps the first method for detecting cerebral pathology in a living patient is **electroencephalography** (EEG). It records the electrical activity of the brain from the placement of electrodes at different locations on the scalp. The site of focal lesion is estimated by comparing graphic representations of brain waves detected from these locations in each lobe of each hemisphere. A lesion is indicated by electrical activity in one location that differs from regular patterns detected at other regions. Although EEG is crude for localizing pathology, it is still useful for distinguishing subcortical from cortical lesions and for estimating severity of damage when a patient is in a coma.

Because EEG is a safe procedure, it has been used extensively in the investigation of normal brain function. A refinement, called the *evoked potential* (EP) or event-related potential (ERP), has some clinical usefulness but also has provided an "exquisite" resolution of the temporal nature of cortical events (Springer and Deutsch, 1998). A computer is used to tease specific neural responses to stimuli out of the complexity of EEG activity. The neural or evoked response appears as a positive or negative spike in the computed wave. Several studies have used the EP to correlate neural responses to hypothesized cognitive stages in word and sentence processing.

Metabolic imaging is used to observe regional activity of the cortex while a person is performing a particular task. **Regional cerebral blood flow** (rCBF) is an indirect measure of metabolism. The procedure capitalizes on an increase of neural activity in a cortical region which causes an increased demand for nourishment and, thus, increased metabolic activity. Blood flow rate increases to satisfy this increased demand. A radioactive compound is injected in the bloodstream or inhaled as a gas. A scanner detects variations in blood flow rate over different regions. The procedure is used to look for activity that may be compensating for infarction.

Single-photon emission computed tomography (SPECT) is an increasingly available and relatively inexpensive procedure that produces a three-dimensional representation of cerebral blood flow. Employing a radioactive tracer nicknamed Tc-99m, investigators can "lock in" brain activity at the time of injection and view that localized activity later. This capability is advantageous for locating epileptic seizure activity as it happens and for detecting neural activity as a patient is performing a cognitive task.

Studies of hypometabolism mentioned earlier were conducted with **positron emission tomography** (PET). The PET scan is a direct measure of metabolism and is more responsive to rapid variations of activity than rCBF studies (Metter and Hanson, 1994). It may detect cortical dysfunction in Alzheimer's disease before cognitive dysfunction can be demonstrated clinically (Gray and Cummings, 1994). Radioactive tracers, called positron-emitting isotopes, are combined either with oxygen or glucose and injected into arteries. After 50 minutes, a rotating scanner detects the rate at which tissue utilizes radioactive nutrients. Metter (1987) noted "the primary limitation for its widespread use is the short half-life of the radionuclides which require the presence of a readily available cyclotron for isotope production" (p. 7). Thus, PET scanning is more expensive than SPECT, limiting its potential for clinical application.

Once called BOLD MRI, **functional magnetic resonance imaging** (fMRI) can detect different oxygen levels in the brain because magnetic properties of oxygenated blood are different from deoxygenated blood. By taking a series of MRI scans, an investigator can identify regions activated while someone is performing a cognitive activity. Springer and Deutsch (1998) reported that fMRI "has revolutionized the study of activated brain function in normal subjects because it can provide data with a temporal resolution of several seconds, can scan activation during any task multiple times, and/or can provide almost continuous information about cerebral activity occurring during changing study conditions" (p. 73).

Transcranial Doppler ultrasound (TDU) is a modified version of ultrasound scanning that examines moving objects such as blood pressure and flow in a cerebral artery. While a patient is reclining in a chair or on an examining table, gel is applied to an area of the head where the bone is thin enough to allow the Doppler signal to enter and be detected (called the transcranial window). A technician directs the signal toward the artery being studied and records detected rates. High flow rates indicate the narrowing of a blood vessel or an arteriovenous malformation. The procedure may also determine if a secondary route of blood flow exists prior to surgery for diseased vessels.

LOCALIZATION AND DISSOCIATION

A specific cognitive dysfunction such as aphasia is possible because the brain is organized into functionally specialized regions and certain neuropathologies can damage one of these regions while sparing others. Our knowledge of regional specialization comes mainly from studies that relate specific dysfunctions to sites of lesion. These studies began in the 1800s, relying on an autopsy to find the damage causing language difficulties. This is called the *lesion-deficit method* for determining the functional responsibilities of areas of the brain. Through the 1970s, the lesion-deficit method was modernized with improved imaging of lesions that can be identified near the time of more comprehensive and standardized evaluation of behavior.

The study of deficits for localizing functions requires the identification of patients with a single impairment. The common term is **dissociation,** which is a pronounced deficit in one task (or a set of tasks) while other performances remain intact or are clearly less impaired. It is as if one function is separated from others. With deficits primarily on language tasks, aphasia is said to be a dissociation of language functions from other abilities. Damage to the left hemispere is suggestive of a left hemisphere role in normal language function. A cognitive neuropsychologist would say that the dissociation indicates that the particular impairment signifies a distinct cognitive process.

There are problems with this simple lesion-deficit approach for inferring the jobs performed by an area of the cortex. One problem is that finding one deficit-lesion relationship does not rule out the possibility that other locations also have a role in the impaired function. For example, discovering that left hemisphere damage causes reading but not drawing deficits does not by itself rule out the possibility that the right hemisphere is also involved in reading. What if right hemisphere damage also causes difficulty with reading tasks?

One solution to this problem is for an investigator to compare the effects of damage in two areas, such as the left and right hemispheres, before concluding that one area is responsible for one function. Continuing with the same example, groups with left and right hemisphere infarcts would be given tests of reading and drawing. If the left damaged group shows the same dissociation but the right damaged group shows good reading and impaired drawing, then we have less ambiguous evidence of a left hemisphere role in reading. Conversely, we would also have evidence that the right brain has a specific role in drawing. This is called a **double dissociation,** which is shown when one patient or group of patients produces a deficit in one task or set of tasks along with no deficit in another task or set of tasks, while another patient or group produces the opposite pattern.

When a cognitive neuropsychologist is searching for evidence of distinct cognitive processes, Ellis and Young (1988) argued that "it would be unwise to regard the search for double dissociations as some sort of royal road to understanding the structure of the mind" (p. 5). Investigators still need to interpret performance on the task or set of tasks that are uniquely deficient.

CLINICAL SYNDROMES OF APHASIA

Aphasic patients are observed to have specific dissociations with respect to linguistic features of language production. For example, some patients have more difficulty finding words (i.e., anomia) than forming sentences (i.e., agrammatism), whereas other patients have more difficulty with sentences than with words. Researchers interested in dividing up the functional responsibilities of the left hemisphere have taken such double dissociations to mean that one part of the left brain deals with word-finding and another part deals with structuring sentences. In either case, a patient displays a particular pattern of deficit, and in this section we shall examine relationships between a pattern of aphasic deficit and site of lesion.

A *syndrome* is a recurring pattern of symptoms. The history of aphasiology is cluttered with systems for labeling different patterns of aphasia. Benson (1979) noted that "the resulting aphasic syndromes represent one of the most confusing aspects of the complex topic of language disturbance" (p. 57). Chapter 1 introduced a broad distinction between nonfluent and fluent aphasias. Nonfluent aphasias tend to be caused by damage in the anterior region, whereas fluent aphasias tend to be caused by damage to posterior regions (Mazzochi and Vignolo, 1979; Naeser and Hayward, 1978). PET studies show that nearly all cases have reduced metabolism in the left temporo-parietal region, indicating that this region is minimally necessary for language processing (Metter and Hanson, 1994).

In the most common classification system, the main syndromes are differentiated according to three key areas:

- severity of *comprehension* deficit
- linguistic features of *spontaneous verbal expression*
- *repetition* ability compared to spontaneous expression

A key symptom may alert a clinician to the likelihood that a patient has a particular syndrome of aphasia. In fact, researchers who are uncomfortable with common classification may classify patients according to the key symptom (e.g., agrammatic aphasia). The syndromes are introduced here to illustrate dissociations within language, show how aphasia varies beyond the nonfluent–fluent dichotomy, and identify most likely sites of damage underlying different types of aphasia.

Broca's Aphasia

Broca's aphasia is named for a 19th century French physician who drew attention to localization of function in the brain. It used to be associated with "expressive aphasia." Agrammatism is the dominant feature, and word-finding is preserved better than sentence formulation. Auditory comprehension is slightly or moderately impaired. The clumsiness of apraxia of speech is likely to show up in the production of words, especially words that are difficult to articulate. The patient is often a good communicator, because the few words produced represent some of the message accurately. Also, our guesses as listeners are within the patient's comprehension ability.

Broca's area is also known as area 44 in the Brodmann numerical system that is used to identify cortical regions objectively or without attributing functional significance to them. Area 44 is located in the third frontal convolution anterior to the pre-central gyrus which distributes impulses to the muscles (see Figure 2.1). Because of this proximity to the primary motor strip, agrammatism is usually accompanied by right hemiplegia and a mild right facial weakness. It has been common to attribute Broca's aphasia to damage simply to Broca's area.

However, chronic agrammatic aphasia is produced by lesions extending from Broca's area to the anterior insula and neighboring anterior temporal and inferior parietal areas. Damage to deeper structures also seems necessary to produce this aphasia, including the posterior internal capsule of tracts between the thalamas and basal ganglia (Levine and Sweet, 1983). Lesions restricted to area 44 can cause an acute Broca's aphasia that may resolve quickly into something else (Kertesz, Harlock, and Coates, 1979). Such smaller lesions produce apraxia of speech or "Broca's area infarction syndrome" (Mohr, Pessin, Finkelstein, Funkenstein, Duncan, and Davis, 1978). Kertesz (1979) stated "there is a spectrum of syndromes produced by Broca's area infarct…the larger lesions produce the full-blown symptom complex of Broca's aphasia" (p. 187).

Global Aphasia

Global aphasia is a severe depression of language ability in all modalities. Some patients may speak noncommunicatively with verbal stereotypes (see Chapter 1). Yet, patients can be alert and aware of their surroundings, and they often express feelings and thoughts through facial, vocal, and manual gestures. The gloomy diagnosis of global aphasia should be reserved for when it can be determined that a patient has very poor language comprehension as well as an inability to speak and write.

The following problems may mask language abilities and give only the appearance of a comprehensive aphasia:

- motor impairments that make it difficult to determine comprehension
- extremely low level of arousal
- extreme disorientation or confusion
- depression or lack of motivation to communicate

The presence of these problems may lead a clinician to conclude correctly that the severity of aphasia is unknown. A diagnosis of global aphasia should be reported after careful consideration, because it can diminish the likelihood of support for speech-language treatment. Clinicians generally keep in mind that diagnosis of any aphasia pertains to how a patient deals with *language,* as opposed to processing other types of stimuli or making other types of responses.

Dissociations in global aphasia may be found in types of words a patient may be able to comprehend. For example, these patients were shown to comprehend famous personal names better than common nouns (Yasuda and Ono, 1998).

CT scans usually expose lesions covering the entire perisylvian region including Broca's and Wernicke's areas (Kertesz, Lesk, and McCabe, 1977; Mazzocchi and Vignolo, 1979; Murdoch, Afford, Ling, and Ganguley, 1986; Naeser and Hayward, 1978). Lesions may also reach deep into white matter beneath the cortex. A few cases have lesions confined to deep structures including the insula, lenticular nuclei, and internal capsule. An exception to pervasive perisylvian damage is an occasional global aphasia with Wernicke's area spared (Basso, Lecours, Maraschini, and Vanier, 1985; Cappa and Vignolo, 1988; Vignolo, Boccardi, and Caverni, 1986).

Wernicke's Aphasia

The most severe form of fluent aphasia is known by other names such as sensory aphasia, receptive aphasia, and jargon aphasia. The patient with Wernicke's aphasia has poor language comprehension, produces jargon, and often lacks awareness of semantic or neologistic paraphasias. The fluent jargon has recognizable sentence structure, indicative of a dissociation of word-finding from fundamental syntactic construction. A patient may continue talking when it is his turn to listen, known as *press for speech.* Sparks (1978) described people with Wernicke's aphasia as having poor "therapeutic set," because they do not realize why they are in the presence of a speech-language pathologist.

The syndrome of severe comprehension deficit and fluent jargon can be found with damage to Wernicke's area (posterior area 22) and neighboring temporal and parietal regions (Kertesz, 1979; Naeser and Hayward, 1978). On a CT scan, damage may look like the medial or posterior lesions of Figure 2.4 (Kirshner, Casey, Henson, and Heinrich, 1989). Often the posterior insula is involved (Mazzocchi and Vignolo, 1979), and in a small percentage of many cases, some frontal lobe damage made the lesions look like they should have caused global aphasia (Basso, et al., 1985; Kirshner, et al., 1989).

Some researchers have tried to distingish among the expressive symptoms that may dominate in the different manifestations of Wernicke's aphasia. A predominance of fluent phonemic paraphasias was related to infarction in Wernicke's area and the inferior parietal area above, whereas lexical (or verbal) paraphasias were related to infarcts in the more posterior angular gyrus and the adjacent occipital area (Cappa, Cavalotti, and Vignolo, 1981). Lesions causing neologistic jargon extended more posteriorly than lesions producing semantic jargon (Kertesz, 1982). Also, exceptional sites of damage have been found with clincial test-based diagnosis of Wernicke's aphasia. CT or MRI scans showed three of five cases to have infarcts in Wernicke's area but damage extended into the middle temporal gyrus. One had damage only to underlying white matter (Dronkers, Redfern, and Ludy, 1995).

Conduction Aphasia

Conversation with someone who has conduction aphasia can go smoothly. We can be surprised during formal testing when the patient's verbal expression deteriorates precipitously when repeating phrases of increasing length and complexity. The identifying characteristic of this disorder is a disruption of *repetition* that is disproportionately severe relative to comprehension ability and spontaneous speech. Free verbal expression is hampered by word finding problems and, especially, by occasional formal and phonemic paraphasias. However, repetition becomes jumbled in a way that is never heard in conversational speaking.

This aphasia is an example of a "disconnection syndrome," meaning that a dysfunction is caused by an impaired connection between structurally intact centers (Geschwind, 1965). These connections, or association tracts, are white axonal fibers running beneath the cortex and connecting one cortical region to another within a hemisphere. The *arcuate fasciculus* is an association tract beneath the left parieto-temporal juncture, and it carries impulses from Wernicke's area for listening to Broca's area for speaking. This connection enables us to repeat and is thought to be damaged in conduction aphasia. Thus, conduction aphasia can be said to be a "subcortical aphasia." It was found in a case of multiple sclerosis in which there was a large white matter lesion in the area of the arcuate fasciculus (Arnett, Rao, Hussain, Swanson, & Hammeke, 1996).

CT scans of individuals with this repetition disorder show anticipated damage to the posterior superior temporal cortex and inferior parietal cortex along with infarction of deep white matter below (Damasio and Damasio, 1980; Murdoch, et al., 1986). As predicted by disconnection theory, posterior temporal damage has been found to spare Wernicke's area (Naeser and Hayward, 1978). Mendez and Benson (1985) noted exceptions in three patients who were without lesions beneath the cortex. Kertesz and his colleagues (1977) speculated that two forms of conduction aphasia may arise depending on whether the lesion is more anterior (a less fluent "efferent conduction aphasia") or more posterior (a more fluent "afferent conduction aphasia").

Anomic Aphasia

Anomic aphasia (or "amnesic aphasia") is often the mildest form of aphasia. It consists of slightly impaired comprehension and fluent, syntactically coherent utterances that are weakened communicatively by a word retrieval deficit. Utterances are vacuous, filled with "generic terms" (indefinite nouns and pronouns) filling the void of concept-bearing content words. An example is the description of how to drive a car in Chapter 1.

Ambiguities can be resolved with situational context and knowledge of the topic. When naming objects, patients retrieve some words quickly or engage in elaborate circumlocution while trying to think of names for other objects. While comprehension is quite good, word recognition difficulties can be detected. The patient may retrieve a word and then for a moment fail to recognize that the word is correct. It might be helpful to keep in mind that all aphasic persons have "anomia" of some kind (the symptom), while only some have "anomic aphasia" (the syndrome).

A specific site of damage responsible for anomic aphasia has been somewhat elusive. The syndrome has been associated with damage to the posterior parieto-temporal juncture (i.e., angular gyrus). A fairly comprehensive structural and metabolic study of 12 patients with mild "anomic aphasia" was conducted by Illes, Metter, Dennings, Jackson, Kempler, and Hanson (1989). All patients had structural damage in the posterior superior temporal gyrus, but the researchers found two subgroups. The most fluent group had good metabolism in both frontal lobes, but a slightly less fluent group had left prefrontal hypometabolism as well as deep damage in addition to the temporal damage. Illes concluded that "an interplay between frontal cortex and neostriatal regions is essential for fluent and well-formed spontaneous language production" (p. 527).

Transcortical Aphasias

The rare transcortical aphasias are distinctive in that *repetition* is much better than would be expected from comprehension and spontaneous speech. Transcortical motor aphasia (TMA) is similar to Broca's aphasia with "a stumbling, repetitive, even stuttering spontaneous output" (Benson, 1979a, p. 84). A patient struggles to answer a question but can repeat a fifteen-word sentence without missing a beat. Lesions are generally located in the frontal lobe, superior and anterior to Broca's area (Rapcsak and Rubens, 1994).

Similarly, transcortical sensory aphasia (TSA) seems like Wernicke's aphasia. Ability to repeat is remarkable, because repetition is nearly impossible in Wernicke's aphasia. Echolalia, in which a person repeats a question instead of answering it, is a prominent feature. Lesions are usually posterior to the common language area. The damage has been picked up with CT imaging at the temporo-occipital border or the watershed area between middle and posterior cerebral arteries.

A mixed transcortical aphasia (MTA) is sort of a combination of TMA and TSA. Language disorder is severe with poor comprehension and meaningless stereotypic utterances. Yet, repetition can be compulsive. MTA is a global aphasia with ability to repeat. It is as if intact mechanisms of speech recognition and production are "isolated" from intentions and meanings generated in the rest of the brain. The literature is inconsistent on the presence of damage in the perisylvian language region. However, diffuse or multifocal pathologies do produce MTA with frontal and parietal damage while sparing the language area.

Caseload

Benson (1979a) concluded that "only about half of the cases of aphasia seen routinely in a clinical practice can clearly be placed into one or another of the syndromes and even this figure is dependent on some degree of diagnostic flexibility" (p. 136). Data on prevalence of syndromes is sometimes divided into cases with unequivocal diagnoses and those with equivocal diagnoses. The low yield of unequivocal diagnoses stems from the fact that many lesions are large or overlap functional regions. Benson added, "In view of the many potential complicating factors ...it is not at all surprising that pure examples of the aphasic syndromes are not common, and in fact it is remarkable that the recognizable syndromes shine through as often as they do" (p. 137). A summary of the syndromes is provided in Table 2.4.

EXCEPTIONAL APHASIAS

As noted previously, traditional diagnosis of aphasia has tied this disorder to etiologies that erupt and damage to the left perisylvian region of the cortex. Chapter 1 removed neurologic causation from the definition of dysfunction, which opens up the possibility of finding aphasias that creep. There are always going to be exceptions to traditional views as long as neuroimaging technology improves and clinical thinking continues to be inconsistent. "Exceptional aphasias" are those that are simply unusual and those that

TABLE 2.4 Summary of the contemporary clinical syndromes of aphasia.

GENERAL CATEGORY	SYNDROME	KEY SYMPTOMS	SITE OF LESION
Nonfluent/anterior	Broca's	agrammatic production	around and including Broca's area
	transcortical motor	like Broca's aphasia but with preserved repetition	prefrontal cortex
	global	poor comprehension, minimal production	posterior & frontal perisylvian language region
Fluent/posterior	Wernicke's	poor comprehension, jargon, press for speech	Wernicke's area (posterior portion of superior temporal gyrus)
	conduction	surprisingly impaired repetition	association tract beneath the temporo-parietal boundary
	anomic	word-finding deficit, empty speech	posterior temporo-parietal boundary (angular gyrus)
	transcortical sensory	like Wernicke's aphasia but with preserved repetition	inferior temporo-occipital border area (perhaps PCA occlusion)
	transcortical mixed	like global aphasia but with preserved repetition	diffuse or multifocal damage in frontal and parietal lobes

could, in some instances, be questionable because of inconsistent definition of dysfunction.

Crossed Aphasia

One unusual aphasia occurs because of individual variation in functional organization of the brain. A few people appear to have a reversed asymmetry with language functions in the right hemisphere and nonverbal functions in the left. Less than four percent of aphasic patients have crossed aphasia, in which right handed individuals have suffered a stroke in the right hemisphere. Researchers want to study cognitive deficits carefully in these cases, wondering if they are indicative of a mirror asymmetry or pure reversal of the norm or are indicative of a more mixed or unusual functional organization.

One review of reported cases indicated that 70 percent of crossed aphasias are a mirror image of typical left hemisphere profiles. Most classical syndromes are possible. Anomalous profiles occur in the remaining 30 percent. The anomalous cases tend to have large right perisylvian lesions but minimal aphasia along with absence of typical right hemisphere dysfunctions. Language deficits focus on phonological processes or lexical-semantic processes (Alexander, Fischette, and Fischer, 1989).

Bakar, Kirshner, and Wertz (1996) studied blood flow and metabolism in three cases. The mirrored expectation of diaschisis in the structurally intact left hemisphere was seen in each patient during the acute phase. In the one patient studied in the chronic period, remote depressions were not detected. The investigation also supported the assumption that exceptional dominance for language in the right hemisphere underlies crossed aphasia.

Subcortical Aphasias

In the review of syndromes, it was noted that cortical damage can be accompanied by subcortical damage (Mazzocchi and Vignolo, 1979). This is due to infarctions that have depth as well as width. "Subcortical aphasias," however, are diagnosed when damage is primarily beneath the cortex in the left hemisphere. Reports of these disorders have raised eyebrows with respect to their implications for neural mechanisms of language as well as for the nature of aphasia.

The key subcortical locations are presented in Figure 2.2. The *internal capsule* is a passage of white motor and sensory fiber tracts squeezed between the thalamus and lenticular nuclei. The *lenticular nuclei* consist of the caudate nucleus and putamen; and both may be referred to collectively as the striatum. These nuclei comprise a substantial part of the basal ganglia in the extrapyramidal motor system. In the literature on subcortical aphasia, an infarct may be identified generally in the basal ganglia or specifically in the putamen or in the capsulostriatum which includes the internal capsule, the caudate, and putamen.

The *thalamus* is the most central nucleus in the cerebrum, consisting of several parts with connections to motor, sensory, and association areas of cortex. Of particular importance are the white fiber connections between the thalamus and prefrontal regions of the cortex (see Figure 1.3), called the thalamofrontal gating system. This system may be responsible for focusing attention (see Chapter 9).

Kirk and Kertesz (1994) compared cortical and subcortical aphasias and found similarities with respect to scores on a standard aphasia test given 7 to 40 days after onset. All subcortical patients were classifiable into aphasia syndromes, but subcortical damage caused more motor and sensory impairments. In general, there is some disagreement over whether forms of subcortical language disturbance are genuine aphasia syndromes or are merely similar to these syndromes. Kennedy and Murdoch (1994) have argued strongly that subcortical damage can produce the same classical syndromes, but they also recognized reservations in using standard clinical tests to establish the true nature of a language disorder. Kirk and Kertesz noted that subcortical language deficits "change dramatically over time," so that diagnosis may be quite different even three months after a stroke (see Chapter 10).

Researchers divide subcortical language disturbances with respect to thalamic and nonthalamic lesions, mainly because these are somewhat distinct neural mechanisms. With a **thalamic lesion,** a patient is likely to have good comprehension and fluent semantic paraphasias and neologisms. Some cases have a transcortical-like sparing of repetition (Murdoch, 1988). In a recent report, two patients with left thalamic infarction demonstrated impairment limited to word retrieval difficulties in spontaneous language and structured naming tasks (Raymer, Moberg, Crosson, Nadeau, and Rothi, 1997). Lesions including the thalamus caused category-specific naming deficits for medical terms and names of celebrities (Crosson, Moberg, Boone, Rothi, and Raymer, 1997; Lucchelli, Muggia, & Spinnler, 1997).

Nonthalamic lesions are also classified as "striatocapsular" or "capsulostriatal" lesions and include the basal ganglia. Researchers in Boston identified syndromes called anterior, posterior, and global capsular/putaminal aphasias (Helm-Estabrooks and Albert, 1991). Anterior aphasias are like Broca's aphasia because of "slow, poorly-articulated speech output" but are unlike Broca's aphasia because of "intact grammatical form" (Naeser, 1988, p. 365). The posterior syndrome is much like Wernicke's aphasia. Fabbro, Clarici, and Bava (1996) studied three patients with lesions confined to the left basal ganglia. Two patients were nonfluent, whereas one presented with fluent spontaneous speech. All produced agrammatic sentences and lexical and semantic mistakes.

One problematic feature of the predominantly neurologically oriented studies of subcortical aphasia is that often no definition of *aphasia* is provided so that we know the criteria for diagnosing symptoms and selecting published cases for review (e.g., Nadeau and Crosson, 1997). It is as if we should assume that everyone agrees on what aphasia is. One reason for skepticism is the apparent interpretation of speech disturbances, especially with damage to the basal ganglia. For example, Alexander and others (1987) looked for "components of aphasic syndromes" that include "ease of speech initiation, articulation, and voice volume" (p. 961). Thus, there is the risk of suspecting that researchers are finding aphasias in apraxia of speech or voice disorders, or in any reduced test score.

There is pronounced disagreement over the complex neural mechanisms that might explain how language disturbance could arise from subcortical lesions (Cappa, 1997; Nadeau and Crosson, 1997; Wallesch, Johannsen-Horbach, Bartels, and Herrmann, 1997). Let us just consider two general possibilities. One explanation supposes that the thalamus and parts of the basal ganglia have a direct role in language functioning so that a lesion impairs that role (e.g., Robin and Schienberg, 1990).

Another explanation need not assume a direct role of subcortical structures in language. Studies of blood flow and metabolism indicate that subcortical lesion is accompanied by remote hypoperfusion creating a penumbral insufficiency for the left perisylvian cortical regions that are directly responsible for language functions (Metter and Hanson, 1994). Return of blood to the cortex may be responsible for the dramatic recoveries observed by Kirk and Kertesz. In general, diagnosis of communicative deficits depends on the time of assessment. This is one reason for considering site of lesion when suggesting a diagnosis and prognosis to a patient's family.

SUMMARY AND CONCLUSIONS

Aphasia occurs because of neuropathologies than can strike regions of the brain responsible for language functions. It is not necessary that the left perisylvian region be the only site of damage for a patient to have aphasia. However, aphasia appears in its clearest form when the left perisylvian region is the only area of damage. Focal neuropathologies include ischemic and hemorrhagic stroke, tumors, and progressive focal atrophies.

Family members, who were likely in a state of shock when the doctor explained what happened, may question the speech-language pathologist about why a particular severity or pattern of language deficit occurred. Armed with knowledge of anatomy and neuropathology, we can help family members and patients understand the effects of size and location of lesion. We may anticipate residual capacities based on our knowledge of intact regions.

Advances in neuroimaging technology reduce the use of clinical evaluation for diagnosing neuropathology. These advances also force revisions in neurological explanation of dysfunction. At one time, the diagnosis of aphasia syndromes was thought to help the neurologist diagnose site of lesion. Currently, the various syndromes simply alert us to the existence of different kinds of acquired language disorders. This individual variation indicates that goals of language treatment can vary from patient to patient.

Charles Dickens suffered a fatal left hemisphere stroke before completing "The Mystery of Edwin Drood" and revealing the solution. It became a Broadway play in which audiences voted on the ending (Rolak, 1993). Martin Exeter's stroke also left some projects unfinished.

CHAPTER 3

CLINICAL ASSESSMENT AND DIAGNOSIS

Complete evaluation of an aphasic patient considers the World Health Organization's levels introduced at the end of Chapter 1. Historically, assessment has been aimed at diagnosing and measuring *impairment.* The evaluation of *disability* and *handicap* had been relegated to informal interviewing and recording basic vocational and social information on a form that might accompany a test of impairment. The emphasis of this chapter is the assessment of language impairment. Standard methodologies for measuring disability have been developing over the past 20 years, motivated partly by the current orientation of health care management (see Chapter 7).

With shifts in rehabilitation settings and reimbursement plans, managed care has also focused the goals of formal evaluation and influenced the time devoted to diagnosing and assessing impairment. For example, when a patient is seen in temporary acute care, goals are tied to survival such as determining if the patient has swallowing problems and needs for communicative assistance. Differentiating speech and language disorders is helpful for discharge planning. A somewhat more detailed analysis of language impairments can be done once a patient is transferred to a rehabilitation unit or center.

This chapter spotlights three major aphasia batteries and a few supplemental tests. In between, it presents some strategies for quick initial evaluation. In covering the comprehensive batteries, the chapter presents what clinicians believe to be the important observations of aphasia.

COMPREHENSIVE NEUROPSYCHOLOGICAL EVALUATION

A clinical neuropsychologist's comprehensive behavioral assessment helps to determine if an aphasic patient has cognitive difficulties other than language deficits. The clinical psychology background of these professionals also delivers a perspective on emotional reactions to stroke and on personality changes. A speech-language pathologist can save assessment time by avoiding tests that overlap with the neuropsychological examination. On the other hand, such cognitive assessment may not be available in some settings.

The core neuropsychological battery is the **Wechsler Adult Intelligence Scale** (WAIS) (Wechsler, 1981). The battery is divided into verbal and performance scales summarized in Table 3.1. Three main scores consist of the Full Scale IQ (FSIQ), and the VIQ and PIQ for the verbal and performance sections. The difference between the VIQ and PIQ, called the *discrepancy score,* is of interest when someone has unilateral brain damage. A patient with left hemisphere damage is likely to have a lowered VIQ relative to the PIQ, and someone with right hemisphere damage is likely to present the reverse (Hom and Reitan, 1990). Several studies have shown that any discrepancy occurs more for men than for women, who tend to have little difference between the VIQ and PIQ no matter which side of the brain is damaged (e.g., Sundet, 1986).

Clinical psychologists begin with the WAIS when using the **Halstead-Reitan Neuropsychological Test Battery** (Reitan and Wolfson, 1985).

TABLE 3.1 Subtests of the Wechsler Adult Intelligence Scale (WAIS). When applied to brain damaged patients, the verbal and performance sections have been interpreted as corresponding roughly to left hemisphere and right hemisphere functions.

VERBAL (VIQ)		PERFORMANCE (PIQ)	
Subtest	*Description*	*Subtest*	*Description*
Information	Answer questions about knowledge generally available in the United States	Digit Symbol	Using a key of number-symbol pairs, write the paired symbol beneath the numbers in 90 secs (i.e., a speed test)
Comprehension	Questions requiring common sense, reasoning, and proverb interpretation	Picture Completion	Tell what is missing from pictures of common objects or scenes
Arithmetic	Verbal math problems} (i.e., "story problems")	Block Design	Using colored blocks, reproduce a pattern shown by examiner or in pictures
Similarities	Explain what a pair of words has in common	Picture Arrangement	Arrange cartoon pictures in a sequence that tells a story
Digit Span	Repeat number sequences forward and backward	Object Assembly	Assemble parts into an object; scored for time and accuracy (timed test)
Vocabulary	Verbally provide the meanings of words increasing in difficulty		

This battery contains the WAIS and additional tests of attention, rhythm, and thinking. A personality inventory and an aphasia screening test are also included. Reitan's company has provided a computerized *Neuropsychological Deficit Scale* for facilitating interpretation of raw scores. Other software transforms scores into an image of the probable site of lesion.

Clinical neuropsychologists also rely on brief examinations. A few short tests have extensive normative data. One is the *Mini-Mental State Examination,* which was mentioned regarding neurological examination in the previous chapter. Another is the *Information-Memory-Concentration Test* (IMC), which was developed in Great Britain along with a version for the United States called the *mIMC* (Katzman, Brown, Fuld, Peck, Schechter, and Schimmel, 1983). Margolin (1992) recommended the *Neurobehavioral Cognitive Status Examination* (NCSE) developed by Kiernan, Mueller, Langston, and Van Dyke (1987). The NCSE is more sensitive to cognitive dysfunction than other short tests. Normal adults can take the test in 15 to 20 minutes, and patients with dementia take a little longer.

APHASIA TESTS

Aphasia tests provide more thorough evaluation of language than neuropsychological testing. Let us review some background regarding purposes, essential characteristics, and worldwide development of these tests.

Diagnostic Decisions

Clinicians answer the following fundamental questions:

- Does the patient have a communicative disorder?
- If so, is the disorder aphasia?

- If so, what kind of aphasic disorder does the patient have?
- Does the patient have other disorders besides aphasia?

Communicative disorder is determined in two ways. One is by comparing a patient's test score to normative standards. The other basis for diagnosing deficit is to compare an individual patient's post-stroke performance with some indication of pre-stroke performance. To increase the likelihood that a deficient score represents a language disorder, tests are constructed to minimize the influence of extraneous factors such as education level, cultural variation, or reasoning skill. For example, we would not evaluate language comprehension by asking a question about who was President of the United States during the Civil War. If a test does not formally consider these factors, a clinician does when interpreting results.

Along with determining whether there is a language deficit, we want to determine whether the deficit represents aphasia. Tests contain features that consider the definitive characteristics of aphasia as we have understood them. For example, aphasia tests are constructed to evaluate language skills in the four major modalities (see Table 1.1). Each modality is tested independently so that nonaphasic modality-specific impairments can be exposed.

The syndromes introduced in Chapter 2 suggest areas of test construction that might help us diagnose types of aphasia. As indicated by the key features distinguishing syndromes, we would be sure to evaluate comprehension at different levels, examine linguistic characteristics of spontaneous verbal expression, and thoroughly examine repetition ability. The main clinical purpose of testing repetition is to determine if a nonverbal patient is stimulable with this task.

To become a little more familiar with aphasia test construction, let us consider a brief informal examination that can be done at beside. If we understand what evaluation is to accomplish, we should be able to do a spontaneous evaluation when a physician surprises us with a patient to see. In addition to information presented so far, all we need is the common objects in a hospital room, a pen, and some paper (Table 3.2). We would have the patient answer some yes/no questions, point to things, and name and describe some other things. If the patient cannot converse, we want to see if he or she can count or recite the days of the week. It may be a bit risky to ask what the day is, because failure or error may be due to comprehension deficit or disorientation in the

TABLE 3.2 A possible bedside examination illustrating the minimal ingredients of an aphasia evaluation.

COMPREHENSION		PRODUCTION	
Listening	*Reading*	*Speaking*	*Writing*
Is your name (Fred)? (No)	*Point to the object on this card*	*Count to ten.*	*Write your name*
Point to the *window* *lamp*	*Do what it says on this card* (e.g., Point to your nose)	*Say Methodist Episocal* *What day is today?* *What do you call this? (e.g., clock, pillow)*	*Write down some things you see in this room.*
Point to the table and ceiling		*Tell me what happened to you.*	
Is Washington DC the capital of France?			

acute period instead of a word-finding problem. Possible ambiguity of diagnosis is why we also ask patients to name common objects and is one reason for preferring more comprehensive and systematic evaluation after diaschisis has cleared.

Standard Testing

The inconsistency of informal testing makes it difficult to measure progress reliably. Henry Head, a British physician, was one of the first to standardize aphasia assessment. He was particularly vexed by one problem. "An inconsistent response is one of the most striking results produced by a lesion of the cerebral cortex" (Head, 1920, p. 89). A patient names an object one moment and fails to name it the next. If we tested naming just once, we might misdiagnose a patient as having severe impairment or no impairment. Head decided that a response had to be observed at least three or four times in what he called "serial tests." He would place a set of common objects (e.g., knife, key, matches) on a table and would ask a patient to point to them by name and then try to name the objects. Head did the same thing for each patient and recorded exactly what was said.

In the 1930s, physicians developed the *Halstead-Wepman-Reitan Aphasia Screening Test* as a quick evaluation of patients at bedside (Halstead and Wepman, 1949). Two hundred were distributed to military neurologists and neurosurgeons during World War II. One version, Form M, could be carried in a shirt pocket; and another version was absorbed into the more comprehensive Halstead-Reitan neuropsychological battery introduced earlier. Other tests in our history include Eisenson's (1954) *Examining for Aphasia* and Wepman and Jones' (1961) *Language Modalities Test for Aphasia* (LMTA).

Hildred Schuell's *Minnesota Test for Differential Diagnosis of Aphasia* (MTDDA) may have been the most widely administered test in the United States and Great Britain in the 1960s and 70s. It could take from two to six hours. It evolved from seven revisions over 17 years, beginning with the first version in the summer of 1948 (Brown and Schuell, 1950). The sixth form was made available to clinics in 1955 on a limited basis for experimental use. The marketed form in 1965 was the eighth version, indicative of the care with which the MTDDA was developed. After Schuell's death in 1970, the test and manual were revised slightly by Sefer (Schuell, 1973).

The MTDDA consists of 46 subtests distributed among five sections. The four language modality sections contain from nine to 15 substests graded from easy to difficult. Commenting on the test's length, Thompson and Enderby (1979) noted that clinicians "tend to avoid any procedure which is cumbersome or seems redundant...Over many test administrations they eventually learn which items seem useful to them" (p. 196). The test has no formal interpretive devices for differentiating among aphasic language disorders, but it does contain graphed profiles of aphasia when accompanied by perceptual or motor disorders.

Schuell (1957) constructed a short test that would take 30 to 35 minutes, but she decided that any short test would be inadequate. Later she suggested establishing a **baseline** and **ceiling** within each section of the full MTDDA (Schuell, 1966). For each modality, a clinician establishes a baseline by starting with a subtest on which the patient should make a maximum of one error. To establish a ceiling, the clinician should stop testing on the subtest producing 90 percent failure and, thus, not spend time on subtests most likely to show severe deficiency. Thompson and Enderby (1979) decided to create a short form by determining the subtests and items that are too easy or too difficult. Their version has only five items per subtest, contrasting with the original 20 to 32 items.

Some legal questions call for a standardized basis for identifying and measuring impairment (Udell, Sullivan, and Schlanger, 1980). Questions of **competency** consider whether a patient is able to function in the best interest of himself or those for whom he or she has been responsible (Porch and Porec, 1977). What is the patient's capacity to stand trial, assume parental responsibilities, live independently, conduct business and personal affairs? Ability to understand one's will, called testamentary capacity, is indicated by assessment of receptive language (Morse, 1968). These issues are important in a specialty of the legal profession called *elder law.*

A second issue deals with **compensation,** which entails determining how much impairment has been sustained. A patient may be seeking compensation from an employer or the government or may be suing a physician and/or hospital because of a surgical accident. In this case, we are called upon for our expertise and data in determining if someone is *malingering.* People pretending to have aphasia make about the same number of errors on both easy and difficult tasks, instead of the aphasic pattern of errors following a hierarchy of task difficulty (Porec and Porch, 1977). Malingerers might show unusual patterns, such as agrammatism without accompanying paralysis or overdoing a particular symptom such as a type of naming error.

International Tests

One of the important developments in American aphasiology over the past 20 years has been an increasing awareness of work being done all over the world (e.g., Holland and Forbes, 1993). Publication of the the journal *Aphasiology* in 1987 has stimulated international dialogue. With respect to assessment, Spreen and Benton (1977) had a plan to create an international test called the *Neurosensory Center Comprehensive Examination for Aphasia* (NCCEA) (see also Benton and Hamsher, 1978). Since then, many countries have either translated batteries that were developed in the United States or have constructed their own tests.

Journals with an international representation publish studies of aphasia diagnosed with tests constructed for a particular language. One prominent examination is the *Aachen Aphasia Test* (AAT) created in Germany (Huber, Poeck, and Willmes, 1984). The AAT was designed to describe impairment in each modality, measure overall severity of impairment, and classify patients according to the major syndromes. The *Montreal-Toulous Aphasia Battery* (Beta version), or the MT-86, was developed in 1986 by Nespoulous and others for evaluating aphasia in a French-speaking population (Beland, Lecours, Giroux, and Bois, 1993). Like the "Cookie Theft" picture in one of the American tests, the MT-86 elicits spontaneous speech and writing with a picture of a bank robbery.

Looking to the Future

Health care managers want health care providers to make efficient use of time. Managers have been especially concerned about broad diagnosis or misdiagnosis sending medical care or rehabilitation down an unproductive garden path. In some instances, more time for initial evaluation can save time down the road with a treatment that is accurately and precisely targeted on a patient's impairment.

Advocates of cognitive neuropsychology (CN) claim to follow an approach to diagnosis that targets specific processing impairments. They have been critical of aphasia batteries, saying they "were not designed primarily with the aim of elucidating the underlying nature of language disorder" (Byng, Kay, Edmundson, and Scott, 1989, p. 72). Goodglass (1989) was sympathetic but also noted that to follow today's CN approach "a painstaking array of experimental procedures is required—one that would be quite impractical in the ordinary course of clinical testing" (p. 94). Kertesz (1989) added, "No doubt recent advances in psycholinguistics and cognitive psychology will find their way into practical aphasia tests, modifying the existing batteries" (p. 100).

One new idea is the *Psycholinguistic Assessments of Language Processing in Aphasia* (PALPA) (Kay, Lesser, and Coltheart, 1992; Lesser, 1995). The stated objective is to evaluate the status of modular processes in the mind's language system, and the test follows a componential analysis defined later in Chapter 4. The PALPA consists of 60 tests, most of which address word-level functions such as recognition, comprehension, and naming. A few tests address sentence "processing" with sentence-picture matching tasks. The theoretical basis for construction and interpretation comes from the analytical case studies of cognitive neuropsychology.

The PALPA's designers emphasized that they relied on a CN-model of word recognition and production mainly to introduce a way of thinking about assessing language disorders, "not because we believe it to be a particularly valid 'model' of language structure" (Kay, Lesser, and Coltheart, 1996b). As of 1996, "we have not carried out psychometrically satisfactory measures of validity or reliability" (Kay, Lesser, and Coltheart, 1996a).

It is hoped that Chapters 4 through 6 clarify the difference between the CN approach and mainstream psycholinguistics. Regarding the latter, Chapter 1 provides an introduction to automatic and controlled processes and the parallel distinction between fast and slow tasks. The PALPA does not make these distinctions by controlling stimulus timing or measuring response time. Nevertheless, the future of testing may move in the direction of enhancing the validity of cognitive diagnosis, especially if we learn that treatments targeted to specific mental processes turn out to be efficacious and efficient (see Chapter 13).

PSYCHOMETRIC CONSTRAINTS: THE PICA

Bruce Porch was disturbed by flexible test administration and vague scoring methods when he embarked on his doctoral dissertation in the late 1950s. He wanted to corral inconsistency by applying psychometric principles that were becoming the rule in educational and clinical psychology. In particular, he wanted to achieve *reliability* for the purposes of measuring progress and comparing patients. After the **Porch Index of Communicative Ability** (PICA) was published in 1967, it became an important tool for the study of recovery.

However, many speech-language pathologists were initially wary about the test's rigidity of administration and reliance on cold numbers for describing patients (e.g., Emerick and Hatten, 1979). Also, it was startling that a 40-hour workshop was needed to learn the complex scoring system. It took a while for clinicians to be comfortable with the PICA's unique methodology. The test has the following salient features:

- relatively small number of subtests given in an unusual sequence
- emphasis on reliability, with very restrictive rules for administration
- complex multidimensional scoring requiring extensive training

Description and Administration

The PICA contains 18 subtests of the four language modalities and other functions. Similar to Henry Head's serial tests, each subtest utilizes 10 common objects arranged neatly on a table (i.e., cigarette, comb, fork, key, knife, matches, pen, pencil, quarter, and toothbrush). The order of subtests is shown in Table 3.3. Auditory, reading, and speech tasks are mixed together in subtests I through XII. Writing subtests are together at the end.

At first glance, order of subtests seems to proceed from difficult to easy, in contrast to other batteries that start with the easiest tasks in each modality. This organization is a product of the use of the same 10 objects across subtests so that functions can be compared without changes in content. Tasks are ordered to minimize a "learning effect" that may come from repeated use of the same objects. That is, if word comprehension were to come before naming, as in other batteries, a patient would have heard the word before the naming test. Thus, minimal linguistic information about objects is given early, and maximum information is deferred. As a result, the sequence does not follow a strict hierarchy of difficulty. Actually, some earlier subtests are likely to be easier than later subtests for many aphasic patients.

Explicit prescriptions for administration apply to the physical conditions of testing as well as what a clinician is to say and do for each subtest. It takes an average of one hour for a well-trained

TABLE 3.3 Order of administering PICA subtests with early and revised categories.

TEST	OUTPUT (1967)	FUNCTION (1981)	TASK
I	Verbal		Describes function of object
II	Gestural	Pantomime	Demonstrates function of object
III	Gestural	Pantomime	Demonstrates function in order
IV	Verbal		Names objects
V	Gestural	Reading	Reads function and position
VI	Gestural	Auditory	Points to object, given its function
VII	Gestural	Reading	Reads name and position
VIII	Gestural	Visual	Matches picture to object
IX	Verbal		Completes sentence with object name
X	Gestural	Auditory	Points to object, given its name
XI	Gestural	Visual	Matches object to object
XII	Verbal		Repeats name of object
A	Graphic	Writing	Writes function of object
B	Graphic	Writing	Writes name of object
C	Graphic	Writing	Writes name to dictation
D	Graphic	Writing	Writes name when spelled
E	Graphic	Copying	Copies name of object
F	Graphic	Copying	Copies geometric forms

Adapted by permission from Porch, B. E., *Porch Index of Communicative Ability: Theory and Development, Volume 1.* Palo Alto, Calif.: Consulting Psychologists Press, 1967.

clinician to give the PICA, but it often takes about 90 minutes. Each of 180 responses is assigned a score based on the multidimensional scoring system shown in Table 3.4. The scale-points reflect degrees of correctness and incorrectness, and there are subtle variations among subtests in the definition of scale-points. The ability to assign scores quickly is learned in the 40-hour "PICA workshops." Diacritical markings provide additional notation for characterizing a response.

Standardization and Interpretation

Whereas an average of one hour is needed for most aphasic patients to take the PICA, 130 neurologically intact adults breezed through in about 30 minutes (Duffy, Keith, Shane, and Podraza,1976). Normal adults had some difficulty in areas that can be influenced by education. Ninety-five percent averaged 12.95 on the graphic subtests, with a mean of 9.63 on writing sentences. Averages for the entire sample are shown in Table 3.5, compared to samples with left hemisphere lesions and probable aphasia.

Reliability is not worth much if a test is not valid regarding what it is purported to measure. The PICA has strong criterion-related validity with respect to other standardized tests but falls short of reflecting natural communicative abilities in daily life (Holland, 1980a; Keenan and Brassell, 1975; Sanders and Davis, 1978). For reliability, Porch (1967) reported inter-examiner and test-retest correlations in the manual. The broader a score's coverage, the more stable it is upon retest two weeks after initial testing.

Mean scores are used for documenting and interpreting performance. The most specific summary score is the individual subtest mean. An average such as 12.25 is called a *response level.* Subtests are grouped according to seven functions shown in Table 3.3. The average for all 180 scores is called the **overall score.** The response level

TABLE 3.4 Multidimensional scoring system of the PICA.

SCORE	LEVEL	DESCRIPTION OF RESPONSE
16	Complex	Accurate, complex, and elaborate
15	Complete	Accurate and complete
14	Distorted	Accurate, complete, but with reduced facility
13	Complete-delayed	Accurate, complete, but slow or delayed
12	Incomplete	Accurate but incomplete
11	Incomplete-delayed	Accurate, incomplete, slow or delayed
10	Corrected	Accurate after self-correction of error
9	Repetition	Accurate after repetition of instruction
8	Cued	Accurate after specified cue
7	Related	Inaccurate but related to correct response
6	Error	Inaccurate
5	Intelligible	Intelligible but not related to test item
4	Unintelligible	Unintelligible, differentiated
3	Minimal	Unintelligible, not differentiated
2	Attention	Attention to item but no response
1	No response	No awareness of test item

Adapted by permission from Porch, B. E., *Porch Index of Communicative Ability: Theory and Development, Volume 1,* Palo Alto, Calif.: Consulting Psychologists Press, 1967.

scores for each subtest, function categories, and overall performance are starting points in using the PICA for differential diagnosis, prognosis, and treatment planning. To improve communication of results, response level scores can be translated into **percentiles** relative to a large sample of aphasic patients. The overall score is more reliable than subtest scores.

In documenting diagnosis of deficit with the PICA, we should recognize that a score of 15 or 16 indicates a level defined by the test and does not necessarily indicate normality (see Table 3.5). Aphasia at the 95th percentile includes scores of 14.44 overall, 15.00 for auditory and reading comprehension, 14.62 for verbal subtests, and 13.46 for written language. These scores are similar to normal, leaving diagnosis of mild aphasia to clinical judgment. Some investigation was undertaken to determine how the test might discriminate between normal and aphasic adults, but this

TABLE 3.5 Normal adults (Duffy, et al., 1976) and aphasic adults (Porch, 1971a, 1981) compared according to classification available when the normals were studied. Aphasia scores illustrate the impact of sample expansion between 1971 (*N* = 280) and (*N* = 357).

	OVERALL	GESTURAL	VERBAL	GRAPHIC
Normal Adults				
Range	13.40–14.99	13.73–15.00	13.48–15.03	11.18–15.03
Average	14.46	14.66	14.55	14.12
Left-Hemisphere Damage				
95th percentile (1981)	14.44	14.74	14.62	13.91
50th percentile (1981)	10.89	12.96	10.77	8.22
50th percentile (1971)	10.64	12.73	11.20	7.50

statistical work does not appear to have been translated into clinical practice (e.g., Brauer, McNeil, Duffy, Keith, and Collins, 1989).

Different data summary forms are provided to help a clinician identify patterns of performance and to facilitate meaningful documentation. Modality-specific conditions, such as motor speech deficits or illiteracy, are revealed by depressions of speech or reading modalities beyond what would be expected with respect to the typical aphasia pattern among modalities. Despite the PICA's symmetry, comparing auditory comprehension and reading is confounded with an addition of prepositions in the reading stimuli (e.g., "Put this card under the fork"). Most of the difference in scores between these two functions appears to be due to the linguistic supplement in the reading stimuli rather than a modality difference per se (Sanders, Davis, and Wells, 1981).

In the studies of reliability, shifts between first and second testing showed a mean improvement of around 0.38 points. This indicates that a subtest shift of 0.40 or more is needed to represent real change as opposed to normal between-test variation. Reliable change scores (i.e., differences between a test and retest) can be determined for general and specific abilities. A 10 percent increase in the overall score is considered to be a reasonable treatment goal, whereas a five percent change "has a limited effect on communicative ability" (Porch, 1981, p. 105).

DIAGNOSING SYNDROMES: THE BOSTON EXAM

Harold Goodglass and Edith Kaplan started developing the "Boston Exam" in the 1960s. The complete **Boston Diagnostic Aphasia Examination** (BDAE) was first published in 1972, and a revised royal blue edition appeared ten years later (Goodglass and Kaplan, 1983). The test did not change, but some of the terminology was adjusted and new norms were obtained.

The BDAE has been used as a basis for documenting syndrome diagnosis. Its 27 subtests put the test between the PICA and the Minnesota test in length, and time of administration ranges from one to three hours. The Boston Exam has the following salient features:

- classification of aphasias into syndromes according to symptom patterns
- analysis of spontaneous verbalization
- the Cookie Theft picture

Description and Scoring

The Boston Exam consists of four major sections, each focusing on a language modality. Auditory and spoken modalities are presented before reading and writing (Table 3.6). The battery is particularly distinctive with its assessment of conversational and expository utterance prior to systematic testing. Conversation is elicted with an interview and discussion of familiar topics. Then a patient is asked to describe the Cookie Theft picture: a kitchen setting in which a child, perched on a tilting stool, is reaching for a cookie jar in a cupboard while a woman, appearing unaware of the crime, is washing dishes over a sink with water running over onto the floor. This picture has been used often in studies of discourse production.

The BDAE places as much emphasis on descriptive analysis as it does on scoring. It follows an orientation to neuropsychological assessment called the "process approach," which shuns scores and prefers description of strategic behaviors leading to response (Kaplan, 1988). This is indicated by the absence of broad summary scores and reliance on pattern of deficit for depicting a patient's disorder. Initial conversational and expository speech are described with a simple aphasia severity rating scale and a rating scale profile of speech characteristics. A subtest summary profile provides a format for depicting pattern of performance (Figure 3.1).

Standardization and Interpretation

A revised normative sample of aphasic patients was assessed between 1976 and 1982, rendering current criticisms of the 1972 sample as being rather obsolete. The revised sample was used to relate raw scores to percentiles. Performance by

TABLE 3.6 Sections and subtests of the Boston Diagnostic Aphasia Examination.

	AUDITORY-ORAL		WRITTEN LANGUAGE	
I. Conversational and Expository Speech	*II. Auditory Comprehension*	*III. Oral Expression*	*IV. Understand Written Language*	*V. Writing*
Interview	Point to objects, actions, letters, numbers, shapes	Oral agility	Identify letters and words	Mechanics (name and address)
Conversation	Point to body parts	Automized sequences	Comprehension of spelling	Alphabet and numbers
Description of Cookie Theft scenario	Commands	Repeat words and phrases	Word-picture matching	Write to dictation
	Complex material	Answer questions	Read sentences and paragraphs	Written naming
		Naming		Picture description
		Word fluency		
		Read words and sentences aloud		

147 normal adults is shown in the test manual (also in Borod, Goodglass, and Kaplan, 1980).

Because of its lack of summary scores, it has been difficult to compare the BDAE to other tests statistically (Holland, 1980a; Ulatowska, Macaluso-Haynes, and Mendel-Richardson, 1976). Comparison to other tests that also classify syndromes is reviewed later in the chapter. There has been some study of the relationship between test patterns and site of lesion. Naeser and Hayward (1978) found agreement between independent classification with the test and predicted site of damage determined with CT scans for 19 subjects.

Cut-off scores were derived from the studies of normal adults. Lowest scores tend to be made by persons over age 60 with fewer than nine years of education. Exceptions to cut-offs for people 60 years of age and older were recommended for measures of nonverbal agility and word fluency (i.e., animal naming). In assessing an elderly client, the cutoff score should be relaxed before it is concluded that performance is disordered.

Diagnosis of syndrome is accomplished by examining the pattern of results on a rating of speech characteristics and a subtest summary profile. The manual provides examples and ranges of performance that are typically seen in cases of Broca's, Wernicke's, anomic, and conduction aphasias. The profile of speech characteristics is a convenient guide for classification (Figure 3.2). The profile describes expression according to the telltale signs of the syndromes. Seven dimensions of extended utterance are compared with auditory comprehension deficit determined during formal testing. Figure 3.2 shows the range around mean performance for two fluent aphasias.

NUMERICAL CLASSIFICATION: THE WAB

At the University of Western Ontario, Andrew Kertesz introduced the Western Aphasia Battery (WAB) as a modification of the BDAE (Kertesz and Poole, 1974). The complete test was published in 1982 for widespread clinical use, following several earlier appearances in studies of recovery and aphasia classification (Kertesz, 1979; Kertesz and McCabe, 1977; Kertesz and Phipps, 1977).

SUBTEST SUMMARY PROFILE

NAME: **J.M.** DATE OF EXAM: **12-9-68**

	PERCENTILES:	0	10	20	30	40	50	60	70	80	90	100
SEVERITY RATING			0					2		3	4	5
FLUENCY	ARTICULATION RATING		1	2		5	6		7			
	PHRASE LENGTH				3	4	5	6	7			
	MELODIC LINE			2	4		6	7				
	VERBAL AGILITY		0	2	5		8	9	11	13	14	
AUDITORY COMPREHENSION	WORD DISCRIMINATION	0	15	25	37	46	53	60	64	67	70	72
	BODY-PART IDENTIFICATION	0	1	5	10	13	15	16	17	18		20
	COMMANDS	0	3	4	6	8	10	11	13	14		
	COMPLEX IDEATIONAL MATERIAL		0	2	3	4	5	6	8	9		12
NAMING	RESPONSIVE NAMING			0	1	5	10	15	20		27	30
	CONFRONTATION NAMING		0	9	28	43		72	84	94	105	114
	ANIMAL NAMING				0	1	2	3	4	6		23
ORAL READING	WORD READING			0	1	3	7	15	21	26	30	
	ORAL SENTENCE READING					0	1		4	7	9	10
REPETITION	REPETITION OF WORDS		0	2	5	7	8		9		10	
	HIGH-PROBABILITY			0	1			4	5	7	8	
	LOW-PROBABILITY						1		2	4	6	8
PARAPHASIA	NEOLOGISTIC	40	16	9	4	2	1		0			
	LITERAL	47	17	12	9	6	5	3	2	1		
	VERBAL	40	23	18	15	12	9	7	4		1	0
	EXTENDED	75	12	5	3	1						
AUTOMATIC SPEECH	AUTOMATIZED SEQUENCES		0	1	2	3		6	7		8	
	RECITING				0					2		
READING COMPREHENSION	SYMBOL DISCRIMINATION	0	2	5	7	8	9					
	WORD RECOGNITION	0	1	3	4	5	6			8		
	COMPREHENSION OF ORAL SPELLING				0	1		3	4	6	7	8
	WORD-PICTURE MATCHING		0	1	4	6	8	9				
	READING SENTENCES AND PARAGRAPHS		0	1	2	3	4	5	6	7		10
WRITING	MECHANICS	1		2		3		4			5	
	SERIAL WRITING		0	7	18	25	30	33	40	43	46	47
	PRIMER-LEVEL DICTATION		0	1		6	9	11	13	14	15	
	SPELLING TO DICTATION						1	2	3	5	7	10
	WRITTEN CONFRONTATION NAMING				0	1	2		6	7	9	10
	SENTENCES TO DICTATION							1	3	6	8	12
	NARRATIVE WRITING			1			2			3	4	5
MUSIC	SINGING		0			2						
	RHYTHM		0					2				
SPATIAL AND COMPUTATIONAL	DRAWING TO COMMAND	0	6	7	8	9	10	11	12			
	STICK MEMORY	0	3	4	6	7	8	9	10	11		14
	3-D BLOCKS		0	2	4	5	6	7	8		10	
	TOTAL FINGERS	0	54	70	81	93	100	108	120	130	141	
	RIGHT-LEFT	0	1	3	4	6	8	9	11		16	
	MAP ORIENTATION (OMITTED)	0	2	5	6	9	11	13		14		
	ARITHMETIC		0	2	4	8	11	14	17	21	27	32
	CLOCK SETTING	0	3	4	6		8	9		12		
		0	10	20	30	40	50	60	70	80	90	100

FIGURE 3.1 The *BDAE*'s subtest summary profile of scores in relation to percentiles for the aphasic population. This is an example of Broca's aphasia with good auditory comprehension, few paraphasias, and expressive problems mainly in repetition.

Reprinted by permission from Goodglass, H., & Kaplan, F., *The Assessment of Aphasia and Language Disorders.* Chicago: Riverside, 1983, p. 78.

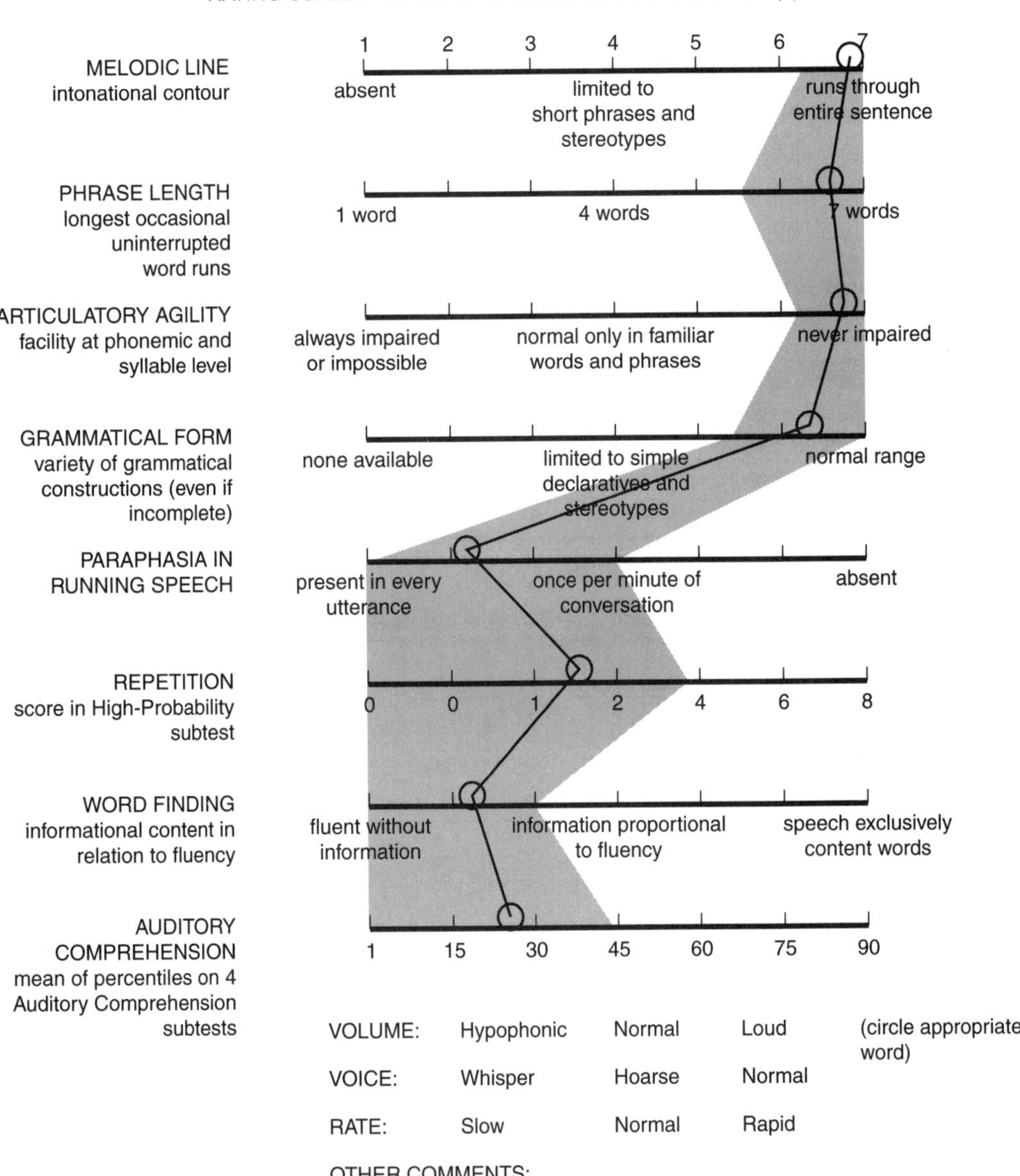

FIGURE 3.2 The Boston Exam's rating scale profiles of speech characteristics for (a) Wernicke's aphasia and (b) anomic aphasia. These syndromes are similar in melodic line, phrase length, articulatory agility, and grammatical form (i.e., fluency). Differences occur with paraphasias, repetition, and auditory comprehension.

Reprinted by permission from Goodglass, H., & Kaplan, F., *The Assessment of Aphasia and Language Disorders*. Chicago: Riverside, 1983, p. 81, 85.

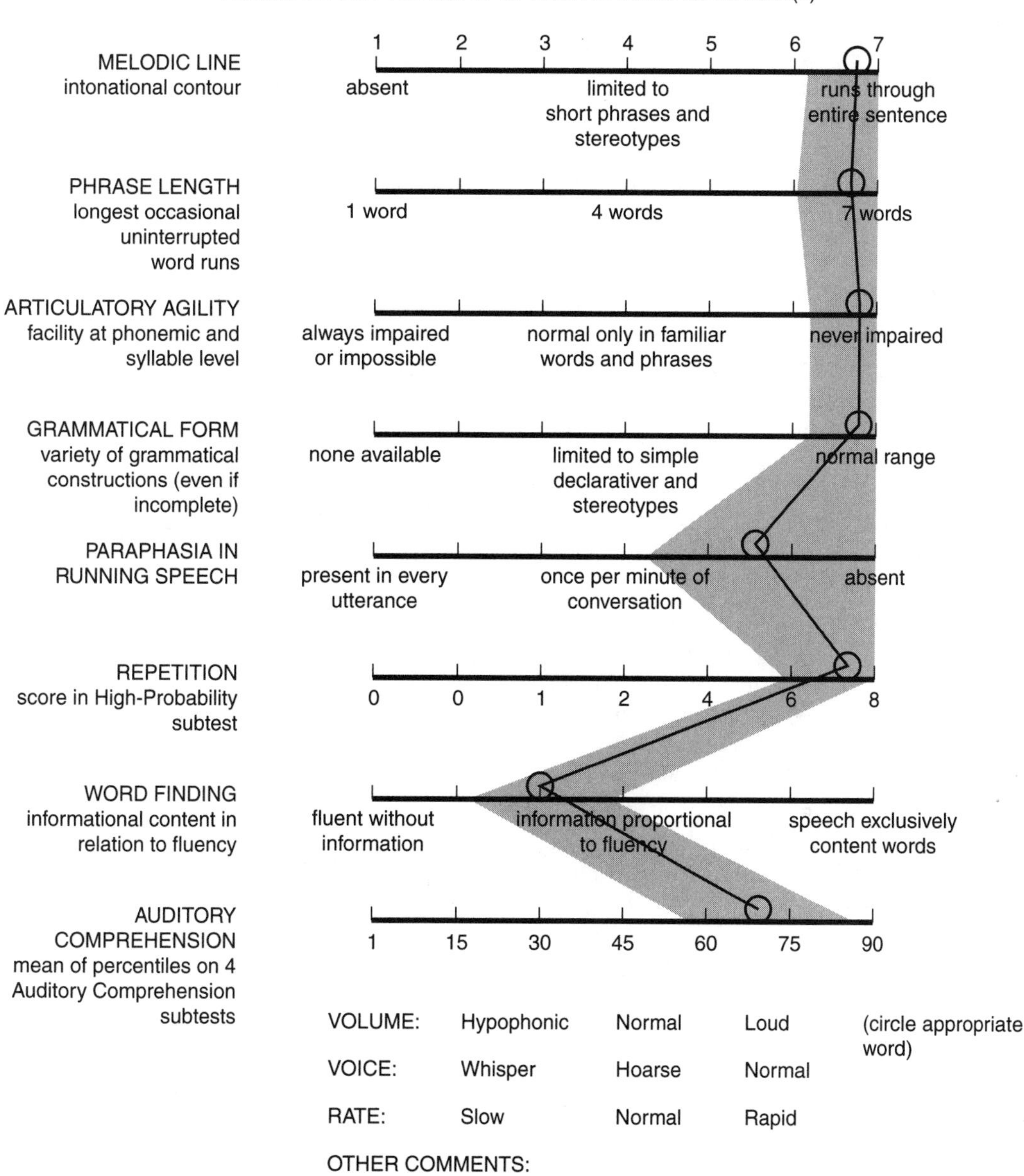

FIGURE 3.2 Continued

Kertesz perceived a problem with definitions of syndromes by different authors. He believed that consistency is possible "only if aphasia types are objectively defined, and classification criteria used in different centers are objectively compared" (Ferro and Kertesz, 1987, p. 374). The "Western" specifies ranges of test scores for key language functions as the basis for classifying aphasias. To this end, the WAB has the following salient features:

- content and administration similar to the Boston Exam
- summary scores including an overall score similar to the PICA
- ranges of scores for classifying aphasias into syndromes

Description and Scoring

The basic battery examines oral language abilities that include auditory comprehension and spoken expression. Visual language and other subtests is an additional section consisting of (V) Reading, (VI) Writing, (VII) Apraxia, and (VIII) Constructional, Visuospatial, and Calculation tasks. The entire test could take as long as the MTDDA, and Kertesz (1982) recommended dividing it into segments across sessions. Organization of the oral and graphic sections are summarized in Table 3.7.

Calculations from test performance and summary scores set this test apart from the Boston Exam. Scores are obtained for the four sections of the oral language test. The spontaneous speech section is rated with two 10-point scales, one for information content and another for fluency. Kertesz (1979) felt that the information content rating is a good estimate of functional communication. The fluency scale is used in classification. For example, 0 to 4 represents levels of nonfluency, and 5 to 10 depicts levels of fluency. The following summary scores have been calculated (see also, Figure 3.3):

- *Aphasia Quotient* (AQ): Used with the test since 1974, the AQ is the summary score for the four sections of auditory-spoken language. Forty percent of the score is derived from the spontaneous speech rating scales. Possible score is 100 (see Shewan and Kertesz, 1980).
- *Language Quotient* (LQ): This is the most recent score developed for this test (Shewan and Kertesz, 1984). The LQ is a composite of all language sections, including reading and writing.
- *Performance Quotient* (PQ): For a while, reading, writing, apraxia, and construction tasks were combined into this score (Kertesz, 1979; Appell, Kertesz, and Fisman, 1982).
- *Cortical Quotient* (CQ): The is the only score besides the AQ that is mentioned in the test manual. The CQ represents performance on all subtests, verbal and nonverbal. The CQ and AQ are the only summary scores examined in reliability and validity studies (Shewan and Kertesz, 1980).

Standardization and Interpretation

Typical scores were reported for 215 aphasic subjects, 63 normals, and 53 nonaphasic brain-damaged patients (Kertesz, 1979). Normals had a mean AQ of 99.6. The tendency for anomic and

TABLE 3.7 Sections and subtests of the Western Aphasia Battery.

AUDITORY-ORAL (AQ)				GRAPHEMIC	
I. Spontaneous speech	*II. Auditory verbal comprehension*	*III. Repetition*	*IV. Naming*	*V. Reading*	*VI. Writing*
Interview	Yes/No questions	*Bed* *Snowball*	Object naming	Comprehend sentences	Name & address
Description of picnic scenario	Word recognition	*The telephone is ringing*	Word fluency	Commands	Write story about a picture
	Follow commands	*Pack my box with five dozen jugs of liquid veneer*	Sentence completion	Words	Write to dictation
			Answer questions	Spelling recognition	

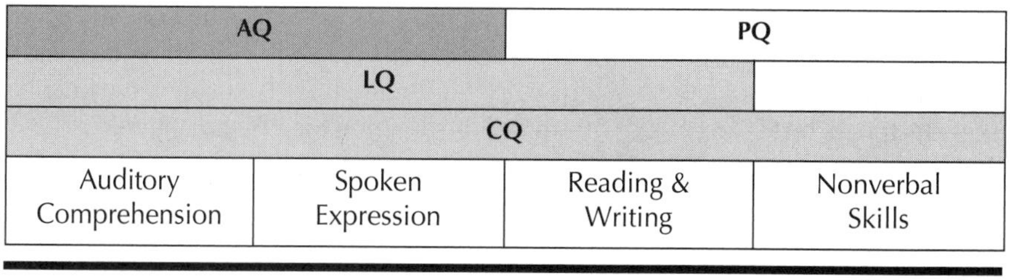

<table>
<tr><td colspan="2">AQ</td><td colspan="2">PQ</td></tr>
<tr><td colspan="3">LQ</td><td></td></tr>
<tr><td colspan="4">CQ</td></tr>
<tr><td>Auditory Comprehension</td><td>Spoken Expression</td><td>Reading & Writing</td><td>Nonverbal Skills</td></tr>
</table>

FIGURE 3.3 An overview of the summary scores for the Western Aphasia Battery.

conduction aphasias to be mild and moderate impairments is indicated in mean AQ's of 83.3 and 60.5, respectively. Broca's and Wernicke's aphasias scored means of 31.7 and 39.0, respectively. Broca's aphasia had the widest standard deviation of all the aphasias. Persons with global aphasia had a mean AQ of 10.5.

Criterion-related validity has been supported by a comparisons to the NCCEA (Kertesz, 1982), PICA (Sanders and Davis, 1978), and the *Lisbon Aphasia Examination Battery*'s quociente de afasia or "quotient of aphasia" (Ferro and Kertesz, 1987). The studies indicated that the WAB assesses aphasia like other batteries. To examine the specific goal of objective classification, Swindell, Holland, and Fromm (1984) compared WAB-derived syndromes to clinical impressions. Swindell found that the test agreed with clinical experience for 54 percent of the aphasic patients studied. Agreement was greater for nonfluent aphasias than fluent aphasias.

Shewan and Kertesz (1980) presented strong reliability, but Trupe (1984) found weak reliability in the content and fluency scales even after clarification and revision of scoring criteria. She concluded that it is difficult to use one fluency scale to characterize behavior consisting of multiple dimensions. She recommended that independent dimensions be rated separately as in the speech characteristics profile of the Boston Exam.

With respect to diagnosis, presence of a language disorder or "aphasia" is identified with an AQ cutoff score of 93.8 (Kertesz and Poole, 1974). In a study of prognostic indicators, aphasic people who surpassed the 93.8 score were considered to be "recovered" (Holland, Greenhouse, Fromm, and Swindell, 1989). Syndromes are identified according to patterns of performance with respect to the fluency scale and scores from auditory comprehension, repetition, and naming subtests (Table 3.8). Conduction aphasia, for example, is recognized by scores that

TABLE 3.8 Criteria for classifying aphasias based on scores from the Western Aphasia Battery.

	FLUENCY	COMPREHENSION	REPETITION	NAMING
Global	0–4	0–3.9	0–4.9	0–6
Broca's	0–4	4–10	0–7.9	0–8
Isolation	0–4	0–3.9	5–10	0–6
Transcortical motor	0–4	4–10	8–10	0–8
Wernicke's	5–10	0–6.9	0–7.9	0–9
Transcortical sensory	5–10	0–6.9	8–10	0–9
Conduction	5–10	7–10	0–6.9	0–9
Anomic	5–10	7–10	7–10	0–9

Reprinted by permission from Kertesz, A., *Aphasia and Associated Disorders: Taxonomy, Localization, and Recovery.* New York: Grune & Stratton, 1979.

are low in repetition relative to higher scores in spontaneous speech fluency and auditory comprehension. One perspective on diagnosis according to these criteria is illustrated in Figure 3.4. The WAB is being used increasingly to characterize patients in neuropsychological case studies.

The WAB was given to persons with Alzheimer's disease (Appell, et al., 1982; Bayles, Boone, Tomoeda, Slauson, and Kaszniak, 1989). When pattern of language impairment was compared with aphasias, it was shown that nonfluent patterns were absent. Appell's subjects were similar to Wernicke's and transcortical sensory aphasias. The WAB was later evaluated for its ability to classify patients as having Alzheimer's dementia, fluent aphasia caused by stroke, or right hemisphere dysfunction (Horner, Dawson, Heyman, and Fish, 1992). The test identified about 73 percent of the cases correctly. The WAB had more difficulty differentiating Alzheimer's dementia from RH dysfunction than fluent aphasia.

Comparing the WAB and the BDAE

Wertz (1983) had serious questions about the validity of the BDAE with respect to its classification of aphasias, and this concern later spread to the WAB. Wertz, Deal, and Robinson (1984) compared the two tests given to the same 45 aphasic patients with single left hemisphere occlusive lesions. There was only 27 percent agreement as to classification of these patients. In a follow-up study, Crary, Wertz, and Deal (1992) performed cluster analyses with each test. They found 38

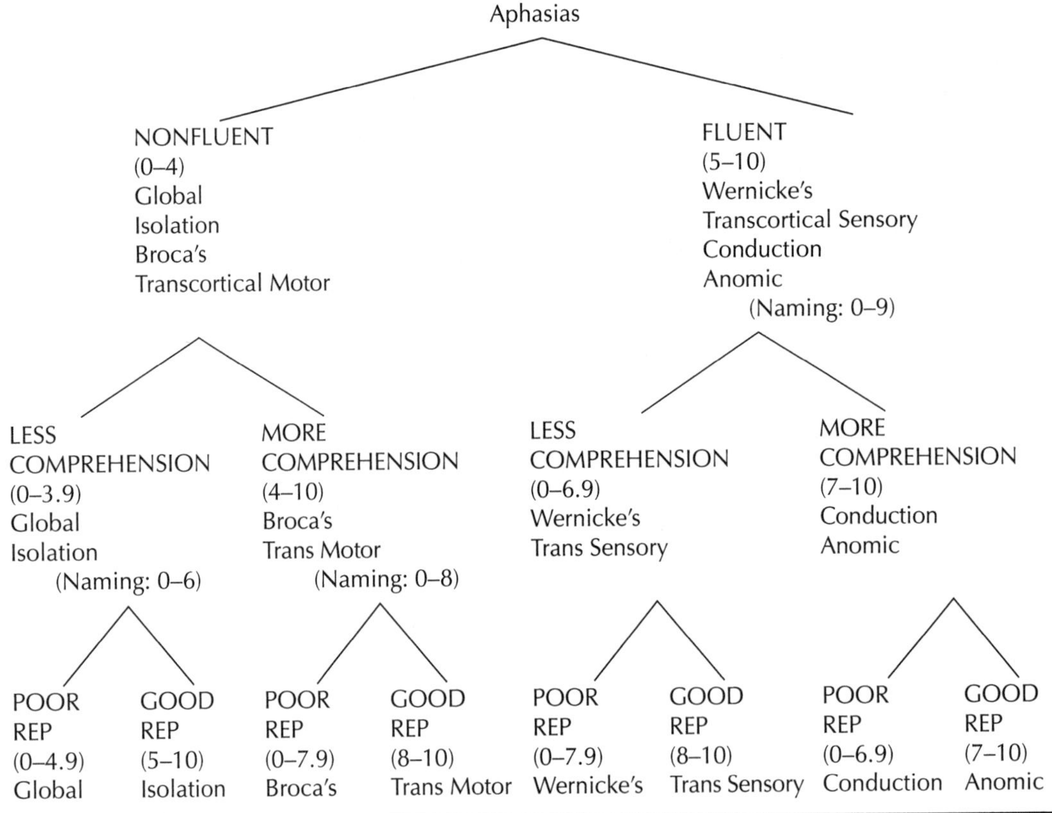

FIGURE 3.4 Decision tree illustrating the manner in which the *WAB* classifies aphasias according to scores for fluency, auditory comprehension, and repetition.

percent agreement between BDAE diagnosis and cluster membership and 30 percent agreement with the WAB, leading to the conclusion that the tests classify aphasias differently.

In Ferro and Kertesz' (1987) comparison of the WAB to the similar Lisbon aphasia test, they found "only a partial overlap" of aphasia types derived from the tests. A major discrepancy was between global and Broca's classifications. The main issue was the amount of comprehension deficit that would turn a nonfluent patient into a global aphasia. Another problematic discrepancy was in diagnosing conduction aphasia.

These studies indicate that score-based diagnosis presents only an appearance of objectivity, because the score definitions are still based on a test author's criteria and scoring is based on an examiner's judgment. Swindell suggested that clinical description be used to supplement scores for documenting diagnosis of a syndrome.

SAVING TIME

A graduate student can prepare for clinical practice by taking what we used to do in three or four hours and figuring out how to accomplish the same goals in 30 minutes. Regarding informal bedside screeening, Brookshire (1997) noted that "an unsystematic approach may lead the examiner to miss important signs and may invalidate comparisons of the patient's performance with that of other patients or with the same patient on subsequent tests" (p. 165). Standard screening protocols ensure that everyone in the clinic does the screening the same way. Large rehabilitation centers are likely to have their own standard protocol, and a few screening tests have been published.

Standardized Bedside Screening

The **Aphasia Language Performance Scales** (ALPS) provides an informal standardized assessment in 20 to 30 minutes (Keenan and Brassell, 1975). The examiner can utilize objects in pockets and a patient's room for assessing comprehension and expression. Modalities are tested with four "scales," each containing a series of items increasing in difficulty.

The **Bedside Evaluation Screening Test** (BEST) comes in a portable kit with a magnetic display board, a few objects, and forms for instant reporting once the test is completed (Fitch-West and Sands, 1987). The test should take less than 20 minutes including the report. It assesses auditory comprehension, reading, naming, repetition, and conversational skills.

Like the ALPS, the **Acute Aphasia Screening Protocol** (AASP) depends on objects reliably found in a patient's room such a pillow, window, and TV (Crary, Haak, and Malinsky, 1989). It should take around 10 minutes. The test begins with a quick check of attention and orientation and then assesses auditory comprehension and basic expressive abilities. The AASP includes a score for conversational style.

Shortened Batteries

Clinicians now commonly administer parts of the Boston Exam or WAB. Crary and Rothi (1989) worked on a short WAB and discovered that four measures would be highly predictive of the standard AQ. These measures are the sequential commands and repetition subtests and the Information Content and Fluency ratings of spontaneous speech. However, considering that the AQ is normally computed based on a weighted formula for 10 scores, it was unclear how an AQ should be computed from these four specific scores.

It may be useful to know whether an overall score from a shortened PICA is equivalent to an overall score obtained from the complete test. A regression analysis determined that 10 subtests and five objects per subtest produces an equivalent overall score (DiSimoni, Keith, Holt, and Darley, 1975). Another short PICA, called the *SPICA,* had similar results (Holtzapple, Pohlman, LaPointe, and Graham, 1989). Only subtests I, VI, VII, and D are presented with the 10 objects; but the overall score from the SPICA is significantly different from the overall obtained with the PICA. Another SPICA with five objects was reliable but had less sensitivity to recovery over four weeks than the complete test (Lincoln and Ells, 1980; Phillips and Halpin, 1978). A shortened PICA may be good for a single assessment but may not be the best means of measuring change.

COMMON SUPPLEMENTAL TESTS

Other tests are continually invented to help us deal with problems that the large batteries do not solve. One problem is posed by patients at each end of the severity continuum. We depend on retained abilities for a starting point in treatment, but a test battery may be so difficult for the most severe aphasia that it does not expose capabilities. Conversely for the most slightly impaired, a test may not be difficult enough to expose deficits that would point to goals of treatment.

The following are the main uses of supplemental tests:

- assess special aphasic populations such as the most mildly or severely impaired
- assess skills not represented in traditional batteries, such as functional communication
- more in-depth evaluation of a language skill, such as reading
- examine psycholinguistic processes according to modern experimental methods

For this chapter, only a few common tests of language functions are introduced. Other supplemental strategies of assessment will be presented in subsequent chapters, mainly because they illustrate how basic research and the health care system can have a direct impact on clinical practice.

Token Tests

The auditory language modality is usually the least impaired in aphasia (see Figure 1.1). Mild comprehension deficits are found in anomic, conduction, and Broca's aphasias. At the University of Milano in Italy, Ennio DeRenzi and Luigi Vignolo felt that it was difficult to detect mild deficits with routine methods available in the 1950s. Later the auditory sections of the PICA and BDAE were found to have low ceilings for aphasic patients, meaning that the challenging end of the tests does not have enough room for mildly impaired patients to show deficit (Morley, Lundgren, and Haxby, 1979).

DeRenzi and Vignolo (1962) created the Token Test to identify and measure subtle comprehension deficits. It was designed so that response would be based on processing language with minimal help from a situation, props, topic, or extraneous verbalization. The test is a series of instructions to identify and manipulate shapes of different shape, color, and size. With contextual factors cleared away, it focuses on the influence of linguistic length and complexity.

Boller and Vignolo (1966) published a complete list of commands, and so their version became the basis for most subsequent versions. The test has five parts. Parts I through IV contain 10 items each, and they differ according to information given about the tokens and length of command. Part V contains 22 commands of varying construction, and the commands are generally more complex than the items in previous sections. The complete test contains 62 items. The following illustrates each part of the 1966 version:

I. Touch the yellow rectangle.
II. Touch the large blue circle.
III. Touch the red circle and the yellow rectangle.
IV. Touch the small yellow circle and the large green rectangle.
V. (1) Put the red circle on the green rectangle.
(11) Touch the white circle without using your right hand.
(20) After picking up the green rectangle, touch the white circle.

The Token Test was introduced in a journal, but incomplete description left it open to modifications. So, investigators have done some tinkering by recommending other shapes, colors, and wording such as "big" and "little" for children (DeRenzi and Faglioni, 1978; Spreen and Benton, 1969; Whitaker and Noll, 1972). The most consistent version has been Boller and Vignolo's 1966 test, but with squares instead of rectangles.

Tokens are arranged in two or four rows depending on the part being given. Several arrangements have been recommended to enhance standardization. DeRenzi and Vignolo (1962) suggested a circles-first arrangement. When all 20 tokens are displayed for Parts II and IV, the top two rows should be circles, large and then small; and the bottom two rows should be rectangles (or squares), large and then small. On the other hand, Spreen and Benton (1969) used a large-small arrangement; large circles and squares formed the first two rows, and small circles and squares formed the last two rows.

Various scoring systems have been used. Originally, errors were counted for each element of each command, with total possible errors being 250. Most clinicians have followed Boller and Vignolo's (1966) recommendation of scoring each command as correct or incorrect and then having a best score of 62 (e.g., Swisher and Sarno, 1969; Gallaher, 1979).

Normative information must be pieced together from many studies (Table 3.9). Aphasic patients with mild comprehension deficit do poorly on Parts IV and V, indicating that initially undetected deficit can be exposed with the Token Test (Morley, et al., 1979; Noll and Randolph, 1978). The test is very difficult for other aphasic persons, who perform much worse than RH-damaged patients and have lower scores than LH-damaged nonaphasic patients (e.g., DeRenzi and Faglioni, 1978; Hartje, Kerschensteiner, Poeck, and Orgass, 1973). Problems with Part V in LHD nonaphasic subjects led to a diagnosis of "latent aphasia" (Boller and Vignolo, 1966). Nonfluent and fluent aphasias score about equally, but specific syndromes differ. Wernicke's aphasia produces more errors than nonfluent aphasia (Mack and Boller, 1979; Poeck and Hartje, 1979).

TABLE 3.9 Some sample scores on the Token Test by different groups (Noll and Randolf, 1978; Swisher and Sarno, 1969).

POPULATION	RANGE	MEAN
neurologically intact adults	48–62	59.7
mild aphasia	18–59	43.5
wide range of aphasia severity	0–58	23

The first abbreviated Token Test became the "Identification by Sentence" subtest of the Neurosensory Center Comprehensive Examination of Aphasia (Spreen and Benton, 1977). There are 39 items instead of 62. A sixth part was added at the low end to provide an easier section so that application can be broadened beyond the original goal of assessing mild deficit. It involves identification by shape *or* color (e.g., Show me a square; show me a red one). A 16-item version was equally capable of deficit identification (Spellacy and Spreen, 1969). Norms were also developed for a 36-item Token Test with a cut-off of 29 for identifying aphasic deficit (DeRenzi, 1979). DeRenzi eliminated the color blue because of problems that elderly adults have in discriminating between blue and green.

Reading Tests

For more thorough examination of a patient's reading capacities, clinical aphasiologists have created printed versions of auditory comprehension tests, borrowed reading batteries from the field of education, or created their own batteries of silent and oral reading tasks. Strategies for diagnosing word-reading deficits have been emerging in cognitive neuropsychology (Chapter 6). The tests are considered when treatment objectives focus on a patient's reading needs, especially for mildly impaired patients wanting to return to jobs requiring reading skill.

Brookshire (1997) reviewed reading assessment extensively, having been particularly interested in paragraph-level tests. Nicholas and Brookshire (1987) used the *Nelson Reading Skills Test* (NRST) to examine inferencing in aphasic adults and also to evaluate the need to read paragraphs in order to answer test questions about them, called **passage dependency.** NRST paragraph tests were found to have better passage dependency than paragraph items in standard aphasia batteries (Nicholas, MacLennan, and Brookshire, 1986), indicating that the NRST is a more valid assessment of text comprehension. Some of the reading tests that Brookshire favors are summarized in Table 3.10.

The **Reading Comprehension Battery for Aphasia** (RCBA) is in its second edition (LaPointe and Horner, 1998). The main test contains ten subtests from word to paragraph levels. Unique sections include a subtest for functional tasks such as reading common signs, a checkbook, and a phone directory. A supplement (RCBA-S) was added for the second edition. It contains seven subtests exploring word level reading in more detail. Subtests include letter discrimination and recognition, word-nonword discrimination, and oral word and sentence reading.

Aphasic patients are often meticulous readers. Van Demark, Lemmer, and Drake (1982) measured an average time of about 45 minutes to administer the main RCBA. They compared 19 nonfluent and seven fluent patients. Both groups had PICA scores indicative of moderate impairment. With a maximum score of 100, the nonfluent group averaged 70.73, and the fluent group averaged 77.85. The mean and range for all subjects were 71.34 and 31 to 97.

The Boston Naming Test (BNT)

The BNT is constructed to detect mild word-finding impairments and can be obtained with the BDAE (Kaplan, Goodglass, and Weintraub, 1983). The test contains 60 line drawings to elicit words of varied familiarity. It begins with simple words that are common in aphasia batteries such as *bed* and *tree,* and at the end it presents infrequent words such as *trellis, palette,* and *abacus.* Certain cues are provided when a patient is slow to respond, and testing stops after six consecutive failures. The score is derived from the total correct with the maximum being 60. Cued and uncued versions of the test proved to be reliable (Huff, Collins, Corkin, and Rosen, 1986).

"Provisional norms" from 84 normal and 82 aphasic adults are included in the scoring booklet. A range of 42 to 60 was found across all normal adult age groups. Normals in their 50s averaged 55.82 in a range of 49 to 59. Because of the high education level of the normal group (15 years) and some of the vocabulary in the test (e.g., *protractor, tripod*), there have been several norming studies of the BNT (Henderson, Frank, Pigatt, Abramson, and Houston, 1998). Race has been an inconsistent factor, but education has been a regular factor. In a study of 323 elderly subjects, Neils and others (1995) found that "institutionalized subjects with a sixth-ninth grade education performed poorly on the BNT regardless of age" (p. 1143). Kimbarow and his colleagues (1996) recommended that clinicians "consider fully the patient's racial and educational background before attributing poor performance to neurological dysfunction" (p. 143).

Nicholas and Brookshire were concerned that some of the pictures are ambiguous, capable of eliciting names other than the ones considered to be correct. They gave the test to 60

TABLE 3.10 Some reading tests from the field of education that have been suggested for use with aphasia.

TEST	READING LEVEL	DESCRIPTION	REFERENCE
Gates-MacGinitie Reading Tests	grades 1–3	word, sentence, and paragraph comprehension	Gates (1978)
Nelson Reading Skills Test	grades 3–9	word and paragraph materials at three reading levels	Hanna, Schell, and Schriener (1977)
Nelson-Denny Reading Test	high school through college	word and paragraph materials	Brown, Bennett, and Hanna (1981)

neurologically intact persons after changing some of the BNT's procedures. They wrote more explicit instructions, established a different cueing procedure, and developed a more elaborate response coding and scoring procedure. The subjects averaged 54.5 which is close to the mean reported by Kaplan (Nicholas, Brookshire, MacLennan, Schumacher, and Porrazzo, 1989).

NOTES ON INTERPRETATION

The details of different aphasia batteries can distract us from our fundamental objectives. In the acute care setting, we are mainly involved in discharge planning. In the rehabilitation setting, we want to plan treatment so that it addresses a patient's communication problems *accurately.* Does the patient have a speech or language disorder? Is the language disorder aphasia? Does the patient have additional problems such as an agnosia, dysarthria, or a low level of arousal? Are clinical findings consistent with the medical diagnosis? Does the medical diagnosis present a favorable prognosis? No matter what test we use, our questions are the same.

A test does not tell us that a person has aphasia. That is, a poor naming score does not always mean that someone has aphasia (see Chapter 4). Instead, we interpret our observations according to what we understand aphasia to be, namely, a disorder of language processing as opposed to hearing loss or a low level of consciousness. An inexperienced clinician may have a tendency to "overdiagnose" a patient who is not talking, especially in the first couple of weeks after onset. The clinician may have the urge to say that someone has one or more of the main communicative disorders studied in graduate school, while forgetting that a patient may be silent for reasons that are unrelated to aphasia (see Chapter 2 on global aphasia). Sometimes it is more accurate to say that we cannot be sure of language abilities (and/or speech abilities) until the patient becomes more alert and has more energy.

We want to determine the status of the four primary language modalities, no matter what test we use; and we want to determine the retained skills that can be useful communicatively. A test battery with 30 subtests does not mean that a patient could have 30 disorders. The 18 subtests of the PICA and the 46 subtests of the MTDDA do not mean that Porch and Schuell disagreed on the number of problems that could be diagnosed with aphasia. We know that aphasic people can have a few specific language disorders in word-finding or sentence construction. In general, any test is harnessed to help us document our clinical observations of fundamental aphasic deficits and/or discover whether a patient has any of these disorders.

So, what do we do with the results, let us say, of 10 subtests and 10 items per subtest? We conduct three levels of comparison summarized in Table 3.11. At the level of basic language functions, we compare listening, reading, speaking, and writing. We look for **common threads** such as problems with language in all modalities. Task comparison is essential because no single task is diagnostic of a disorder. For example, a low repetition score could be indicative of a hearing loss, short-term memory deficit, or motor speech disorder. In task comparison, we look for common threads such as difficulties only in tasks requiring lengthy verbal input or only in tasks requiring speech output. Within a single task, comparing items may direct us to specific problems for focusing treatment. A patient may make comprehension errors with particular sentence structures or may make particular types of errors in naming tasks.

As we identify specific language problems, we are starting to plan for language treatment. We **prioritize** with respect to a patient's communicative needs as well as the time we have. What will a patient be most motivated to work on? What is most likely to improve in the next month or so? What problems can the family help us with? For some patients, improving comprehension (e.g., yes-no response) goes a long way to improving communicative interaction. For some patients, reading or writing skills are relatively unimportant.

There are some things to avoid. As Head suggested decades ago, we should avoid quick

TABLE 3.11 Levels in analysis of aphasia batteries or supplemental tests.

COMPARISON	DEFINITION	DIAGNOSTIC ISSUES
function	comparing status of language modalities	• aphasia vs. sensory loss, agnosias, or motor speech disorders
task	comparing task performances within a modality	• level of language impairment such as words, sentences, or discourse/text • impairment of a specific process such as word-retrieval
item	comparing specific items within a task	• impairment of a specific linguistic feature such as verbs or passive sentences • impairment of a semantic category such as living things or vegetables

diagnosis based on too few observations. A sampling of 10 items per test is considered the minimum for establishing a baseline level of deficit. Also, we should avoid letting a test do our thinking for us. Diagnosis should be based on a collection of information. For example, the cut-off of 93.8 from the WAB does not diagnose aphasia or language disorder by itself. Someone without brain damage can score an AQ of 92.5. A test score is important for documentation that supports a thoughtful diagnosis. The study by Swindell and others (1984) showed 46 percent disagreement between the WAB and informed observation for diagnosing syndromes. Thus, this test does not necessarily tell us the type of aphasia a patient might have.

Diagnosis is based on a logical alignment of medical information and clinical observations.

MARTIN EXETER'S INITIAL REPORT

Martin Exeter was transferred to the Rehabilitation Unit at Pocumtuck Medical Center five days after his stroke. His first day of rehabilitation included brief evaluations by a clinical neuropsychologist and physical therapist. A social worker met with family members for a few minutes. Besides his wife Jackie, his daughter Julianna and son Peter were present. Martin and Jackie were married in their early thirties. Julianna was a sophomore in college and came home as soon as she heard the news. Peter was a junior in high school.

The speech-language clinician met the family to review her findings in initial assessment (Figure 3.5). The family wanted to know more about strokes and aphasia and the future. The clinician explained that they would have to wait and see how he was doing near the end of his inpatient stay, but his progress to date indicated that his aphasia should not keep him from taking care of himself at home. The clinician could not say at this time exactly how many inpatient sessions would be covered by their insurance, but she stressed the importance of their support. Each family member wanted to know what they could do to help, and the clinician assured them that their help would be very important in his language treatment. The clinician also wanted to observe the family's interaction styles with Martin before making specific recommendations.

Julianna said she wanted to quit school to be with her father for a while. The speech-language clinician advised her that quitting school would not be necessary for her father's language rehabilitation, but she would have to decide for herself. Jackie did not want Julie to quit school. The clinician asked Julie if she knew how quitting school would make her father feel, and Julie indicated that she would not tell him and hoped her mom and brother would keep it from him, too. The clinician thought that Julie's observations of how

POCUMTUCK MEDICAL CENTER SPEECH-LANGUAGE PATHOLOGY		
Name: Martin Exeter	Location: Rehabilitation Unit	Date: 4-17-93

INITIAL EVALUATION SUMMARY

Dr. Exeter is a 55-year-old male who suffered an ischemic stroke on April 10, 1993. He is a professor at the university. After five days in acute care at this hospital, he was referred to the Rehabilitation Unit by Dr. Irving Waxman.

History

Medical diagnosis was a thrombotic stroke causing aphasia and moderate hemiparesis on the right side. There were no sensory deficits. A CT scan showed an area of infarction in the region of the left middle cerebral artery distribution, specifically in the inferior left frontal lobe sparing part of the 3rd frontal convolution but extending into the inferior parietal region and superior temporal region. After two days, Dr. Exeter became aware of his surroundings and was able to recognize hospital staff and family.

While in acute care, he was evaluated briefly by Patricia Burns, speech-language pathologist, who determined that Dr. Exeter has a severe aphasia, mild dysarthria, and no swallowing difficulties. He was able to answer a few simple questions, but was still in an acute confusional state at the time of evaluation. He was able to gesture most basic needs, and by the fourth day was able to produce a few words communicatively. It was recommended that he be transferred to the Rehabilitation Unit for further evaluation and determination of post-acute rehabilitation needs.

Subjective Observation

During initial interview, Dr. Exeter was attentive and cooperative. Normal conversation was overwhelming, but he understood simple instructions. He was still limited in verbal expression. He became somewhat agitated when he could not express himself.

Objective Language Evaluation

Dr. Exeter was given selected portions of the Boston Diagnostic Aphasia Examination to evaluate auditory-oral language abilities:

In auditory comprehension, he scored 64/72 for word comprehension, 10/15 for following commands, and 5/12 for answering questions about short paragraphs. Body part identification was not administered. In general, he had difficulty with the most complex material.

In verbal expression, he described the Cookie Theft picture producing six nouns, one verb, and one 2-word phrase that were appropriate. He scored 84/114 for picture naming and 20/30 for answering simple questions with one word. He was able to repeat short common words. He scored 4/16 in repetition of short phrases and sentences, a task that elicited more language than he could produce spontaneously.

Conclusions

Dr. Exeter has some functional comprehension and limited agrammatic verbal production. He can communicate most basic needs. His speech and test results conform to a pattern of severe but still evolving Broca's aphasia. Apraxia of speech is evident when repeating complex words and sentences. This diagnosis is consistent with site of lesion and accompanying hemiparesis. While individuals with this type of aphasia often make excellent progress, it is too soon to predict Dr. Exeter's outcome. However, his rapidly improving comprehension, relatively young age and good health, and motivation are all positive signs that he can progress a substantial degree.

Recommendations

(1) Dr. Exeter should receive language treatment to improve auditory comprehension, word-finding efficiency, and phrase length.

(2) Reading and writing abilities should be evaluated, especially because these skills are important to him with respect to his professional interests.

(3) The speech-language pathologist should meet with family members to answer questions and introduce them to the rehabilitation process.

FIGURE 3.5 Summary of Martin Exeter's initial speech and language evaluation in the Rehabilitation Unit.

her father gets along in the hospital the next few days would help her make her decision.

Peter was quiet. The clinician asked him what sort of things he and his father did together. Peter started to answer but then left the room. Jackie said that Martin would take Peter to sporting events at the university. The basketball team was surprisingly good this year. They were looking forward to playing golf in the summer. Peter would want to know if his dad would be able to play golf again.

SUMMARY AND CONCLUSIONS

The three comprehensive batteries reviewed in this chapter were published in a span of 15 years, between 1967 and 1982. No new battery was published in the United States in the subsequent 18 years. Evidently a need had been satisfied during the earlier period. Table 3.12 provides a historical perspective on most of the tests introduced here, especially in their relationship to other developments in clinical aphasiology. The motivation for developing new tests is likely to come from at least two sources, namely, changes in health care management and discoveries about the nature of aphasia that make a difference in rehabilitation. Many of these assessment methods are presented in the following chapters.

Insurance companies do not tell speech-language pathologists to take 30 minutes for evaluation. Instead, time for evaluation is prioritized given a limit on the number of sessions that will be reimbursed. Clinicians have had to re-evaluate what is minimally needed to classify a patient for reimbursement and get therapy started. Fundamental diagnoses can be accomplished in an informal evaluation. Tests become important for documentation of deficit and setting baselines from which to measure progress. Time consuming reading and writing tests are not necessary to distinguish speech and language disorders and to identify language problems vital to everyday communication. Clinicians may use Schuell's baseline-ceiling approach to compress a large aphasia battery.

Beyond the initial evaluation, "diagnostic therapy" mines more useful discoveries about a patient as clinical interaction moves on. Refinements of diagnosis can be a problem-solving component of the treatment process.

TABLE 3.12 A chronology of assessments along with certain clinical developments.

DECADE	TESTS	CLINICAL THEORY AND RESEARCH
pre-1940s	• Head's serial tests for aphasia • IQ tests for neuropsychology	• case studies to prove localization theories • Weisenberg & McBride's clinical studies
1940s	• Schuell starts MTDDA	
1950s	• Eisenson's test • Research edition of MTDDA	• Wepman's central-transmission distinction
1960s	• Token Test • PICA	• Porch's test-based statistical prognosis
1970s	• BDAE	• lesion localization of syndromes • Wertz questions PICA-based prognosis
1980s	• WAB • functional measures (Chapter 7)	• Wertz questions test-based classification • model-based cognitive neuropsychology • functional communication
1990s	• PALPA	• impairment, disability, handicap • managed care

Chapter 4

INVESTIGATING APHASIA IN GENERAL

As a psychologist at the university, Martin Exeter's specialty was cognitive psychology. Long ago he learned that if he told people only that he was a psychologist, they would seek his help for emotional problems or make a joke about it. Experimental psychology is different. He enjoyed thinking scientifically and testing theories of the mind in the laboratory. His research dealt with language comprehension, and for most of his career he had not realized that psycholinguistic processes were a clinical concern. While preparing for his lecture in Europe, he was beginning to learn a little about aphasia.

One thing Dr. Exeter liked about experimental psychology is that, because nothing is really certain, there is a great opportunity to discover something. As a cognitive disorder, there is little that is certain about aphasia. The next few chapters deal with how discoveries are made about the underlying nature of acquired language disorders. Chapters 4 through 6 focus on aphasic impairments, and Chapter 7 explores communicative disability.

The present chapter focuses on deficits that are common to most people with aphasia, including problems of comprehension and word-finding. Clinical implications are as follows:

- development of new supplemental assessments and measurement strategies
- new insights about language disorder that may focus treatment strategies

As part of the scientific foundation for clinical studies of word-level processing, we shall pay more attention to the automatic level of processing and the activation of stored information in lexical and semantic systems.

BASIC RESEARCH IN CLINICAL APHASIOLOGY

We support our beliefs about clinical practice (e.g., diagnosis) with personal experience, expert opinion, and experimental research. Research can expand our viewpoint from personal experience but sometimes does not support expert opinion. Speech-language clinicians rely on a basic understanding of research in order to evaluate experimentally supported clinical claims. Three general topics in this section include styles of research, experimental design, and the influence of disciplines on the study of language disorder.

Data-Driven and Theory-Driven Research

There are two approaches to observing the effects of stimulus manipulations on responses, namely, data-driven and theory-driven approaches. To say that something "drives" a study is to state the primary motivation and background for designing an experiment.

Brookshire (1983) stated that the goal of research is "to demonstrate that manipulation of certain (independent) variables under controlled conditions affects other (dependent) variables in predictable ways" (p. 342). This turns out to be the goal of data-driven or empirical research. The following are examples of empirical questions:

- What is the effect of utterance complexity on pointing to pictures?
- What type of errors does a patient make in an object naming task?

A theoretical interpretation is sometimes added after an empirical study, called *post-hoc analysis.*

For example, in a publication of a study of puzzle-solving, the concept of resource allocation was introduced as the best explanation after results were presented (Selinger, Walker, Prescott, and Davis, 1993; also, Cannito, Hough, Vogel, and Pierce, 1996; Nicholas and Brookshire, 1995).

In a comment on data-driven studies of aphasic comprehension, Tyler (1988) suggested that "researchers have, on the whole, been primarily interested in whether a patient (or group of patients) has difficulty with particular types of linguistic information, but they rarely attempt to locate the source of the difficulty in a particular aspect of the comprehension process" (p. 376). In theory-driven research, a researcher uses a theory of mechansims between a stimulus and response in order to arrange appropriate stimulus-response pairings and predict the effects. The following are examples of theoretical questions:

- Does stroke cause a loss of semantic information from long-term memory?
- Can the syntactic processing mechanism be uniquely impaired in aphasia?

Predictions establish a foundation for testing the validity of a theory. The author of a publication explains how a theory generated the experimental design and how results can be interpreted accordingly. Obtaining data becomes a means to an end, rather than an end itself. A theoretical account contributes to the **internal validity** of a study or whether we can establish a causal relationship between internal events and responses.

Empirically speaking, we ask whether a response pattern can be attributed to characteristics of a stimulus. Theoretically speaking, we ask whether a response pattern can be attributed to an hypothesized hidden condition or process.

Clinical Research Designs

Planning an experiment involves consideration of design and procedure. With respect to design, any study consists of at least one comparison such as comparing two subjects with a particular procedure or comparing two procedures with one subject. This is similar to clinical diagnosis in which we compare a patient's test score to a normal score. Also, we compare a patient's performances on numerous tasks to discern a common thread among the different scores.

In research, deficient or intact skills are identified with a between-subject design when one group of subjects is neurologically intact (Table 4.1). A comparison between brain-damaged and neurologically intact groups is less straightforward than a comparison between two neurologically intact groups. Two normal groups

TABLE 4.1 Basic experimental designs and the empirical questions they answer.

DESIGN	COMPARISON	BASIC QUESTIONS	EXAMPLES
between-subject	brain-damaged vs neurologically intact	What deficits are caused by brain damage?	trauma patients vs normal subjects
	brain-damaged vs brain-damaged	What behaviors can be linked to a specific neuropathology or site of lesion?	anterior vs posterior infarct
within-subject	task A vs task B	Is there a pattern of retained and impaired language abilities in an aphasic patient?	comprehending words vs naming objects
	item A vs item B	Can a patient have problems finding some words but not others?	abstract vs concrete words

are expected to be alike in every respect except for the variable being studied. This assumption underlies use of the traditional t-test for comparing the average scores of two groups. However, this assumption does not usually apply when one group has brain damage (see Clark and Ryan, 1993, Duffy and Myers, 1991). Group description has improved over the years, increasing our confidence that two groups are homogeneous except for the variable being studied (Obler, Goral, and Albert, 1995).

A within-subject design is employed for learning as much as we can about one group or a single case. An investigator may want to discover a unique pattern of performance among tasks or among items within a task. A single case is often examined when an investigator wants to use a large number of tasks to answer a very specific question. A group of subjects is preferred to increase the likelihood that results can be applied to a population. In either type of study, an informative subject description helps us determine the **external validity** or generalizability of findings to other patients (Brookshire, 1983).

Interdisciplinary Influences

Like other domains of communicative disorders, aphasiology draws upon basic sciences for frameworks about language functions and methods for studying them. Aphasiologists have varying experience with these sciences. A speech-language pathologist may have been mentored primarily in speech science, neurology, linguistics, or cognitive psychology.

Human language function is studied in two intimately related fields. **Linguistics** is the study of the structure of language. Linguistic research is the logical examination of words and sentences. In the 1960s linguists and experimental psychologists began to work together, forming the discipline of **psycholinguistics.** The data of psycholinguistics comes from people processing words and sentences in a laboratory. The initial question was whether linguistic theories have "psychological reality" as a characterization of human knowledge.

Cognitive neuropsychology (CN) also has the goal of developing theories of normal language processing. CN is distinctive because it relies on brain damaged subjects, but it is divided between two approaches. In one, investigators study aphasia at word- and sentence-levels with psycholinguistic methods generally applied to groups of subjects (e.g., Caplan, 1988; Zurif, Gardner, and Brownell, 1989). Psycholinguists become interested in aphasia in order to "extend the range of observations" that bear on language systems (Dell, et al., 1997). In the other approach to CN, investigators rely solely on single cases to test models of functions primarily at the single word level (e.g., Coltheart, Sartori, and Job, 1987; McCarthy and Warrington, 1990).

The aphasia laboratory is like a kitchen crowded with many chefs, each advocating a favorite approach to the study of behavior, the brain, and cognition (Table 4.2). Moreover, two disciplines dealing with the same problem are often oblivious to each other's accomplishments. Sometimes this results in different terms for the same thing or different things labeled by the same term. A science reporter attended an interdisciplinary conference on memory and found the disciplines to be like warring tribes suspicious of each other's customs (Johnson, 1991). LeDoux and Hirst (1986) edited a book in which psychologists and neuroscientists took turns writing about perception, attention, memory, and emotion. The book was to be "a pioneering attempt...to force scientists who are working on the same problem but from different perspectives to address each other." A cooperative approach has not yet fully replaced a somewhat competitive approach.

LANGUAGE-SPECIFIC DISORDER

Jackie Exeter had said that Martin could not talk but his mind was OK. While many aphasic patients appear to have problems only with language, clinicians have long wondered whether

TABLE 4.2 Disciplines that provide clinical investigators with experimental paradigms for the study of language impairments.

DISCIPLINE	ORIGIN	DOMAIN	PRINCIPAL METHOD
linguistics		form and structure of language	logical analysis of sounds, words, and sentences
behavioral psychology	experimental psychology	stimulus-response relationships	learning experiments; empirical research
cognitive psychology	experimental psychology	mental representations & processes in cognition	group studies of task accuracy and response time
psycholinguistics	cognitive psychology	mental representation & processes in language functions	group studies of task accuracy and response time
clinical neuropsychology	clinical psychology	cognitive dysfunctions caused by brain damage	group studies of standardized test performance
cognitive neuropsychology	cognitive psychology	mental representation & processes in cognition (including language)	case studies of brain-damaged persons; many tasks presented

other "intellective" deficits hover around the edges of language disorder. Other impairments could be general (e.g., attention) or function-specific (e.g., visuospatial processes).

Language and Intelligence

As indicated in Chapter 3's introduction to the WAIS, patients with LHD are likely to have a Verbal IQ that is lower than the Performance IQ. How do aphasic patients do with the nonverbal or performance subtests? Does a lower VIQ mean that the PIQ is normal? In the first report of IQ tests with aphasic patients, Weisenburg and McBride (1935) found that aphasic people frequently have nonverbal cognitive deficits in addition to language impairment. With a German version of the WAIS, Orgass and Poeck (1969) found a mean PIQ of 80 in thirty subjects, which was below the mean of 100 and significantly less than nonaphasic persons with LHD or RHD.

The reduction of PIQ indicates that aphasic patients can have difficulties beyond their language disorder. Hom and Reitan (1990) compared groups with LHD, RHD, and multi-infarct brain damage on the Halstead-Reitan battery which includes the WAIS. They found that the three brain-damaged groups did not differ with respect to having "significant impairments in abstraction and reasoning, attention and concentration...and flexibility of thought (p. 651). Thus, any cortical damage appears to have some effects on general cognitive functions.

Raven's (1962) **Coloured Progressive Matrices** (RCPM), which is often used by speech-language pathologists, is thought to be a predictor of general intelligence. Tasks increase in difficulty from completing simple geometric designs to reasoning with a subtle pattern of figures. In a study of a large group of aphasic subjects, those with severe comprehension deficit were well below nonaphasic brain-damaged groups. Moderate-to-mild aphasias were comparable to RHD subjects (Kertesz and McCabe, 1975).

Vigilance and Allocation of Attention

Malcolm McNeil and his colleagues have argued that certain characteristics of aphasic behavior cannot be explained soley with respect to impaired language mechanisms (McNeil and Kimelman, 1986; McNeil, Odell, and Tseng, 1991). One of these characteristics is the variability or inconsistency of language behavior, such as naming an object one moment and not naming the same object a few moments later. McNeil suggested that a possible explanation lies in the influence of a multifaceted attention mechanism on the language system.

To understand the influence of attention on language behavior, it is useful to be introduced to cognitive theory of attention (Haberlandt, 1994; Solso, 1991). Attention mechanisms are part of the support system for all cognitive skills such as language comprehension, visuospatial orientation, reasoning, and so on. Attention operates at different levels and in different ways (Table 4.3). The base level is simple arousal or being "awake," as if the brain provides a level of "psychic energy" so that a person can function. Once aroused, our minds operate at levels of awareness from a foggy stupor to a clear "consciousness" of our surroundings, thoughts, and memories. Impairment at these levels is common with traumatic brain injury and can also occur with bilateral stroke in the thalamus and adjacent structures.

Two clinical research teams became interested in McNeil's ideas about aphasic variability. One team studied the effect of divided attention on sustained attention (Erickson, Goldinger, and LaPointe, 1996; LaPointe and Erickson, 1991). These investigators compared performance of an auditory vigilance task alone to performance of the same task in a dual-task condition. In one study, the vigilance task was verbal, involving listening to a series of words. In the other study, the vigilance task contained a series of tones. In both studies, aphasic subjects could sustain auditory attention; but, unlike a control group, vigilance was reduced when subjects had to sort cards at the same time. Another team also showed that aphasic individuals can differ from normals in attention to auditory stimuli (e.g., Peach, Rubin, and Newhoff, 1994). Thus, an aphasic patient may have some problems with verbal and nonverbal attention, especially under conditions of competing processing demands.

Semantic Memory

Semantic memory contains our information about the world. Its core is universal in the sense that most people have the same basic knowledge of living and nonliving things. Fringes of world knowledge vary according to locale, culture, and expertise. Psychologists are most interested in *natural* universal knowledge or, namely, how it is really stored in our heads (with "imperfections").

TABLE 4.3 Levels and types of attention. Selective and divided attention are discussed later in the chapter.

LEVELS AND TYPES	FUNCTION	ASSESSMENT
arousal	state of consciousness; primitive wakefulness	gross motor response to sensory stimulation
awareness	assumes arousal; from stupor to clear perception of surroundings	answer questions
selective attention	focus; resistence to distraction; managing limited resources by selection	two stimuli or tasks; response to one (e.g., dichotic listening)
sustained attention	vigilance or concentration; maintaining focus on one stimulus for a period of time	a series of stimuli and response to one
divided attention	allocating limited resources to multiple processes or tasks	two stimuli or tasks; response to both (dual task paradigms)

In discussions of aphasia, agnosia, and other disorders later in this text, we shall deal with a variety of views about how semantics fits into the processing system. Researchers tend to agree that semantic memory is central to language processing because of its role in comprehension and the meaningful use of words.

If our stored knowledge were to contain every object that we ever encountered, we might have difficulty recognizing new or unusual versions of common objects. Instead, semantic memory stores concepts. A **concept** is the simplest unit of world knowledge and may be defined as the mental representation of a class of objects or actions. Concepts are stored separately from words. For this text, a concept will be represented in brackets. The concept [hat] may be a universal element of knowledge, but the word for it varies from language to language and is stored in lexical memory (e.g., *chapeau, cappello, hoed,* or *hat*).

Investigators agree that concepts are organized in some way. The prevailing view in psycholinguistics is that our knowledge store takes the form of a **semantic network.** In the spatial metaphor used to characterize this network, a concept is represented as a **node** connected to other nodes. A streamlined example is shown in Figure 4.1. A network permits a general category like [vehicle] or a general attribute like [red] to be recorded once. A network depicts the relatedness among concepts according to a distance metaphor. Related concepts are close together like "neighbors" in the network, and less related concepts are more distant from each other. Relative distances between concepts lead to predictions of processing times from one node to another.

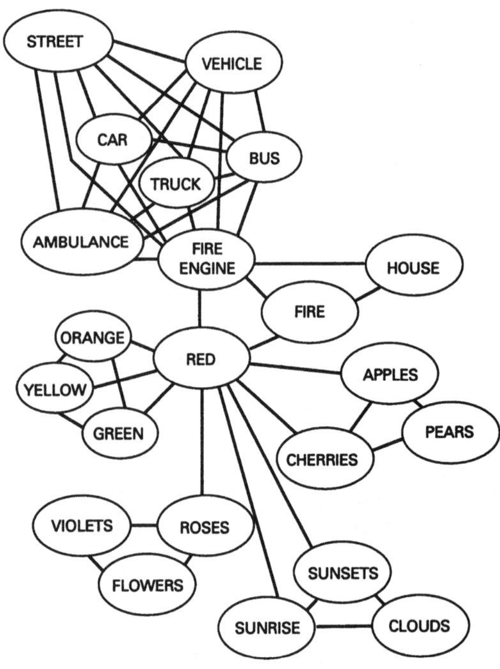

FIGURE 4.1 A simple semantic network suggestive of semantic relatedness or "distance" between concepts.

Reprinted by permission from Collins, A. M., & Loftus, E. F., A spreading-activation theory of semantic processing. *Psychological Bulletin,* 82, 1975, p. 412. American Psychology Association, publisher.

A clinical evaluation of conceptual knowledge is to have patients match or sort *objects* (not words) according to common categories. Researchers also address semantic memory through word-sorting tasks. Using words, however, can fog the window to concepts, because words necessarily involve contact with lexical memory. Some aphasic patients are normal when sorting objects into semantic categories (Milton, Wertz, Katz, and Prutting, 1981), but many others exhibit deficits and do worse than persons with right hemisphere damage (Cohen, Kelter, and Woll, 1980; Gainotti, Carlomagno, Craca, and Silveri, 1986; Grossman and Wilson, 1987). Thus, as with nonverbal intelligence and vigilance, there may be subtle changes in semantic memory for some persons with aphasia.

Later we shall consider whether semantic memory accounts for some comprehension and word-finding deficits. Moreover, matching and sorting tasks provide an incomplete examination of conceptual knowledge. In these "slow tasks," conscious problem solving strategies may be overlaid upon the automatic activation of concepts, and automatic processing may still expose strengths in a semantic network. The neglect of automatic processing will be corrected shortly.

Food for Thought

A language-specific disorder is most evident when a patient has difficulty with verbal tasks and relative success with nonverbal tasks. An aphasic patient knows what he or she wants to say but just cannot think of the words for it. The patient seems to get along when words are not needed. However, in clinical neuropsychological evaluations and in studies of vigilance and conceptual knowledge, some areas outside of the language system are shown to be statistically deficient relative to normal levels of performance.

Thinking back on the definitional points raised in Chapter 1, deficits beyond language in aphasic patients can mean at least two things:

- aphasia is more than a language disorder; thus, aphasia is not what Darley thought it was
- aphasia can be accompanied by other disorders; thus, aphasia is still what Darley thought it was

Clinical aphasiologists tend to agree with Darley. When one patient has problems in other areas besides language, it does not necessarily mean that the difficulties stem from damage to a single functional system. Aphasia can be accompanied by hemiplegia, visual field deficit, mild dysarthria, and/or apraxia of speech. Co-occurrence of word-finding deficit and hemiplegia, for example, does not mean that these are the same disorder. Similarly, aphasia can also be accompanied by and influenced by other cognitive deficiencies. Thus, one patient may require different types of rehabilitative treatment.

WORD PROCESSING

The clinical test of word comprehension is to present a word auditorily or visually and have a patient point to a picture. Nearly all aphasic patients have difficulty comprehending language at some level, but many do not have problems understanding single words. About 45 percent of aphasic subjects make no errors or are within normal range in a picture pointing task (Schuell and Jenkins, 1961; Varney, 1984). A substantial deficit with individual words indicates severe receptive disorder.

If we are to understand comprehension disorder in cognitive terms, we should consider what happens mentally in a clinical word comprehension task. Initially, the mind represents the stimulus, and the representation undergoes different levels of processing introduced in Table 4.4. The goal of accessing meaning can be impeded because of a problem early or late in the process. An elderly aphasic person could have a hearing loss or visual impairment that existed prior to stroke. So that these problems do not interfere with assessing comprehension, we should make sure that such patients are wearing a hearing aid or glasses.

Speech Perception

Perception results in the mental representation of a stimulus, called a **percept.** Investigators have explored the possibility that aphasic people have a problem forming a percept of the speech signal, which might explain some comprehension deficits. Speech perception is assessed two ways:

- *discrimination* in which subjects make same-different judgments regarding CV-syllable pairs (e.g., /pa/, /ba/) or nonsense word pairs (e.g., ursit, ursat)
- *identification* or "labeling" in which a patient points to a letter for the phoneme.

Discrimination is easier for aphasic people, and labeling errors may be caused by a language deficit instead of a speech perception problem (Blumstein, Tartter, Nigro, and Statlender, 1984; Riedel and Studdert-Kennedy, 1985). Most aphasic patients are within normal range for discrimination. Most of those with a deficit improve to normal

TABLE 4.4 Functional levels of word processing beginning with sensation and concluding with comprehension.

FUNCTIONAL LEVELS	SUBJECTIVE EXPERIENCE	PROCESS	ASSESSMENT
Sensation	*I hear something.*	Initial detection of acoustic signal from the environment	audiometric tests
Perception	*I hear the sound /metaphysics/.*	Mental representation of a lexical stimulus, called a percept	discrimination identification
Recognition	*It sounds like a word. I've heard that word before.*	Activation of word in lexical memory (match percept to lexical representation)	word-naming lexical decision
Comprehension	*I know what that word means.*	Activation of concept in semantic memory (match lexical representation to concept)	point to picture

perception within four months after a stroke (Franklin, 1989; Varney, 1984). For others, deficits are stable over the first year (Gow and Caplan, 1996).

Is the speed of syllable production just too fast for some aphasic listeners? In early studies, aphasic subjects perceived the order of two sounds only when there was enough time between them. Normal intervals were too quick (Swisher and Hirsch, 1972; Van Allen, Benton, and Gordon, 1966). However, Riedel and Studdert-Kennedy (1985) found no support for the strong theory that the main deficit in aphasia is a problem with perceiving rapid auditory stimuli.

Perception and comprehension are compared to determine whether there is a relationship between impaired perception and aphasic comprehension deficit. In one study, 14 aphasic subjects with impaired perception also had deficient word comprehension, but 8 of 12 with the worst word comprehension had normal perception (Varney, 1984). Therefore, to explain many deficits of word comprehension, we need to look beyond the representation of the stimulus.

Word Recognition

Hearing a word like *metaphysics* may induce a sense of recognition but not full comprehension. Recognizing something means that we have had some prior experience with an object or word and that a representation of this experience was stored somewhere. Recognition occurs when we match a percept to the stored representation. If we saw an object just a few seconds ago, then the stored representation may be active in working memory. However, usually we recognize people, places, and things with reference to a representation stored long ago in long-term memory. For recognizing common objects, we activate concepts stored in semantic memory. For recognizing words, we activate the lexicon stored in lexical memory.

Because word recognition requires contact with the mental lexicon, recognition tasks are employed to study lexical memory. As indicated in Chapter 1, our mental lexicon contains what we know about words. This includes what a word sounds like (phonology) and looks like (orthography). We may think about our knowledge of a word's form when we read a foreign word and realize we do not know its pronunciation or when we realize that there are words we use but do not know how to spell. Word form is represented as what is called a **lexeme.** Knowledge of words also includes their grammatical categories such as knowing that *bank* can be a noun or a verb. Grammatical knowledge is called a **lemma** (Levelt, 1989). There are different viewpoints on the organization of this information, and one includes the notion that lexemes and lemmas are stored in a network much like semantic memory.

The recognition tasks used to study access to the lexicon are "fast tasks." A **lexical decision task (LDT)** is usually used with aphasic patients. Most studies of normal adults employ visual word presentation. Usually a word or nonword (e.g., BOOK or CHOT) is shown on a computer until a subject presses a YES or NO button indicating if the letter-string is a word. The nonword is a structurally possible word, but researchers are mainly interested in response to the real word. It normally takes just over half a second (600 milliseconds) to respond to common words (Forster and Chambers, 1973). In one study, aphasic subjects were as fast as normal controls and, also like the controls, responded faster to common words than rare words (Gerratt and Jones, 1987). The results indicated that aphasic people are able to match the percept of a stimulus to a lexeme.

The instant of recognition is quicker than 600 milliseconds (msec). Psycholinguists want to locate the instant of matching a percept to a lexeme within this time frame. The goal is to determine what happens in the so-called *pre-lexical* period up to activating the stored lexeme. Afterward, response time is consumed by a *post-lexical* phase involving at least the motor processes for pressing the button. Various experiments supported an estimate that lexical access normally occurs within 100 to 300 msec after stimulus presentation (McCrae, Jared, and Seidenberg, 1990).

A **lexical priming task** focuses on the first 300 msec. In this paradigm, pairs of words are presented, one after the other. A **prime** (e.g., LOOK) is presented prior to the test-word, now called the **target** (e.g., BOOK). Subjects just listen to or look at the prime. They make the usual lexical decision response only to the target. Investigators are particularly interested in subconscious response to the prime, which can be inferred from the prime's influence on the target. A **priming effect** is indicated by a faster response for related prime-target pairs (e.g., LOOK-BOOK) than for unrelated pairs such as RAISE-BOOK. The prime is assumed to activate lexical neighbors in a network so that a related target is "primed" for access. In studies of neurologically intact adults, an interval much less than 300 msec is placed between the prime and target so that fast pre-lexical automatic activation can be studied.

The word pair LOOK-BOOK is related phonologically or orthographically. An effect of this relationship is called **form-priming.** At McGill University, Shari Baum directed studies in which she presented such prime-target pairs auditorily (Gordon and Baum, 1994). Initially, the interstimulus interval was 500 msec, which is much longer than what normal adults need for form priming to occur. Only nonfluent subjects had a phonological priming effect. Later, Baum found form-priming in fluent and nonfluent aphasic subjects at a shorter interstimulus interval of 250 msec (Leonard and Baum, 1997). These results indicate that aphasic persons can activate related "lexical candidates" in less than 300 msec.

In current psycholinguistic research, form priming occurs in normal subjects when the interval between prime onset and target onset is only around 50 msec (e.g., Lukatela, Frost, and Turvey, 1998). An investigator presents the prime so fast that it is not recognized consciously. Yet, the prime still has an influence on recognizing the target, similar to the influence of a "subliminal" frame in a film. These so-called masked primes provide an experimental mechanism for observing the effects of automatic processing as defined in Chapter 1.

Word Comprehension

In comprehending a word, we rapidly activate a concept in semantic memory. Knowledge of concepts and knowledge of what a word means are slightly different things (also keeping in mind that knowledge of word meaning and word form are different things). Regarding meaning, we may have conceptual knowledge of a [river's edge] stored in the semantic network, and we may know about [tilting an airplane]. Additionally we are likely to know that *bank* refers to these concepts as a noun or a verb. Many of us may also know about a [series of oars on a boat] having witnessed crew races. However, we may not have known that *bank* refers to a series of oars. Knowledge of word meaning is represented as a pointer or connection between a lexeme in lexical memory and a concept in semantic memory. Sometimes learning a meaning for a word means making a connection between a known lexeme and a known concept.

As mentioned earlier, the *clinical* examination of word comprehension has consisted of "slow tasks" in which a patient takes time pointing to an object in an array of pictures. With this task, researchers have tried to isolate the central disorder by using pictures for words that are phonologically or semantically related to the correct choice (Gainotti, Caltagirone, and Ibba, 1975; Schuell and Jenkins, 1961). Aphasic subjects made more semantic errors than phonological errors. When foils were varied according to semantic relatedness, errors tended to be the picture most related to the correct one (Pizzamiglio and Appiciafuoco, 1971). These results indicate that aphasic word comprehension disorder lies in lexical-semantic relationships as opposed to phonological encoding.

In clinical studies, lexical-semantic structure is commonly studied with **word-sorting** and other metalinguistic tasks. Patients group words on their own or according to categories stated by an examiner. When sorting words into requested categories, nonfluent and fluent subjects have exhibited knowledge of categorical and functional organization (McCleary, 1988). In one study, a group of aphasic subjects was able to match "high importance" attributes to a noun (e.g., *wings* to *bird*) but were deficient in matching "low importance" attributes (e.g., *sings* to *bird*) (Germani and Pierce, 1995). When deficits appear, they usually occur in posteriorly damaged fluent aphasias (e.g., Grober, Perecman, Keller, and Brown, 1980; McCleary and Hirst, 1986). Investigators started wondering if fluent aphasias are uniquely deficient in the lexical-semantic system.

To determine if a deficit in semantic or lexical-semantic knowledge contributes to a word comprehension deficit, studies include a comparison between a word comprehension task and a metalinguistic semantic task with words or objects. In one study, eight of 16 aphasic subjects were identified as having deficient word comprehension (Chertkow, Bub, Deaudon, and Whitehead, 1997). Three of these 8 were "nonverbally preserved" according to a task involving objects, whereas five were diagnosed as being "nonverbally impaired." Thus, a conceptual deficit may or may not accompany word comprehension problems.

Now let us turn to what is likely to happen in our heads when we hear or see a word like *bank*. This was Martin Exeter's nitch in the field of psycholinguistics. Like other experimental psychologists, he recruited students to be subjects. He had them sit in front of a computer and look at words flashing on the screen. He wanted to figure out what happens as we activate meanings for words automatically or without conscious effort, called the "click of comprehension" (Foss and Hakes, 1978).

Dr. Exeter was fascinated by Collins and Loftus' (1975) paper detailing how activation of a concept automatically spreads to nearby nodes in semantic memory and how this **spreading activation** accounts for a variety of experimental results. In a semantic priming task, a prime such as BANK precedes a lexical decision target such as MONEY. The decision is usually faster with a semantically related prime than with an unrelated prime (e.g., BABY). This difference is called the **semantic priming effect.** The prime BANK is presumed to activate nodes in its conceptual neighborhood, so that it is likely that the related target is active before it is presented. With an unrelated prime, it can be said that a subject's mind is somewhere else when the target is presented (i.e., in an area about babies).

Dr. Exeter and his colleagues published scores of studies that refined procedure. The prime-target interval for visual stimuli, called the *stimulus onset asynchrony* (SOA), became a crucial means of identifying and measuring automatic processing. Semantic priming can occur with as little as a 16 msec SOA (Simpson and Burgess, 1985). One problem was the use of an unrelated prime as the control or baseline condition. A baseline should not activate a particular area of the semantic network, and so a **neutral prime,** such as *XXXX,* became a common part of the priming procedure. Neutral primes allow for a more precise measure of the following (Neely, 1976):

- **facilitation,** when target recognition is faster with a related prime than a neutral prime
- **inhibition,** when target recognition is slower with an unrelated prime than a neutral prime

In preparing for his lecture in Europe, Martin Exeter discovered that clinical researchers were measuring facilitation relative to an unrelated prime rather than a neutral prime. Therefore, they were probably overestimating the amount of facilitation occurring in their subjects.

In aphasiology, early studies of semantic priming contained long intervals such as 500 msec (Blumstein, Milberg, and Shrier, 1982). Chenery, Ingram, and Murdoch (1990) compared groups of high- and low-comprehending subjects. Both groups showed semantic priming despite being impaired in a slow metalinguistic task of semantic judgments about word-pairs. Baum (1997) found semantic priming to be consistent in nonfluent subjects but inconsistent in fluent subjects. Because of the long prime-target intervals, these studies could not determine if spreading activation in semantic memory is as rapid in aphasia as it is when the brain is neurologically intact. Nevertheless, the capacity for activation of concepts demonstrated that clinical tasks of word sorting "tend to overestimate the extent to which a patient is impaired" (Tyler and Moss, 1997, p. 296).

More specific questions can be pursued with semantic priming. Tyler and Moss (1997) compared priming with abstract word-pairs (e.g., *value-worth*) and concrete word-pairs (e.g., *boat-ship*) in a subject called DrO who had a fluent aphasia with mild word-finding difficulties. The patient displayed a semantic priming effect for abstract and concrete words in the visual modality with a 500 msec prime-target interval. However, he was primed only for concrete words in the auditory modality with a 200 msec interval. Further investigation revealed that DrO had an auditory processing deficit along with his aphasia. A modality-effect might have been related to the fact that more time was allowed in the visual modality for unusually slow spreading activation to occur. Yet, why would the effect be isolated to concrete words? Tyler and Moss proposed that concrete words are more likely to overcome a noisy input system because they possess more semantic features than abstract words.

SENTENCE COMPREHENSION

When comprehension is tested with stimuli much longer than a single word, the impression is that all cases of aphasia have a comprehension deficit to some degree (Basso, et al., 1978; Smith, 1971). Sentence comprehension is assessed several ways clinically. Patients choose a picture from a set, follow instructions with objects or tokens, answer yes-no questions, and verify the truth of a sentence relative to a picture. This section on sentence comprehension deals with this type of clinical evaluation and the manipulation of linguistic variables such as structural complexity, agent-object reversibility, and canonicity. Automatic sentence processing is discussed in the following chapter.

Structural Complexity

Clinical researchers have been interested in general factors such as sentence length and complexity. Increasing the length of sentences can make them harder for aphasic people to comprehend (Lasky, Weidner, and Johnson, 1976; Weidner and Lasky, 1976). However, the effect of length is not straightforward. Longer sentences can also be easier, which happened when information was added from *Which one is the knife?* to *Which one is the knife that cuts?* (Clark and Flowers, 1987; also, Gardner, Denes, and Weintraub, 1975; Pierce and Beekman, 1985). Length sometimes adds facilitative informational redundancy.

For mildly impaired aphasic patients, comprehension difficulty may not show up until sentences are both long and complex. The Token Test reveals deficit in over 90 percent of aphasic patients (DeRenzi, 1979). In focusing on the role of syntax, researchers tested the hypothesis that aphasic persons comprehend sentences of the same length differently because of structural differences. In one study, Token Test commands were adjusted in order to examine syntactic complexity while controlling for length (i.e., *b* is more complex that *a* at each length):

(1a) Touch the red circle.
(1b) Touch each yellow circle.
(2a) Touch the small blue circle and the small red circle.
(2b) Before you touch the green square, touch the white circle.

Complexity reduced comprehension of short sentences. However, *1b* also required more visual scanning of tokens besides being more complex syntactically. Similarly, structurally less complex *2a* has a more complex response than *2b,* indicating that mode of response in a task may obscure possible effects of linguistic variables (Curtiss, Jackson, Kempler, Hanson, and Metter, 1986).

The influence of early psycholinguistics can be seen when structural complexity was defined systematically according to linguistic theory. Initially researchers addressed an assortment of grammatical features such as word order, negation, verb tense, and prepositions (Lesser, 1974; Parisi and Pizzamiglio, 1970). Then, Shewan and Canter (1971) focused on passive and negative sentences. Three levels of syntactic complexity were identified according to number of transformations that were thought to modify basic subject-verb-object order (*3a*). The next structural level contained a single change which was either a passive or negative transformation (*3b*), and the third contained two transformations (*3c*).

(3a) The girl is reading a book.
(3b) The dogs are not chasing cats.
(3c) The milk was not drunk by her.

This comparison set the foundation for developing a clinical test called the **Auditory Comprehension Test for Sentences** or ACTS (Shewan, 1979). The ACTS contains 21 test sentences. Each sentence is read to a patient who responds by pointing to one of four pictures. Three picture foils are based on systematic changes in the test sentence to facilitate error analysis. It takes about 15 minutes to determine effects of word familiarity, length, and syntax. A maximum score of 21 is based on number of correct responses, and error analysis identifies position of error in the sentence (i.e., first or second half) and grammatical category of error (i.e., primarily nouns or verbs).

Early studies addressed a very general question as to whether aphasic patients have a "quantitative" or "qualitative" difference from normal comprehension. A quantitative deficit is indicated by more errors than normal subjects. A qualitative deficit is suggested by an order of structural difficulty that differs from normal adults. The findings were that aphasic subjects differ from normal in number of errors and response speed but do not differ according to order of difficulty (Parisi and Pizzamiglio, 1970; Shewan and Canter, 1971). This led to the conclusion that aphasic comprehension is an inefficient normal mechanism rather than a processing anomaly that does not occur in a normal language system.

Complexity is also increased by adding a subordinate clause to a main clause. Despite the fact that *4a* is longer than *4b, 4a* is structurally simpler than *4b* with its center-embedded clause. The longer sentence is generally easier for aphasic people to understand (Goodglass, Blumstein, Gleason, Hyde, Green, and Statlender, 1979).

(4a) The man was greeted by his wife, and he was smoking his pipe.
(4b) The man greeted by his wife was smoking a pipe.

Butler-Hinz, Caplan, and Waters (1990) found a similar result. However, when verifying sentences with embedded clauses against a picture, four moderate to severe aphasic subjects demonstrated an ability to comprehend (Ni, Shankweiler, Harris, and Fulbright, 1997). These apparently conflicting results indicate that the demonstration of a comprehension deficit may be partly a function of the task and not the structure per se.

Word Order and Thematic Roles

When testing comprehension of single nouns, a patient does not have to detect a functional role for that noun. However, comprehending simple declarative statements entails figuring out who is doing what to whom. In a sentence, a noun becomes an agent or recipient of an action, an instrument, or a location. In linguistic terms, this means figuring out the thematic roles played by the nouns in sentences like *5a*.

(5a) The nurse kissed the girl.
(5b) The girl drank the milk.

The order of nouns around a verb is one clue to their thematic roles. To assess the ability to capitalize on word order, clinical researchers employ **reversible sentences** in which the agent and recipient can be switched while preserving common sense. With respect to *5a,* agent-recipient order is the only difference between related pictured options (e.g., *The girl kissed the nurse* or *The nurse kissed the girl*).

For aphasic subjects, reversible sentences like *5a* are more difficult to understand than nonreversible statements like *5b* (Heeschen, 1980). In nonreversible statements, a semantic clue or constraint appears to be helpful. That is, the reversed option is implausible (i.e., milk cannot drink). Without such semantic aids, word location becomes paramount for understanding reversible sentences. The **reversibility effect** has became a central finding in studies of aphasic sentence comprehension, especially in the study of Broca's aphasia (see Chapter 5).

A patient may get a good score for nonreversible sentences merely by rejecting the absurdity of an implausible option instead of engaging in good syntactic processing. **Plausibility** may be a factor in reversible statements like *6b* in which the event is theoretically possible but unlikely, if not absurd.

(6a) The policeman arrests the thief.
(6b) The thief arrests the policeman.
(7) The woman greeting her husband was smoking a pipe.

Aphasic subjects find comprehension easier when sentences correspond to their world (6a) than when sentences represent implausible events (6b) (Deloche and Seron, 1981; Heilman and Scholes, 1976; Heeschen, 1980; Kudo, 1984). In one study, plausibility did not matter when sentences like *4b* became simply less probable as in *7,* according to Goodglass and others (1979). Many aphasic individuals seem able to use their knowledge of the world to facilitate sentence comprehension.

Canonicity

Early research determined that reversible passives like *The girl is kissed by the nurse* are harder for aphasic people to comprehend than reversible actives like *5a* (e.g., Pierce and Wagner, 1985; Shewan and Canter, 1971). The problem with passives is often attributed to word order, because thematic roles are reversed from straight-shooting active statements. The agent-action-recipient sequence in actives is known as the *canonical order* for thematic roles in English (see Chapter 6 for other languages). Investigators wondered if difficulty with the passive exception is the tip of an iceberg, because there are other structural exceptions to canonical order.

Researchers have fiddled with sentences to determine whether aphasic difficulty can be attributed to the more general canonicity and not just to the passive exception. One trick is to create reversible clefted sentences such as *8a* and *8b.*

(8a) It was the woman that shot the man.
(8b) It was the farmer that the painter kicked.

In a study by Ansell and Flowers (1982), mildly aphasic subjects had more difficulty with *8b* than

8a, even though sentence structure is essentially the same. In fact, the canonical *6a* was understood almost without error. Let us call this finding the **canonicity effect.** The key factor seems to be the deviation from canonical order in which, like passives, the recipient of the action is located before the verb and agent.

David Caplan (1987) argued that traditional forms of testing do not permit the study of important syntactic and semantic features. He preferred an **enactment procedure** in which subjects manipulate toy animals in response to instructions. Toy animals include a monkey, frog, elephant, goat, cow, rabbit, and sometimes a bear and donkey. More types of errors are possible with this procedure, permitting more specific identification of difficulty. Caplan employed a *Thematic Role Battery* extensively to assess the ability to assign thematic roles to noun phrases in a variety of simple and complex reversible sentences. In one study, 14 structures generated a battery of 168 items (Waters, Caplan, and Hildebrandt, 1991).

Caplan found that patients can understand a variety of syntactic structures but comprehension gets worse as syntactic complexity increases. In particular, sentences preserving the canonical order of English (*9a*) were easier than deviations from canonical order (*9b*) (Caplan, Baker, and Dehaut, 1985).

(9a) The elephant hit the monkey that hugged the rabbit.
(9b) The elephant that the monkey hit hugged the rabbit.
(10) The frog hit the monkey and patted the elephant.

In *9b,* the recipient of *hit* (elephant) appears before the agent. Except for the most severely impaired, aphasic people use word order to comprehend but have difficulty when a sentence deviates from canonical order (Caplan and Hildebrandt, 1988). Complexity effects were replicated with a two-picture choice task, indicating that Caplan's findings are robust across test procedures (Caplan, Waters, and Hildebrandt, 1997).

EXPLAINING SENTENCE COMPREHENSION DEFICIT

Let us recall Tyler's (1988) comment at the beginning of this chapter in which she wrote about extensive interest in discovering aphasic response to a variety of linguistic variables but little interest in locating the source of difficulty in the comprehension process. Complexity, reversibility, and canonicity effects describe results but do not explain them. That is, we should want to know what happens in the mind to cause these effects, because the disorder is in the patient's brain. Since 1988, interest has been shifting from empirical description to testing theoretical accounts of comprehension patterns.

A Language Disorder

It may seem obvious to suggest that impairment resides somewhere in the language comprehension system. Researchers tried to uncover language processing problems by manipulating linguistic components of stimuli, such as syntactic or semantic features. Caplan (1987) suggested that "syntactic comprehension impairments are often independent primary disorders of sentence processing" (p. 323), rather than a result of some peripheral or general feature of cognition such as short-term memory. He also concluded that the syntactic processor is not impaired in an "all-or-none" fashion but rather is impaired partially.

However, proposals of a disordered language processing mechanism have been more common in the study of syndromes. Especially in the study of Broca's aphasia (see Chapter 5), investigators have borrowed seriously from psycholinguistic paradigms for examining the obligatory processes of sentence comprehension. The rest of this section deals primarily with explanations of aphasia in general. With this perspective, investigators have turned to peripheral or general features of cognition.

Auditory Processing

As with words, explaining comprehension deficits begins with mental representation of the auditory stimulus. It was noted earlier that speech perception is not necessarily related to word comprehension deficit, but some still wondered if perception is related to sentence comprehension problems. In a comparison of perception to sentence comprehension, some patients with impaired perception passed a comprehension test; others with good perception had poor sentence comprehension (Carpenter and Rutherford, 1973). Other researchers found minimal relationship between speech perception and comprehension (Baker, Blumstein, and Goodglass, 1981; Gandour and Dardarananda, 1982; Miceli, Gainotti, Caltagirone, and Masulo, 1980). Shewan (1982) concluded that explanations of language comprehension problems on the basis of perceptual disturbances "are no longer widely accepted" (p. 61).

Brookshire (1997) has speculated that a variety of perceptual and memory-related disorders cause problems with sentence comprehension in aphasia. These disorders were applied to interpretation of the **Revised Token Test** (RTT). Before considering some of Brookshire's hypotheses, let us examine the RTT and its role in the study of auditory processing.

McNeil and Prescott (1978) borrowed principles of PICA construction to reduce inconsistencies in the family of Token Tests. The RTT contains 10 sections balanced with 10 commands per section. A 15-point multidimensional scoring system is applied to each element of each command. The RTT takes around 30 minutes to administer, and computation of results also takes a lot of time. A project was undertaken to determine if a shortened RTT yields the same information as the full test (Arvedson, McNeil, and West, 1985). A "five-item" version was predictive of the overall score from the complete test. Arvedson suggested that the short version is substitutable in order to obtain the overall score, but she was cautious about more specific analyses with the short RTT.

One general question has been whether the auditory processing system in aphasia is fast enough to handle the normal rate of speech. Comprehension sometimes improves when rate is reduced or when pauses are inserted, indicating that aphasic auditory processing has slowed down (Blumstein, Katz, Goodglass, Shrier, and Dworetsky, 1985; Poeck and Pietron, 1981; Weidner and Lasky, 1976). However, two- or five-second pauses did not matter for complex commands in other studies (Hageman and Lewis, 1983; Liles and Brookshire, 1975), and pauses did not help for a picture pointing task (Blumstein, et al., 1985). With the RTT, Brookshire and Nicholas (1984) found inconsistencies with reduced rate and four-second pauses and recommended that "previous reports of the effects of pauses and slow rate upon aphasic listeners' comprehension should be interpreted with caution" (p. 327).

McNeil and Prescott suggested that the RTT helps us look for Brookshire's peripheral deficits. The analysis involves looking for patterns of scores across items in a subtest such as *tuning-in* (i.e., gradually improving from the first to tenth item), *intermittent processing* (i.e., fluctuating across items) and *tuning-out* (i.e., declining scores across items). At first, only the intermittent pattern was clearly evident (McNeil and Hageman, 1979). When the RTT was repeated in two days, those who were intermittent were consistently intermittent; but other patterns were inconsistent (Hageman and Folkestad, 1986; Hageman, McNeil, Rucci-Zimmer, and Cariski, 1982). Since these studies, Brookshire's patterns of deficit have been relatively ignored.

Short-Term Memory

In Chapter 1, short-term memory (STM) was identified as a temporary storage component of working memory. For a long time, it was thought that comprehension depends on a person's **immediate memory span.** Moreover, aphasic patients have had difficulty when asked to repeat a series of numbers or words of increasing length (Albert, 1976; Black and Strub, 1978; Cermak and Moreines, 1976; DeRenzi and Nichelli, 1975; Tanridag, Kirshner, and Casey, 1987). Although this deficit can occur for different reasons, the hypothesis is that a short memory span constricts comprehension for some patients.

To determine if memory span is related to sentence comprehension, clinical investigators compare STM and sentence comprehension performances. Studies have indicated that semantic processing (i.e., number of content words in the Token Test) may lean on STM, but syntactic processing of complex sentences does not relate to memory span (Martin and Feher, 1990). In general, memory span does not seem to be related to comprehending single sentences. Caplan and Waters (1990) concluded that it may come in handy when context needs to be reviewed after an erroneous interpretation initially. Similarly, an immediate memory span may be more crucial for discourse comprehension when previous information needs to be stored temporarily to help in interpretation of the currently processed sentence.

Working Memory and Resource Allocation

The entire cognitive workload is managed in working memory (WM). Attention helps to manage the resources utilized for any task (Table 4.3). **Focused attention** is studied by presenting two different stimuli or tasks and having subjects concentrate on one of them. **Divided attention** is studied with a dual-task paradigm. A subject is asked to perform two tasks at the same time, one being the main skill being studied and the other being a distractor task. The main task is often one that can be done well. If an aphasic person has a resource allocation deficiency, performance on the main task would be reduced in a dual-task condition when it would not be reduced normally.

In the 1990s, there have been several proposals that aphasia includes a reduction of WM capacity. In one approach, investigators demonstrate that aphasic patients are deficient in managing simple concurrent tasks and then speculate that the deficit could be responsible for well-known comprehension problems observed elsewhere (LaPointe and Erickson, 1991; Peach, Rubin, and Newhoff, 1994; Tseng, McNeil, and Milenkovic, 1993).

The proposal also surfaces as an explanation of structural complexity effects across all cases of aphasia. One version is supported by experiments in which a general pattern of aphasic comprehension deficit was simulated with normal adults (Miyake, Carpenter, and Just, 1994). Aphasia-like complexity effects were observed in normal adults when sentences were presented at an excessive speed or when subjects had low working memory spans. The investigators claimed to have shown how known comprehension deficits can be induced by a reduced WM capacity. A subsequent computer simulation of aphasia was also used to support this claim (Haarmann, Just, and Carpenter, 1997).

Another version of capacity theory came from Caplan and Hildebrandt (1988) who explained syntactic difficulties as a reduction of a resource system *specializing in syntactic processing*. Later, Caplan and Waters (1996) used a dual-task paradigm to test the hypothesis more directly. They selected aphasic patients who performed above-average on a sentence-picture matching task and who had a clear complexity effect. Then, while responding to each item in the comprehension test, subjects repeated a sequence of digits within their digit spans. The effect of syntactic complexity was not increased in the dual-task condition, leading Caplan and Waters to conclude that WM capacity may not be a factor for some patients.

A brief debate over the role of WM in comprehension and aphasia has transpired between the Caplan-Waters team (1995; Waters and Caplan, 1996) and the Carpenter-Just group (Just, Carpenter, and Keller, 1996; Miyake, Carpenter, and Just, 1995). Caplan and Waters contended that WM operates with independent system resources including one for syntactic processing, whereas Carpenter and Just claimed that WM operates with a single resource pool. Caplan and Waters (1995) suggested that Carpenter and Just's simulations do not resemble aphasia in important respects. Each research team has stated that the other conducted invalid experiments and misinterpreted the opposition.

In an unusual twist to this fray, Martin (1995) drew attention to the possibility that language comprehension deficits could be caused by damage to a "component" of the language processing system instead of by a WM problem. In response, Miyake, Carpenter, and Just (1995) referred to component processes as "procedural knowledge" (a term not used by Martin) and then proceeded to criticize Martin for proposing a "partial-loss-of-knowledge" problem. However, equating component processes and procedural knowledge is atypical in psycholinguistic research.

Why might aphasic individuals have problems with dividing attention? Murray, Holland, and Beeson (1997) evaluated two possibilities. One is a reduced "sense of effort" or perception of task difficulty that might cause a person not to allocate resources in a difficult task. Another possibility is a reduced perception of accuracy (or lack of awareness of errors) that might cause someone to ignore the challenges of a task. Murray's aphasic subjects were normal in monitoring their accuracy but had problems perceiving task difficulty after making lexical decisions under single task, selective attention, and divided attention conditions. Thus, aphasic people may not engage allocation strategies because of difficulty anticipating the effort required in certain linguistic processing conditions.

OBJECT NAMING

All aphasic people have some kind of difficulty with word-finding, which is most often researched, assessed, and treated with an object-naming task (or "confrontation naming"). Geschwind (1967) wrote that "we are speaking of naming in the narrower sense and not of word-finding in the flow of speech" (p. 97). Object-naming places word-finding under a microscope in which we can examine mistakes with respect to a clear target. As indicated late in Chapter 3, naming errors may signify a disorder but do not necessarily signify aphasia. Geschwind wrote of aphasic misnaming and nonaphasic misnaming, implying that misnaming may be caused by an impaired language system or by another impairment.

Process-Model of Naming

Causes of deficits can be hypothesized according to a process-model for the naming task. Process-models begin with processing the stimulus and end with the motor response for this task. One researcher proposed what happens in between: (a) "the first step is the identification of the object as a member of a category whose stored representation provides a good match with the stimulus object" (b) "Once a category representation has been activated, then the corresponding label is retrieved" (Brownell, Bihrle, and Michelow, 1986, p. 50). This section provides an introduction to the discipline of cognitive neuropsychology (CN).

The CN-model of spoken naming in Figure 4.2 consists of independent processing components (in boxes) and the routes between them. This model operates serially, that is, with each process informing the next process in order from the top down. **Object recognition** activates a concept in the **semantic system** which then points to the **phonological output lexicon** guiding speech production. For writing, lexical representation is the *orthographic output lexicon.* Cognitive neuropsychologists tend to agree on the existence of a semantic and a lexical component, although terminology may vary slightly (e.g., "conceptual system," "speech output lexicon"). CN-models may become a basis for the clinical diagnosis of disorders affecting naming. Such models are the basis for interpreting results of the PALPA (see Chapter 3).

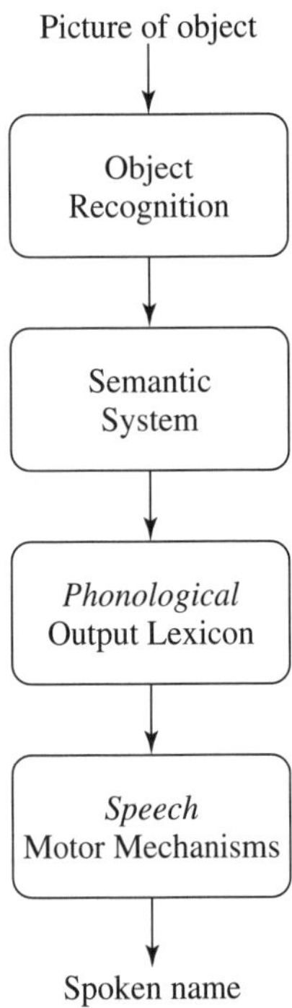

FIGURE 4.2 A typical model of object naming. Components are represented similarly elsewhere (e.g., Figures 3.4, 7.1). As suggested with Figure 2.9, diagnosis entails determining the impaired component that is responsible for misnaming.

(Reprinted by permission from Bruce, C. & Howard, D., Why don't Broca's aphasics cue themselves? An investigation of phoneme cueing and tip of the tongue information. *Neuropsychologia,* 26, 1988, p. 261. Pergamon Press, publisher.

Diagnosis is said to entail looking for location of the "functional lesion" responsible for misnaming. Is it in the semantic system or the phonological output lexicon? Before trying to answer these questions, we should realize that no single task leads to a diagnosis, because, like naming, each task utilizes multiple processes. Similarly, a single error can have different interpretations. Naming errors do not correspond precisely to syndrome diagnosis (LeDorze and Nespoulous, 1989; Mitchum, Ritgert, Sandson, and Berndt, 1990). The strategy in CN, called **componential analysis,** entails comparing performances on a few tasks (Table 4.5). Like analyzing a test battery, an investigator looks for common threads among deficient and intact performances. The assessment is truly theory-driven, in that the investigator selects combinations of tasks that should logically help to determine the status of components in the model.

Modality-Specific Impairment

Sensory impairments result in weak input to the cognitive processes of recognition and knowledge activation. For example, blindness closes the visual door to central language processes. When an aphasic patient has severe visual problems, we test word-finding by entering another door, that is, by providing input to another modality. Impairment at the level of recognition is called agnosia, and implications of this disorder for naming are discussed in Chapter 6.

One alternative to visual naming is called *naming to description* or definition, whereby the stimulus to name is presented auditorily. A stimulus might be "It is good for telling time and can be worn on your wrist." Visually intact aphasic patients make more errors when naming to description than when naming pictured objects (Barton, Maruszewski, and Urrea, 1969; Goodglass and Stuss, 1979). Therefore, naming to description may overestimate word-finding impairment for visually impaired patients.

Semantic or Lexical Impairment?

Aphasia has been quite broadly diagnosed as involving a "lexical-semantic" impairment. Now, the central question has become whether the impairment lies in either the semantic system or the lexical system. Earlier in this chapter, semantic and lexical memories were described as being interconnected parts of a storage network. One challenge has been to tease apart effects of the semantic and lexical systems when designing experiments. Distinguishing a deficient semantic

TABLE 4.5 Differential diagnosis of naming difficulties based on a process-model of object-naming similar to Figure 4.2. Diagnosis of disorder is suggested with respect to component of principal deficiency.

PROCESS COMPONENT	DISORDER	RELATED TASKS
object recognition	visual agnosia	match examples of an object; demonstrate use of object
activation of semantic memory	dementia or aphasia	object classification; word-picture matching
activation of lexical memory	aphasia	object-naming
phonetic programming	apraxia of speech	complex word repetition
motor execution	dysarthrias	oral mechanism examination

system from deficient lexical access is akin to distinguishing between misnaming because we do not know what an object is and misnaming because we cannot find its name.

A deficient semantic system is thought to send poor conceptual input to the output lexicon. From earlier in this chapter, we should be familiar with findings of intact semantic structure in some aphasic patients but not others. Investigators have found damaged semantic systems in a variety of neurological disorders including Alzheimer's dementia. It was noted in Chapter 2 that some progressive fluent aphasias have been labeled as having semantic dementia (see Chapter 6). A few experimental designs are used to see if a naming impairment can be attributed to a deficient semantic system.

One type of experiment is to compare naming errors to word comprehension. For example, Gainotti and his colleagues (1981) made this comparison with different types of aphasic patients. Comprehension was tested for error type, such as word form or semantic relationship. Although number of semantic comprehension errors were related to word-finding difficulty in general, they found an inconsistent relationship between type of naming error and type of word comprehension problem. They concluded "that different mechanisms may produce anomia and that only some forms of word-finding defect may be due to a breakdown of the semantic systems" (p. 20).

Another exploration of the semantic system is to compare naming to metalinguistic tasks such as object-sorting, which is similar to the strategy for studying word comprehension mentioned earlier in this chapter. Goodglass, Wingfield, and Ward (1997) studied rapid decisions about categorical relationships between objects as well as about semantic relationships between words and objects presented with a computer. Although aphasic subjects were slower than normal on these tasks, performance did not predict naming performance.

A third type of evidence is the discovery of category-specific naming deficits, especially when a patient has a comprehension problem with the same conceptual areas. Broad dissociations have been seen with a variety of neuropathologies, mainly with respect to living and nonliving things (Caramazza, 1988). As indicated in Chapter 2, patients with thalamic lesions have been found to have problems specifically with medical terms and celebrities. This phenomenon is discussed in Chapter 6 with respect to testing theories of semantic memory. Nevertheless, like naming information in one modality but not others, it is difficult to say that the word-retrieval mechanism is broken when it works for a wide range of conceptual areas. The dissociating variable is semantic.

Investigators also examined object familiarity by comparing the naming of common or "high-typical" examples of a category (e.g., *kitchen* chair) to uncommon or "low-typical" examples (e.g., *beach chair*) (Brownell, et al., 1986). Normally, a basic name is elicited by highly typical examples (e.g., *chair*). Low-typical examples tend to elicit more subordinate labels than basic names (e.g., *beach chair*). Aphasic subjects followed this pattern. They had difficulty producing subordinate names but conveyed the low-typical concepts with compensatory strategies. Instead of saying "racing car," a nonfluent patient would say "car, goes fast." Fluent patients provided an attribute without the basic name. Because of this object recognition ability and communicative flexibility, Brownell concluded that the semantic system was intact. He located damage in the activation of particular lexical forms.

In general, we cannot say that damage to the semantic system is an essential element of aphasia. People with aphasia have trouble finding words despite good input from the semantic system. As Brownell indicated, the disorder can be isolated to the lexical system. However, some aphasic people can have damage to the semantic system that is related to word-finding. Future research should determine the nature of the semantic problem (i.e., knowledge loss or access problem) and its relationship to word-finding difficulty.

Lexical variables pertain to characteristics of words per se, such as frequency of use and grammatical category. Common words are easier for an aphasic person to retrieve than rare words (e.g., Gardner, 1973). Grammatical category is usually studied by comparing nouns and verbs. For some patients, nouns are more difficult. Others display more difficulty with verbs, and others show no difference (Basso, Razzano, Faglioni, and Zanobio, 1990; Berndt, Mitchum, Haendiges, and Sandson, 1997; Williams and Canter, 1987). Berndt found that selective noun deficit is associated with severe word-finding disorder, and selective verb deficit can occur in fluent and nonfluent aphasias.

One indication of partial access to lexical form is the **tip-of-the tongue state** in which properties of a correct word are conveyed instead of the word itself. Barton (1971) instructed aphasic subjects to point, upon naming failure, to the target word's first letter, number of syllables, and "big" or "small" for indicating size of the target word. Subjects guessed these properties accurately over 60 percent of the time in spite of being unable to say the word. It was as if an object activated the concept and parts of lexical form. In another study, some aphasic subjects were less successful in reporting features of unspoken words, and a few others could not do it at all (Goodglass, Kaplan, Weintraub, and Ackerman, 1976).

Psycholinguistic Study of Naming

CN-models have been criticized for ignoring details about representation of information and how processes work in semantic and lexical systems (Rapp, Hillis, and Caramazza, 1993; Seidenberg, 1988). Psycholinguists put word-finding within a spreading activation network and consider that lexemes are stored so that they can slide quickly into sentences.

There are two fundamental positions on the naming process in psycholinguistics. One position is that semantic and lexical processes operate in a **serial** fashion. Activation spreads sequentially from semantic memory to lexical memory (Schriefers, Meyer, and Levelt, 1990). The other position is that the two systems are more **interactive,** meaning that they operate simultaneously or "in parallel" (Dell and O'Seaghda, 1992).

Schriefers and others (1990) compared serial and interactive predictions of naming latencies using a *picture-word interference task.* This task incorporates principles of priming research. In the interference paradigm, a drawing of an object (e.g., a dog) is presented and a potentially interfering word is superimposed on the picture. A subject's job, however, is only to name the picture. Schriefers was interested in effects of the incidental word on naming times. Some words were semantically related to the picture (e.g., *cat*). Other words where phonologically related (e.g., *fog*). Other words were unrelated, and neutral strings were imposed to detect interference. Schriefers also varied the interval between presenting objects and words. Because semantic and phonological interference effects occurred independently and at different intervals, Schriefers suggested that picture naming is a serial operation from semantic activation to lexical activation.

Lyndsey Nickels at Birkbeck College in London has conducted experiments comparing serial and interactive models in predicting relationships between certain variables and paraphasias (Nickels, 1995). The imageability rating of words was considered to be a semantic variable. Word length was a lexical variable. Word familiarity was thought to be related to both semantic and lexical modules. The interactive version predicts that all variables would affect both types of errors. A serial model is more selective, predicting imageability to be related to semantic errors and length to be related to phonological errors. Results supported the serial model.

Gary Dell proposed that word-form retrieval, called *lexical access,* requires two steps *after* semantic activation (Dell, Schwartz, Martin, Saffran, and Gagnon, 1997). In a spreading activation system, a concept cannot map to a word form directly as in Figure 4.2. Grammatical mediation is indicated by a high frequency of normal phonologically unrelated word-finding errors within the same syntactic category (e.g., nouns for nouns, verbs for verbs). Therefore, the first step is lemma access or mapping a concept onto grammatical information such as syntactic category. The second step is lexical access or mapping the lemma onto phonological form. According to Dell, processing evolves as a series of "jolts" from semantics to sound. Not everyone is happy with this idea. Caramazza (1997) argued that an intermediate lemma stage is unnecessary.

The work of Dell, Schwartz and others (1997) has relied mainly on a highly sophisticated statistical analysis of naming errors by normal and aphasic adults. Their central proposal was the *continuity thesis* which states that aphasic naming errors are not qualitatively different from errors made by nonaphasic speakers. There are two possible explanations. One is that neuropathology damages representations at each level, and the other is that it reduces transmission of activation between intact levels of the network. A patient could also have both problems.

The **Philadelphia Naming Test** (PNT) arose out of Dell and Schwartz's work (Roach, Schwartz, Martin, Grewal, and Brecher, 1996). The unique contribution of this test is its error analysis and interpretation. The PNT consists of 175 nouns of different frequency and syllable lengths. Pictures are presented on a computer, and naming latencies are measured. The goal is to analyze errors according to "what they reveal about the mental processes underlying normal and pathological word retrieval" (pp. 129–130).

Deloche and his colleagues (1997) provided a brief commentary on written naming. Relatively few systematic studies have been conducted with aphasic groups, and fewer have been done comparing written and spoken naming. Deloche advised that "the mechanisms of written naming disturbances cannot be simply deduced from the results of studies on oral naming" (p. 220). Although error terminology corresponds to paraphasias to some degree, a few types of naming (or spelling) errors are not errors in speech because of unique features of the orthographic code (e.g., writing "sause" for *sauce*).

PRODUCTIVE WORD-FINDING

So that clinicians may address a full range of word-finding conditions, Chapey, Rigrodsky, and Morrison (1977) argued that "divergent thinking" should be considered in addition to the "convergent thinking" in object naming tasks. Confrontation naming converges on one idea and one response. In a divergent mode, we generate a quantity and variety of responses.

Word Fluency

The word fluency task involves producing a number of words to a single stimulus. Two types of word fluency tasks include producing words starting with a letter or words belonging to a conceptual category such as vegetables or countries. The task provides an opportunity for a different kind of qualitative analysis of word-retrieval based on lexical-semantic connections. Letter-fluency tasks induce generation of words from a lexical base by having patients fish for commonalities of form. The categorical-fluency task induces generation of words from a semantic base.

In a **categorical or semantic word fluency** task, a patient is asked to produce members of a semantic classification, often as many as possible in 60 seconds. The task has also been called "category generation" (Hough, 1989), "category naming" (Grossman, 1981), "word-naming" (Joanette, Goulet, and Le Dorze, 1988), or a "controlled-association task" (Cappa, Papagno, and Vallar, 1990). In assessment, there is usually a limit of around 60 seconds for producing as many words as possible. Speed maximizes the number of words produced, but still the task can be highly strategic in the mind of the speaker.

Grossman (1981) used 10 categories such as sports, birds, furniture, tools, clothes, and weapons. Normal adults produced 14.66 words per category. Nonfluent aphasic patients produced 5.29 words, and fluent patients produced 6.71. These levels are fairly consistent. In another study, normal adults averaged 13.51 words per category; and mildly impaired fluent aphasic persons produced 6.76 (Adams, Reich, and Flowers, 1989). The skill fluctuates as normal adults average 22.5 animal names in a minute period but display a range of 9 to 41 words (Borod, Goodglass, and Kaplan, 1980; Goodglass and Kaplan, 1983). Persons with right hemisphere damage were also impaired, indicating that word fluency is sensitive to any brain damage.

Grossman examined the succession of words produced to a category like birds. Responses were given scores identified with prototypicality bands extending from the most typical members of a category to the least typical members. Bands were defined according to ratings of typicality determined by Rosch (1975). Ideal members of a category were assigned a 1.00 (e.g., "robin"), whereas the most peripheral instances or items not belonging to a semantic field were assigned a 7.00 (e.g, "fish"). Normal adults and persons with right hemisphere damage produced most of their responses from three bands between 1.00 and 2.99 (Grossman, 1981). Nonfluent aphasic subjects produced prototypical examples as the normals did.

The **letter word fluency** task was introduced by Borkowski, Benton, and Spreen (1967). They obtained data on production of "as many words as you can in 60 seconds" that begin with a letter. Six letters were difficult for normal adults; J elicited 4.83 associations. Moderate difficulty was observed with N (8.23). Easy letters for normal adults went into the FAS test, with these three letters eliciting 10.22 to 11.50 words from persons without brain damage. The FAS test became a common test and part of one aphasia battery (Spreen and Benton, 1969). Damage to the left or right hemisphere caused a large drop in production.

Persons with LHD did worse than those with RHD only for difficult letters. Persons with LHD, RHD, and bilateral damage were impaired in another study; and a discriminant analysis showed that only 48 percent of patients could be classified as to side of lesion using this method (Wertz, Dronkers, and Shubitowski, 1986). At around seven words per letter, the task did not clearly distinguish nonfluent and fluent groups studied by Collins, McNeil, Lentz, Shubitowski, and Rosenbek (1984). Fluent aphasias produced more words in another study (Bayles, Boone, Tomoeda, Slauson, and Kaszniak, 1989).

In general, word fluency tasks present a challenge for any brain damaged person, and we might be tempted to consider this test strategy for measuring progress in word-finding. However, five administrations of the category test over a two-week period showed that word fluency can be quite variable with acute and chronic aphasia (Boyle, Coelho, and Kimbarow, 1991). A sample of individual ranges includes 1 to 8 words or 14 to 23 words for foods. For some patients, performance varied depending on the category used, such as 8 to 10 for animals and 9 to 17 for foods. This lack of consistency suggests that a single word fluency test is not a good diagnostic tool and that the value of word fluency is limited for measuring progress.

Words in Discourse

Words are produced naturally in an extended flow of interrelated words, often elicited by picture description. In a comparison with object-naming, the two procedures were equally successful in eliciting nouns for nonfluent and fluent subjects (Basso, et al., 1990). For action-naming or verb-finding, mildly impaired cases did better with description, leading to the conclusion that "performance on a single word confrontation-naming task may not be highly predictive of performance in connected speech" (Williams and Canter, 1987, p. 132). Goodglass, Hyde, and Blumstein (1969) thought that object-naming does not sample lexicon used in conversation. Naming tends to elicit "picturable" concrete words whereas conversation contains more nonpicturable words such as animal, time, year, wife. Aphasic subjects used more nonpicturable than picturable nouns in spontaneous speech.

Speaking rate differentiates nonfluent from fluent aphasias. Normal rate in words per minute (wpm) has been considered to be 100 to 175 wpm (Howes, 1964; Kerschensteiner, Poeck, and Brunner, 1972). Syllables per minute discriminated normal from aphasic groups (Yorkston and Beukelman, 1980). Normal elderly adults produced 193 syllables per minute. Mildly aphasic patients produced 121 syllables per minute. Kerschensteiner used the following categories to characterize variation among aphasic patients:

very slow—0 to 50 wpm
slow—51 to 90 wpm
normal—above 90 wpm

Of forty-seven aphasic subjects, 17 were very slow, 13 were slow, and 17 were normal.

Quantification of elements is useful for measuring subtle progress in discourse production. Because counting number of units is biased by size variations among speech samples, most researchers utilize ratios (Table 4.6). A **type-token ratio** (TTR) is the number of different categories of items (i.e., types) relative to the total number of items produced (i.e., tokens). For measuring diversity of vocabulary, the TTR would be the number of different words relative to the total number

TABLE 4.6 A sample of ratios for measuring word production in spontaneous speech.

MEASURE	RATIO	APPLICATION
type-token ratio	different words relative to total words	patients with limited productive vocabulary
anomia index	pronouns relative to total nouns	vagueness in anomic aphasia
function word deletions	omissions of closed class words relative to total utterances	grammatical deficits; free grammatical morphemes
function word substitutions	substitutions of closed class words relative to total function words	grammatical deficits; free grammatical morphemes
inflected verbs	verbs with inflectional endings relative to total verbs	grammatical deficits; bound morphemes

Hier, Hagenlocker, and Shindler, 1985; Prins, Snow, and Wagenaar, 1978; Saffran, Berndt, and Schwartz, 1989.

of words. As variety of vocabulary increases, this TTR increases. The ratio is sensitive to sample size; "generally speaking the smaller the number of words spoken the larger the type-token ratio" (Fillenbaum, Jones, and Wepman, 1961).

Marshall (1976) studied conversational behaviors as "a situation whereby the aphasic, unprompted by the clinician, illustrates that he is unable to retrieve a word and initiates some effort to do so without assistance from the clinician" (p. 445). These efforts included semantic and phonemic paraphasia, circumlocution, indefinite terms (e.g., "the one," "stuff"), and taking or requesting more time. Taking more time was the most frequent precursor to retrieving a word. **Unassisted self-correction** was studied for a variety of tasks such as confrontation naming, answering questions, and sentence completion (Marshall and Tompkins, 1982). Types of self-correction follow:

- *cued corrections* when a patient produced a related response prior to the target response,
- *effortful corrections* when a patient produced a series of partial responses leading to the target response,
- *immediate corrections* when a patient quickly provided the target response.

Subjects classified as low-verbal engaged in as much self-correction as high-verbal subjects, but the more severely impaired were less successful. The less impaired subjects had more immediate self-corrections.

SUMMARY AND CONCLUSIONS

This chapter introduced some supplemental tests and some research strategies that have not yet found their way into clinical application. Most of the supplemental assessment procedures are summarized in Table 4.7.

Since 1960, basic research in clinical aphasiology has changed from a predominance of data-driven studies to the appearance of a steadily increasing number of theory-driven studies. Theory-driven research started out with tests of whether aphasia is a loss of knowledge or breakdown of process. Now, the research makes a distinction between automatic and controlled processing. Investigators figure out ways of doing

TABLE 4.7 Supplemental tests and measures introduced in Chapter 4.

FUNCTION	TEST	DESCRIPTION
intelligence	Coloured Progressive Matrices (CPM)	visuospatial recognition and reasoning; nonverbal predictor of overall IQ
auditory comprehension	ACTS	brief sentence comprehension test
	Revised Token Test	more structurally systematic and standardized version of the Token Test; multidimensional scoring
	memory span tests	immediate repetition of digit or word sequences of increasing length
naming	Philadelphia Naming Test	picture naming with cues and error analysis
words in extended speech	word fluency tests	producing a number of words to a single stimulus
	word production ratios	quantification of word-types in extended utterance

studies that can address these distinctions in a valid manner.

In teaching cognitive paradigms to future specialists in cognitive-communicative disorders, two points stand out as being the most difficult:

- *Short-term memory is not the same as working memory.* STM is the temporary holding "buffer" in the processing system, and one approach to assessment is the memory span test. WM encompasses the entire processing "workspace," including a buffer to shelve some pertinent materials temporarily. One approach to assessing WM is the dual-task paradiagm in which a subject does two things at once.
- *Knowledge and process are interrelated but different aspects of a functional system.* Knowledge, such as the semantic network, is a "fixed" *structure* characterized by spatial metaphors. Spreading activation is a *process* occurring in a region of the network, and its duration can be measured. The "distance" between nodes in a network (i.e., their relatedness) is predictive of processing time, but distance (or relatedness) is an attribute of structure, not process.

What do we do when faced with multiple theories of the same thing? Is this a bad scientific situation? Focusing on one theory would certainly make learning aphasiology easier, and some researchers tend to advocate a single theory and then set out to prove it. However, when there are truly alternative explanations of something, other researchers set out to compare them in order to find the truth. For the sake of truth, it is better to know when an issue is not yet resolved and the nature of options left standing through the systematic evolution of research.

Chapter 5

INVESTIGATING SYMPTOMS AND SYNDROMES

Strokes cause aphasias. This chapter sharpens our focus on some symptoms and the syndromes introduced in Chapter 2. The syndromes characterize qualitative differences among aphasic patients. These differences make us wonder whether a single strategy for treating aphasia is appropriate (and most efficient). The study of whether syndromes represent impairment of a distinctive psycholinguistic process has the following clinical implications:

- more specific diagnosis leading to more specialized treatments
- methods of assessing automatic, obligatory processing

We shall examine some features of language processing covered in the previous chapter and other features not covered. New features include syntactic processing, the short-term buffer in working memory, and production of phonological form. Some features are more prominent in the study of some syndromes than others. Broca's aphasia has been the most scrutinized syndrome. Grodzinsky (1991) called it "the flagship of the neuropsychology of language." After an extensive presentation on Broca's aphasia, the chapter returns to stage-theories of naming as a thematic current throughout the study of fluent aphasias.

AGRAMMATISM

So far, we have focused on production of words and have ignored the grammar of language production. Once researchers train their sights on grammar, they think about Broca's aphasia. Agrammatism is the definitive feature of this syndrome. Perhaps to avoid formal classification systems, many investigators prefer to say that these patients have "agrammatic aphasia."

Symptoms of Agrammatism

To look for problems with grammar, we must elicit sentences. Spontaneous speech is usually obtained through complex picture description or an interview. More restrictive procedures include the following:

- describe pictured actions or object locations
- complete a sentence or short story
- create a sentence given a noun or verb
- describe the actions of a clinical investigator

Once sentences are elicited and transcribed, they are analyzed with respect to the presence or absence of known features of grammar. A few guides have been developed to help us identify specific problems and to facilitate measurement of grammatical deficit (Table 5.1). These scales attend to lexicon, grammatical morphology, and syntactic structure. For example, LARSP was created for children and was the first formal guide to be applied to aphasia (Kearns and Simmons, 1983). Other scales have a particular emphasis such as grammatical morphology (Miceli, Silveri, Romani, and Caramazza, 1989) or phrase structure (Byng and Black, 1989). These orientations are indicative of the two broad features of grammar that are examined, namely:

- grammatical morphology or lexical characteristics (e.g., closed-class words)

TABLE 5.1 Analytical methods and measurements applied to the grammar of aphasic spontaneous speech production.

ANALYSIS	AUTHORS	SAMPLING	DESCRIPTION
LARSP (Language Assessment, Remediation and Screening Procedure)	Crystal, Fletcher and Garman (1976)	conversation	developmentally-based profile of word classes and syntactic structures
SUMLARSP	Edwards, Garman and Kent (1993)	2 conversations 2 story-telling tasks	modified LARSP; improved utterance segmentation and clausal analysis
SSLA (Shewan Spontaneous Language Analysis)	Shewan (1988)	picture description	profile of variables similar to Boston Exam; includes speaking rate, articulation rating
grammatical morpheme measures	Miceli, Silveri, etal (1989)		free and bound grammatical morpheme omission and substitution
grammatical measures	Saffran, Berndt, and Schwartz (1989)	fairytale; first 150 words of narrative	counts and ratio measures of lexicon, morphology, and sytactic structure
predicate-argument analysis	Byng and Black (1989)	same as Saffran, except for unlimited amount	counts of phrase and predicate-argument structures; related to production theory
computer analysis	Thompson, Shapiro, Tait, et al. (1995)	Cinderella story	more types of sentences, embedded clauses, verbs and verb arguments

- syntax or structural characteristics (e.g., word order).

Historically, agrammatism (in English) has been thought to be "telegraphic" because of **omissions of grammatical morphemes.** These morphemes include *function words* (e.g., articles, conjunctions) and *inflectional endings* marking subject-verb agreement, verb tense, and case for nouns and conjugational forms in languages other than English. Closed- and open-class words are said to be free morphemes, because they stand alone. Inflections must be attached (i.e., bound morphemes).

For examples, let us look at a couple of descriptions of the Boston Exam's Cookie Theft picture:

- function word omission: "Mother washing dishes...water flows sink."
- inflection omission: "The mother is wash dish...the water flow from the sink."

Neat dissociations like this are rare, however. Usually agrammatism contains a mixture of function word and inflectional omissions.

The prominance of grammatical morpheme omission in the diagnosis of agrammatism is indicated in a division of nonfluent subjects into two groups in a study by Saffran and others (1989). An agrammatic group of nonfluent aphasias tended to omit grammatical morphemes, and nonagrammatic nonfluent patients were judged to produce a full range of grammatical morphemes.

Tesak and Niemi (1997) wondered if agrammatism is really like "telegraphese" or what Gardner (1974) called "telegramese." The importance of this question is derived from theories of agrammatism stating that patients with Broca's aphasia choose a "telegraphic register" as an adaptive strategy for dealing with their disorder. Tesak and Niemi compared agrammatism in four languages to telegrams written by a large group of normal subjects. One clear characteristic of normal telegraphese was an omission of function words ranging from 61 percent in Dutch to 77 percent in German. In agrammatism, there were 7 percent omissions in Swedish and 66 percent omissions in Dutch. Therefore, similarity between agrammatism and telegraphese depends on the language.

Types of grammatical morphemes can be dissociated from each other, although not in a clear-cut manner like the earlier examples of Cookie Theft descriptions. In particular, function words can disappear without omissions of inflectional endings (Saffran, et al., 1989). Miceli's 20 agrammatic subjects were inconsistent in the co-occurrence of impaired functors and inflections. A more significant variation in agrammatic production appears when Broca's aphasia is examined in languages other than English. Although comparison of languages is a topic of Chapter 6, it is important to note here that **grammatical morpheme substitution** occurs in other languages more than it does in English. Thus, omission can no longer be considered to be a definitive characteristic of agrammatism. After studying agrammatism in Italian, Miceli redefined the term as referring to "the omission of freestanding grammatical morphemes with or without the substitution of bound grammatical morphemes" (Miceli, et al., 1989, p. 450).

Regarding structural or syntactic characteristics of agrammatism, two problems are considered most frequently. One is the **simplification** of sentence structure. In general, agrammatic patients do not use subordinate clauses as much as neurologically intact adults (Bastiaanse, Edwards, and Kiss, 1996). Instead of embedding a phrase with modifiers, an agrammatic patient sequences ideas as a series of simple structures. For example, instead of constructing a noun phrase such as *a large white house,* a patient may say "a large house, a white house." A patient might say "girl tall and boy short" instead of *the girl is taller than the boy* (Gleason, Goodglass, Green, Ackerman, and Hyde, 1975).

The other possible symptom is a **structural error** such as an illegal word order. For example, English does not allow utterances like "man the" or "ing-walk," but such errors do not appear to occur with aphasia (Bates, Friederici, Wulfeck, and Juarez, 1988).

Errors can be difficult to detect, because a string of words can be ambiguous structurally. Let us consider "ball hit boy." This could be an order error for an intended active sentence or an omission of function words from an intended passive sentence. Because word order can be reversed legally (e.g., passive sentences), an error is detected when there is evidence that a particular structure was intended (e.g., "ball hitting boy"). In one study, subjects with Broca's aphasia reversed noun phrases 40 percent of the time when the phrases were alike in animacy (e.g., "The sink is in the pencil") (Saffran, Schwartz, and Marin, 1980). In Byng and Black's (1989) study, three-element utterances were nearly always in NVN order. Errors such as NNV were not observed, and the investigators concluded that reversal errors are rare.

Saffran and others (1980b) observed **omission of main verbs** in agrammatic sentences. Then, a few studies found that action-naming was more difficult than object-naming in Broca's aphasia (e.g., Williams and Canter, 1987; Zingeser and Berndt, 1990). A special failure to activate verbs could have implications for sentence structure because of grammatical information carried by verbs.

The grammatical information (or "lemma-level" representation) is known as *predicate-argument structure,* in which the verb is the predicate and attached noun-phrases are its arguments. To simplify this linguistic construct considerably, let us think of the difference between transitive and intransitive verbs. Transitive verbs (e.g., *eat*) specify that they can take on themes (or "direct objects"). Intransitive verbs like *sleep* cannot take on a direct object. Verb-argument structure specifies the "frames" that can accompany a verb.

Further study showed that not all agrammatic patients have problems producing main verbs, and the problem is not exclusive to nonfluent aphasias (Berndt, Mitchum, Haendiges, and Sandson, 1997; Miceli, et al., 1989). Patients that have a special verb-finding problem tend to use common vague verbs in narration (e.g., *get, do, have*) and tend to simplify sentence structure more than patients with minimal verb retrieval problems (Berndt, Haendiges, Mitchum, and Sandson, 1997). Also, there is more variability. Some agrammatic patients produce more verbs in isolation than in sentences, and others produce more verbs in sentences than in isolation.

With Broca's aphasia, producing transitive verbs is easier than intransitive verbs (Jonkers and Bastiaanse, 1997). Also, putting verbs in sentences becomes harder with greater complexity of a verb's argument structure (Thompson, Lange, Schneider, and Shapiro, 1997). We shall return to argument structure later with respect to sentence comprehension.

Because of exceptions to an old definition of agrammatism and because of more variation than is implied by the old definition, some aphasiologists have questioned whether agrammatism is a legitimate entity. Miceli and others (1989) were adamant, declaring that data "can no longer be ignored just for the obstinate protection of a fictional category of dubious theoretical value" (p. 475). Caplan (1991) suggested that variability of grammatical morpheme production in Broca's aphasia is indicative of the complexity of sentence formulation. In his opinion, agrammatism is an appropriate classification, and we just have to learn more about the intricacies of grammatical processes and be more flexible in defining agrammatism.

Grammatical Knowledge

Initially, researchers attributed agrammatism to a vaguely specified dissociation of syntax from other linguistic components of language (Caramazza and Berndt, 1978). It was called the "no-syntax hypothesis" (Kolk and Van Grunsven, 1985). One problem with this hypothesis was that it was unclear as to whether it refers to syntactic knowledge ("competence") or syntactic processes ("performance").

Might elements of language be missing because of a "loss of grammar" or erasure of grammatical knowledge stored in long-term memory? A common strategy for evaluating the grammatical store is to compare performance on a number of different tasks. Schnitzer (1978) wrote that "a deficiency which affected all of the linguistic abilities would have to be either a remarkable coincidence or (more likely) a deficiency in the linguistic competence underlying all modalities" (p. 347). Caplan (1985) added that "disturbances found only in one language task have been considered to be disturbances in performance, sparing competence, while disturbances found in all language-related tasks reflect a disturbance of the central set of representations, that is, of competence" (p. 133). Success with any one language task indicates that knowledge is retained to some degree.

When studying a function such as verbal expression, the investigator might include a **metalinguistic task** to examine an area of knowledge. Such tasks require conscious judgments about language or about a language function, as in editing what someone has written. Common metalinguistic tasks include the following:

- word-sorting: arranging words or phrases into a sentence
- grammaticality judgment: given a pair of sentences, choosing the correct one
- grammaticality judgment: given one sentence, deciding whether it is "good" or "bad"

Metalinguistic tasks have been employed extensively, partly because they involve "shallow processing" (Linebarger, Schwartz, and Saffran, 1983a) or may circumvent processes of comprehension and expression tasks (Baum, 1989).

The most common metalinguistic task for grammar is *grammaticality judgment.* Patients do not usually have to comprehend fully or produce a sentence. The task is simply to detect errors or violations of linguistic rules. The ability of agrammatic subjects to detect morphological and syntactic violations of all sorts has been demonstrated repeatedly in many languages (Branchereau and Nespoulous, 1989; Devescovi, Bates, D'Amico, Hernandez, Marangolo, Pizzamiglio, and Razzano, 1997; Linebarger, Schwartz, and Saffran, 1983a; Shankweiler, Crain, Gorrell, and Tuller, 1989; Wulfeck, Bates, and Capasso, 1991). Exceptions may occur with complex sentences or demanding processing conditions (Haarmann and Kolk, 1994).

Grammaticality judgments support the view that people with Broca's aphasia retain the representation of phrase structure and grammatical morphology in long-term memory. Bates, Wulfeck, and MacWhinney (1991) concluded that linguistic competence remains intact for Broca's and Wernicke's aphasias. Berndt and Caramazza (1980) long ago decided that, instead of a loss of syntax, "disruption of the syntactic processing mechanism undermines the Broca patient's ability to utilize syntactic information in all language performances that require syntactic analysis" (pp. 272–273).

Garrett's Theory of Sentence Production

Schwartz, Lingebarger, and Saffran (1985) noted that "it is one thing to describe agrammatism in syntactic terms and quite another to locate the responsible deficit in a mechanism that constructs syntactic representations" (p. 86). In order to explain sentence production behavior with a cognitive mechanism, we need some idea of what the mechanism is and how we go about evaluating it.

In search of a mechanism, investigators turned to Garrett's (1984) serial theory of sentence production for interpreting patterns of expressive disorder. Figure 5.1 summarizes processing subsystems and levels of mental representation computed by each process. Formulation begins with an idea and ends in two motor stages, namely, "regular processes" for speech programming and "coding processes" for execution of

PROCESSES	REPRESENTATIONAL LEVELS	DESCRIPTION
Inferential	Message	idea to be conveyed (activation of semantic memory)
Logical & Syntactic	Functional	conceptually specified slots for content words and specification of thematic roles of agent, recipient, and so on (like deep structure)
Syntactic & Phonological	Positional	syntactic frame (e.g., grammatical morphemes) and phonological form of words inserted into the frame (like surface structure)
Regular Phonological	Phonetic	programming movement sequences
Motor Coding	Articulatory	executing movement

FIGURE 5.1 Stages of sentence production according to Garrett (1984). In drawings of Garrett's model, the processes on the left are shown to generate the representational levels on the right.

movement. Each representation informs the next process in sequence. The absence of a stimulus processing component indicates that this is a general theory rather than a task-specific model. It was mainly intended to account for normal errors or "slips of the tongue."

This model is more subtle than one that would have semantics, syntax, and the lexicon ordered in a row. For example, there is a syntactic component in two levels. Syntactic and lexical-semantic components are formulated interactively within each of these levels, making it possible for different language disorders to be caused by damage at one level. Also, the semantic and lexical components of naming theories discussed in Chapter 4 have been associated with the two linguistic levels of Garrett's theory (Brownell, et al., 1986; LeDorze and Nespoulous, 1989).

Focusing on omission of function words, Garrett (1984) proposed that agrammatism is caused by a damaged positional level mechanism because this is where function words are selected. Also, evidence of intact functional level formulation is demonstrated by retention of basic canonical structure and logical location of agents and other thematic roles around a verb. Omission and substitution of grammatical morphemes as well as structural simplification have been interpreted as damage to the positional level (Caramazza and Berndt, 1985; Ostrin and Schwartz, 1986).

An impaired functional level was suggested by Maher, Chatterjee, Rothi, and Heilman (1995). Their patient WH was left-handed with a right hemisphere infarction and resulting aphasia. His speech was fluent with poor syntactic structure and omission and substitution of grammatical morphemes. Diagnosis was partly a process of eliminating the positional level as being disturbed. Words were well-formed, and WH could produce grammatical morphology in constrained tasks. WH's functional level problem was inferred from errors in placing agents and recipients around a verb (i.e., "a word-order problem"), especially in word-sorting tasks. It was characterized as a failure in mapping logical thematic roles onto canonical structure.

Linguistic studies of agrammatism tend to isolate problematic features of grammar without establishing a clear identity with a cognitive theory. Linguistic theories are classified cognitively as **representational theories.** That is, they appear to capture the product of a formulation process. Two versions postulate a limitation on generation of a phrase structure or "syntactic tree." Caplan (1985) wrote of an "impoverished syntactic representation." People with agrammatism do not construct a hierarchical tree and, instead, activate a canonical linear subject-verb-object form through which any idea is conveyed. According to a slightly different view, agrammatic productions are the result of an "underspecified syntactic representation." A complete tree is formed but some terminal nodes are missing (Grodzinsky, Swinney, and Zurif, 1985).

Adaptation and Resource Allocation

Goodglass (1976) entertained the possibility that effort of production, especially with the frequent burden of apraxia of speech, results in the elimination of less salient words such as functors. Thus, telegraphic utterance is an adaptive "economy of effort." If patients did not have motor problems, they would produce complete sentences. However, patients with little apraxia omit grammatical morphemes, and economy of effort does not accout for substitution errors.

Kolk and Heeschen (1990) differentiated impairment symptoms attributable to a damaged processor (i.e., negative symptoms) from adaptation symptoms attributable to compensatory adjustments by the cognitive system (i.e., positive symptoms). They claimed that some symptoms of agrammatism are due to adaptation that is either *preventive* (before formulation is started) or *corrective* (after mistakes are made). Omissions were considered to be adaptive symptoms (e.g., telegraphic strategy) and substitutions are impairment symptoms. They were particularly interested in variability in a patient's agrammatic behavior with respect to the sentence production task. Task-dependent changes included reduction of grammatical morpheme omission in picture description relative to conversation, and increased substitution rates for picture description. This variability was considered to reflect some conscious use of strategy (Hofstede and Kolk, 1994).

Kolk and Heeschen's theory of impairment, called *synchrony reduction,* was that agrammatic patients are slow to activate structural representations. This slowness reduces the synchrony required to combine elements of a sentence and, thus, makes complex structures difficult to produce. Task-effects pointed to consideration of reduced working memory capacity and the resulting reduction of resources available for complex formulation operations. That is, picture description supposedly requires fewer resources than conversation, thus, reducing the need to form a telegraphic strategy of omission. Strategic ellipsis (e.g., "more milk," "too late") was thought to be a preventive strategy intended to avoid computational overload that would occur if a complete sentence were attempted (Kolk and Heeschen, 1992).

COMPREHENSION WITH AGRAMMATISM

Broca's aphasia is the clearest example of what used to be broadly termed "expressive aphasia." Auditory comprehension has been said to be "good" or "relatively preserved," at least relative to the overt agrammatism in language production. However, the *Boston Diagnostic Aphasia Examination* specifies a range from the 50th to 90th percentile for auditory comprehension (Goodglass and Kaplan, 1983). According to the *Western Aphasia Battery,* a patient can be between 4 and 10 points for this function (Kertesz, 1982). The manual for the ACTS shows where Broca's aphasia ranks relative to a maximum score of 21 and other syndromes (Shewan, 1979):

- anomic aphasia 14.8
- Broca's aphasia 12.5
- Wernicke's aphasia 9.7

Therefore, clinical measures indicate that substantial comprehension impairment can occur with Broca's aphasia, and it is in the middle of the pack relative to other syndromes.

Asyntactic Comprehension

Early attempts to uncover a specific disorder focused on distinguishing between lexical and syntactic factors in comprehension. The most frequently cited study is Caramazza and Zurif's (1976) comparison between reversible (*1a*) and nonreversible (*1b*) statements presented to subjects with Broca's or conduction aphasia. Because comprehension was thought to be relatively good with these syndromes, structurally complex sentences were used to increase the likelihood that aphasic subjects would make revealing errors.

(1a) The girl that the boy is chasing is tall.
(1b) The apple that the boy is eating is red.

Subjects chose interpretations from two pictures. Sometimes the foil differed according to a lexical element and, other times, according to a reversal of agent and recipient.

Two findings have had a tenacious influence. First, subjects with Broca's aphasia had particular difficulty with reversible statements (*1a*). Second, they made more thematic role order errors than lexical errors. Caramazza and Zurif concluded that people with Broca's aphasia can use semantic or pragmatic constraints to comprehend thematic roles (e.g., apples do not eat) but are impaired when they must rely on the syntactic feature of word order. Interpretation was consistent with the "no-syntax" hypothesis as applied to agrammatism (Caramazza and Berndt, 1978). Suspicion of a special word order problem grew with studies showing particular difficulty with passive sentences (Samuels and Benson, 1979; Schwartz, Saffran, and Marin, 1980a) and mostly order errors when errors were made, even with reversible active sentences (Gallaher and Canter, 1982).

Sherman and Schweickert (1989) tried to deal with problems in Caramazza and Zurif's design by controlling for complexity, reversibility, and plausibility. Results reinforced Caramazza and Zurif's conclusions. For plausible events, reversible sentences led to more errors than nonreversibles. Plausibility was easier than implausibility, indicating again that people with Broca's aphasia process semantic constraints to overcome limitations with syntax.

People with Broca's aphasia acquired a reputation for having difficulty with word order when it is the main cue to thematic roles. Some researchers started to identify Broca's aphasia according to an "inability to interpret other than simple active structures or semantically constrained sentences" (Rosenberg, Zurif, Brownell, Garrett, and Bradley, 1985, p. 292; also, Shapiro and Levine, 1990). This "asyntactic comprehension" disorder would come to be diagnosed basically as

- deficit with noncanonical reversible sentences (e.g., passives)
- significantly more order errors than lexical errors.

These criteria for identifying agrammatic comprehension can vary slightly, such as requiring only that a patient have a deficit with reversible sentences in general. Particular investigators may add a qualification that patients do well on word comprehension and grammaticality judgment tasks (Saffran, Schwartz, and Linebarger, 1998).

Processes of Sentence Comprehension

The main task for the sentence comprehension system is thematic role assignment or, namely, figuring out who is doing what to whom. Like word comprehension, everyday sentence comprehension is the result of automatic obligatory processes. According to Tyler (1987), core processes operate on a *principle of optimal efficiency* by assigning "an analysis to the speech input at the theoretically earliest point at which the type of analysis in question can be assigned" (p. 146). Core processes are supplemented with capacity-consuming controlled processes.

Sentence comprehension is assumed to rely on three subsystems: a lexical processor, a syntactic processor, and a semantic or interpretive processor (Figure 5.2; Cairns, 1984; Garnham, 1985). At least, these components identify lines of specialized investigations of comprehension. That is, some researchers focus on lexical access in sentences. Other researchers specialize in the assignment of syntactic structure to regions of sentences. Others are more interested in the ultimate interpretation of sentences, especially in a narrative context.

Some fundamental questions are entertained in most studies of normal adults. One is whether each processor, especially lexical access or syntactic parsing, operates as an autonomous subsystem. For example, does parsing occur without influence from lexical access or interpretations of nearby sentences? The manner in which one processor informs another is a regular theme in studies of a processing subsystem. One hypothesis is that the three processors are somewhat autonomous and operate serially. Figure 5.2a indicates that the parser is not left totally on its own. Another hypothesis is that all components are interdependent and operate in an interactive or parallel fashion (Figure 5.2b).

Two general strategies are used to study sentence comprehension. Most clinical assessments consist of **off-line** procedures in which subjects respond after a sentence is presented. The procedures include the slow tasks of sentence-picture matching, sentence verification, and following directions. Response latency usually allows for a great deal of controlled processing to occur. The off-line approach measures the cumulative result of all processes or the *final interpretation* of a sentence.

On-line procedures, on the other hand, examine processing as it occurs "in real time." It is important to note that just any measure of response time (RT), especially after a sentence is presented, is not definitive of the on-line approach. In on-line studies, subjects respond to a point within a sentence, usually before its presentation is completed. RT is indicative of relative processing load at that point. Inference about a process itself is based on the success of a theory of the process predicting processing loads at key locations. The approach is said to detect *intermediate interpretations* within a

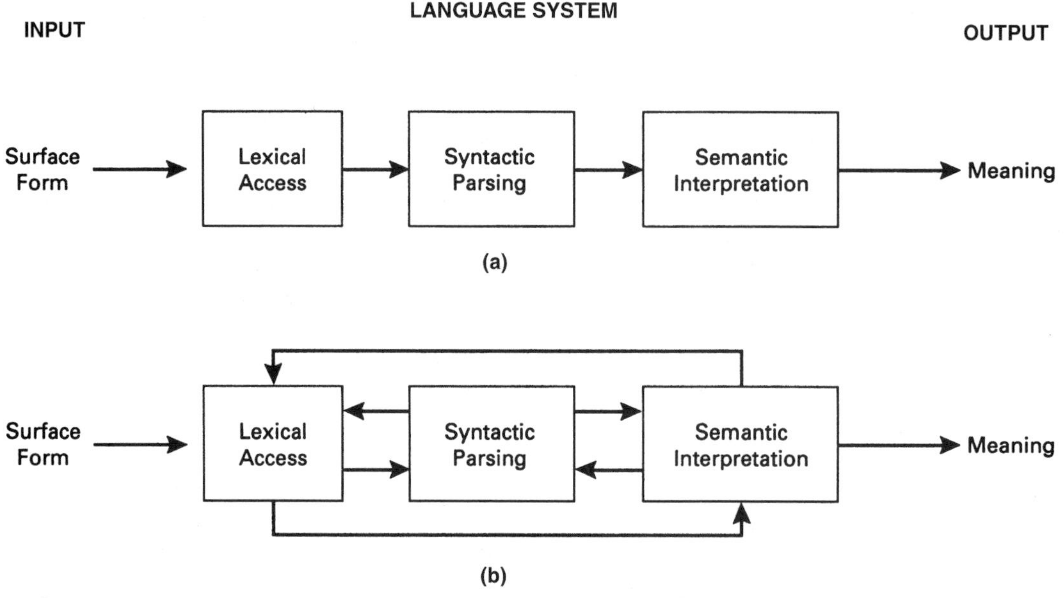

FIGURE 5.2 The major subsystems of sentence comprehension arranged according to serial theory and the preferred interactive-parallel theory.

sentence. Many on-line techniques are used to study lexical access or syntactic parsing in normal adults, but the approach has seen limited duty in the study of aphasia so far. Some examples are provided in the next two sections.

Lexical System

The primed lexical decision task introduced in Chapter 4 provides a look at the lexical processor in isolation. For now, let us consider the simple activation of meaning for Broca's aphasia. One of the early basic findings pertained to comparison between slow semantic tasks such as word relatedness judgment and the fast priming task. Aphasic subjects who were impaired in semantic judgment accuracy demonstrated semantic priming with LDTs (e.g., Milberg and Blumstein, 1981). This *automaticity effect* indicated that automatic semantic processing can be intact while controlled processing is impaired and, therefore, diagnosis of semantic problems depends on examination of both levels of processing.

Milberg and Blumstein (1981) were left with a surprising result, however. Patients with Broca's aphasia did not have a semantic priming effect. This result appeared to contradict the syntax-semantics dissociation proposed in the 1970s. These investigators decided to look more closely at the automaticity of semantic processing in Broca's and Wernicke's aphasia (Milberg, Blumstein, and Dworetzky, 1987). Subjects with Broca's aphasia again had no semantic priming effects. The researchers concluded that agrammatic patients have a lexical-semantic impairment at the automatic level of processing, which came to be known as the **automaticity hypothesis.**

Milberg and Blumstein's research design suffered some criticism (e.g., Baum, 1997; Hagoort, 1997; Ostrin and Tyler, 1993). One problem appeared to be the complexity of the task, because they used paired primes (e.g., SHORE-BANK) before targets (e.g., RIVER). Katz (1988) simplified the task by presenting semantically ambiguous one-word primes (e.g., BANK) for targets such as MONEY or RIVER. This time, agrammatic subjects displayed semantic priming for both meanings of BANK. This result was indicative of a basic finding in psycholinguistics, namely, that ambiguous nouns normally activate multiple meanings automatically (Simpson and Burgess, 1985).

Another problem with the early work was that Milberg and Blumstein relied on a long prime-target interval of 500 msec which, as discussed in Chapter 4, can allow for controlled processing to obscure capabilities at an automatic level. Shorter intervals have been used in more recent studies. Tyler and others (1995) inserted 200 msec. Hagoort (1993, 1997) initially compared 100, 500, and 1250 msecs and, later, intervals of 300 and 1400 msec. Subjects with Broca's aphasia displayed semantic priming at the short intervals. In cognitive terms, patients exhibited spreading activation to related concept nodes in a semantic network within 100 msec. The results led these investigators to reject Milberg and Blumstein's automaticity hypothesis for this syndrome.

In a sentence, an ambiguous word activates multiple meanings instantaneously, even when prior context is suggestive of one interpretation (Seidenberg, Tanenhaus, Leiman, and Bienkowski, 1982; Swinney, 1979). This was evidence that lexical-sematic access operates as an autonomous or "encapsulated" system. Subtle features of on-line research indicated that context selects interpretation a few syllables (or milliseconds) later. So, how do psycholinguists determine such things?

Swinney, Zurif, and Nicol (1989) borrowed a common on-line procedure to study multiple meaning activation in aphasia. In this case, an ambiguous word like *plant* is presented as a prime in a spoken sentence such as *2*.

(2) The gardener was responsible for watering every plant * on the enormous estate.

While listening to a sentence, aphasic subjects made a visual recognition decision about letter-strings (e.g., TREE or FACTORY or an unrelated word) shown immediately after the ambiguous prime (*). This auditory presentation of a sentence along with an on-line visual lexical decision is called **cross-modal priming.** Subjects with Broca's aphasia were primed only for primary meanings (i.e., TREE), unlike normal adults who are primed exhaustively for both dominant and secondary word-meanings (i.e., TREE and FACTORY). Swinney concluded that patients with Broca's aphasia are slow in the autonomous access of meanings.

The proposal that exhaustive access is merely delayed should be tested with another LDT a few syllables later (Caramazza and Badecker, 1991). To check this out, Swinney's study was followed with a similar one that placed lexical decision five syllables after the ambiguous word (e.g., *plant*). Again, subjects with Broca's aphasia were primed only for the primary word (Prather, Love, Finkel, and Zurif, 1994). It is still possible that these patients are slow to activative multiple meanings automatically, if they activate multiple meanings at all. Because priming was isolated to the meaning consistent with context, it appears that context penetrates the lexical system early in Broca's aphasia.

In addition to word-meaning, the lexical processor feeds grammatical information to the syntactic processor. This information is carried by free grammatical morphemes (i.e., function words), the morphological structure of words (i.e., inflections), and the argument structure of verbs. Researchers have wondered if patients with Broca's aphasia have as much trouble using grammatical morphemes in comprehension as they do for production. In the following paragraphs, this question is considered before addressing verbs.

A simple LDT was used for comparing access to open- and closed-class words (Bradley, Garrett, and Zurif, 1980). Diagnosis of deficit hinged on normal subjects, who had a frequency effect for open-class words but not for closed-class functors. Subjects with Broca's aphasia did not exhibit this difference. The investigators proposed a **lexical hypothesis** stating that agrammatic comprehension is an impairment in accessing function words. However, several investigators could not replicate the frequency effect with normal adults, thereby, weakening the basis for claiming that aphasic patients are different (e.g., Petocz and Oliphant, 1988; Taft, 1990). Gordon and Caramazza (1983) could not replicate Bradley's findings for aphasic subjects.

Studies had subjects comprehend sentences in which functors matter for interpretation. Heilman and Scholes (1976) presented sentences like *3* in a picture-choice task with word-order and lexical foils.

(3a) She showed her baby the pictures.
(3b) She showed her the baby pictures.

In these sentences, position of *the* carries information about thematic roles of other words. Subjects with Broca's and conduction aphasias had difficulty making word-order decisions. Elsewhere, subjects with Broca's aphasia uniquely failed to distinguish definite and indefinite articles (Goodenough, Zurif, Weintraub, and Von Stockert, 1977). Consequently, Broca's aphasia developed a reputation for being insensitive to free-standing grammatical morphemes. However, there was seemingly contradictory evidence because of appropriate response to sentences like *Bill walking the dog* and *Bill the walking dog* (Caplan, Matthei, and Gigley, 1981).

The on-line task of **word-monitoring** was used to test the lexical hypothesis in real time. In this task, subjects are instructed to press a response key when they hear a predetermined word as they are listening to a sentence. Like other on-line tasks, response time is considered to be indicative of processing load at the location of the target word. Agrammatic subjects' response was slower to function words than content words, in contrast to normal controls (Friederici, 1983; Swinney, Zurif, and Cutler, 1980; Tyler and Cobb, 1987).

Accessing verbs may have a more direct influence on structural parsing because of the information that verbs carry about predicate-argument structure, discussed earlier in the chapter. Lew Shapiro was interested in the influence of verb complexity according to the number of noun-phrase argument structures that can be attached to a verb. In particular, he looked for evidence of automatic activation of all possible argument structures, much like the multiple activation of lexical meanings illustrated by Swinney's research.

To test the multiple activation idea, Shapiro used Swinney's cross-modal priming procedure. Let us first look at the stimuli used for manipulating verb complexity.

(4a) The happy officer *put* * the new suit on * the shelf.
(4b) The sad girl *donated* * the new suit to * the charity.

The verb *put* is simpler than *donated,* because *put* takes on a single argument structure consisting of a theme (*new suit*) and location (*on the shelf*). On the other hand, *donated* allows two possible structures indicated partly by the optionality of location in *4b.* Verbs like these were presented auditorily in similarly structured sentences (Shapiro and Levine, 1990).

Shapiro and Levine were interested in what happens at the site of the verb. Subjects made visual lexical decisions at the verb in one condition and "downstream" in another condition. Subjects with Broca's aphasia performed normally in that processing time varied with complexity at the point of contact with verbs, indicating that these patients activated multiple possibilities allowed by a verb. This effect dissipated downstream in a manner similar to what happens when mulitple meanings are activated. Fluent aphasic subjects were not sensitive to argument structure. Another study also showed that patients with Broca's aphasia were sensitive to properties of verbs on-line, whereas patients with Wernicke's aphasia were impaired (Shapiro, Gordon, Hack, and Killackey, 1993).

In sum, different proposals have been put forth regarding the nature of lexical processing in Broca's aphasia. Most evidence requires more replication. Lexical-semantic access by itself may not be as slow as once thought, but the possibility remains that meaning activation in sentences is damaged. The notion of delayed lexical access was targeted at grammatical morphemes. So far, word-monitoring has provided some on-line evidence that function words are problematic in sentences.

Syntactic System

Syntactic parsing is the assignment of structure to a string of words. For now, let us just get a better idea of what syntax or structure refers to and, thus, consider what it means to assign structure to a sentence. Ambiguous sentences like *5* illustrate the role of structure in conveying who is doing what to whom:

(5) They fed her dog biscuits.
 (a) They fed (her dog) biscuits.
 (b) They fed her (dog biscuits).

Sentence *5* is a **global ambiguity,** because the whole sentence has two plausible interpretations. Either the dog ate biscuits, or "she" ate dog biscuits. The parse establishes "attachments" among words. Is *dog* attached to *her* (*5a*) or *biscuits* (*5b*)? In conversation, such ambiguities are normally resolved with prosodic cues. Subjects with Broca's aphasia were found to have difficulties using stress and juncture to comprehend sentences like *5* (Baum, Daniloff, Daniloff, and Lewis, 1982).

To study parsing, researchers like to present structural ambiguities without such cues. Soon, we shall examine how linguists and experimental psychologists have combined to study what happens when we are faced with a structural ambiguity. Until then, let us examine how the syntactic component of comprehension has been viewed in aphasiology.

Friederici (1988) proposed that parsing is impaired in Broca's aphasia based on evidence of intact knowledge and on-line tests of sensitivity to grammatical morphology. However, the early word-monitoring studies could have been indicative merely of recognition processes without implications for structural assignment. In a more recent use of word-monitoring, the target word was placed immediately after inflected or uninflected words appearing in either a grammatical or ungrammatical context (Friederici, Wessels, Emmorey, and Bellugi, 1992). In general, subjects with Broca's aphasia displayed some deficient sensitivity to omitted inflection as a function of context, leading Friederici to conclude that syntactic information associated with inflection is not activated fast enough.

The theory of slow syntactic activation was supported by **syntactic priming** studies. Baum (1988) compared grammatical primes (e.g., *It's true that the boys*) and ungrammatical primes (e.g., *It's true that the boy*) presented prior to a target (e.g., *play*). Syntactic priming did not occur for subjects with Broca's aphasia as it did for normal controls with 500 msec between stimuli. Haarmann and Kolk (1991) varied SOA and presented primes like *We can* and targets like TALK or NOSE. Aphasic subjects were facilitated at 1100 msec intervals but not at 300 or 700 msec. Additional evidence was provided by Blumstein, Milberg, Dworetzky, Rosen, and Gershberg (1991).

Tyler and her colleagues (1995) conducted a word-monitoring study leading to a different conclusion. Patients with Broca's aphasia listened to sentences with syntactic violations, such as *6.*

(6) They went into London chose to CARPETS and curtains.

The experimenters placed target words immediately after a violation or after the correct version in another sentence. The aphasic subjects were sensitive to the violations, indicating that this study provides "no evidence supporting the claim that Broca patients are slow to access syntactic information in general or the more specific claim that they are slow to access members of the closed class" (p. 152).

Another approach to studying syntactic processing "in real time" involved the presentation of **filler-gap** constructions. Sentence *7* is a stimulus used in a study by Zurif, Swinney, Prather, Soloman, and Bushell (1993).

(7) The man liked the *tailor* with the British accent *who* claimed to know the queen.

Minimizing linguistic obfuscation, let us simply consider that *who* represents a gap linked to its antecedent *tailor* (or "filler"). Subjects were placed in another cross-modal priming task to examine reactivaton of an antecedent in a timely fashion to interpret *who* (i.e., to fill the gap). In this case, *who* was a prime for a decision target (e.g., *clothes* or *weight*). Semantic priming relative to the unrelated target would indicate that *tailor* is activated at the gap location. Zurif and Swinney found that subjects with Wernicke's aphasia displayed priming (i.e., filled gaps), but those with Broca's aphasia were not primed (i.e., did not fill gaps). The deficit in Broca's aphasia was interpreted as being a parsing (or attachment) problem in which a concept is not reactivated at a gap.

Blumstein and others (1998) attempted to replicate Zurif's findings with a modified priming task in which the sentence and lexical decision target were both presented auditorily. The priming sentence and lexical target were distinguished by having different speakers present them. One reason for doing this was to bypass aphasic reading deficits for the lexical decision component of the task. Blumstein obtained a result that was nearly the opposite of Zurif and Swinney's. Subjects with Broca's aphasia evidenced reactivation at the gap site, whereas those with Wernicke's aphasia did not.

Linguistic representational theories have been proposed to account for agrammatic comprehension. How such theories fit into a cognitive framework is unclear, but for this discussion it is assumed that they depict the result of a parsing operation. Caplan and Futter (1986) proposed a **linearity hypothesis** stating that agrammatic patients use a linear (or canonical) agent-action-recipient order to assign thematic roles for a sentence. This is why difficulty occurs with sentences structured differently.

Grodzinsky (1986, 1989) disagreed with Caplan by claiming that patients do generate hierarchical representations. Instead, impairment is an incomplete structural representation. For example, in linguistic theory of passives, a "trace" that designates thematic role is said to be left in the wake of movement of NPs from their canonical position. Grodzinsky's **trace-deletion hypothesis** states that agrammatic patients delete traces from structural representations and end up assigning thematic roles randomly.

As promised, we can now turn to the psycholinguistic study of normal parsing. To determine if structure is autmatically assigned "at the earliest possible point," researchers present sentences that are structurally ambiguous at a particular location (like presenting a semantically ambiguous word somewhere in a sentence). This is called a **local ambiguity.** Sentence *8* is one example.

(8) The steel ships are transporting is expensive.

As we read left to right, we may discover that *the steel ships* has two possible interpretations. It could be a noun-phrase agent for *transporting;* or, as we learn downstream, it could be broken up into two noun-phrases with *the steel* as the subject of *expensive.* In a local ambiguity, one of the possible interpretations is erroneous. A local ambiguity creates a **garden-path (GP) sentence** in which a reader could be led astray initially. Psycholinguists have wondered if the syntactic parser makes mistakes and then corrects. If so, we can answer the question of whether an automatic parser acts autonomously.

Lynn Frazier's theory of parsing stimulated the study of garden path phenomena (e.g., Frazier and Rayner, 1982). Consistent with Tyler's assumption of optimal efficiency, the hypothesis was that the parser autonomously assigns a complete structure at the earliest opportunity (even without clear input from lexical access). The parser also assigns the simplest structure. Finally, a listener or reader revises the structural assignment if it turns out to be incorrect. In sum, automaticity and autonomy lead a parser into making a lot of mistakes and corrections.

GP sentences are used to test whether structure is applied judiciously to a whole sentence or, instead, is slapped on as soon as a few words enter the system. Many of these studies rely on duration of eye-fixation as the measure of relative processing load. The crucial comparison is between a garden-path sentence and a disambiguated counterpart such as *The steel that ships are transporting is expensive.* The critical element for measurement is the point at which an error can be recognized in the GP sentence (i.e., *is expensive*).

The central finding by Frazier's research team (known as "the Amherst group") was that fixation in the critical region is longer for sentences like *8* than for disambiguated control sentences. The additional time indicates that a subject is "garden-pathed" into an erroneous *initial parse* and has to revise in order to assign the *ultimate parse.* Thinking of the possible interactive influence of other components such as lexical-semantic access, Ferreira and Clifton (1986) stated that "it is important to distinguish between initial and eventual use of nonsyntactic information" (p. 348). They explained that "if the syntactic processor (or parser) is modular, it should initially construct a syntactic representation without consulting nonsyntactic information sources, such as semantic or pragmatic information or discourse structure" (p. 348). The Amherst group published numerous demonstrations of an initial parse reacting on its own, beneath our conscious control.

Other psycholinguists argue that the initial parse is not autonomous. Instead, it is "constraint-based," influenced by lexical and broader interpretive components. Accordingly, the Amherst group's findings are considered to be an accident of experimental design. Lexical activation (e.g., verb-argument structure) keeps the initial obligatory parse from being erroneous (MacDonald, Pearlmutter, and Seidenberg, 1994). Parsing can also be "discourse-driven" or informed by narrative context (Altmann, Garnham, and Henstra, 1994). However, others indicate that the "garden-path theory" cannot be ruled out, because differences in experimental procedures have coincided with differences of theory (Ferreira and Henderson, 1990; Mitchell and Corley, 1994). What these studies have in common is that they employ sentences with local structural ambiguities and on-line procedures. This is different from clinical studies in which it is claimed that off-line sentence-picture matching, sentence repetition, and grammaticality judgment are a way of assessing the parsing mechanism (e.g., Romani, 1994).

In sum, there is a lack of evidence that addresses the agrammatic patient's on-line assignment of syntax to local structural ambiguities in sentences. Instead, the priming paradigm has been directed at specific contingencies at the ends of sentences, indicating some delay of processing. On-line procedures (i.e., word-monitoring, cross-modal priming) have addressed "sensitivity" to grammatical morphemes in context and the ability to fill gaps. Such studies were assumed to measure activation of syntactic structure. So far, structural issues have been considered most explicitly in linguistic theories of linearity or trace-deletion based mainly on off-line procedures.

Semantic Interpretation

Semantic processing can be confused by bad information from damaged components of the system. For Broca's aphasia, the semantic constraint hypothesis states that intact semantic processes are a source of controlled or strategic adaptation to these limitations. Another possibility, suggested first by Schwartz and others (1980a), also stipulates that lexical and syntactic processes are intact but that asyntactic comprehension is actually based on an impairment in the final interpretive operation of assigning thematic roles. This is called the **mapping hypothesis,** and it has taken on some clinical importance because of the promotion of "mapping therapy" (see Chapter 13).

The mapping hypothesis states that patients with clinical evidence of asyntactic comprehension fail to assign thematic roles to normally realized syntactic representations (Linebarger, 1990). With respect to the serial model of Figure 5.2a, the impairment can be said to be *between* the syntactic parser and semantic interpretation, where a mapping operation superimposes "who is doing what to whom" on a successful parse. Put more simply, the mechanism coordinates sentence meaning with sentence form. Empirical support for the mapping hypothesis is based on the claim that there is evidence of intact parsing despite the clinical evidence of sentence comprehension problems (i.e., difficulty with reversible sentences, role reversal errors dominating lexical errors).

Grammaticality judgments have been the main source of support for the mapping hypothesis

(Linebarger, 1990; Linebarger, Schwartz, and Saffran, 1983). Success with grammaticality judgment in many studies suggested to Linebarger that the parser must be intact. Linebarger and Schwartz's own research showed that agrammatic patients were successful in making plausibility judgments about a variety of sentences (e.g., *The worm swallowed the bird*) but had difficulty when NPs were moved away from canonical positions (e.g., *We saw the bird that the worm swallowed*). Thus, agrammatic patients activate syntactic structure and can assign thematic roles, but they have difficulty with mapping them onto each other. Schwartz and her colleagues (1987) also proposed variants of the mapping theory, namely, a "procedural" version specifying difficulty in assigning thematic roles to syntactic categories and a "lexical" version specifying inadequate predicate-argument information.

The main argument against the mapping hypothesis pertains to its reliance on off-line grammaticality and plausibility judgments as the basis for concluding that the syntactic parser is intact. The previous section showed how parsing is studied in psycholinguistics. Swinney and Zurif (1995) suggested that to diagnose the status of parsing, an experimenter should specify what a parser does and then design an experiment that addresses its characteristics. An experiment should also distinguish between a mapper and a parser in real time. At least, an investigator should consider that parsing has an automatic component and then test this characteristic accordingly.

In addition, Linebarger's use of the term "mapping" could be confusing for a couple of reasons. One is that the term is often employed as a generic metaphor for any instance of superimposing one type of information onto another. For word comprehension and production, phonological representations are said to "map onto" semantic representations and vice versa (e.g., Franklin, Howard, and Patterson, 1995). Moreover, the index in the 1100-page *Handbook of Psycholinguistics* contains no item for a distinct mapping process (Gernsbacher, 1994). The proposal that a distinct thematic mapping operation exists appears to come mainly from Linebarger's work. Although one aim of cognitive neuropsychology is to use dissociations to discover normal processes, a mapping process (at least, by this name) is not yet identified by an independent body of research with normal adults (as opposed to the large body of independent work on lexical access and syntactic parsing).

Working Memory and Resource Theory

A reduction of working memory capacity is becoming a regular theme for explaining language deficits. As indicated in Chapter 4, the idea has been applied to aphasia in general, and the hypothesis has been tested by simulation studies using computers and normal adults. One aspect of the theory is that a specific symptom, such as agrammatism, is not caused by a damaged component of a processing system. Instead the reduction of overall processing capacity may target one system more than others, such as the relatively demanding sentence processing systems. This would give the appearance of a damaged component.

Several investigators have suggested that resource theory accounts at least partially for comprehension deficits in Broca's aphasia (e.g., Haarmann and Kolk, 1994; Swinney and Zurif, 1995). Using a sentence-picture matching task, Friederici and Frazier (1992) found an interaction between syntactic structure and processing demands of the task for agrammatic subjects. The processing demands were manipulated by presenting pictures with a sentence or delaying the pictures after the sentence. The interaction was interpreted as the limitation of processing resources affecting syntactic processing more than lexical processing.

Summary and Conclusions

Broca's aphasia is a swaggering flagship in a contentious sea. Theories of comprehension and production can be divided generally into linguistic theories and psycholinguistic theories. General agreement is found with respect to the status of linguistic knowledge or competence. People with Broca's aphasia have not lost their knowledge of lexical and syntactic features of the language they speak. Thus, investigators agree that impairments should be identified with processing. They tend to reject notions of a totally demolished device in favor of some form of partial impairment, at least, for most patients of this type.

The menu of explanations is shorter for expressive agrammatism than for comprehension. Agrammatism may be a problem either at Garrett's positional level or may be the result of reduced working memory capacity. The situation is more complex for comprehension (see Table 5.2). Some say the problem is slow lexical activation, and others say it is not slow. Some point to damaged parsing. Others claim that parsing is fine, and thematic mapping is impaired instead. While findings appear to be contradictory, such as response times at gaps, we should take a deep breath and realize that all sorts of methods are just being introduced. Blumstein and her colleagues (1998) concluded that "at this time we have yet to come up with a definitive explanatory basis for the syntactic comprehension deficits of Broca's aphasia" (p. 167). This is important for the clinical consumer of research to realize in case someone claims to have the answer.

ANOMIC APHASIA

Sometimes called amnesic aphasia, anomic aphasia is the mildest form of acquired language disorder. It gets relatively little attention in basic clinical research. Wernicke's aphasia is studied much more frequently as a fluent contrast to Broca's aphasia.

Anomic aphasia is nearly the opposite of agrammatism. Comprehension seems unimpaired until we give the Token Test or assess reading. Whereas content-bearing words are produced and function words are problematic in agrammatism, function words are produced normally and content-bearing words are problematic in anomic

TABLE 5.2 Summary of the investigation of asyntactic comprehension. The pattern of symptoms consists of more difficulty with noncanonical sentences (e.g., passives) than canonical sentences (e.g., actives), more difficulty with thematically reversible than nonreversible sentences, and more thematic-order errors than lexical selection errors. Only component-based theories are included. We should not forget the working memory hypotheses.

COMPONENT	THEORY	SHORT DEFINITION	METHOD
lexical	automaticity hypothesis	slow activation of meaning in semantic memory	semantic priming cross-modal priming
	lexical hypothesis	insensitivity to function words	word-monitoring
syntactic	no-syntax hypothesis	general problem with structural knowledge or processing	off-line comprehension tests
	impaired parser	slow assignment of structure	syntactic priming
	linearity and trace-deletion hypotheses	simple or incomplete structural representation	off-line comprehension tests
semantic	mapping hypothesis	impaired assignment of thematic roles to intact parse	off-line comprehension tests & grammaticality judgments

aphasia. A patient fills word-finding gaps with generic terms and circumlocutions. Anomic aphasia is usually associated with a posterior lesion sparing Wernicke's area, but the same general characteristics can be observed after frontal lesions. A "frontal anomic aphasia" may be studied in comparison to posterior anomic aphasia (e.g., Kohn and Goodglass, 1985).

Divided Attention

Patients with frontal and posterior anomic aphasic can have attention problems while performing simple clinical tasks (Murray, Holland, and Beeson, 1995). Without a competing distraction, tasks of semantic categorization, grammaticality judgment, and sentence completion are done almost normally. However, patients drop below normal performance under focused and divided attention conditions as defined in Chapter 4. In a later study of spontaneous picture description, a group with mild fluent aphasia (mostly anomic) had performance decrements in the dual-task condition that normal controls did not have (Murray, Holland, and Beeson, 1998).

The studies of attention and resource allocation indicate that mildly impaired patients should be assessed in optimal conditions to determine their peak capabilities. On the other hand, identifying the deficit may be important for functional communication, because some of these excellent communicators become distressed over language processing problems that arise when they are trying to get a ticket at an airport or participate in a gathering of friends.

Language Comprehension

Anomic aphasia has been examined rarely with lexical-semantic access paradigms. Chenery, Ingram, and Murdoch (1990) compared high- and low-comprehending aphasic subjects in a semantically primed lexical decision task. The high-comprehending group consisted of mostly anomic aphasia. This group was able to make controlled semantic judgments and displayed semantic priming with a 500 msec prime-target interval. Both performances indicated that semantic memory is largely intact and it can be activated normally when given plenty of time.

Some patients have a peculiar problem with abstract words. One case, DRB, had difficulty comprehending abstract words in the auditory but not visual modality (Franklin, Howard, and Patterson, 1994). Tyler and Moss (1997) studied another patient, DrO, who progressed from jargonaphasia to a someone with mild word-finding problems. This case exhibited semantic priming for abstract and concrete words in the visual modality but only for concrete words in the auditory modality. Further analysis indicated that DrO had a general auditory processing deficit that may have been left over from the earlier jargon phase. Why would there be this selective semantic activation in the auditory modality? Tyler and Moss thought that it has something to do with a slow activation of phonological representations coupled with a normally lower activation level of less rich representation of abstract words compared to concrete or highly imageable words.

Regarding sentence comprehension, patients exhibited a normal sensitivity to function words in one study but had difficulty with inflections in a highly inflected language (Goodenough, et al., 1977; Smith and Bates, 1987). Peach, Canter, and Gallaher (1988) compared subjects with anomic and conduction aphasia in comprehending thematic information in active sentences. Both groups were accurate around 70 percent of the time and, like patients with Broca's aphasia, made significantly more subject-object order errors than lexical errors. Therefore, patients with anomic aphasia have a comprehension deficit. In clinical testing, it is most likely to be displayed with the Token Test and reading tests.

Word-Retrieval

In general, naming accuracy with anomic aphasia is equivalent to Broca's aphasia, except when posterior and anterior anomic aphasias are separated (Table 5.3). The more frequently recognized posterior form has a more severe naming deficit than the anterior form. Groups do not differ in fre-

TABLE 5.3 Object-naming scores for the major syndromes.

	KOHN AND GOODGLASS (1985)	WILLIAMS AND CANTER (1982)	
		High-Frequency Words	*Low-Frequency Words*
Maximum score	85.0	20.0	20.0
Broca's	50.4	11.7	12.5
Anomic (posterior)	42.9	12.1	10.9
Anomic (anterior)	54.5		
Conduction	59.4	10.0	6.8
Wernicke's	39.1	7.8	6.1

quency of semantic paraphasias, so that this error by itself does not appear to differentiate type of aphasia. People with anomic aphasia are better in retrieving verbs (Miceli, et al., 1984; Williams and Canter, 1987). Anomic aphasia is distinctive in the use of circumlocutions when intended words are difficult to access (Kohn and Goodglass, 1985). Good comprehension enables these patients to perform about equally when naming verbal descriptions and naming objects (Goodglass and Stuss, 1979).

Those of us who are neurologically intact occasionally have a person's name on the tip of our tongue. We may say that it is a long name and begins with a certain sound. We may report the number of syllables. Do aphasic people enter a tip-of-the-tongue or TOT state? If so, what does it tell us about the word retrieval system? Beeson and her colleagues in Arizona looked at these questions with respect to naming famous people. Before examining what happened, let us consider again the framework used for explaining naming or word-finding problems.

The framework continues to be two-stage theories of word-finding that separate a lexical (or phonological) level from a semantic level (e.g., Figure 4.2; Schriefers' and Dell's work in Chapter 4). People with anomic aphasia exhibit two behaviors that are informative regarding the status of this system. One is the presence of word-finding gaps filled by generic terms such as *something* or *that thing over there.* The other is circumlocution, which is indicative of intact semantic activation (i.e., the concept to be conveyed) and a general capacity to retrieve lexical forms.

Ellis, Kay, and Franklin (1992) provided a guide for distinguishing between impairments at the semantic and lexical levels of word production. An impairment of the semantic system should result in word-finding problems because the semantic system informs the lexical system. As indicated in Chapter 4, pervasive semantic deficits in comprehension and object classification should be indicative of a problem in this system. Another clue would be word-finding deficits that are unique for particular semantic categories. We would suspect a disorder confined to the lexical system when object-sorting and word comprehension are relatively intact.

Case studies have demonstrated this approach to diagnosis. Case EST had a deep left temporal meningioma (Kay and Ellis, 1987), and case DRB had a left middle cerebral artery infarction (Franklin, Howard, and Patterson, 1995). These cases performed well in word comprehension and in object sorting and matching according to semantic categories, indicating that conceptual knowledge was intact. EST recognized famous faces but had trouble naming them (Flude, Ellis, and Kay, 1989). His impairment was diagnosed as a reduction of "the amount of activation reaching the (intact) speech output lexicon from the (intact) semantic system" (Ellis and Young, 1988, p. 122).

With an approach that differed from Nickels' procedure reported in the previous chapter, a case of severe anomic aphasia was used to test the serial and interactive versions of two-stage theories (Laine and Martin, 1996). The investigators explored effects of semantic and phonological relatedness on naming errors with a *multitarget naming task.* A picture contained six drawings of objects that had either a semantic relationship, a phonological relationship, a mixture of these relationships, or both relationships. The subject was asked to name each object in each picture; but because of severity of naming deficit, some practice trials were conducted to encourage enough responses for analysis. Errors indicated a sensitivity to both types of relationhip, such as semantic relatedness producing more semantic errors. It was concluded that results supported an interactive model of naming.

What about the TOT state with anomic aphasia? When a patient could not name a famous person in Beeson's study, the patient was asked a series of questions about the person and the name (Beeson, Holland, and Murray, 1997). A group with anomic aphasia was compared to groups with Broca's and conduction aphasia. Performances with Broca's and conduction aphasia were similar with 64 to 70 percent ability to provide semantic information and 25 to 30 percent ability to identify the first letter of the first or last name. Patients with anomic aphasia were quite different. They were more accurate naming than the other groups (i.e., 60 percent accuracy). When they could not name, they produced semantic information 91 percent of the time but could identify the first letter only 7 percent of the time. These patients had a fairly intact semantic system but an occasional serious difficulty accessing an entire lexical form, or "access to phonology was more of an all-or-none phenomenon with the anomic group" (p. 333).

CONDUCTION APHASIA

The principal basis for diagnosing conduction aphasia is the severity of repetition impairment relative to the high level of auditory language comprehension and fluent spontaneous production. The main linguistic symptom is the occurrence of word production errors that sound like the intended word (i.e., formal and phonemic paraphasias). In some patients, these errors are sparse until the patient is asked to repeat, and errors increase as sentence length increases and familiarity decreases (Goodglass and Kaplan, 1983).

Researchers have been curious about either the demonstrative repetition deficit or the phonological mistakes in spontaneous speech. Because of the repetition deficit, neurological theory put conduction aphasia into the category of *disconnection syndrome,* meaning that a connection between functional "centers" is damaged (Geschwind, 1965). Good comprehension and fluent sentence production indicated that auditory and speech centers are intact. The auditory center just could not send impulses to the speech center.

Language Comprehension

There have been several reports of asyntactic comprehension with conduction aphasia. Suspicion of syntactic comprehension deficit began with studies showing groups with conduction aphasia performing like those with Broca's aphasia (Caramazza and Zurif, 1976; Goodglass, et al., 1979; Heilman and Scholes, 1976). In Peach and others' (1988) study, subjects with conduction aphasia were very much like Broca's aphasia in comprehending active sentences. Peach concluded that these syndromes along with anomic aphasia demonstrate a syntactic comprehension deficit, despite the fact that only one has agrammatic expression.

Asyntactic comprehension was also reported in case studies. Case MC had trouble comprehending passives and center-embedded relative clauses (Caramazza, Basili, Koller, and Berndt, 1981). Case EA identified thematic roles in active reversible sentences but made order errors with passives and locatives. It was decided that EA could map thematic relations onto basic NVN structure but had the agrammatic patient's problem when relying on order information in noncanonical sentences (Friedrich, Martin, and

Kemper, 1985). How can at least two clinical syndromes have apparently the same comprehension deficit? In the next section, we shall examine the case of EA a bit further with respect to the role of short-term memory in processing grammatical features of a sentence.

Repetition and the STM Question

The unique deficit of repetition was purported initially to demonstrate the distinctiveness of memory stores through a "selective impairment of short-term memory" (Shallice and Warrington, 1977). As indicated in Chapter 1, STM is now considered to be a component of working memory. It is identified as a **short-term buffer.** Input buffers retain stimulus representations briefly so that currently processed information can be related to previous input. Output buffers hold onto activated word forms while output processes act upon them. Some CN-models of word-level functions contain specialized buffers in addition to phonological and orthographic processors (e.g., Hillis and Caramazza, 1992).

A fundamental issue is the nature of representation in a buffer. According to Baddeley (1986), a buffer for auditory-oral processing has two components: a *phonological store* of recent input that decays over time and an *articulatory loop* that rehearses information we want to keep around for a while (also, Shelton, Martin, and Yafee, 1992). Isolated memory span deficit signifies impaired phonological encoding and is considered to be evidence for "fractionation" of a phonological buffer from an articulatory buffer in working memory.

Impairment of a phonological buffer is illustrated by two cases. Each suffered a stroke with resulting symptoms of conduction aphasia. Case PV perceived speech normally in discrimination and rhyme judgment. She repeated single words but could not repeat digit and word sequences longer than three items. Retention time for subspan lists was reduced (Vallar and Baddeley, 1984). Case EA had an auditory digit span of 1.5 and displayed no recency effect for retaining items at the end of long lists. A deficit of phonological encoding was indicated when phonologically similar letters were harder to retain than phonologically dissimilar letters (Friedrich, Glenn, and Marin, 1984). Both cases had longer spans for visual stimuli, thereby, locating the problem in the auditory system.

When memory span was considered to be a gross indicator of processing capacity, researchers wondered about the impact of deficient "STM" on auditory language comprehension. As indicated previously, processing capacity is now examined with respect to working memory and resource allocation, and automatic processing is thought to take up little room in working memory. With respect to the revised role of STM, the question is worded in terms of whether the phonological buffer is necessary for sentence comprehension.

To examine the role of the short-term buffer, let us look at the comprehension abilities of PV and EA. PV could comprehend long sentences of around 16 words. Impairment became apparent when verification of long sentences was made unusually difficult. She displayed a variety of syntactic comprehension and judgment abilities except when anomalies occurred between widely separated elements in stories (Vallar and Baddeley, 1987). EA, on the other hand, was one of the cases with conduction aphasia shown to have asyntactic comprehension. Contrary to the typical pattern in aphasia, performance improved from auditory stimuli to reading (Friedrich, et al., 1985).

Friedrich and others (1985) concluded that EA's phonological buffer impairment could not account for her pattern of sentence comprehension. Comprehension processes continued to operate despite the short-term memory disorder. EA's clinical performances seemed to reflect "an inability to maintain and co-ordinate different levels of processing simultaneously" (p. 409). Thus, Friedrich appeared to entertain the possibility that EA had a limitation in managing resources in working memory. Another possibility was based on the assumption that "a phonological code...is the primary means by which important syntactic markers are represented" (p. 409). With her phonological buffer impairment, EA was not encoding grammatical morphemes.

Phonological Output Processes

Sound-related errors can be a distraction when listening to someone with conduction aphasia. A traditional approach to classification is to refer to all sound-related errors as phonemic paraphasias. In Chapter 1, Table 1.3 displays a system in which formal paraphasias are real words (e.g., *laser* for *razor*) and phonemic paraphasias are nonwords (e.g., *slazer*). The sound-relatedness of errors suggest that word-finding in conduction aphasia is different from the word-finding disorder in anomic aphasia. Conduction aphasia does not seem to involve the "all-or-none" retrieval found in anomic aphasia.

Again, two-stage theories of semantic and lexical processing become a framework for diagnosis. Best (1996) analyzed a case who produced real-word sound-related errors (i.e., formal paraphasias). MF had anomic aphasia according to interpretive guidelines of the *Western Aphasia Battery.* However, "had he scored only one less word correct on the repetition subtest, he would be classified as having conduction dysphasia" (p. 448). Again, imageablity and word-length were considered to be variables that could separate semantic impairment from lexical impairment. Unlike Nickels' findings reported in Chapter 4, there was not a clear separation of semantic and lexical effects, indicating that neither serial or interactive theory could account fully for MF's word-finding errors.

Studies of conduction aphasia tend to concentrate on the lexical stage of phonological output. Blumstein (1973) compared the conversational speech of patients with conduction, Broca's, and Wernicke's aphasia. She concluded that the groups were identical in the kind of phonemic errors produced. Perhaps influenced by this work, subsequent studies left the impression that any sound-level error was being called a phonemic paraphasia.

Because some of Blumstein's patients were fluent and others were nonfluent, researchers began to wonder if the widespread use of "phonemic paraphasia" was obscuring important differences in the speech of patients with different aphasias. This has been a particular concern regarding Broca's aphasia, which can be accompanied by motor system impairments of apraxia of speech (AOS) and/or mild dysarthria. There could be different levels of impairment associated with the distinction between phonemic and phonetic levels of speech production.

The ability to diagnose disorders at the phonemic and phonetic levels is partly a function of level of observation (Canter, Trost, and Burns, 1985). The usual clinical strategy is *perceptual analysis* which involves classifying what we hear. *Acoustic analysis* records the speech signal with devices such as a spectrograph. Parameters of acoustic analysis include sound duration and voice onset time (VOT) for voiced sounds. Both of these approaches observe the external result of the production mechanism. *Internal analyses* depend on observing structures or events within the speech mechanism, such as evoked potentials in the brain stem, muscle contraction, or velar movement. As observation gets further from neurological events, the chance of misdiagnosis increases. Thus, the opportunity for error is greatest in perceptual analysis. Researchers thought that errors across syndromes in Blumstein's study sounded alike but were not necessarily the same disorder internally.

Many researchers set out to obtain relevant observations. Spectrographic measures showed longer sound duration in subjects with Broca's aphasia than in the fluent aphasias (Williams and Seaver, 1986). Synergy in VOT was found with fluent aphasias but was lacking in Broca's aphasia or patients with diagnosis of AOS (Blumstein, Cooper, Goodglass, Statlender, and Gottlieb, 1980; Itoh, Sasanuma, Tatsumi, Murakami, Fukusako, and Suzuki, 1982). Velar movement was asynchronous in nonfluent aphasia, whereas timing was normal in fluent aphasias (Itoh, Sasanuma, Hirose, Yoshioka, and Sawashima, 1983). This sample of results indicates that nonfluent aphasia is accompanied by a disruption of the motor system, whereas motor function in fluent aphasias is normal.

Clinicians do not normally have such laboratory support. So, can we hear differences in the speech of nonfluent and fluent aphasias? Table 5.4 is a summary of some differences uncovered in research. Two research teams studied naming and word repetition in Broca's, conduction, and Wernicke's aphasia (Canter, 1988; Canter, et al., 1985; Manoi, Fukusako, Itoh, and Sasanuma, 1983). Conduction aphasia had more substitution errors taken from elsewhere in the same word, called transpositions. Buckingham (1989) called them "linear ordering derailments" that can be anticipatory (e.g., *papple*) or perseverative (e.g., *gingerged*). Speech with Broca's aphasia contained more transitional disruptions from one sound or syllable to the next. Errors increased as a function of motoric complexity in Broca's speech but not in fluent aphasias. All groups made one-feature errors, namely, an incorrect sound close to the target; but three-feature errors were more likely in fluent aphasia.

At Boston University, Kohn and Smith (1990) have been working on ideas about what happens to phonological output processing in fluent aphasias with many sound-related errors. In an extensive analysis of CM, they found that some errors were unlike normal errors. A few interactions occurred across several words in an utterance. In word-interactions, a segment of one word is "copied" into another word. Kohn interpreted these behaviors as an "inability to clear a phonemic output buffer." That is, pieces of lexical items activated for previous production remain stuck in this temporary holding region of working memory.

Later, Kohn and Smith (1995) distinguished two types of phonological difficulty that are indicative of two stages in phonological output processing. The first stage is the activation of a stored "underspecified" *lexical-phonological representation.* Damage to this stage is indicated by greater difficulty in repeating and reading nonwords than real words. The lexical representation is sent to the second stage which consists of sequential *phonemic planning* "from left to right." Damage to this stage, along with intact lexical activation, should cause errors that preserve or simplify the phonological structure of targets. Kohn and Smith found that fluent patients with lexical activation disorder made segmental errors with no

TABLE 5.4 Differential diagnosis of phonological disorders, including the terminology used to designate functional levels. (Garrett's terminology (Figure 5.1) is represented in boldface.)

DISORDER	CNS LOCATION	FUNCTIONAL LOCATION	SPEECH SYMPTOMS
Conduction aphasia	Posterior cortex	**Phonological process (positional level)** Pre-motor stage	Fluency More errors in final position Sequence errors Transpositions anticipatory perseverative No distortions
Apraxia of speech	Anterior, pre-motor cortex	**Regular phonological processes (phonetic)** Pre-articulatory or motor programming Sub-phonemic	Laborious More errors in initial position Transition errors Distortions and substitutions
Dysarthria	Motor cortex and below	**Motor coding process (articulatory)** Execution	Varied distortion and substitution Respiratory and phonatory deficit Impairment at all functional levels

position constraints, whereas fluent patients with phonemic planning disorder made errors that increased systematically from left to right.

In sum, phonemic errors in conduction aphasia are diagnosed as a disorder at a "pre-articulatory" phonemic level in the language system, whereas AOS is a disorder in the articulatory or motor system. Like dysarthria or hemiplegia, AOS can accompany agrammatic aphasia because of site of lesion. AOS contributes to the nonfluency of these cases. Perhaps, we can say that the person with AOS produces an accurate lexical representation with difficulty, whereas conduction aphasia involves an inaccurate lexical representation produced smoothly. With respect to conduction aphasia, disorder underlying repetition deficit may converge on the disorder underlying phonological errors on the basis of phonological processing (Kohn, 1984). That is, there may be a common disorder underlying impairment of a phonological input buffer and a phonological output buffer.

WERNICKE'S APHASIA

Wernicke's aphasia is the most severely impaired fluent syndrome, caused by a lesion in the posterior superior region of the temporal lobe. It is characterized by jargon and severe comprehension deficit. According to Mitchum and others (1990), neologisms are so characteristic that Wernicke's aphasia is one of the few syndromes that can be identified by object-naming errors alone. Also, because of poor recognition of deficit, patients are not at all self-conscious about their neologisms and other paraphasias. The term *jargonaphasia* is seen frequently in a presumed reference to patients with Wernicke's aphasia.

One curious finding in surveys of aphasic populations is a tendency for people with Wernicke's aphasia to be older (i.e., in the 60s) than people with Broca's aphasia (i.e., in the 50s). Coppens (1991) reviewed these studies and the many explanations inspired by this finding. One of the more reasonable explanations is a selection bias in the studies, attributable to a tendency for fluent aphasias to survive longer because lesions are smaller and a tendency for Wernicke's aphasia in the acute stage to have the same pattern of deficit through the chronic stage.

Word Comprehension

When syndromes are compared in tests of comprehension, this group usually makes the most errors along with global aphasia. Because of the severity of comprehension deficit, it is appropriate to focus on word comprehension in Wernicke's aphasia.

A patient may be with a group of people and act as if he does not even hear the conversations. Proximity of the lesion to the primary auditory area, as well as severity of deficit, led researchers to suspect that the processing of linguistic stimuli does not go beyond speech perception. The deficit appears to be like "pure word deafness" (Kirshner, Webb, and Duncan, 1981). Yet, speech perception deficits are not specific to this syndrome and are often not sufficient to reduce language comprehension substantially (Basso, et al., 1977; Blumstein, et al., 1977; Miceli, et al., 1980). Nevertheless, variation of lesion size and location may create an "auditory-predominant" subgroup in which auditory processing is substantially below reading (Heilman, Rothi, Campanella, and Wolfson, 1979; Kirshner, Casey, Henson, and Heinrich, 1989).

A loss or disorganization of semantic memory might reduce comprehension at the word level and produce paraphasias. In an object classification study, Wernicke subjects were impaired in relating objects according to action, function, and physical attributes (Cohen, et al., 1980). In another study, subjects were shown three objects (e.g., apple, banana, pear) and, when ready, were then shown a series of test-objects one at a time (e.g., peach, chair). They had to press a button indicating whether a test-object belonged to the class of objects presented initially. Wernicke's aphasia did not exhibit a unique problem, indicating that semantic content and structure are preserved (Koemeda-Lutz, Cohen, and Meier, 1987).

Part of the surprising findings in Milberg and Blumstein's early work with semantic priming was that subjects with Wernicke's aphasia had the priming effects that did not occur for Broca's aphasia (Milberg, et al., 1987). Yet, Wernicke subjects also had many more errors making lexical decisions, and they performed much worse than Broca subjects in making judgments about the semantic relatedness of word-pairs. In Hagoort's (1993) study with shorter SOAs (prime-target intervals), Wernicke's subjects were primed like those with Broca's aphasia. Thus, the semantic system with Wernicke's aphasia may be intact structurally and at the automatic level of processing. Difficulties occur with slow tasks examining conceptualization at the controlled or strategic level.

Sentence Comprehension

Wernicke's aphasia has been swept up with Broca's aphasia in efforts to determine if aphasias include a broad double dissociation of semantic and syntactic functions. The general hypothesis regarding Wernicke's aphasia has been that it might be a problem in the semantic domain while syntactic capacities remain intact. In this section, we shall consider sentence comprehension as before with respect to the lexical component and then the syntactic component.

Regarding activation of word-meaning in sentences, four Wernicke subjects were quite different from subjects with Broca's aphasia with the cross-modal semantic priming procedure (Swinney, et al., 1989). The Wernicke subjects seemed to be like normal adults, accessing multiple meanings automatically when the LDT was located right after the ambiguous prime. In the follow-up study in which the LDT was located five syllables after the ambiguous prime, the Wernicke subjects continued to show activation of both meanings (Prather, et al., 1994). This is unlike Broca's aphasia but is also unlike neurologically intact adults, indicative of a unique problem with Wernicke's aphasia. The problem appears to be a failure of context to bias or "penetrate" lexical access for the correct interpretation of the ambiguous word. It is as if the lexical-semantic system is stuck in a modular mode.

Regarding structural aspects of sentences, early studies showed that Wernicke's aphasia, while more severely impaired generally, does not differ from other syndromes in the relative difficulty of syntactic forms (e.g., Parisi and Pizzamiglio, 1970). Caramazza and Zurif (1976) were "perplexed" about the performance pattern of five Wernicke subjects in their pivotal study revealing asyntactic comprehension. These subjects performed well on the task and had equal difficulty with syntactic and semantic factors. Caramazza and Zurif wrote frankly about an issue that may pertain to other studies: "The good level of performance in the Wernicke's patients may have been due simply to a bias in the selection of patients; since patients had to have enough comprehension skills to be able to understand our instructions and perform the experimental task, we likely included only very mildly impaired, atypical Wernicke's aphasics" (p. 579).

Like other aphasias, processing canonical order appears to be preserved in Wernicke's aphasia (Bates, et al., 1987a). Shapiro and others (1993) concluded that these patients, unlike Broca's aphasia, are impaired in activating verb-argument structures. The two studies of gap-filling leave us with findings that are as contradictory for Wernicke's aphasia as they are for Broca's aphasia. Zurif and others (1993) found that subjects with Wernicke's aphasia filled gaps, but those with Broca's aphasia did not. Blumstein and her colleagues (1998) obtained nearly the opposite result. The jury will be out for a long time regarding sentence comprehension in Wernicke's aphasia, because people with this syndrome should be difficult to test with sophisticated psycholinguistic procedures.

Word-Retrieval

In clinical tests of object-naming, patients with Wernicke's aphasia make more errors that the other syndromes (Table 5.3). Nouns are easier than verbs in picture description as well as naming (Williams and Canter, 1987). Patients also appear less likely to exhibit the tip-of-the-tongue state (Goodglass, Kaplan, Weintraub, and Ackerman, 1976). Unlike other syndromes, naming to description is more difficult than object naming, perhaps, because of auditory comprehension deficit (Goodglass and Stuss, 1979). Kohn and Goodglass' (1985) naming study indicated that these patients do not differ from others in number of semantic and phonemic errors. Neologisms appear to set them apart (Mitchum, et al., 1990).

Jargon consists of fluent verbalization containing lexical semantic and unrelated paraphasias and sublexical neologisms. We were introduced to this form of aphasia with Gardner's (1974) sample in the first chapter. It has complete sentences with lots of functors and inflections that seem to be in the right places. The sample is hard to interpret with one neologism (i.e., "repuceration") and words like "barbers" that have no apparent connection to context. Because of its minimal neologisms, we would refer to this sample as semantic jargon.

Unrelated and semantic errors indicate that people with Wernicke's aphasia can activate the lexicon. A semantic problem was indicated by the number of semantic paraphasias being correlated with number of semantic errors on a word-comprehension test (Gainotti, 1976). Rinnert and Whitaker (1973) inventoried relationships between semantic paraphasias and targets and compared them to normal word associations. Sixty percent of error-targets corresponded to association norms for the error or the target. It was concluded that "semantic confusions are more like than unlike normal word associations" (p. 66). Thus, semantic errors may come from an intact semantic structure, which is consistent with normal semantic priming effects. A case study led to a *lexical activation hypothesis* stating that flow of activation is reduced between semantic and phonological systems (Ellis, Miller and Sin, 1983).

In his study of word fluency, Grossman (1981) examined the succession of words produced to a category like birds (see Chapter 4). In contrast to nonfluent subjects, patients with Wernicke's aphasia were likely to produce words in the most distant bands of a category and words that did not belong in the category. Patients started producing examples of high typicality and progressed to examples of low typicality. They "often cross the borders around a referential field" (p. 327). Word fluency makes room for strategic processing, and patients with Wernicke's aphasia may be having difficulties using controlled word-finding strategies.

Neologisms tend to contain phonological sequences that are permissible in a patient's language. Exceptions are forms like "chpicters." More examples come from samples provided by Buckingham and Kertesz (1976):

- "I appreciate that farshethe, because they have protocertive" (p. 66).
- "I would say that the mik daysis nosis or chpicters" (p. 70).

Investigators have distinguished two types. **Target-related neologisms** retain some phonological similarity to the target and could be roughly the same as sublexical phonemic paraphasias. **Abstruse neologisms** have little relationship to the target.

Buckingham (1981) asked "Where Do Neologisms Come From?" They could be an extreme manifestation of phonemic paraphasias, called the *conduction theory* (Kertesz and Benson, 1980). For the culprit to be a faulty phonological mechanism, a patient should produce a mix of phonemic paraphasias, neologisms, and ambiguous transformations. Also, the patient should not at the same time be producing other lexical paraphasias "or we could never, in principle, rule them out as possible inputs to the phonemic transformations" (Buckingham, 1981, p. 50). This theory was ruled out at first, because subjects exhibited no "middle ground" (Buckingham and Kertesz, 1976). Later, Buckingham (1987) would "not rule out the possibility that some bizarre lexical productions could stem from severe phonemic paraphasia" (p. 383).

Another proposal was that a patient has "anomic aphasia" but fills empty lexical slots with neologisms, called a *masking theory* (Buckingham, 1981). This would be an automatic or subconscious adjustment in the production system. When lexical activation fails, neologisms become "strings of well-formed phonemes or syllables that fill in the gaps and compensate for words not retrievable from the lexicon" (p. 198). Later, Buckingham (1987) suggested that a *random generator* of syllabic segments produces neologisms. In the context of masking theory, the random generator is assumed to fill gaps left by an underlying anomia. A lesion results in an abnormal process in addition to a damaged normal process.

Buckingham's ideas are similar to Kohn and Smith's stages of phonological output processing used to interpret sound-related errors in conduction aphasia. Abstruse neologisms could arise from damaged lexical activation. Target-related neologisms could arise from damaged phonemic planning (Kohn and Smith 1994). If the latter is so, related errors should show the serial position effect from left to right found with conduction aphasia. In a study of neologistic naming errors, data did not conform to the discrete predictions of the theory. That is, related and remote neologisms did not differ with respect to serial position of phonemic errors (Gagnon and Schwartz, 1997).

Sentence Formulation

In a study of picture description, Wernicke subjects generated as many words as normal subjects (Gleason, Goodglass, Obler, Green, Hyde, and Weintraub, 1980). These aphasic subjects produced many more verbs than nouns and used more indefinite "pointing" words (e.g., this, here) than normals and Broca's subjects. Schwartz (1987) suggested that the syntactic aspects of language formulation are relatively spared in jargonaphasia and, thus, are dissociated from lexical aspects.

There have been relatively few linguistic studies of syntax in jargon. It is a tough corpus, because it can be hard to tell a syntactic error from a semantic one. The inexquisite syntax spoken by neurologically intact persons also confounds interpretation. Picking over grammar in jargon leaves us wondering what can be called a deficit. Yet, the classical idea was that jargonaphasia contains a symptom of commission called **paragrammatism.** This term was suggestive of a neat definitional opposite to agrammatism. According to definition, paragrammatism is the substitution of grammatical morphemes *in fluent utterance.* Having incorporated this notion in the Boston Exam, Goodglass and Kaplan (1983) stated that in paragrammatism "most inflections and small grammatical words fall smoothly into place, but with unsystematic substitutions or omissions of both grammatical morphemes and lexical words (i.e., nouns, verbs, adjectives), and tangled grammatical organization" (p. 7).

The logical notion of paragrammatism has run into a couple of problems. One is that some of the symptoms of commission suggested by this classification do not appear or are hard to find in fluent aphasias. In particular, the phrase level order errors not found in Broca's aphasia were also not found in Wernicke's aphasia in the comparison of English, Italian, and German (Bates, et al., 1988).

The other problem is that people with Wernicke's aphasia exhibit some of the characteristics of agrammatism. In Gleason's study of discourse, these patients used fewer and simpler structures than normal controls. Phrases were sequenced instead of embedded. Because of the similarity of grammatical mistakes in Wernicke's and Broca's aphasias, many investigators have come to argue that there is no difference in syntactic disorder (Heeschen, 1985) or that the traditional distinction needs "conceptual realignment" (Goodglass and Menn, 1985). "We conclude that the contrast between agrammatism (attributed to Broca's aphasia) and paragrammatism (attributed to Wernicke's aphasia) has been greatly exaggerated" (Bates, et al., 1991, p. 137).

Kolk and Heeschen (1990) applied their theory of resource limitations to sentence production in Wernicke's aphasia. Because of their lack of awareness of their jargon, people with Wernicke's aphasia do not employ adaptive strategies. This idea was related to differences in sentence repetition. Patients with agrammatism have more of a mixture of omissions and substitutions than in spontaneous speech, whereas those with jargon have no task effect (Heeschen and Kolk, 1988).

MARTIN EXETER'S APHASIA

In the acute period, Martin Exeter appeared to have severe aphasia. His early confusion included problems with understanding what people were saying to him. He could not answer their questions. When questions required a simple nod for "yes" or a frown for "no," he would often indicate yes for no and no for yes. His CT scan indicated to the doctors that the global condition would probably be temporary. Then, even in his first week in the rehabilitation unit, his language comprehension started improving and he was saying more words. His aphasia was taking on the appearance of Broca's aphasia. A brief aphasia test indicated that he was able to understand simple sentences. His aphasia would change more in the next few months.

During the two weeks or so after his stroke, Martin's "comprehension" was splitting between an improving recognition of what was going on around him and a persistent difficulty with understanding language. It was not until Martin started language treatment that the speech-language pathologist began analyzing his comprehension more than the initial assessment was able to do. The 10 minutes to administer Shewan's *Auditory Comprehension Test for Sentences* showed that passive sentences were difficult for him. He made mostly thematic role order errors. He was able to name more than half the pictures shown to him. He could produce only one or two words with a great deal of effort when answering a question. He used nouns, adjectives, and sometimes a verb.

Occasionally, instead of making the effort to answer, he would say "I can't talk any more" surprisingly easily. When he got especially frustrated, he would blurt out "I don't want to do that anymore." A graduate student getting experience at the hospital asked if this meant that Martin had fluent aphasia. The speech-language pathologist explained that these were only automatic phrases that he says a lot. The student was asked to notice the nature of his propositional speech. His usual conversation consisted only of a painstaking word here or there.

SUMMARY AND CONCLUSIONS

One approach to reducing health care costs is for a rehabilitation team to "develop more specific therapies for disabilities..." (Dobkin, 1995). The opportunity for more specific language therapies is suggested by an increase of precision in the observation of behavior and in the diagnosis of a patient's disorder. In the clinic, we may need to look more closely, for example, at the phonological configuration of sound-related naming errors. The difference between Chapters 4 and 5 indicates that diagnosis has changed from generalizations about aphasia to the identification of an impairment underlying specific aphasic symptoms.

Along with the absence of new supplemental tests in this chapter, a prominently displayed development is the on-line examination of sentence comprehension. If this paradigm is giving us a better idea of what is going wrong in a patient's language system, then assessment procedure may be supplemented accordingly some day. Clinical professionals will be especially responsive if psycholinguistic paradigms identify impairments reliably and the diagnosis makes a difference in treatment accuracy and efficiency.

Asyntactic comprehension is one example of a clinical pattern with multiple explanations in the literature. The asyntactic pattern of a canonicity effect and order errors could be caused by an impaired language processor or reduced working capacity. No single theory has overwhelming support, especially in the absence of comparisons to alternatives. As Blumstein stated, we do not yet know what causes asyntactic comprehension. This lack of definite answers excites scientists and annoys clinicians. We should be patient, however, considering that theories of normal processes are being refined based on hundreds of studies with thousands of young adults. We should not be too demanding of a few pioneering studies with a few aphasic subjects.

However, one promising development in aphasiology is illustrated in a study at the University of Maryland School of Medicine by Berndt, Mitchum, and Wayland (1997). They compared predictions from three different theories of asyntactic comprehension, and then let the chips fall where they may. The three theories were the trace-deletion hypothesis, a grammatical morpheme filter hypothesis, and the increasingly visible capacity constraint hypothesis. Although the capacity constraint hypothesis was most consistent with the results, the conclusions are not really all that important at this point. What is important is that the investigators did not appear to be invested in proving one theory, and hopefully they started a trend.

CHAPTER 6

SPECIAL INVESTIGATIONS

Like a box of chocolates, this chapter contains an assortment of topics. It expands on some previous topics and delves into others not yet covered. The chapter has two main themes. One is the case study approach to testing models of word-level processing. We can give our diagnostic problem-solving skills a good workout by contemplating issues in cognitive neuropsychology. The manifestation of aphasia in various languages is the other principal theme. We shall compare aphasia among different languages and examine the bilingual patient.

MODALITY-SPECIFIC NAMING PROBLEMS

According to traditional diagnosis of aphasia, language impairment should be observed in all major modalities. A problem with naming along with normal language comprehension would be indicative of something else. By turning our attention to nonaphasic misnaming we return to perception and recognition, this time with respect to objects as the stimulus rather than words. Agnosia is a problem in recognizing a stimulus, and failure to recognize an object visually is called **visual object agnosia.** Someone with this disorder can still recognize an object by touching it or hearing a characteristic sound. Visual agnosia may also cause someone to misname an object.

An Expanded Model for Naming

Studies of fluent aphasia expanded the naming model (see Figure 4.2) with more detail regarding phonological output processing in the lexical stage (e.g., lexical activation and planning). Now, we examine expansion at the other end. In the study of neurologically intact or nonaphasic brain-damaged persons, investigators use the naming task to assess object recognition. Correct naming indicates that a person has knowledge of the object.

Regarding the early stages of a naming model, Ellis and Young (1988) believed that "modern studies of agnosia demand a richer type of theory" (p. 33). Ellis and Young's choice of theory is outlined in the model for object-naming in Figure 6.1. This model adds an early sensory stage for initial representation and a couple of perceptual processes preceding recognition. Other processes leading to a naming response are nearly duplicated in the two figures. Without boxes, the model shows representations that are computed by presumed processes. It indicates that perception is more complex than indicated in Chapter 4.

Stages of the model were borrowed from Marr's (1982) influential theory of visual perception, and these stages are briefly defined in Table 6.1. The perceptual process computes a representation of a stimulus (or percept). A viewer-centered representation is "photographed" from the viewer's perspective. An optional three-dimensional object-centered representation is an "objective" 3-D description independent of a viewer's vantage point. It is computed when an object is in an unusual or unfamiliar position with respect to the viewer.

Recognition matches a percept to a "structural description" of like objects already stored in LTM. The stored representation, called a **recognition unit,** is not likely to be a particular object, because we do not remember every pencil, chair, or car we have seen. Instead, the recognition unit represents generalizable physical characteristics of a

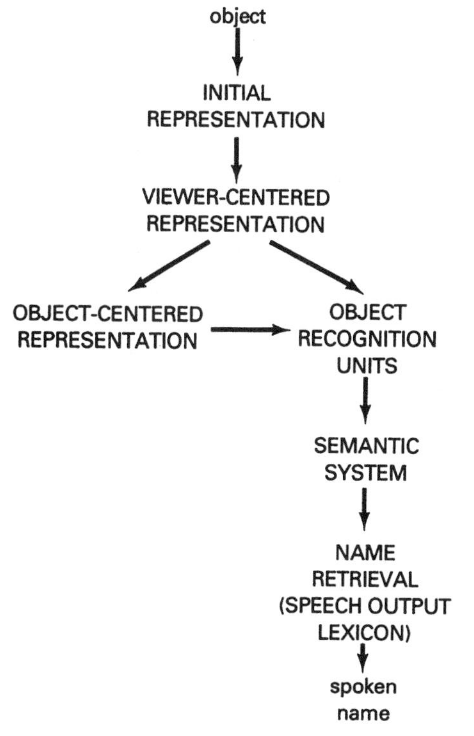

FIGURE 6.1 A model of object recognition when assessed with a naming task. Emphasis is on perception, a component omitted from the naming model in Figure 4.2. This model shows mental representations computed by implied process.

Reprinted by permission from Ellis, A. W., & Young, A. W., *Human cognitive neuropsychology.* Hove, UK: Lawrence Erlbaum, 1988, p. 31.

class of objects such as all pencils, chairs, and cars. Strict recognition is a "pre-semantic" function in the sense that someone need not yet activate conceptual information, especially when recognizing an unusual object or a word like *hubris.* Now, let us see what this theory has to say about visual agnosia.

Types of Agnosia

Over a century ago, Lissauer provided a framework for identifying two types of visual agnosia according to the distinction between perception and recognition:

- **apperceptive visual agnosia,** or insufficient percept or representation of a stimulus; that is, a perceptual deficit that causes recognition difficulty.
- **associative visual agnosia,** failure to relate a good percept to a representation of the object in memory; that is, a recognition problem without perceptual deficit.

If we apply the perception-recognition distinction to the other modalities, it is logically possible for a patient to have apperceptive tactile agnosia, associative tactile agnosia, and so on (Goldberg, 1990). The main point is that a patient may fail to recognize an object for different reasons, one being a perceptual deficit.

Evidence for an object-centered stage of perception comes from a type of apperceptive visual agnosia caused by *right hemisphere damage.* Patients with right parietal lesions usually have no difficulty with the clinical naming test. However, they have been found to make naming errors when objects are presented in an unusual viewpoint (Layman and Greene, 1988). The ability to match objects in the same view is preserved, but it can be difficult to match an object in a typical view with the same object in an unusual view (Warrington and James, 1986). This has something to do with a patient's ability to take a multidimensional perspective of a stimulus so that an atypical appearance can be related to the more typical recognition unit (see discussion of imagery in Chapter 8).

The classical form of agnosia is associative agnosia or impaired recognition with good perception. A patient fails to name objects by sight but matches and copies objects, and names them when presented in other modalities. A **miming task,** in which a patient demonstrates the use of an object, is commonly used to assess recognition in case studies. It is also part of the PICA (see Chapter 3). Dissociation of recognition from perception tends to be caused by *bilateral occipital lesions*

TABLE 6.1 Definition of the stages in the naming model of Figure 6.1.

PROCESS	REPRESENTATION	DESCRIPTION
visual analysis	initial	a 2-dimensional "primal sketch" of an object according to an observer's vantage point
perception	viewer-centered	fills out the percept as a nearly 3-dimensional or "2½-D" sketch according to an observer's vantage point
	object-centered	optional stage; a "3-D" percept independent of vantage point; generalizable to an object in any position
recognition	object recognition unit	relating the percept to a general image or recognition unit; "I've seen the object before"
	semantic system	activating meaning in relation to an object percept; "I know what the object is"

(Bauer and Rubens, 1985). A few cases with left occipital damage have also been reported.

Associative agnosia is often defined a bit differently, namely, as an inability to relate an object (or its percept) to the object's "meaning" (e.g., McCarthy and Warrington, 1990). A patient has difficulty accessing knowledge about a class of objects. The association of this agnosia with semantic deficit is reflected in the following remark:

> *"A class of neuropsychological syndromes exists which can be conceptualized as 'cortical amnesias,' or more accurately, 'amnesias for general knowledge.' These syndromes are rare but well-known, and they are referred to as associative agnosias or asymbolias. It has been argued that, in spite of their traditional designation as forms of agnosia, these syndromes can be naturally understood as deficits of semantic memory" (Goldberg, 1990, p. 468).*

However, when looking at the model in Figure 6.1, we can see that this approach to defining recognition (and associative agnosia) skips over the recognition unit stage in which one can recognize without "knowing."

A pre-semantic recognition unit is needed when sensing that we have seen an object before without necessarily knowing what it is or what it means. Recognition memory involves accessing an episodic representation of a prior experience. If we saw the object a few seconds ago, its representation may still be in a working memory buffer to be matched to the second percept of the object. If we saw an object a few months ago and remember that we saw it, the percept has been matched to a recognition unit in long-term episodic memory.

One method for assessing pre-semantic object recognition is like the lexical decision task. In an *object decision task,* a subject must identify whether an object is meaningful or meaningless. A case with left occipital damage had an object recognition impairment demonstrated this way. It was described as a disorder of "access to the stored structural descriptions for objects" (Davidoff and De Bleser, 1994).

Recognition memory is tested by presenting a series of items, repeating some of them, and asking a subject if an item was seen or heard before. This task is used for studying episodic memory or learning. In one study, a series of abstract designs was presented to groups with left-hemisphere and right-hemisphere strokes (Trahan, Larrabee, and Quintana, 1990). Subjects were asked to identify a design as "new" or "old." Both groups were deficient, but those with RH-dysfunction performed worse than those with LH-dysfunction.

Investigators have disagreed over whether the perception-recognition dichotomy is sufficient to capture the variations among individual cases (e.g., Warrington and Rudge, 1995). For example, let us consider the following comment on apperceptive agnosia:

> *Rather than classify patients who have recognition deficits at later stages of object recognition as having true apperceptive agnosia and those with defects at the earlier stage as pseudo, we suggest that perhaps apperceptive agnosia should be divided into subtypes (e.g. apperceptive agnosia perceptual subtype, apperceptive agnosia-impaired structural representations subtype, etc.)...the perceptual subtype may have to be further subdivided (e.g. apperceptive agnosi-form discrimination subtype) (Heilman and Bowers, 1995, p. 179).*

Humphreys and Riddoch (1987) dealt with the varied patterns of deficit by identifying five types of agnosia. Some of these types represent what others consider to be variations of apperceptive or associative agnosias (Table 6.2).

Optic Aphasia

Someone with optic aphasia has severe difficulty naming visually presented objects but a preserved ability to name objects by touch, sound, or from auditorily presented description. So far, this seems like a visual agnosia, but the difference is that the patient with optic aphasia recognizes objects visually (Davidoff and De Bleser, 1993). Also, the patient is conversationally fluent with intact auditory language comprehension. Nearly all cases are deficient in reading aloud, showing that spoken word production is impaired only for visually presented objects and words (Campbell and Manning, 1996). Most cases have focal lesions in the left occipital lobe.

Optic aphasia indicates that a single-modality naming deficit does not necessarily diagnose a sensory disorder. We still have to evaluate object recognition without verbal response, usually with tasks of miming object use and sorting objects. Optic aphasia is compared to agnosias and regular aphasia in Table 6.3.

Some are skeptical about whether this is a true aphasia because of the belief that an aphasia should entail naming difficulty regardless of modality of nonverbal stimulation (Goodglass, Barton, and Kaplan, 1968). The other side of this doubt is that optic aphasia might still be a visual object agnosia, despite claims that perception and recognition are intact. More specifically, some believe that a case of apparent optic aphasia can be really an associative agnosia (e.g., Riddoch and Humphreys, 1987), especially considering that some tests of perception and recognition show "good" but imperfect performance. Campbell and Manning (1996) noted "some fragility of visual processing" in one case with test scores above chance but outside the normal range.

TABLE 6.2 Approximate alignment of two classifications of agnosias relative to the object naming model in Table 6.1.

WARRINGTON'S AGNOSIAS	HUMPHREYS & RIDDOCH'S AGNOSIAS	LOCUS OF DYSFUNCTION	SITE OF LESION
apperceptive	shape	initial representation	bilateral occipital (primary visual area)
	integrative	viewer-centered perception	right occipito-parietal; bilateral occipital
	transformation	object-centered perception	right parietal
associative	semantic	object recognition	bilateral occipital (association area)
	semantic access	semantic system	bilateral posterior; LH

TABLE 6.3 A comparison of disorders causing misnaming of visually presented objects.

	OBJECT PERCEPTION	OBJECT RECOGNITION	VISUAL NAMING	TACTILE NAMING	AUDITORY NAMING
apperceptive visual agnosia	impaired	impaired	impaired	intact	intact
associative visual agnosia	intact	impaired	impaired	intact	intact
optic aphasia	intact	intact	impaired	intact	intact
aphasia	intact	intact	impaired	impaired	impaired

Campbell and Manning also suggested that optic aphasia is problematic for the serial naming model, because there is nothing in it that localizes impairment. Perception is intact as shown by object matching. Recognition and the semantic system seem intact as shown by object categorization and sorting. Lexical access for language production is intact as indicated by naming to other modalities and good word fluency. Thus, the model has to provide for word-finding with respect to a specific input modality. If it turns out to be a valid entity, optic aphasia may expose a feature of language function that we did not know about 20 years ago. The language system may contain components that are friendlier to some modalities than others.

MORE COGNITIVE NEUROPSYCHOLOGY

As indicated in Chapter 4, cognitive psychology and cognitive neuropsychology have the same goal, which is to determine the nature of normal cognition. The main difference is that cognitive psychology relies on neurologically intact subjects, usually in large groups, whereas cognitive neuropsychology (CN) relies on neurologically impaired subjects, often as case studies. A single case is often used to test a *process model* depicting the mental processes that take place when a *particular task* is performed. CN has already influenced the previous discussion of agnosias and the introduction to naming in Chapter 4. The two main topics are semantic memory and reading.

Semantic Memory

Let us examine two related questions. Both pertain to the manner in which impairments of the "semantic system" are diagnosed. The first question relates to the use of category-specific deficits to diagnose disorders of the semantic system. The other question addresses whether brain damage shows that we have one semantic memory or several semantic memories.

Some investigators believe that deficits in specific conceptual categories are indicative of a degradation of an area of the conceptual store. In turn, such deficits indicate that semantic memory is organized into conceptually coherent regions. One commonly observed **category-effect** occurs in comparisons between living and nonliving things across a variety of tasks. In cases of viral encephalitis, this *animacy effect* manifested as severe impairment for animals, foods, and plants, and much better performance with inanimate objects (Sartori, Job, Miozzo, and Zago, 1993; Silveri, and Gainotti, 1988; Sheridan and Humphreys, 1993; Warrington and Shallice, 1984).

Funnell and Sheridan (1992) were suspicious of some of these results because living things are often less familiar than nonliving things. When they controlled for familiarity with a case of traumatic brain injury, they found a familiarity effect but no animacy effect. Hillis and others (1990) noted that Silveri and Gainotti's case had more difficulty with wild animals than domestic animals, which may be one basis for an effect based more on education or cultural experience than on the selectivity of brain damage.

Two research groups have been arguing over a more fundamental feature of the semantic system. A group in the United States has favored a **unitary semantics** position which states that a single semantic memory, as shown in Figure 6.2a. is sufficient to account for the effects of brain damage (Caramazza, Hillis, Rapp, and Romani, 1990; Rapp, Hillis, and Caramazza, 1993). A group in England has favored a **multiple semantics** position which states that we possess more than one semantic memory as indicated in Figure 6.2b (Shallice, 1987, 1988b, 1993; McCarthy and Warrington, 1990; Warrington, 1975; Warrington and Shallice, 1984). Warrington's research team has been prolific in diagnosing neurological dysfunctions according to the multiple semantics view.

The main support for multiple semantic memories has been the dissociation between object processing and verbal processing observed in agnosias, aphasias, and other disorders (Shallice, 1988a; McCarthy and Warrington, 1990). After Warrington's (1975) original study of two cases with Alzheimer's dementia, the principal evidence came from a comparison between *cued definitions* tasks. Patients were asked for definitions to a picture cue or a spoken word cue. Aphasia, with its greater impairment with words, was diagnosed as a dysfunction of a verbal semantic system (e.g., Warrington and McCarthy, 1983). Associative agnosia, with a greater deficit given object cues, was diagnosed as an impairment in a visual semantic system (e.g., McCarthy and Warrington, 1986).

Some investigators were critical of Warrington and Shallice's evidence and conclusions. Riddoch and Humphreys examined data that Warrington (1975) used to diagnose dissociations in cases AB and EM (Riddoch, Humphreys, Coltheart, and Funnell, 1988). AB, who was diagnosed with a visual semantic deficit, had an overall visual task score (112/160) that was similar to the verbal score (109/160). EM, diagnosed with a verbal deficit, had a verbal score (104/160) that was inferior to the visual score (132/160). Thus, a dissociation was not really evident with AB. All scores were deficient relative to normal controls, indicative of a disorder that was broader than a single domain. Humphreys and Riddoch (1988) argued that data could be explained by appealing to structural descriptions in recognition units instead of a distinctive visual semantic memory.

The Caramazza-Hillis team has probably come down hardest on multiple semantics theory. They have been especially critical of the empirical basis for Warrington and Shallice's claims, such as relying mainly on the cued definitions task rather than a wider variety of tests. The case in Italy, who had difficulty with wild animals, was presented visual and verbal semantic memory tests in which one was biased to wild animals and the other was biased to domestic animals (Hillis, Rapp, Romani, and Caramazza, 1990). Thus, the effect could have been due to familiarity rather than a difference between visual and verbal memory stores.

Finally, outside the debate over semantic systems, other investigators in England have identified a disorder of semantic memory called **semantic dementia** (Graham, Lambon Ralph, and Hodges, 1997; Hodges, Patterson, and Tyler, 1994; Snowden, Griffiths, and Neary, 1996). Like primary progressive aphasia (see Chapter 2), it is caused by non-Alzheimer lobar degeneration. Semantic dementia has the following characteristics:

- progressive comprehension deficits with words, not sentences
- progressive severe naming deficit
- surprisingly mild word-finding difficulties in effortless spontaneous speech
- intact phonological and grammatical features of utterances
- surface dyslexia and agraphia
- intact episodic memory, visuospatial skills, and nonverbal problem-solving

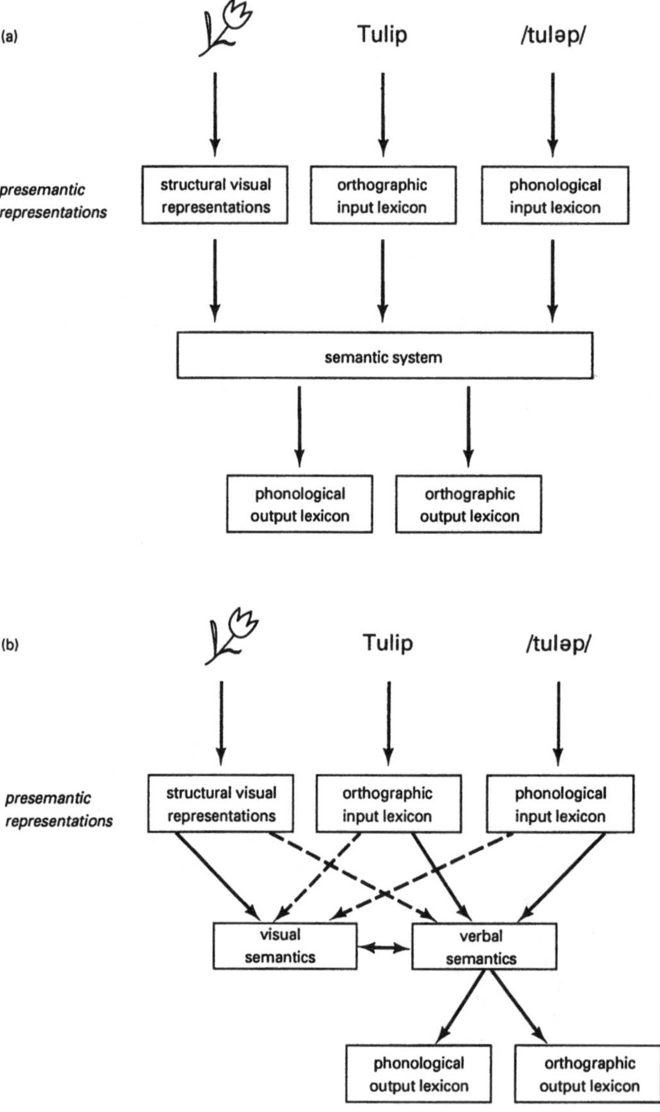

FIGURE 6.2 Relationships among lexical, visual, and semantic representations often proposed in cognitive neuropsychology. Two hypotheses have been debated: (a) semantic memory is independent of lexical and visual-object representations; (b) semantic memory is divided into visual and verbal forms.

Reprinted by permission from Hillis, A. E., Rapp, B. C., Romani, C., & Caramazza, A., Selective Impairment of semantics in lexical processing. *Cognitive Neuropsychology, 7,* 1990, pp. 194, 223. Lawrence Erlbaum, publisher.

A speech-language pathologist might diagnose these symptoms as a fluent aphasia. One exception to most aphasias, however, is the problem comprehending words but not sentences. Also, deficits are not solely in the verbal domain. Patients with semantic dementia have face recognition problems early in the disease and are deficient in picture-based tests of semantic knowledge. The latter extension of semantic difficulties led to the label for this disorder, even though Hodges and others (1994) claimed to have adopted the term semantic dementia "to describe a form of progressive fluent aphasia" (p. 507).

Reading Words

Word reading may be the "flagship" of single-case cognitive neuropsychology. *Reading aloud* is the pivotal task. As with all task-related models, reading models are suggestive of hypotheses about the impaired component that could be responsible for a pattern of performance on a variety of tasks. When an impairment can be identified, the models indicate alternative routes to successful reading. Reading problems are especially important to aphasic patients who want to use a computer at home and who are particularly fastidious about their spelling.

Figure 6.3 identifies common components of a CN-model for reading aloud without the usual connecting arrows. CN-models usually contain two routes from visual input to spoken response. In the primary or **lexical-semantic route,** a percept of the stimulus activates the lexicon (i.e., input-related form), which activates semantic memory, which then activates the lexicon again (i.e., output-related form) to guide speaking. A "nonlexical" or **conversion route** by-passes the semantic system, providing a capability for reading an unfamiliar word aloud (e.g., *Pocumtuck*).

PRIMARY ROUTE	ALTERNATE ROUTE	DESCRIPTION
visual analysis	visual analysis	perception percept formation or stimulus representation
orthographic input lexicon		recognition activating stored orthographic representation or "word-form unit"
	grapheme-phoneme conversion	recoding of orthographic percept into phonological representation according to regular spelling-to-sound conversion rules
semantic system		comprehension activating a concept in semantic memory related to orthographic or phonological form
phonological output lexicon		activating a phonological form related to the concept
acticulatory mechanism	acticulatory mechanism	motor speech processes

FIGURE 6.3 Stages in dual-route models employed to account for reading words aloud. Normally an arrow is drawn from one stage to the next. In this basic version, one route activates semantic memory, whereas the alternate route activates a recoding or conversion mechanism that bypasses semantic memory.

The ability to pronounce unfamilar words or nonwords depends on a rule-based spelling-to-sound conversion mechanism, called "phonological reading."

Clinical investigators try to identify a component of the reading process that is responsible for symptom patterns in acquired dyslexias. In componental analysis, researchers manipulate stimulus variables and record spoken reading errors called **paralexias.** Stimulus variables and types of errors are shown in Table 6.4. Some variables relate strictly to word form such as whether a string of letters is a real word, a nonword, or a "pseudoword" that comes close to being a real word. Other variables pertain to the semantic system such as a word's concreteness or imageability. Assessment includes administering other tasks such as word repetition to determine if a disorder is specific to one input modality.

One approach to diagnosis is to relate core performance patterns to a classification of dylexias (e.g., McCarthy and Warrington, 1990). Research often entails finding cases with basic symptoms of a category and then doing futher analysis to explain the symptom pattern according to the process model. Classification begins with a general distinction between *peripheral dyslexias* and *central dyslexias,* roughly corresponding to the distinction between sensory and cognitive levels of function (Shallice, 1988). Except for "pure alexia" (or alexia without agraphia), these types of dyslexia are usually one part of a more pervasive disorder such as aphasia or attentional impairments.

The most common classification system is summarized in Table 6.5. In peripheral dyslexias, reading problems are caused by impairments outside the reading system. Central dyslexias are dis-

TABLE 6.4 Symptoms observed in reading aloud as a function of word characteristics and paralexic error.

	SYMPTOM	DEFINITION	EXAMPLES
stimulus factors	word superiority effect	real words more accurate than nonwords	*clean* better than *blean*
	grammatical category effect	difference between content words and function words	*tree* better than *the* *the* better than *tree*
	concreteness or imageability effect	concrete words more accurate than abstract words	*camera* better than *danger*
	regularity effect	regular words more accurate than irregular words	*mint* better than *pint* *cove* better than *love*
paralexias	visual	looks like word	"plant" for *planet* "camping" for *campaign*
	phonological	sounds like word	"cambane" for *campaign*
	regularization	pronouncing an irregular word according to regular grapheme-phoneme conversion rules	"hayve" for *have* "sue" for *sew*
	inflectional (morphological)	changes structure, not grammatical category	"plant" for *plants* "running" for *run*
	derivational (morphological)	changes structure and grammatic category	"strange" for *stranger* "territorial" for *territory*
	semantic	similar meaning	"coast" for *seashore* "tear" for *crying*

orders of the reading process and can be a component of aphasia. The following are key characteristics of these impairments:

- In **phonological dyslexia,** there is a severe difficulty pronouncing nonwords, and familiarity is a strong factor. This disorder indicates that "the processes for pronouncing known words must be separable from those for pronouncing unknown words" (Ellis and Young, 1988, p. 211).
- In **surface dyslexia,** spelling-sound regularity is a strong factor. Nonwords and function words can be read aloud by the aforementioned phonological reading mechanism.
- **Deep dyslexia** is the reverse of surface dyslexia in the sense that nonwords and function words are harder to read than real content words. A patient makes a lot of semantic errors. Sometimes errors are visually mediated, such as reading *sympathy* as "orchestra." This error may have been accessed via the percept "symphony." There are a couple of opinions as to the model-based cause of deep dyslexia.

When a component process is impaired or a route is blocked, persons with acquired dyslexias appear to use compensatory strategies for reading aloud or for reading comprehension. A common

TABLE 6.5 Types of dyslexia. Central dyslexias consist of phonological, surface, and deep types.

CLASSIFICATION	SYMPTOMS	DIAGNOSIS
Visual (peripheral)	• visual paralexias • reading one letter at a time	• possibly "pure alexia" • usually left occipito-parietal lesion
Attentional (peripheral)	• visual errors with the left or right side of words • cannot name parts of visual arrays but can name them in isolation	• attentional neglect of the left or right side of a word • right or left parietal lobe lesion (see Chapter 8)
Phonological	• word superiority effect (real words much easier than nonwords) • good nonword repetition (auditory input) • can pronounce irregular words	• impaired conversion route, whereas orthographic and phonological lexicons per se are intact • usually left posterior lesion
Surface	• strong regularity effect • regularization errors • no semantic errors • nonwords and functors better than content words	• damage to lexical or semantic stages of the primary route • usually left posterior lesion
Deep	• mainly semantic errors • visual and derivational errors • strong word superiority effect • content words better than functors • concreteness effect	• impaired grapheme-phoneme conversion, or • damage to mapping input to semantics or semantics to output • left hemisphere lesion, including fronto-temporal lesions

strategy is called **letter-by-letter reading.** The key observation is an abnormally slow reading time, noted specifically by a large increase in reading latency as word length increases. It can take up to three or four seconds to read 3-letter words and a two-to-three second increase for each additional letter. A letter-by-letter reader is often identified as someone with pure alexia (or alexia without agraphia) or vice versa. However, reading one letter at a time is observed with various types of dyslexia. Other compensatory strategies include the following:

- *reading by sight* to compensate for the spelling-sound conversion problem in phonological dyslexia
- *reading by sound* to compensate for semantic route damage in surface dyslexia

Others take another route to diagnosis, bypassing classification of dyslexia and relating results of evaluation directly to components in a process-model (e.g., Hillis and Caramazza, 1995a, 1995b; Tainturier and Caramazza, 1996). Hillis and Caramazza (1992) claimed that classification is abitrary and is "not informative with respect to the nature of damage that underlies the reading disorder" (p. 250). They argued that classification-based studies are "empirically inadequate" mainly because of incomplete testing biased to a classification. Also, classified cases can have different explanations (e.g., Berndt, Haendiges, Mitchum, and Wayland, 1996), which can make it difficult to choose a reading therapy based on a classification (Price and Humphreys, 1992). Hillis and Caramazza advocated that "all theoretically relevant aspects of performance in language and other cognitive tasks should be considered in determining the level of impairment for every patient" (p. 251).

To maintain an objectivity in case studies, investigators often avoid reporting diagnostic classification of aphasia syndrome and location of lesion. As a result, it can be difficult to relate the case to others in the clinic. Also, there does not seem to be a fixed relationship between dyslexia classification and diagnostic categories of aphasia. Table 6.6 shows some of the case studies in which an aphasia syndrome was diagnosed along with a diagnosis of the patient's reading difficulty. Different types of aphasia can have the same reading impairment; and one type of aphasia, such as Broca's aphasia, can have different types of reading impairment. Thus, we cannot take a short-cut to diagnosing a reading impairment, such as diag-

TABLE 6.6 A guide to finding case studies when clinical syndrome was diagnosed.

	CASE	DYSLEXIA CATEGORY	SOURCE
agrammatic	DE	phonological	Patterson (1978)
or Broca's	JH	surface	Watt, Jokel, and Behrmann (1997)
	HH	deep	Laine and Niemi (1997)
	VS	deep	Nolan and Caramazza (1983)
	BL	deep	Nolan and Caramazza (1982)
anomic	PR	peripheral	Price and Humphreys (1993)
	EW	peripheral	Price and Humphreys (1992)
	MS	phonological	Friedman (1996)
	EST	surface	Kay and Patterson (1985)
conduction	BR	phonological	Friedman (1996)
Wernicke's	MP	surface	Behrmann and Bub (1992)
transcortical	JD	phonological	Farah, Stowe, and Levinson (1996)
sensory	TL	phonological	Friedman, Beeman etal (1993)

nosing Broca's aphasia and then assuming that the patient has a particular reading disorder.

Psycholinguists are not particularly interested in developing models for specific tasks and are more interested in testing general theories of reading for any reading task. Thus, there is little regard for speech output processes when studying word recognition and comprehension with a lexical decision task (Crowder and Wagner, 1992; Rayner and Pollatsek, 1989). Psycholinguists have tested the idea that a grapheme-phoneme conversion mechanism can come before activating the mental lexicon for reading unfamiliar words, rather than being a mechanism that bypasses lexical and semantic components (e.g., Figure 6.4). A common method is form priming, in which the prime is imperceptible consciously (e.g., Lukatela, et al., 1998).

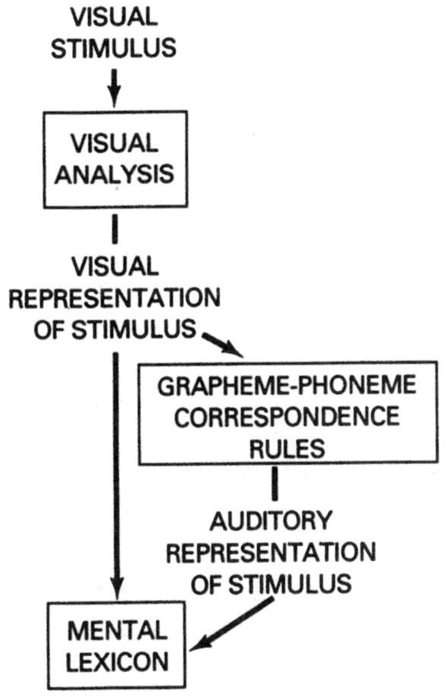

FIGURE 6.4 A theory of printed word recognition in which a representation of a stimulus is related to a representation of the lexical item in the mental lexicon. Sometimes the graphemic representation is first automatically recoded into a phonemic code.

Reprinted by permission from Garnham, A., *Psycholinguistics: Central topics*. London: Methuen, 1985, p. 60.

Findings with the slow controlled tasks of CN-based case studies may differ from findings with fast tasks designed to study automatic obligatory processes. Bub (1995) found a case of pure alexia who displayed the expected slow letter-by-letter reading for a semantic judgment task but not for a lexical decision task.

UNIVERSAL APHASIA

The brain is, of course, a universal structure, and strokes are the same across cultures. However, aphasiology in the United States has been built upon what Bates and Wulfeck (1988) called an *anglocentrism* in which aphasia has been studied mainly with respect to its appearance in English (also, Niemi and Laine, 1991). Universal mechanisms of aphasia are more likely to be determined by comparing different languages. Most interest has been directed at grammatical features, with separate investigations of grammatical morphology and syntactic structure.

A few research teams have compared languages directly, called **cross-linguistic research** or comparative aphasiology. One team compared Broca's and Wernicke's aphasias in English, Italian, and German for comprehension and production (Bates and Wulfeck, 1989). A second team focused on production in a project called the Cross-Language Agrammatism Study (CLAS I) involving 14 languages (Menn and Obler, 1990). CLAS II was formed more recently, and the team published a comparison of Swedish, French, German, Polish, and English (Ahlsén, Nespoulous, Dordain, Stark, Jarema, Kadzielwa, Obler, and Fitzpatrick, 1996). Also, since CLAS I, smaller teams have formed such as one comparing Dutch, German, Swedish, and Finnish (Tesak and Niemi, 1997) and another comparing English and Japanese (Menn, Reilly, Hayashi, Kamio, Fujita, and Sasanuma, 1998).

Language Comprehension

As we know from the study of sentence comprehension, universal thematic roles of agent and recipient are conveyed through linguistic cues such as word order and grammatical morphemes. English speakers rely a great deal on word order to signify agents and recipients of an action, whereas other Indo-European languages rely on a more intricate system of grammatical morphemes as well as word order for signaling thematic roles. For example, Italian signifies thematic role with inflectional case-marking of nouns such as accusative (i.e., recipient role) and dative (i.e., indirect object or goal). French employs more determiners than English, such as distinguishing gender of nouns.

First, let us consider inflectional endings or case-markings. Studies have shown that retention of grammatical knowledge is similar across languages (e.g., Wulfeck, Bates, and Capasso, 1991). In a comparison of Turkish and Hungarian, subjects across three syndromes were impaired in using case markings to comprehend (MacWhinney, Osman-Sagi, and Slobin, 1991). As in studies with English, subjects with Wernicke's aphasia had more difficulty than Broca and anomic subjects. The use of morphology to signal attachment (i.e., subject-verb agreement) was impaired in Broca's and Wernicke's aphasia in English, Italian, and German (Bates, Friederici, and Wulfeck, 1987a). With other languages, subjects with Broca's aphasia show difficulty with inflection but no problem in the use of semantic information (e.g., Smith and Bates, 1987; Smith and Mimica, 1984).

Aphasic patients retain a capacity for processing fundamental canonical order in many languages (Bates, et al., 1987a; MacWhinney, et al., 1991). We know that English speakers have difficulty understanding noncanonical expressions (e.g., passives). In English, the fundamental thematic sequence is subject-verb-object (SVO) as in *Mother bought bread.* In Japanese, canonical order is subject-object-verb (SOV) as in *Mother bread bought.* This difference gives an investigator an opportunity to test whether comprehension difficulty is related to a particular surface form or to the more universal attribute of canonicity no matter what the form is. Hagiwara and Caplan (1990) found that sentences with the Japanese canonical SOV order were understood with less difficulty than deviations from this order. This suggests that canonicity is a more important factor than surface structure.

Researchers have compared word order and inflections for sentence comprehension. In an order-dependent language like English, word-order errors were easier to identify than inflection errors; whereas in an inflection-dependent language like Italian, inflectional errors were easier to identify (Wulfeck, Bates, and Capasso, 1991). Regarding Italian, asyntactic comprehension appears to affect inflection more. In a pattern opposite of that found in English, German and Italian patients relied on word order cues in an apparent compensation for morphological deficit (Bates, et al., 1987a). In Turkish and Hungarian, switches of order did not pose a problem when case markings were available (MacWhinney, et al., 1991).

Language Production

Cross-linguistic researchers suspected that agrammatism would be manifested differently depending on the importance of grammatical morphemes in a language. Perhaps, the most striking discovery was the variability of agrammatism among languages and among patients within languages. This was surprising to English-speaking aphasiologists who had become comfortable with thinking of agrammatism as a symptom of omission. Patients with Broca's aphasia substitute grammatical morphemes more often in other languages. Substitution errors for inflections and function words occur in German (Bates, Friederici, and Wulfeck, 1987b), Hungarian (MacWhinney and Osman-Sagi, 1991) Italian (Miceli, et al., 1989), French (Nespoulous, et al., 1988), and Hebrew (Grodzinsky, 1984). Omissions do occur more often in English than in other languages.

Tesak and Niemi (1997) found that the ratio of omission to substitution is quite variable among languages with 66 to 1 percent in Dutch and 7 to 4 percent in Swedish. The range is from nearly complete absence of substitution to equal

TABLE 6.7 A sample of small-scale cross-linguistic comparisons to English.

ENGLISH AND	SUBJECTS	KEY FINDING	REFERENCE
French	nonfluent aphasia	sensitivity to morphological grammatical markings in comprehension similar in the two languages	Nicol, Jakubowicz, and Goldblum (1996)
Chinese	Broca's aphasia fluent aphasia	morphological and syntactic limitations comparable in English and the Cantonese dialect of Chinese	Yiu and Worrall (1996)
Japanese	varied aphasias	in narration, pragmatic positioning of protagonist at beginning of sentences, called empathy, is preserved in both languages	Menn, Reilly, Hayashi, et al. (1998)
Dutch, French	Broca's aphasia	negative sentences more difficult than positives for French and English, not for Dutch; linguistic form of negation differs from Dutch, indicating the linguistic form is the problem instead of negation per se	Rispens, Bastiaanse, et al. (1997)
Dutch, Hungarian	fluent aphasia	some structural simplification of verbal expression in all languages, especially in using subordinate clauses	Bastiaanse, Edwards, and Kiss (1996)

rates of substitution and omission. Table 6.7 summarizes other relatively recent findings.

The occurrence of morphological substitutions in Broca's aphasia has implications for the traditional dichotomy between agrammatism and paragrammatism (i.e., ommission vs. substitution). Substitution errors, which are difficult to detect in English, occurred with similar frequency in Broca's and Wernicke's aphasia in German (Bates, et al., 1987b). In studies of German and Dutch aphasias, Heeschen and Kolk (1988) detected differences in spontaneous speech in which Broca's aphasia has a higher proportion of omissions to substitutions, whereas Wernicke's aphasia has a mixture or a predominance of substitutions.

Regarding structural characteristics of sentence production, cross-linguistic studies addressed the status of word order in picture descriptions (Bates, Friederici, Wulfeck, and Juarez, 1988). Phrase-level morphological sequence errors, defined early in Chapter 5, did not occur in English, Italian, and German for either Broca's or Wernicke's aphasia. To study preservation of canonical order, three-element productions were examined. Canonical SVO order was used 81 percent of the time across syndromes and the three languages. Order around a preposition was correct across syndromes and languages about 70 percent of the time. These results were well above chance, and aphasic subjects did not differ from normals. The canonical order of SOV also appeared to be preserved in Turkish speakers (Bates and Wulfeck, 1988). Resiliance of canonical order appears to be a universal feature of aphasia. Sometimes, canonical order is overused as a "safe-harbor," especially for speakers of Italian and German.

American Sign Language

American Sign Language (ASL) for the deaf is expressed in a visuospatial mode and possesses grammatical features akin to spoken languages. "Despite the important differences in form, signed and spoken languages clearly share underlying structural principles. Like spoken language, sign language exhibits formal structuring at the lexical and grammatical levels, similar kind and degree of morphological patterning, and a complex, highly rule-governed grammatical and syntactic patterning" (Poizner, Klima, and Bellugi, 1987, p. 21).

Researchers at the Salk Institute for Biological Studies in California examined a small group of deaf persons who suffered single strokes in the left or right cerebral hemisphere. Subjects with left hemisphere-damage had disorders similar to the aphasias observed in spoken languages (e.g., lexical and grammatical deficits). Those with right hemisphere-damage did not exhibit language problems. The conclusion was that "the left cerebral hemisphere in humans may have an innate predisposition for the central components of language, independent of language modality" (Poizner, et al., 1987, p. 212).

ASL codes grammatical information spatially. Because the right hemisphere is specialized for visuospatial processing, the Salk team has been interested in comparing the effect of left and right hemisphere lesions on spatial coding in this language (Hickok, Say, Bellugi, and Klima, 1996). This question is explored in Chapter 8 on right hemisphere dysfunction.

Musical notation could also be considered to be a code with arbitrary symbols and a syntax. After a left hemisphere stroke, the composer Ravel recognized musical patterns but had difficulties reading musical notation, naming notes, and finding their location on the keyboard of his piano (Alajouanine, 1948). These observations provide additional input to the question of a universal aphasia. Our definition and understanding of aphasia has to be compatible with impairments of ASL and other formal languages.

APHASIA IN BILINGUAL INDIVIDUALS

Half the people of the world use at least two languages. Grosjean (1989) defined bilinguals as "those people who use two or more languages in their everyday lives" (p. 4). He has taken a wholistic view of people who speak two languages. A bilingual person "cannot be decomposed into two separate parts...rather, he or she has a unique and specific linguistic configuration" (Grosjean, 1989, p. 6).

Does aphasia affect a bilingual person's languages equally or differently? In a review of cases reported over several decades, Albert and Obler (1978) found that each language seemed to be impaired. Languages differed in severity of aphasia in 80 percent of the cases. In another retrospective study, Paradis (1977) found that 41 percent seemed to have aphasia equally between the two languages spoken, twice the proportion reported by Albert and Obler. Paradis noted other studies reporting as high as 90 percent having similar deficit across two languages. In a controlled study, accuracy and latency of object-naming did not differ in two languages for a group of 10 aphasic bilinguals (Vogel and Costello, 1986). In another study, there was no significant difference on verbal subtests of an aphasia battery (Porch and de Berkeley-Wykes, 1985). Therefore, the answer to our question may await building a large body of controlled comparisons, but it appears that languages may be impaired equally or differently in bilingual aphasia.

Investigators have wondered if there is a simple basis for a difference in aphasia between languages. Long ago Ribot and Pitres thought that differences should occur for different reasons

(Paradis, 1977). The **rule of Ribot** ("primacy rule") stated that the native or first-learned language should be less impaired, which was supported in a study of some word-level tasks (Junque, Vendrell, Vendrell-Brucet, and Tobena, 1989). On the other hand, the **rule of Pitres** stated that the most frequently used language should be less impaired because of "habit strength." However, research has been unable to support one rule or the other as a broad generalization. **Alternating aphasia** is an unusual pattern in which expression with one language is impaired one day, and the other language is impaired the next day, and so on (Paradis, Goldblum, and Abidi, 1982). The likely pattern can be complicated by a dissociation between comprehension and expression. Good comprehension can be retained in two languages, while verbal expression is severely impaired in one language.

Bilingualism is hard to study. Early case studies and the retrospective reviews of 20 years ago are considered to be "primitive" (Solin, 1989; Zatorre, 1989). Albert and Obler (1978) suggested that their data "cannot be taken to represent that which would be seen in a systematically tested population of polyglot aphasics" (p. 141). They were skeptical of their proportions based on case studies because patients with a discrepancy between languages were probably the more interesting to report. More importantly, bilinguals vary in (a) proficiency in the second language, (b) age of learning the second language, (c) manner of learning the second language (e.g., naturally or formally), (d) context of learning the second language (e.g., where it is predominant), (e) affective factors such as cultural attitudes toward a language, and (f) linguistic relationship between languages because some languages are more similar than others (Obler, Zatorre, Galloway, and Vaid, 1982).

Also, the language behavior of a "stable bilingual" varies according to the situation. When bilingual people converse with monolingual people, bilinguals enter a **monolingual mode** in which they deactivate the language not known by the monolinguals. When conversing bilinguals share the same two languages, the conversants enter a **bilingual mode** in which they activate both languages. An aphasic bilingual is likely to display different behaviors depending on the interactional mode necessitated by a clinician's linguistic status. Failure to consider the conditions in which multiple languages are evaluated has been one weakness in the study of aphasia's intrusion on the bilingual's linguistic skill.

A diagnostic problem is to distinguish aphasia from normal bilingual behavior. Bilingual behavior may be seen as abnormal to a monolingual clinician who is not familiar with bilingual behavior. One feature of bilingual behavior is **language mixing,** which occurs mainly in a bilingual mode. Mixing is "any case in which elements from one language are used in the context of another language" (Perecman, 1984). The concept of "interference" appears in the literature, but linguists prefer the broader notion of mixing which can be quite intentional. The language chosen for conversation between bilinguals is the base language. Once the base language is chosen, another language is mixed in by *code-switching* (i.e., reverting completely to the other language for a word, phrase, or sentence) or by *borrowing* a word from the other language and integrating it with the base language such as a French speaker using "weekend" or "brunch" including attachment of French inflection.

Perecman (1984) estimated that language mixing occurs in less than 10 percent of multilingual aphasias and more often in Wernicke's aphasia than other syndromes. She tried to differentiate aphasic language mixing from nonaphasic mixing. "Lexical-level mixing," such as word borrowing, occurs in normal and aphasic bilinguals. In an object-naming task, some patients occasionally name in the unsolicited language (Vogel and Costello, 1986). Perecman claimed that "utterance-level mixing" is a phenomenon of aphasia as opposed to normal language use; patients respond in a language that is different from the one in which they are addressed.

Another capacity of bilingual persons is **spontaneous translation** which is an immediate unsolicited translation of one's own or someone else's utterance into another language. Perecman (1984) determined that few aphasic bilinguals engage in spontaneous translation. One patient who repeated sentences in another language could not translate on request.

Grosjean (1985, 1989) was concerned about Perecman's analysis, especially regarding the notion that utterance-level mixing is necessarily a sign of disorder. Responding in another language may normally occur in conversation depending on the pragmatic application of code-switching rules when the bilingual mode is appropriate. Grosjean suspected that impairments might occur in the management of languages with respect to linguistic status of a communicative partner, such as (a) using the wrong base language with a monolingual interlocutor, (b) extensive code-switching with a monolingual, (c) language mixing while reading a monolingual text, and (d) failing to switch or translate upon request. Therefore, utterance-level mixing is a pragmatic violation when a monolingual clinician is speaking to a bilingual client but may be quite natural when a clinician is bilingual. Data does not appear to be available on the extent to which these behaviors occur in aphasic persons when speaking to monolingual and bilingual clinicians.

Grosjean (1989) had some suggestions for the evaluation of bilingual aphasic persons (see also Paradis and Libben, 1987). First, we should determine the following information about a patient's bilingualism prior to brain injury, perhaps, by interviewing a family member:

- Relative ability in each language (linguistic level, style, reading, writing)
- Situations and purposes for which each language was used (home, work, recreation)
- Persons with whom each language was used (family, friends, colleagues)
- Situations and people when in a monolingual mode
- Situations and people when in a bilingual mode
- Amount and kind of mixing when in the bilingual mode (code-switching, borrowing)
- Translation abilities

This information leads us to assessment and treatment that are appropriate for a particular language used by the bilingual patient. For example, we should not assess for aphasia in reading and writing in a language not used for these purposes. We should employ work-related content with the language used at work.

When evaluating each language, we obtain samples of language behavior in conversation and formal tests. Each language should be examined in each interactional mode, remembering that the abilities of a bilingual person in each language are not the same as abilities of two monolingual persons. In the monolingual mode, conditions should lead to a deactivation of the language not being used, which is likely to occur when the examiner does not know the other language. Pretending not to know the other language "is rarely foolproof" (Grosjean, 1989).

With an English and Spanish speaking patient, for example, a monolingual English speaking person should do one evaluation and a monolingual Spanish speaking person should do the other evaluation. A family member may be enlisted to translate and administer the aphasia test in the language not known by the clinician (e.g., Paradis and Goldblum, 1989). In a study of object naming, clinicians placed 30 minutes to two days between tests (Vogel and Costello, 1986). The clinicians claimed that 15 to 20 minutes seemed too brief to minimize interference (or maximize deactivation of one language). Thirty minutes to one hour was sufficient for most subjects.

For obtaining behavior samples in the bilingual mode, the patient should feel comfortable code-switching and borrowing. Again, a bilingual family member or friend may be sought. Grosjean (1989) recommended that we learn about how aphasia has affected the special skills used in this mode such as whether the patient uses the "wrong" language when speaking to a bilingual family member or friend, mixes languages to the same extent as before, and mixes in the same way as before. Has the ability to translate languages changed? We know relatively little about aphasia in bilinguals evaluated this comprehensively, so that clinicians have an opportunity to contribute to our knowledge in this area through this assessment strategy.

SUMMARY AND CONCLUSIONS

This chapter dealt with two general areas of special investigation. One is the case study approach in cognitive neuropsychology, which provides strategies for diagnosing misnaming, semantic problems, and reading aloud. Occasionally unusual diagnostic categories are proposed, such as optic aphasia and semantic dementia. The other area of special investigation pertains to the appearance of aphasia in different languages, including what comparative aphasiology has to say about the fundamentally universal nature of aphasia and what we might expect regarding patients who speak more than one language.

Some of the diagnoses in cognitive neuropsychology may be confusing to those of us who come from the perspective of another discipline. This is not a bad point to ponder. After all, CN is an evolving science. Its value for rehabilitation is to provide a basis for aiming treatment at a clearly impaired component of cognition. Some misnaming will be treated by targeting lexical access and/or formulation. Other misnaming will be treated by targeting recognition of objects. Still other misnaming will be treated with a hearing aid or glasses. The approach may sharpen our ability to

TABLE 6.8 A chronology of outside influences on clinical aphasiology.

DECADE	DISCIPLINE	KEY APHASIA REFERENCES
pre 1900	• Medicine/Neurology (localization)	• Broca in 1861; Wernicke in 1874
pre 1940	• Educational psychology (testing)	• Weisenburg and McBride (1935)
1940s	• Clinical neurology	• Goldstein (1942); Luria (1966)
1950s	• Clinical/Counseling psychology • Experimental design & statistics	• Eisenson (1949); Wepman (1951) • Schuell and Jenkins (1959, 1961)
1960s	• Structural linguistics • Behavioral psychology • Neoclassical neurology	• Goodglass and Mayer (1958) • Brookshire (1967); Holland (1970) • Geschwind (1965)
1970s	• Speech and hearing sciences • Clinical psychology (test theory) • Transformational linguistics • Cognitive neuropsychology	• Shankweiler and Harris (1966); Swisher and Hirsch (1972) • Porch (1967) • Shewan and Canter (1971) • Shallice and Warrington (1970)
1980s	• Psycholinguistics (automaticity) • Psycholinguistics (on-line) • Neurolinguistics	• Milberg and Blumstein (1981) • Swinney, Zurif and Cutler (1980); Tyler and Cobb (1987) • Caplan (1987); Grodzinsky (1986)
1990s	• Cross-linguistics	• Bates and Wulfeck (1989); Menn and Obler (1990)

infer the hidden impairment from observable data. The downside is that CN has yet to provide a consistent theory and a consistent set of rules that everyone follows for designing assessments and interpreting raw data.

Cross-linguistic studies have pointed out two universal characteristics of aphasia, namely, problems with comprehending exceptions to canonical structure and difficulties with grammatical morphemes in Broca's aphasia and, perhaps, Wernicke's aphasia as well. Regarding the latter, the symptom is not necessarily omission or substitution in a particular case. Variation among languages is manifested in the use of grammatical morphemes. Omission is more characteristic of agrammatism in English than in other languages.

Chapters 4 through 6 surveyed basic clinical investigation of the nature of aphasia and some related problems. The many explanations for the same thing can be blamed partly on the multidisciplinary study of aphasia. Table 6.8 summarizes most of these influences according to a chronology of when various disciplines were introduced in the study of aphasia. This chronology is suggestive of how aphasiology has evolved over the past 100 years.

CHAPTER 7

FUNCTIONAL COMMUNICATION AND DISCOURSE

Thinking of aphasia in terms of disability and handicap leads us to its functional implications. Since Audrey Holland (1975) pointed out that aphasic people communicate better than they talk, we have paid attention to how well a patient conveys thoughts and feelings regardless of language ability. Most of the present chapter deals with communication, thereby, focusing on disability.

Aphasia threatened Martin Exeter's career as a professor. He had to cancel his lecture in Europe. However, it did not take long for his vocational prospects to be put aside, because daily living demanded his total concentration for the first few months after his stroke. Daily living included the ability to communicate his wishes and ideas. It included connecting with his wife, children, and friends. In addition, if he could communicate better, then perhaps he could salvage at least parts of his career.

NONVERBAL MODALITIES

One option for maximizing functional communication is to supplement or replace impaired language functions with another means of communicating, especially for the acute period following stroke or for chronically severe or global aphasia. This section identifies capacities for nonverbal communication when someone has aphasia. For now, we shall focus on behaviors elicited in formal conditions that determine a patient's capacity. Later in the chapter, we shall examine more natural communicative conditions in which gesturing accompanies speech.

Assessing Limb Movement

Limb apraxia is a disorder of skilled movement (or **praxis**) that cannot be attributed to paralysis. A movement, such as brushing teeth, can be performed in natural circumstances but not when a patient is asked to perform the action. Thus, the disorder may not be experienced until it is diagnosed in the clinic (DeRenzi, Motti, and Nichelli, 1980). Limb apraxia occurs mainly when there is damage to the left parieto-temporal lobe boundary (DeRenzi and Lucchelli, 1988). Because of this posterior location, patients with this disorder often do not have hemiplegia.

Evaluation is usually done in conditions of imitiation, movement on command, and natural or spontaneous movement. Movements are classified according to *transivity,* such as transitive actions upon objects (e.g., dialing a phone) or intransitive actions without objects (e.g., an OK sign), and according to *complexity* such as a single movement (e.g., drinking) or a sequence of movements (e.g., making coffee). Clinical researchers often study transitive movements as **pantomime** or pretended movement without the object in hand (i.e., "mime").

To facilitate diagnosis, researchers have categorized movement errors, especially for mimed transitive gestures such as combing, hammering, erasing, or smoking. Rothi and others (1988) looked for content errors (e.g, wrong pantomime), temporal errors (e.g., wrong sequence of movements), and spatial errors (e.g., unusual amplification of movement). In a comparison of aphasic subjects to normal controls, several error types were never or rarely produced by any subject.

These included unrelated, sequencing, amplitude, and unrecognizable errors.

One observed spatial error is the use of **body-part-as-object** (BPO), such as puffing on a finger when asked to mime smoking a cigarette. The BPO error differs from what Raymer and others (1997) called **body-part-as-tool** (BPT) errors in which someone actually uses a body part as the tool. Examples of the latter include using a straightened finger as a toothbrush or pencil when miming the appropriate action, as opposed to pretending to hold the toothbrush or pencil. In comparisons among brain damaged groups and normal controls, researchers have reached opposite conclusions regarding whether BPT responses are symptoms of deficit (e.g., Duffy and Duffy, 1989; Haaland and Flaherty, 1984; McDonald, Tate, and Rigby, 1994). That is, normal adults do these things, too. Subsequent research demonstrated that a truly pathological BPT error occurs only after a patient is reinstructed to pretend to hold the tool (Raymer, et al., 1997).

Duffy and Duffy's (1989) **Limb Apraxia Test** (LAT) is one device for assessing praxis. The LAT relies on the imitation task in order to specify response parameters precisely, minimize verbal instruction, and minimize the influence of cognitive problems that may appear when making movements on command. The test also avoids conventional intransitive gestures. Eight subtests are constructed according to the following factors:

- movement with and without objects
- simple (i.e., one to three components) and complex (i.e., four to six components)
- sequenced (i.e., complete movement) and segmented (i.e., one component at a time).

Scoring is based on the PICA's model of a multidimensional system. A control group showed that there is no difference between left and right hand performance of the tasks. Sixty-eight percent of LHDs performed beneath the range for normal controls.

The **Test of Oral and Limb Apraxia** (TOLA) by Helm-Estabrooks (1991) evaluates movement a little differently from the LAT. The section on oral apraxia instructs a patient to perform nonrespiratory actions with the mouth such as "Lick a lollipop" and respiratory actions such as "Cough" and "Blow out a candle." Oral and limb movements are observed first upon command and then by imitation. Transitive and intransitive gestures are compared. An early version of this test was correlated with a rating of spontaneous gesture, indicating that TOLA may be predictive of natural gestural use (Borod, Fitzpatrick, Helm-Estabrooks, and Goodglass, 1989).

The Question of Asymbolia

Two origins of miming deficit have been considered when it occurs with aphasia (Wang and Goodglass, 1992). One possibility is that pantomime deficit is a manifestation of limb apraxia. The other possibility is that language and pantomime deficits are part of a broad disorder that could be called "asymbolia." In 1870, Finkelnburg described the case of a pious Catholic woman who could not initiate the sign of the cross and another case of a violinist who was able to play by ear but could not read musical notation (cited in Duffy and Liles, 1979).

Some gestures are more symbolic than others. Comparable to verbal language, a symbolic gesture has a somewhat arbitrary relationship to its referent. For example, a salute does not share physical characteristics with a referent, and yet its meaning is known by a community. On the other hand, gestures can be a natural expression of emotion, such as a clenched fist or a frown. The physical similarity between a gesture and its referent is known as the gesture's *iconicity.* Iconic gestures, such as pantomime, are replicas of their referents. *Intentionality* is another variable, and aphasic patients retain unintentional or subpropositional emotional expression or reaction (Buck and Duffy, 1980; Gardner, Ling, Flamm, and Silverman, 1975). The question is whether aphasia necessarily includes deficit with intentionally or propositionally symbolic behavior such as appropriate use of the "OK" sign.

Investigators tried to separate cognitive and motor factors in gesture production. Duffy and Duffy (1981) found that miming the use of objects was correlated with severity of aphasia and that apraxia contributed little to pantomime performance. In another study, aphasic subjects without limb apraxia were impaired for imitating American Indian Sign Language (Amer-Ind) and American Sign Language (ASL) (Daniloff, Fritelli, Buckingham, Hoffman, and Daniloff, 1986). ASL contains many arbitrary symbols, but Amer-Ind is loaded with pantomimic representations of referents.

Because of the possibility of a motor confound, many investigators decided to study **pantomime recognition.** It also provided an opportunity to determine whether a central disorder can be inferred from coexisting receptive and expressive deficit. To assess recognition, a researcher produces a pantomime, and a subject identifies the referent in a set of pictures. Evidence of asymbolia with aphasia came from a group mean deficit (Duffy, Duffy, and Pearson, 1975), correlation with a measure of overall language ability (Duffy and Duffy, 1981), and correlation with receptive language ability (Ferro, Santos, Castro-Caldas, and Mariano, 1980). Aphasic patients also had more difficulty recognizing pantomime than facial emotion (Walker-Batson, Barton, Wendt, and Reynolds, 1987), and posteriorly damaged subjects had particular difficulty verifying a mimed action that was physically similar to an action on an incorrect object (Lambier and Bradley, 1991).

The studies mentioned so far relied on the average performance of an aphasic group. When the number of aphasic subjects below a cut-off score was computed, the proportion of subjects with recognition deficits varied from 41 to 74 percent (Gainotti and Lemmo, 1976; Seron, Van Der Kaa, Remitz, and Van Der Linden, 1979; Varney, 1982). Range of aphasic scores in Duffy and Duffy's study overlapped considerably with the normal range. Some studies showed no relationship between pantomime recognition deficit and severity of aphasia (Daniloff, Noll, Fristoe, and Lloyd, 1982; Feyereisen and Seron, 1982). Therefore, many aphasic persons do not have pantomime recognition deficit, indicating that this problem is not a necessary component of aphasia.

Meanwhile, other researchers claimed that pantomime deficit in aphasic patients is a movement disorder or a manifestation of limb apraxia (Goodglass and Kaplan, 1963; Kertesz, Ferro, and Shewan, 1984). Like Duffy and Duffy (1981), Wang and Goodglass (1992) found pantomime recognition and production to be correlated with each other and with auditory comprehension, but, unlike the Duffy findings, pantomime abilities were not correlated with severity of aphasia. Wang and Goodglass were concerned about use of the PICA in the Duffy study as a measure of aphasia, because this battery contains subtests of gesturing with objects. Wang and Goodglass also found a strong correlation between miming and a measure of motor praxis. Using a sophisticated analysis of their own data, Duffy, Watt, and Duffy (1994) concluded that pantomime impairment has both a symbolic and motoric basis.

Most investigations of the asymbolia question have relied on pantomime as an example of symbols. Because pantomime may not be truly symbolic because of its iconicity (Peterson and Kirshner, 1981), the issue of whether aphasia is a sweeping asymbolia may not be clearly resolved by this research. Moreover, a clinician is concerned about the communicative avenues available to aphasic persons. The research shows either that pantomime can be one option with little training for some patients or that pantomime has to be trained for other patients.

To determine whether miming is available, a test of pantomime was developed. The **Assessment of Nonverbal Communication** (Duffy and Duffy, 1984) contains two tests of recognition and two tests of production. For recognition, a videotaped demonstration can be obtained for maximizing consistency of presentation. Response is made with a choice of four pictured objects. One expression test models the naming task in that the examiner shows a picture of an object, and the patient demonstrates its use. Finally, in a "referential abilities" test, the patient's gesture is evaluated by a third person who must decide what was conveyed by choosing one of four pictures. One foil is an object that would be used in the same location in space as the correct object, thereby requiring a precise gesture.

Drawing

Although many of us would say we are not artistic, most of us can draw to some degree. Because the right hemisphere is thought to be responsible for visuospatial skills, we might expect aphasic patients to have retained whatever drawing skill they had. However, right hemiplegia can restrict the usually preferred side for writing and drawing. This may be one reason why 30 to 40 percent of patients with left or right hemisphere strokes have some degree of drawing deficit as tested by copying tasks (e.g., Arena and Gainotti, 1978; Carlesimo, Fadda, and Caltagirone, 1993).

The next chapter has a discussion of drawing from the perspective of right hemisphere dysfunction. One point in that chapter is that drawing difficulties with LHD are different from those with RHD. Patients with LHD generally include accurate details and preserve the overall structure of an object, but they draw slowly and very simply (e.g., Gainotti, and Tiacci, 1970; Swindell, Holland, Fromm, and Greenhouse, 1988). What is important for the present discussion is whether drawing with aphasia is recognizable or can convey meaning to an observer.

In one study, clinicians examined copying and sketching ability of three severely aphasic individuals with right hemiparesis and little drawing experience. The patients were right-handed and drew with the left hand. All three produced intelligible copies and sketches of objects. The wives of two of the subjects were surprised with their husbands' newly discovered artistic skills. The study demonstrated that drawing can be a communicative option (Kashiwagi, Kashiwagi, Kunimori, Yamadori, Tanabe, and Okuda, 1994).

PRAGMATIC LANGUAGE

The traditional clinical concern with relating words to objects is not the whole story regarding the language system. Taking a communication perspective, we must consider the language system as it operates in natural context. For example, we might consider how a process-model of naming operates when people are talking to each other or how a model of reading works when thumbing through a phone book. The study of natural language use is called **pragmatics.** Relevant observations consist of language behavior in relation to context.

The language system's contexts have been said to be **external** to a speaker, such as a communicative situation, and **internal** which consists of world knowledge and emotional states. Functional tasks rely on these contexts in different ways. Conversation is more *situation-dependent,* because many referents exist in the participants' surroundings. Reading is more *knowledge-dependent,* because interpretation depends heavily on the reader's knowledge (and imagination). "Rarely can we look around the room to make sense of what we have just read in a book" (Smith, 1982, p. 82). The plausibility effect (Chapter 4) is one indication of how world knowledge facilitates language comprehension.

Let us focus on the messages expressed or understood in real-world language use. There is "a gap between the semantic representations of sentences and the thoughts actually communicated by utterances" (Sperber and Wilson, 1986, p. 9). A **speaker's meaning** can differ from the literal or acontextual semantic representation of a sentence called **sentence-meaning** (Searle, 1979). In a notorious murder case in England, a teenager's life hinged on his intent when he said "Let him have it, Chris" to a friend pointing a gun at a policeman. In this case, meaning lies in the speaker's intent and a listener's interpretation. Ambiguity is created by the situational context. Did the speaker mean "give him the gun" or "shoot him"?

How do we study or evaluate the exchange of hidden intentions? A solution to this problem includes finding some clear differences between sentence- and speaker-meanings that can be presented in experiments. One approach to distinguishing these meanings was Searle's (1969) contention that the basic unit of communication is the *speech act.* Speech acts include asserting, greeting, warning, and requesting. When we politely ask "Can you open the door," we are making a request rather than literally asking about someone's ability to open the door. The act of requesting is part of speaker-meaning, and patients can produce speech acts mainly because it does not take much verbalization to greet, warn, request, and so on (Ulatowska, Allard, Reyes, Ford, and Chapman, 1992).

Indirect speech acts have been investigated with aphasic subjects in the form of indirect requests. In one study, video vignettes contained a situation followed by a request (e.g., "Can you open the door?"). Another actor made either an appropriate response to speaker-meaning or a pragmatically inappropriate literal response (i.e., "Yes"). A mixed group of aphasic subjects usually responded to speaker-meaning, indicating that they had an ability to relate the situation to the utterance (Wilcox, Davis, and Leonard, 1978). This ability was unrelated to clinical measures of literal comprehension. Other investigators have supported the conclusion that aphasia does not impair the capacity to make nonliteral interpretations (e.g., Foldi, 1987).

Inference is the general psycholinguistic mechanism for making nonliteral interpretations. A relatively simple type of inference is to add information not explicitly stated in a sentence, called an elaborative inference. An example is to hear "The woman stirred the coffee" and think of [spoon]. Such inferences have been put to the test of whether they arise in spreading activation of semantic memory during comprehension (e.g., Dosher and Corbett, 1982). Inference is also considered to be a mechanism used in the comprehension of metaphor, a topic that we visit with respect to the study of right hemisphere dysfunction in Chapter 8.

DISCOURSE AND TEXT

"Discourse" has been used to refer to numerous things, but here the term refers broadly to units of language larger than a sentence (e.g., Carroll, 1999). Monologue and dialogue are examples of discourse and share features of processing simply because each entails dealing with strings of sentences. Dialogue is called *conversational discourse.* For reading and writing, this level of language use is known as *text.* We can continue to think about pragmatics, because language is normally used at the level of discourse, and the discourse itself provides a linguistic context in which single words and sentences are usually understood and produced.

The ensuing discussion is going to be about what makes discourse different from words and sentences. Its special qualities come from interrelationships among statements known broadly as **coherence.** A conversation of alternating single sentences makes sense because the statements are about a single topic holding them together. Coherence is studied at two closely related levels. The local or *microstructural level* pertains to the overlap of meaning between sentences. This local level overlap is known as **cohesion.** It is the minimum level of discourse and needs only pairs of statements to be studied. The global or *macrostructural level* pertains to broad themes and structural schemes. It is necessarily invoked with a length of three or more statements.

One type of cohesive device in microstructure is **anaphora,** which is a lexical unit that refers to information presented previously. One type of anaphora is the pronoun, which can serve the function of *coreference.* That is, a pronoun and antecedent can refer to the same referent. Lexical coreference occurs when a noun, such as a superordinate term, refers back to a specific or subordinate term. In *1,* the determiner or definite article *the* signals that a particular *vehicle* should already be known to a reader or listener.

(1) A bus came roaring around the corner. The vehicle hit a pedestrian.
(2) We checked the picnic supplies. The beer was warm.

In *2,* the noun-phrase *The beer* seems to refer back to something in the previous sentence, but there is no explicit antecedent for it. A reader or listener makes what is called an instantiation inference in which beer is assumed to be among the picnic supplies. When coreference and inference come together, it is called a **bridging inference.** In comprehending discourse, a bridge is often needed when a distant antecedent has vanished from the short-term buffer (Fletcher and Bloom, 1988; Lesgold, Roth, and Curtis, 1979).

Macrostructure is the "upper limit of structural organization" where an entire discourse or text is held together (Stubbs, 1983). The topic or **theme** of a discourse contributes to coherence at this level, as every statement is expected to be related to the overall theme in some way. For example, a text may be about nuclear disarmament or a conversation may be about uncle Fred. Also, types of discourse possess an overall **structure** leading to expections for what comes next. The following are some discourse types:

- **narrative,** or a story which is commonly said to have a beginning, middle, and end
- **exposition,** such as a lecture; may include research presentation with methods, results, and so on
- **procedures** or **routines,** telling how to perform the steps of a task, such as making a sandwich
- **description,** or a characterization of an event or scene

Communicative competence includes knowledge of these forms. Besides clinical studies of picture description, narration or story-telling is the most frequently studied form of discourse, perhaps, because its structure is more apparent and familiar than the other forms.

Story grammars are theories of our knowledge of narrative structure. These grammars, which Toolan (1988) called a deep structure, specify story-telling functions and how they are organized. Thorndyke's (1977) hierarchy branches into functions of *setting, theme, plot,* and *resolution.* Then, *plot* branches into multiple *episodes,* and an episode contains a *subgoal, attempt,* and *outcome.* Stein and Glenn's (1979) grammar has a plot-starter called the *initiating event.* We may recognize a setting such as "Once there was a wily fox who lived in a forest." A plot is initiated when "one day the fox left the forest to explore a henhouse in a nearby village." Studies of reading time and recall support the notion that a story grammar has psychological reality (Mandler, 1987).

Like a theory of any cognitive function, a minimal account of discourse comprehension contains a knowledge structure and a processing system. Semantic memory has to contain more than object-concepts, and so the network is broadened to account for knowledge of complex situations generally known as **schemas.** For example, we have a schema for weddings. Our schema for narrative structure (i.e., story grammar) lets us know when someone is telling us a story about a wedding. Processing is constrained by what is called the **bottleneck problem.** That is, only small chunks of a discourse can squeeze into working memory as we listen or read. Theories of comprehension propose different levels of representation for holding onto previous input temporarily and for accumulating a representation of the entire discourse (e.g., Haberlandt and Graesser, 1990; van Dijk and Kintsch, 1983).

APHASIC DISCOURSE PRODUCTION

Aphasic discourse production is evaluated for somewhat different reasons. One is to determine the nature of impaired word-finding and syntax in a natural productive circumstance (i.e., "spontaneous speech"). The other reason is to determine a patient's abilities with respect to discourse-specific functions. When evaluating discourse, we should consider the method for *elicitation* and the method for *analysis* somewhat independently. For example, we can elicit a narrative (i.e., discourse-level) but analyze only word-finding (i.e., word-level).

Elicitation Method

Stimuli and instructions determine whether a patient's discourse is a narrative, procedure, or description (Table 7.1). The types of discourse in the table are produced as **monologue,** that is, with the

TABLE 7.1 Methods for eliciting different kinds of monologue. Description has been the most commonly elicited form in clinical evaluation.

	VISUAL STIMULUS	INSTRUCTION
description	complex picture	*Tell me everything you see in this picture.*
procedure	none	*Tell me how you make a sandwich.*
narration	complex picture	*Tell me a story about this picture.*
	picture sequence	*Tell me the story being told in these pictures.*
	none	*Tell me the story of Cinderella.*

patient talking and the clinician listening. Description, narration, or exposition can also arise in **dialogue** such as an interview (e.g., *I'd like to ask some questions about your job*) or a conversation (e.g., *What do you think about the President's problems*?). In some studies, an interview is said to be the means for studying conversation.

The early clinical discourse research could be somewhat confusing. The main problem is that varied types of discourse were called "narrative." Ehrlich (1988) asked subjects to tell "everything you see happening..." in a complex picture and called the result "narrative discourse." On the other hand, others instructed patients to tell a story about a picture when the goal was to elicit a story (Liles, Coelho, Duffy, and Zalagens, 1989). Mentis and Prutting (1987) asked for procedures but called the result narrative. Exposition was not studied by name, but it could have occurred in interviews with "minimal interviewer involvement" (Glosser and Deser, 1991).

Clinical researchers have been interested in whether the condition for eliciting discourse makes a difference in observations of language production. The concern is whether standardized test conditions are valid with respect to the way an aphasic person talks in natural circumstances. In one study, a test of describing object functions was compared to conversation (Roberts and Wertz, 1989). Utterances and clauses were longer and word-finding was more accurate in conversation, but syntactic structures were formed better in the object-function test. Another study showed that some discourse conditions such as describing pictures of the Kennedy assassination elicit more words than describing the Cookie Theft picture (Bottenberg, Lemme, and Hedberg, 1987). Thus, a full picture of sentence-level capacities may require observation in formal and natural conditions and with different topics.

Discourse Analysis

First, the transcript of a patient's discourse is parsed into units for various purposes, one being to have a frame of reference for computing density of different forms like number of words per sentence or number of sentences per episode in a story. Also, investigators like to have a basis for examining meaningful relationships among elements of a discourse. The most common units are listed below:

- **sentence:** a syntactic unit containing a subject and predicate
- **T-unit:** a syntactic unit containing a main clause and attached subordinate clauses
- **p-unit (proposition):** an informational unit defined either as (a) a predicate and its arguments or (b) a smaller unit roughly associated with each verb and modifier

A sentence may be the most ambiguous of the three. Mentis and Prutting (1987) divided spoken narratives into sentences according to pauses and intonation, which may not correspond to punctuation in text or a transcript of spoken narration. Several others have utilized T-units (e.g., Liles, et al., 1989; Ulatowska, Freedman-Stern, Doyel, and

Macaluso-Haynes, 1983). An example might be the following: *The heroic policeman who apprehended the thief turned over his weapon before the investigation began.* The ambiguity of syntactic units is that this could be a sentence or a T-unit containing the equivalent of two or three sentences.

Psycholinguists tend to use either "surface" or "deep" propositional units. Surface p-units contain a predicate and its arguments as spoken or written (e.g., Stein and Glenn, 1979). The result is a list of statements regarding the descriptive states or action-related events in a story (e.g, *the policeman apprehended the thief; the investigation began*). Others use smaller propositions as minimal units of meaning (e.g., Kintsch, 1994). These deep p-units are based on the linguistic assumption, for example, that *heroic policeman* is a statement that is equivalent to the deep structural *policeman is hero.* A transcription is likely to contain more deep p-units than surface p-units.

Choice of units can be related to the level of analysis. For example, surface p-units may be recorded with little regard for grammatical precision because of an interest in examining the ability to tell a story. Levels are designated broadly as "within-sentence" **microlinguistic analysis** of lexical and grammatical forms (see Table 5.1) and "between-sentence" **macrolinguistic analysis** of the unique properties of discourse at microstructural and macrostructural levels. These levels of analysis are summarized in Table 7.2.

In a cohesion analysis, the first thing to look for is the presence of cohesive elements such as pronouns and nouns preceded by *the.* Investigators may stop there (e.g., Bloom, Borod, Obler, Santschi-Haywood, and Pick, 1995). However, other researchers look for a **cohesive tie** between an element and an antecedent. Incomplete ties are noted when an antecedent cannot be found. In a study of interviews with fluent aphasic patients, they produced a normal number of cohesive elements but also produced more incomplete cohesive ties than controls, indicating that pronouns and definite articles were difficult to interpret (Glosser and Deser, 1991).

Narration has been employed to study global themes and structure. With a story-recall task, Gleason and others (1980) found aphasic patients were deficient in number of thematic statements. They tended to reiterate major themes and omit details. In another study, patients displayed intact narrative form and did not differ from controls in the number of actions expressed. They were deficient in producing certain components such as setting, resolution, and evaluation (Ulatowska, Freedman-Stern, Doyel, Macaluso-Haynes, and

TABLE 7.2 Basic types of discourse analysis.

LEVEL	ANALYSIS	MEASUREMENT APPROACH	REFERENCE
Microlinguistic	informativeness	counting main concepts	Nicholas and Brookshire (1993)
		counting deep propositions	Joanette, et al. (1986)
	grammar	counting omissions and substitutions of grammatical morphemes	Haravon, Obler, and Sarno (1994)
Microstructural	cohesion	counting cohesive elements (e.g., pronouns) and clear connections to antecedents (i.e., cohesive ties)	Lemme, et al. (1984)
Macrostructural	story grammar	rating scale of narrative organization	Bottenberg, et al. (1987)

North, 1983). Bloom and others (1995) rated stories according to accuracy, completeness, logic, and whether they had a beginning, middle, and end. They found overall story structure to be preserved but coherence reduced in other respects.

We might imagine that fluency distinguishes syndromes of aphasia with respect to microlinguistic features. Early research distinguished narrative styles in Broca's and Wernicke's according to word-finding and grammatical characteristics (Gleason, et al., 1980). More recently, Christiansen (1995b) compared Broca's, conduction, and Wernicke's aphasias with narrative production and comprehension tasks. She evaluated production by rating the relevance of propositions in stories told from cartoons. Fueled by their press for speech, patients with Wernicke's aphasia were distinctive in producing more irrelevant statements than the other patients. Those with Broca's and conduction aphasia were more coherent.

Then, Christiansen (1995a) focused on mildly fluent aphasias. She compared syndromes according to the occurrence of so-called coherence violations, namely, information gaps, repetitive propositions, and irrelevant propositions. The patient groups displayed different kinds of problems. Those with mainly word-finding deficits of anomic aphasia produced mostly information gaps and fewer propositions than the other groups. Patients with conduction aphasia produced more repetitions than other violations, which was considered to be a compensation for grammatical difficulties. Those with mild Wernicke's aphasia produced more irrelevant propositions than other violations and seemed to produce more description than narration.

Clinical analysis of discourse production is in its infancy as investigators experiment with methods for getting at cohesion and overall coherence. Aphasic sentence-level language deficiencies can mask capacities at the discourse level, but aphasia also seems to attack local level discourse functions directly such as coreferential cohesion. Yet, we do not know if poor cohesion is secondary to word-finding deficit or an impairment of a process unique to establishing cohesive ties. People with aphasia produce recognizable narrative structure. That is, someone with anomic or Broca's aphasia can tell a good story with circumlocutory or agrammatic statements. Generally, aphasia seems to impair microlinguistic parameters while preserving macrolinguistic parameters.

Informativeness

Some aphasiologists are interested in measuring the informativeness of discourse. They look for the presence of predefined content units without regard to their relationships to each other. Measurements address the density and rate of content production in narration and other types of discourse. The main objective is to have a reliable measure that discriminates aphasia from normal performance.

Initially, Yorkston and Beukelman (1980) divided Cookie Theft descriptions into content units the size of a word or short phrase. A content unit was considered to be "a grouping of information that was always expressed as a unit by normal speakers" (p. 30), such as *cookies, from the jar, mother,* and *in the kitchen.* A mildly aphasic group did not differ from normal elderly subjects in amount of information, but these patients were much less efficient with 18.7 units per minute compared to the control group's 33.7 units per minute. Other investigators supplied profiles for severely impaired patients according to this method (Craig, Hinckley, Winkelseth, Carry, Walley, Bardach, Higman, Hilfinger, Schall, and Sheimo, 1993).

At the Veterans Administration Medical Center in Minneapolis, Linda Nicholas and Robert Brookshire worked on improving content analysis. In particular, they wanted a system that is not tied to a particular picture and can be used with any stimulus. They started by counting the most informative words in a narrative, which they called **correct information units** (CIU) (Nicholas and Brookshire, 1993). The basic measures were the percent of words that are CIUs and the number of CIUs per minute. These measures separated aphasic patients from normal controls.

Later, the investigators determined that obtaining 300–400 words from four or five stimuli lead to the most reliable informativeness score (Brookshire and Nicholas, 1994).

Nicholas and Brookshire turned their attention to a more elaborate system for identifying **main concepts,** still being especially concerned with establishing a reliable measure that is sensitive to deficit (Nicholas and Brookshire, 1995). Main concepts are statements that form a "skeletal outline" of the essential information in pictured stories. One study showed that aphasic patients produce fewer complete and accurate concepts and more incomplete and inaccurate concepts than neurologically intact individuals. Other researchers counted units of particular kinds of information in a narration (Bloom, Borod, Obler, and Gerstman, 1992).

Do Nicholas and Brookshire's measures correspond to impressions of informativeness? Doyle and others (1996) asked volunteers to rate the informativeness of several narratives produced by aphasic patients. The investigation indicated that the CIU and main concept measures are strongly related to the subjective judgments and, thus, are valid measures of perceived informativeness.

DISCOURSE COMPREHENSION WITH APHASIA

Tests of discourse-level comprehension have been used mainly for identifying subtle comprehension deficits. The usual clinical method is to read a paragraph to a patient or ask a patient to read a paragraph. Then we ask questions about what was just heard or read, thereby, testing recall as well as comprehension. In aphasia batteries, many questions can be answered without having heard or read the paragraphs (Nicholas, MacLennan, and Brookshire, 1986). This off-line approach differs from on-line comparisons of information load at specific points in a text. For example, in a "moving window" paradigm, portions of a text are shown one at a time. A subject presses a button causing one portion to disappear and the next one to appear (e.g., Haberlandt and Graesser, 1990).

Few studies have targeted microstructural comprehension of cohesive devices. Chapman and Ulatowska (1989) presented short vignettes in which two characters were introduced in the first sentence and a subsequent sentence referred back to one of the characters in *3.*

(3) The customer shouted angrily at the waitress that the meal was awful.
The waitress was new at the job and did not know how to respond.
or
She was new at the job and did not know how to respond.

Subjects were given response cards showing the two characters and were asked questions such as "Who was new at the job and did not know how to respond?" Aphasic subjects responded less accurately with the pronominal anaphor than the lexical anaphor (see also Kahn, Joanette, Ska, and Goulet, 1990).

Let us take a few minutes to consider how pronominal cohesion can be studied psycholinguistically. That is, how might one study mental processes of referential connections? Chang (1980) presented multi-propositional sentences like *4* as primes.

(4) Bill and Mary went to the store and he bought some milk.

Immediately following the sentence, either BILL or MARY was shown as a target. Subjects had to press a yes-no button indicating whether the name had appeared in the sentence. Of course, the correct answer is the same with each target. However, decision for the correct referrent was reliably faster (e.g., BILL).

The faster decision to BILL can be explained according to spreading activation theory. The pronoun reactivates the antecedent so that this concept has a greater activation level relative to MARY by the time of target-decision. Mental response to the pronoun could be like the recognition process of matching a stimulus to a representation already stored in memory. In this case, the antecedent is "nearby" in working memory. As indicated below, the second proposition is currently active in working memory, and the

Bill and Mary went to the store	he bought some milk
buffered (STM)	active

previous statement is stored in a temporary buffer so that the antecedent can be found. Pronoun interpretation might require a "scanning" mechanism that goes back through the buffered information.

The concept of **The Discourse Comprehension Test** is similar to analysis of informativeness in production (Brookshire and Nicholas, 1993). The test contains 10 stories played to patients on a tape recorder, and each story is followed by eight yes-no test questions. Some test questions address **main ideas** considered to be central to the theme of the story, and other questions address **details** peripheral to the story-line. Inferencing is assumed to be assessed by presenting questions about information either explicitly stated or implied in a story.

Aphasic patients made more errors than neurologically intact subjects on the Discourse Comprehension Test. Yet, normal and aphasic groups displayed the same pattern with respect to type of question. Both groups did better with main ideas than details and did better with explicit information than with implied information (Nicholas and Brookshire, 1995). In another study, patients with Broca's and conduction aphasias performed poorly in recalling main ideas. Those with Wernicke's aphasia were within the normal range, a finding that was surprising considering their poor sentence comprehension and reduced coherence of narrative production (Christiansen, 1995b).

Nicholas and Brookshire (1995) found both quantitative and qualitative similarities among aphasia, RHD, and traumatic brain injury. They noted that "this does not necessarily mean that the underlying reasons for their performance deficits are the same" (p. 78). As introduced in Chapter 4, theory-driven clinical research is designed to discover observational methods that direct us to underlying impairment. Nicholas and Brookshire acknowledged that "evaluation of the underlying reasons...would appear to be a productive area for future research" (p. 78).

CONVERSATION

The dynamic interaction of natural conversation differs from formal clinical interactions. For example, tests and treatments tend to have a patient either comprehending repeatedly or producing utterances repeatedly; whereas participants take turns talking in the give-and-take of conversation. This section covers three distinctive aspects of conversation:

- exchange of new information
- management of turn-taking
- use of multiple modalities

The study of conversation has slightly different orientations. Besides our interest in how aphasia appears in a natural activity, we want to know whether patients' have any difficulty with the unique features of conversation.

New Information

Conversation is conducted as if there were a tacit agreement or "social contract" between participants. Grice (1975) called it the **principle of cooperation.** According to Grice's "maxims," a speaker tries to be informative, truthful, relevant, and concise; and a listener assumes that this is what the speaker is trying to do. Let us focus on the informativeness maxim as we turn our attention to **shared responsiblities** of participants in a conversation. More specifically, we shall pay more attention to a clinician or others engaged in conversation with an aphasic person.

The informativeness maxim gives us another way of examining speaker-meaning. It states that a speaker tries to convey **new information** in addition to rehashing information a listener already knows. Comprehension is said to be a process of relating new information to information already known, called given or old information. A speaker uses linguistic devices to help a listener identify what is new and what is old. For example, a pronoun signals that we are referring to information that a listener should already know from a previous utterance, the situation, or knowledge of the world. When a speaker estimates what a listener already knows, a speaker is said to be assuming the point-of-view of the listener.

Conditions can be devised to observe a patient conveying new information. A blunt procedure is to put a barrier between a patient and a listener so that the listener does not see the patient's stimuli. Another method is to provide both participants with their own set of pictures of slightly differing events. Aphasic patients can be quite good at verbalizing information about one picture that is distinctive enough for listeners to choose the same picture (Busch, Brookshire, and Nicholas, 1988). Another approach is to switch listeners, so that a patient may talk to one who is already familiar with a message or another who is unfamiliar with the message. Thus, we try to minimize or control a **listener's prior knowledge** of a patient's topic or meaning. Also, we may record the *listener's* comprehension accuracy in addition to recording the patient's expressive behavior.

A new information condition necessarily leads to more shared responsibility for exchanging messages. That is, some **communicative burden** shifts to the listener who now has to figure out what the patient means. Marshall and his colleagues (1997) used an interactive task to study severely impaired patients. The patients transmitted messages to a listener who paraphrased, verified, and questioned until the message was understood. Groups of raters recorded the patients' communicative efficiency and the communicative burden assumed by the listener (e.g., amount of questioning). The severely impaired patients varied in communicative efficiency, and lower efficiency seemed to be associated with increases in the listener's burden.

Another dimension of listener-knowledge is captured in the **familiarity of a listener** to a speaker. Clinicians, spouses, and strangers contribute differently with respect to world knowledge and communicative strategies. Stimley and Noll (1994) had familiar and unfamiliar examiners administer the four verbal subtests of the PICA to aphasic patients. The patients scored significantly better on the most difficult subtests with the unfamiliar examiner. One explanation was that a patient may reduce effort assuming that the familiar clinician already knows some things about the patient's communicative style. In Marshall's experiment, ratings differed according to the amount of information the raters knew about the messages. One explanation was that prior knowledge of messages may make clinical observers more attentive to the particulars of how messages are conveyed (Marshall, et al., 1997).

Familiarity of a listener may not affect a patient's story-telling behavior (Bottenberg and Lemme, 1991; Brenneise-Sarshad, Brookshire, and Nicholas, 1991). In a study of conversations with patients who had Broca's aphasia, Doyle and others (1994) manipulated familiarity of the communicative partner, conversational method (i.e., open topic and constrained topic), location (i.e., at home or a simulated home environment), and number of participants (i.e., dyad or triad). Only conversational method affected the use of statements, requests, answers, and ambiguities.

In general, investigation of shared information has suffered from the absence of clear connection between the experimental manipulations and the measure of patients' behavior. The measure is often one that has already been developed for general purposes. Explanation can be facilitated with a study derived from a theoretical framework that links the measure to variables. That is, a framework would indicate why chosen independent variables *should* affect the chosen dependent variables.

Conversational Management

Now, we consider interactive characteristics of conversation. Clinical investigators have borrowed methods from sociolinguistics and anthropology or have invented their own approaches.

Generally attention is given to the local management system of turn-taking or the global structure of any conversation whether it be face-to-face or over the telephone. Like trying to tame a wild horse, clinicians are working on reliable methods of observation directed by frameworks specifying structural features of conversation.

An **ethnographic approach** is taken by Simmons-Mackie and Damico (1997). Their goal is to study aphasia in its natural state without preconception. Experiments are unrestricted interpersonal interactions so that data can be "authentic" as a sampling of the real world. Patients interact with family, friends, clinicians, or strangers. Although Simmons-Mackie and Damico look for certain categories such as compensatory behaviors, their analytic orientation is to scrutinize the data repeatedly without formalized measurement procedures. One technique, called lamination sessions, invites several professionals to comment on the data to provide different perspectives. "Within this methodology the collection and close examination of natural data suggest patterns which implicate theory" (p. 763).

Mild-to-moderately impaired aphasic people tend to conform to conversational rules. In the typical conversation, speaker-turns rarely overlap (i.e., simultaneous talking), and gaps between speakers often span less than a second. This precision stems from an inherent predictability of a speaker-turn enabling a partner to anticipate when a switch from speaking to listening will occur. We may be concerned about the comprehension deficit and press for speech of Wernicke's aphasia. However, these patients also appear to be sensitive to turn-taking conventions (Schienberg and Holland, 1980).

There are different types of turn-sequences (Levinson, 1983). One is the **adjacency pair** in which a speaker-turn (first part) is followed by a predictable response from the other speaker (second part). For example, a greeting is followed by a greeting; an answer follows a question. Other types of turn-sequences may encompass three or four turns. One of these is the **repair-sequence,** in which a speaker's turn is modified because it failed to convey a message. We might anticipate that repairs are frequent in conversation with an aphasic person, because either the patient or another speaker does not get a point across.

Lubinski, Duchan, and Weitzner-Lin (1980) referred to repairs as "hint-and-guess" sequences in conversation with aphasic patients. A patient's speaking turn consists of a hint, and a listener guesses the patient's intent. The patient may attempt a repair in the third turn of the sequence. A repair may be self-initiated (without prompting) or other-initiated (with prompting). It may be a self-repair by the patient or an other-repair by another participant. Neurologically intact adults prefer self-initiation and self-repairs. Other-repairs are rare; and when they occur, they are usually modulated with prefaces such as "You mean…?" or addendums such as "…, I think."

Ferguson (1994) studied precursors of repairs in conversations between aphasic patients and either familiar individuals living with the patients or less familiar individuals who were visiting the patients. In particular, she looked for *trouble-indicating behavior* by either participant, such as commenting about a word-finding problem or failing to continue in the conversation. Then she examined types of repair, called *repair trajectories.* Of course, normal subjects indicated more trouble and used more repairs when interacting with aphasic partners compared to interacting with other normal partners. Visiting subjects made more other-repairs than subjects living with the aphasic participants, indicating that unfamiliar partners are more likely to seek a "speedy remedy" for trouble.

Conversational Gesturing

Gesturing serves at least two functions during conversation. As discussed early in this chapter, one function is communicative with either the automatic gestures that show emotion or the volitional gestures that express ideas. Gestures are also used for signaling conversational moves, thereby, regulating an interaction. Clinical researchers are especially interested in severely nonfluent or global aphasias for whom gesturing may be considered to be a compensatory behavior (Simmons-Mackie and Damico, 1997).

Simmons-Mackie and Damico (1996) employed their ethnographic approach to identify **discourse markers** that nonfluent aphasic people employ in managing conversational interaction. They observed the following markers in two patients:

- initiation or alerting (e.g., raised finger indicating desire to begin or maintain a speaking turn)
- termination or reorientation (e.g., hand clasp to end a failed communicative attempt)
- participant role request (e.g., eye gaze and body movements to relinquish speaking turn)
- affiliation or politeness (e.g., "Is good" as a response to an offer)
- truth level (e.g., "I don't know" amidst trying to convey something)

Other research has shown that severely nonfluent patients indicate when they are not comprehending, and they signal for help from a clinician (Herrmann, Koch, Johannsen-Horbach, and Wallesch, 1989).

Researchers have also studied whether communicative gestures arise naturally in communicative situations. Severely aphasic patients displayed better gestural ability in a new information condition than in a formal test of limb apraxia (Feyereisen, Barter, Goossens, and Clarebaut, 1988). Yet, communicative use of gesture decreased when a barrier was placed between patients and partners, indicating that patients are sensitive to the viability of gesture as a communicative option (Glosser, Wiener, and Kaplan, 1986). In conversational interactions, patients with Broca's aphasia used more gesture than neurologically intact persons (Le May, David, and Thomas, 1988; Smith, 1987). Gesturing style in Broca's and Wernicke's aphasia corresponded to the nature of their verbal expression (Duffy, Duffy, and Mercaitis, 1984).

In developing the **Boston Nonvocal Communication Scale,** Borod and others (1989) measured spontaneous use of gestures during "informal activities," especially when interacting with others. Seven types of behavior were rated on a four-point scale for frequency of occurrence. Behavioral categories included greetings, pointing, indicating yes or no, and using pantomime or drawing to communicate. Spontaneous gestures were used less often by a globally aphasic group than by other groups.

More recently, aphasic patients were videotaped while describing a complex picture to someone who had not seen it. Then they were asked questions to create a more interactive condition (Hadar, Wenkert-Olenik, Krauss, and Soroker, 1998). The researchers tracked gestures that supplemented meaning conveyed with language. Also, aphasic patients were divided into some unusual categories (i.e., conceptual, semantic, and phonologic groups). The findings indicate that patients with conceptual deficits beyond aphasia gestured differently from normal controls. Pantomimes were sometimes unrelated to associated words. Patients with deficits restricted to word-finding gestured most like controls.

OVERALL FUNCTIONAL STATUS

At rehabilitation centers, a patient's functional independence is commonly rated soon after admission and at discharge. Professionals generally use rating scales to assess *activities of daily living* (ADL), and these scales encompass the domains of several rehabilitation services. Subscale ratings are usually obtained for each activity or function. A full-scale score addresses overall dysfunction. One of the original rating scales is the **Barthel Index** for ten activities of daily living including ambulation, feeding, bathing, and dressing (Fortinski, Granger, and Seltzer, 1981; Mahoney and Barthel, 1965). Current scales are used to track progress, measure functional outcomes, and assist in determining costs of rehabilitation.

A national task force developed the **Functional Independence Measure** or **FIM** (State University of New York, 1990). It is a widely used multidisciplinary scale intended to measure overall severity of disability or "burden of care." It consists of 18 items classified into the following six subscales:

- self-care (eating, grooming, bathing, dressing, toileting)
- sphincter control (bladder and bowel management)
- mobility (bed, chair, toilet)
- locomotion (walking or wheelchair, stairs)
- communication (comprehension, expression)
- social cognition (interaction, problem solving, memory)

These subscales are grouped into *motor* and *cognitive* domains with communication and social cognition included in the latter. Each member of the rehabilitation team uses a fairly reliable 7-point scale for rating abilities in his or her domain (Hamilton, Laughlin, Granger, and Kayton, 1991). The speech-language pathologist rates functional comprehension and expression, reserving lowest ratings for "complete dependence on a helper" and highest ratings for independence requiring "no helper" (also, see Chapter 10).

The **Rehabilitation Outcome Measure** (ROM) was developed to be more discipline-friendly than the FIM (Chiaromonte, 1996). In contrast to the FIM's single scale for all rehabilitation professions, the ROM has separate 7-point scales for speech-language pathology, occupational therapy, or physical therapy. The scale for SLP is worded generally from "profound" to "moderate" to "independent." The OT scale is worded from "total assistance" to "minimal assistance" to "total independence." Also, in contrast to measuring two broad communicative functions with the FIM, the ROM's scale for SLP distinguishes between language and speech and can be applied to nine deficit areas including reading, writing, voice, and swallowing.

Regarding assumptions underlying the FIM and similar constructs in rehabilitation, Holland (1998) expressed some concern regarding "a health care climate that is driven by notions of independence" (p. 846). She reasoned that this climate may appear to be contradictory to the communication domain in which cooperation is inherent to conversation. "The behaviours involved in conversation, by definition, are functionally *interdependent*" (p. 846). This realization becomes especially important for functional treatment (see Chapter 12). For the aphasic adult, a communicative independence "is being able to hold up one's end of a conversational interchange" (p. 846).

ASSESSMENT OF FUNCTIONAL COMMUNICATION

Although functional assessment has been mandated by legislation and payment providers (Frattali and Lynch, 1989), some devices have been around since before the mandates. The main idea is to ensure that services are helping a patient progress in activities that are essential for daily living and, thus, maximize independence from the health care system. Newer methods are influenced by the currently reduced time for assessment.

Communication Profiles

The **Functional Communication Profile** (FCP) is a rating scale for mostly language functions of "everyday urban life" (Sarno, 1969). A clinician estimates (or predicts) abilities in five categories: Movement, Speaking (e.g., saying nouns, noun-verb combinations), Understanding (e.g., for conversation, television, movies), Reading, and Other (e.g., writing, calculation). Functional performance is defined as the use of language "without assistance, cues, or artificial conditions." The estimates are obtained from informal interviews and formal test performances. While the interview is freshly in mind, each item is rated on a nine-point scale. The FCP has been used to study recovery not detected by a traditional aphasia test (Sarno, et al., 1971; Sarno and Levita, 1979).

Prutting and Kirchner (1987) devised a **pragmatic protocol** that addresses 30 features of conversation. It has sections for rating verbal aspects (e.g., topic selection and initiation, turn-taking behaviors), paralinguistic aspects (e.g., intelligibility, prosody), and nonverbal aspects (e.g., proximity, posture, gesture). Each behavior is rated as appropriate, inappropriate, or not observed. Profiles were reported for 11 LHDs and 10 RHDs in 15 minutes of conversation with a familiar partner.

Communicative Abilities in Daily Living (CADL)

Audrey Holland's CADL presents familiar situations for examining interpersonal interaction and response to communicative problems such as making an appointment, shopping at a store, or reading the speedometer. Peformance is scored according to communicative adequacy. Many items pertain to the numerous visual symbols and signs that we rely on in everyday life. Holland (1980a) wanted "to incorporate both more natural language activities and a more natural style in an effort to more closely approximate normal communication" (p. 47).

The test contains a series of 68 items organized within a series of situations; and, within each situation, items are arranged according to the natural sequence in which behaviors would occur. It begins with two items for social greetings between a patient and clinician occurring away from the test site. It proceeds to a brief interview and then to role-playing a trip to the doctor's office. Subsequent situations are presented with drawings, photographs, and props. Functional problems include driving, shopping, and using a telephone. The test takes 35 to 40 minutes.

Scoring is done with a three-point scale applied to each item. A score of 2 is given when the patient conveys a message in any manner. Failure to convey a message is scored 0. A 1 is an "in the ballpark" response. The maximum score is 136 points. We can develop a profile of abilities according to ten categories of functional behavior, such as the following:

- Speech acts (i.e., items that call for informing, explaining, negotiating, requesting, and warning)
- Utilizing verbal and nonverbal context (e.g., What do you do when the gas gauge reads empty?)
- Social conventions (e.g., end of the test, reaction to clinician's saying, "I'm sorry this all took so long")
- Nonverbal symbolic communication (e.g., recognition of facial expression)
- Humor, absurdity, metaphor (e.g., Look at these cartoons. Which one is funny?)

Functional Assessment of Communication Skills (ASHA-FACS)

In 1992, the American Speech-Language-Hearing Association sponsored the development of a supplemental measure of functional communication for obtaining outcome data with adults. The developers especially wanted to assess the areas of disability and handicap, or the use of language and other communicative skills in activities of daily life. The result is the **ASHA Functional Assessment of Communication Skills** (ASHA-FACS) which covers four domains summarized in Table 7.3. A field test version with 44 items was

TABLE 7.3 Domains assessed with the ASHA FACS. Only some of the 44 items are listed under the domains (Frattali, et al., 1995).

SOCIAL COMMUNICATION	COMMUNICATION OF BASIC NEEDS	DAILY PLANNING	READING/WRITING/ NUMBER CONCEPTS
Uses names of familiar people	Recognizes familiar faces or voices	Tells time	Understands signs
Explains how to do something	Expresses feelings	Dials the telephone	Follows written directions
Participates in telephone conversation	Requests help	Keeps appointments	Writes or types name
Understands nonliteral meaning and intent	Responds in an emergency	Follows a map	Completes forms
			Makes money transactions

described for initial publication (Frattali, Thompson, Holland, Wohl, and Ferketic, 1995).

To obtain observations, the clinician becomes familiar with a patient's communicative behavior and solicits judgments of family members and other caregivers. Each of the items is rated according to two scales. One is a 7-point Scale of Communicative Independence. The other is a 5-point Scale of Qualitative Dimensions of Communication, which is intended to assess the nature of functional deficit. As reported in 1995, a second pilot test had produced data on 32 patients with aphasia due to stroke and 26 patients with traumatic brain injury. One study found that the ASHA-FACS and the Western Aphasia Battery are strongly correlated (McIntosh, Ramsberger, and Prescott, 1996).

Experimental Assessments

The **Amsterdam-Nijmegen Everyday Language Test** (ANELT) has been revised a couple of times during the course of its development (Blomert, Kean, Koster, and Schokker, 1994; Blomert, Koster, Van Mier, and Kean, 1987). It is a measure of verbal communicative abilities exhibited in verbally presented functional scenerios like the following:

- The kids on the street are playing football in your yard. You have asked them before not to do that. You go outside and speak to the boys. What do you say?
- You have an appointment with the doctor. Something else has come up. You call up and what do you say?

Verbal responses are evaluated according to an A-scale for understandability of the message independent of linguistic form and a B-scale for intelligibility of an utterance independent of content or meaning. Two equivalent versions of the test (i.e., ANELT I and ANELT II) permit measuring progress without the bias of a learning effect.

The **Communicative Effectiveness Index** (CETI) attempts to reach into a patient's daily life (Lomas, Pickard, Bester, Elbard, Finlayson, and Zoghaib, 1989). A family member or friend is asked to rate communicative ability for 16 situations that had been determined to be most important to family members. Situations include getting someone's attention, having coffee-time visits and conversations, conveying physical problems such as aches and pains, starting a conversation with people not close to the family, and conversing with strangers. Ratings are based on a scale with respect to "not at all able" at one end and "as able as before stroke" at the other end.

Another approach to measuring pragmatic skills, similar to parts of the CADL, comes from observing real-life interactions that some have decided to call *service encounters.* In such encounters, information, goods, or services are exchanged in face-to-face interaction or over the telephone. Togher, Hand and Code (1997) evaluated patients making two types of telephone calls. One task was to call a bus service for information that would be helpful for organizing a group outing. Another task was to call the police to find out how a brain injured person gets a driver's licence reinstated. As we might gather from the tasks, the patients had a relatively high level of language ability, in these cases, after traumatic brain injury (Chapter 9).

Transcripts of the service encounters were assessed with a Generic Structure Potential (GSP) analysis. This analysis begins with dividing the conversations into speaking turns (or "moves"). The turns are classified as to the presence of obligatory elements in the encounter, such as a greeting, service request, service enquiry, closing, and goodbye. Other elements may be predictable deviations from the type of patient being evaluated. Togher looked for incomplete, unrelated, or inappropriate reponses. The investigators found that their patients differed from controls who engaged in the same encounters.

MARTIN EXETER'S FUNCTIONAL SKILLS

Jackie Exeter quickly discovered that Martin could communicate better than he could talk even during his acute hospitalization. It made sense to try writing at first, but this effort showed that aphasia affects both modalities. Many residual communicative sensitivities were drawn from an intact right hemisphere and intact structures involved in new learning and memory of his life before his stroke. For example, just a few days after the stroke, it was evident that he knew where he was and recognized his family and friends. Doctors and nurses became familiar quickly. A few words referred to Europe and his job.

Communicative intent was apparent when considering words, left-handed gestures, and slightly asymmetrical facial expressions. He gave a "thumbs up" to his worried son, Peter. When Julianna showed up in his room for a second visit, Martin frowned a little and muttered something that sounded like "school" and a question. When she said she would go back to school as soon as she knew he was OK, Martin smiled. As the days became weeks, he could get across basic needs, but his language impairment was keeping him from conveying details. Jackie had to ask many questions. Sometimes listeners were not sure if he

TABLE 7.4 Functional tests and measures introduced in this chapter.

CATEGORY	ASSESSMENT DEVICE	AUTHOR	DESCRIPTION
nonverbal abilities	Limb Apraxia Test (LAT)	Duffy & Duffy (1989)	imitated movements
	Test of Oral and Limb Apraxia (TOLA)	Helm-Estabrooks (1991)	requested and imitated movements
	Assessment of Nonverbal Communication	Duffy and Duffy (1984)	pantomime recognition and production
discourse	correct information unit analysis	Nicholas & Brookshire (1993,1995)	counting informative words and main concepts
	Discourse Comprehension Test	Brookshire & Nicholas (1993)	comprehension of main ideas and details
overall functional screening	Functional Independence Measure (FIM)	State University of New York (1990)	multidisciplinary rating scales for severity of disability
	Rehabilitation Outcome Measure (ROM)	Chiaromonte (1996)	more discipline-friendly scales for severity disability
functional communication	Functional Communication Profile (FCP)	Sarno (1969)	predictive rating of language skills in natural conditions
	informal pragmatic protocol	Prutting & Kirchner (1987)	ratings of verbal and nonverbal behaviors in conversation
	Communicative Abilities in Daily Living (CADL)	Holland (1980a)	testing that includes role-playing and functional problems to solve
	ASHA Functional Assessment of Communication Skills (ASHA FACS)	Frattali, Thompson, Holland, Wohl, and Ferketic (1995)	rating scales of four areas of functional activities

was talking about the present, past, or future unless the topic became apparent. Martin made a great deal of progress over the months after the stroke. Long-term progress in communicative abilities is reviewed at the end of Chapter 10.

SUMMARY AND CONCLUSIONS

In presenting disabilities caused by aphasia, this chapter addressed areas of communicative ability that are either spared or somewhat disrupted by language-specific impairment. Topics included nonverbal communication, the processing of words and sentences in context, and conversational skills. Some of these topics set up ensuing discussions of pragmatic disorders in the next two chapters. Table 7.4 summarizes functional assessments that were also introduced.

The chapter began by reviewing the communicative impact of deficits beyond the language system. Most patients are able to tap into nonverbal processes for recognition of information and expression of basic needs. Many can gesture and draw. However, severe aphasias are accompanied by difficulties in using symbolic gestures and drawing. Linguistic deficits can also reduce the informativeness of discourse and disrupt its microstructural cohesion. On the other hand, intact schemas in semantic memory and knowledge of narrative organization contribute to communicative competencies remaining after left-hemisphere stroke. Aphasic people follow the rules for managing conversational interaction. There is a great deal to build upon for treatment designed to maximize a patient's functional communicative capacities. In general, when a speech-language pathologist attends to a patient's communication with family and others, the clinician establishes a link between the patient's progress and its relationship to communicative contexts (see Chapter 12).

CHAPTER 8

RIGHT HEMISPHERE DISORDERS

In 1974, Associate Supreme Court Justice William O. Douglas suffered a stroke in the right side of his brain (Gardner, 1982). Because he could talk and write, he appeared to recover rapidly. He checked himself out of rehabilitation and was anxious to resume work, claiming his weakened left arm was injured in a fall. Upon returning to the Court, he insisted he was the Chief Justice. In court "he dozed, asked irrelevant questions, and sometimes rambled on." After being asked to resign, "he came back to his office, buzzed for his clerks...asked to participate in, draft, and even publish his own opinions separately; and he requested that a tenth seat be placed at the Justices' bench" (p. 310).

For a long time, persons with nondominant or right hemisphere strokes were not referred to speech-language clinics, because their primary disorders are related to nonverbal cognitive systems and they do not display the word-finding and grammatical deficits associated with aphasia. Now, these patients may be referred for the following reasons:

- The patient has a swallowing problem or motor speech deficit.
- Someone with an old right-hemisphere infarct has recently suffered a left-hemisphere stroke.
- The patient has communicative difficulties caused by right-hemisphere stroke.

Justice Douglas' rambling talk and failure to appreciate situations might have put him in the third category.

The chapter begins with standard clinical assessment of language behavior and investigation of language processing. Then, many of the areas of nonverbal cognitive impairment are introduced, and later discussion turns to influences of some of these primary impairments on language behavior. Finally, the chapter presents areas of pragmatic difficulty in the use of language. As we go along, some new information about aphasia is provided in comparison to right hemisphere dysfunction (RHD).

LANGUAGE EVALUATION

A speech-language clinician might begin evaluating someone with a right hemisphere stroke by administering familiar tests of language ability that were designed for assessing aphasia. Our standard language tests assess mostly word-and sentence-level abilities. Hiram Brownell has studied language abilities with RHD extensively at Boston College. His perspective was that "RHD patients are most often nonaphasic in that they can normally process most words and sentences in isolation" (Brownell, 1988, p. 248).

Aphasia Batteries

The *Western Aphasia Battery* was given to 53 nondominant hemisphere damaged patients (Kertesz, 1979). This mostly RHD group had an average aphasia quotient (AQ) of 92.9, which is slightly beneath the cut-off score of 93.8 for language impairment but well above the 53.5 average for stroke-induced aphasia. The RHDs' standard deviation around the mean was 8.0 compared with 29.9 for the aphasic group, an indication that RHDs are more homogeneous on a language evaluation. Many were normal, but others were somewhat below the cut-off.

On the *Porch Index of Communicative Ability,* RHDs had an average overall score of 13.03 compared with 11.12 for an aphasic group (Wertz and Dronkers, 1994). Porch and Palmer (1986) produced conversion tables according to the subtest categories. Table 8.1 displays a few scores at the same percentile levels for RHDs and aphasic LHDs, indicative of the general severity levels of each group. As severity of deficit increases, the difference between aphasia and RHD becomes more pronounced for actual response level. A difference in auditory comprehension does not appear until severe overall impairment (25th percentile). A difference in verbal expression becomes pronounced at a higher level (50th percentile) favoring the RHDs. Above the 60th percentile, RHDs' spoken language falls in the normal range.

Also in Table 8.1, comparative deficit is reversed for the nonverbal test of copying shapes (subtest F) in which RHDs have lower scores. Their drawing difficulty is especially striking, considering that these patients are not likely to have paralysis of their preferred (right) hand, while many aphasic people attempt to draw with their weakened preferred (right) hand.

A French battery was given to a group with RHD (Joanette, Lecours, Lepage, and Lamoureux, 1983). Contrary to the traditional aphasia battery, some language tasks were comparable to complex verbal subtests in intelligence tests such as verbal reasoning and producing sentences from abstract nouns (e.g., *cleverness, competition*). The RHD group was deficient in 34 of 47 subtests, and most exhibited difficulties with something.

In general, RHD does not allow patients to escape difficulty with some language-related activities, especially when overall dysfunction is severe and the language system is challenged (see Myers, 1999; Tompkins, 1995). Some patients will score below an aphasia test's cut-off for language impairment that some might say is diagnostic of

TABLE 8.1 Response levels from 94 right-hemisphere-damaged patients (Porch and Palmer, 1986) compared with 357 left-hemisphere-damaged aphasic patients (Porch, 1981) at percentiles determined for each group. Copying shapes is subtest F, in which RHDs have lower scores than LHDS.

		OVERALL	AUDITORY COMPREHENSION	VERBAL	WRITING	COPYING SHAPES
90th	RHD	13.99	15.00	14.59	13.21	13.8
	LHD	14.04	15.00	14.35	13.18	14.5
75th	RHD	13.47	15.00	14.24	11.94	12.8
	LHD	12.89	15.00	13.50	11.05	14.0
60th	RHD	12.95	14.87	13.92	10.66	12.1
	LHD	11.71	14.60	12.30	9.23	13.3
50th	RHD	12.60	14.80	13.73	9.82	11.7
	LHD	10.89	14.25	10.77	8.22	13.0
40th	RHD	12.34	14.66	13.45	8.90	11.2
	LHD	9.96	13.60	8.90	7.33	12.4
25th	RHD	11.32	14.15	12.56	7.50	9.9
	LHD	8.38	11.70	6.04	6.29	11.1
10th	RHD	9.33	11.30	10.30	5.63	7.3
	LHD	6.15	8.05	3.75	4.98	8.0

aphasia. However, we should be reminded of a point in Chapter 3 stating that we do not allow a test to do our diagnosing for us. Someone with RHD makes mistakes on language tasks for reasons other than having a language disorder or aphasia, and the reader should identify these reasons in this chapter (also, see discussion of agnosia in Chapter 6). The next two sections give us some idea of how these patients do with words and sentences in isolation, and what investigators have thought of these performances.

Language Comprehension

One source of information about specific language skills comes from investigators who quietly use RHDs as a control group in studies focusing on aphasia. Unfortunately the RHDs are often ignored in discussion of results, despite the fact that they sometimes perform almost as poorly as the aphasic subjects (e.g., Chenery, et al., 1990).

Patients have displayed good word comprehension, showing mild deficit when presented with four semantically similar picture options (Couglan and Warrington, 1978). Their few errors were related in meaning and occurred when there was a diagnosis of an additional general mental deficiency (Gainotti, Caltagirone, and Miceli, 1983). These results have led to speculation that RHD can affect the lexical-semantic system in a unique way (e.g., Hagoort, Brown, and Swaab, 1995). A few studies displayed little hint of deficient semantic structure in a variety of sorting or semantic judgment tasks (Gainotti, et al., 1986; Grossman and Wilson, 1987; Koemeda-Lutz, et al., 1987), whereas one study showed judgments as deficient as aphasic subjects (Chenery, et al., 1990).

Investigators have also begun to study the automatic obligatory level of word processing. Leonard and Baum (1997) studied activation of lexical information with the auditory form-priming task introduced in Chapter 4. Like aphasic subjects, RHDs had a pronounced priming effect for combined phonological-orthographic relatedness with a 250 msec interval between a prime and a lexical decision target. For semantic priming, which detects spreading activation in the semantic network, a control group of mostly RHDs exhibited priming at a generous 500 msec interval (Chenery, et al., 1990). However, the status of automaticity needs to be examined at much shorter prime-target intervals.

Another study tapped into the region of semantic memory storing concepts of famous people. Schweinberger (1995) compared RHDs and LHDs with a visual priming task and a 455 msec prime-target interval. A prime was a name like *Lennon,* and the related target was *McCartney.* To look for facilitation, a famous target was preceded by an unfamiliar name considered to be a neutral prime. To look for inhibition, *Travolta* was one prime and *Carter* was the unrelated target. Overall, RHDs were faster than LHDs. RHDs exhibited facilitation relative to neutral primes, but LHDs were not facilitated. When the prime was the face of a related person instead of the name, RHDs were not facilitated; whereas LHDs were primed slightly. This finding anticipates an area of interest discussed later in this chapter, namely, the ability of RHDs to recognize faces.

RHDs usually do not have a deficient short-term memory span (Tanridag, et al., 1987) and display little or no difficulty following Token Test instructions (e.g., Boller and Vignolo, 1966; Hartje, et al., 1973; Swisher and Sarno, 1969). They may have difficulty arranging words into a grammatical sentence (Cavalli, DeRenzi, Faglioni, and Vitale, 1981), but grammatical judgment tasks indicate that they possess fundamental linguistic knowledge (Grossman and Haberman, 1982; Schwartz, et al., 1987). Problems may arise with sentence comprehension when determining thematic roles in passive sentences (Heeschen, 1980; Hier and Kaplan, 1980).

Language Production

RHDs tend to name common objects effectively (Boller, 1968; Newcombe, Oldfield, Ratcliff, et al., 1971; Porch and Palmer, 1986). A statistical deficit has been uncovered, for example, with normal controls naming 18.4 of 20 objects correctly and RHDs naming 16.8 (Diggs and Basili, 1987). In another study, RHDs were compared to nonaphasic LHDs with a variety of language tasks (Vallar, Papagno, and Cappa, 1988). None of the RHDs were below normal cut-off scores. The nonaphasic LHDs were deficient mainly with naming, indicating that LHD, whether or not it causes aphasia, is more likely to cause naming problems than right hemisphere damage.

As indicated in Chapter 4, one method for investigating whether there is a semantic basis for naming deficits is to see if the deficit is related to metalinguistic tasks. Germani and Pierce (1995) compared RHDs and LHDs with a word sorting task which involves relating lexical and semantic knowledge. With the Boston Naming Test, RHDs were significantly less impaired than LHDs. Both groups were unimpaired when sorting according to "important" attributes (e.g., book-chapters), but both groups were impaired when sorting according to less important attributes (e.g., book-pictures). Unlike the aphasic subjects, RHDs displayed no relationship between sorting and naming scores. Thus, RHDs retain a high level of naming ability and common lexical-semantic knowledge.

Word-finding problems appear with divergent word fluency tests (Boller, 1968; Borkowski, et al., 1967; Wertz, et al., 1986). RHDs had more difficulty with semantic fluency than with first-letter fluency (Joanette and Goulet, 1986). In another study of semantic fluency, RHDs generated fewer words than normal controls (Grossman, 1981). Joanette's patients were deficient quantitatively only after the first 30 seconds (Joanette, Goulet, and Le Dorze, 1988). RHDs generated more clusters of related items than aphasic subjects, again indicating better use of semantic knowledge (Grossman, 1981). Compared with aphasic subjects, the items in clusters were less central to a category (e.g., "waterskiing, sailing, swimming" for SPORTS, instead of *baseball* or *football*).

Glosser and Goodglass (1991) studied word associations by asking RHDs to say the first word that comes to mind when given another word. Response latency was measured with a stopwatch. On a number of dimensions, this clinical group was unimpaired. They were normal in number of high-frequency or popular words produced and in response speed. However, RHDs sporadically produced idiosyncratic or "pragmatically deviant" words that were not produced by normal controls, such as saying "snake" in response to *memory,* "substitute" to *because,* or "mile" to *salty.*

People with RHD tend to be fluent conversationalists. Clinical investigators find more problems with lexical-semantics than with phonology and syntax (Cappa, et al., 1990). Reduced productivity in word-fluency only after 30 seconds indicates that problems arise with processes that are "less automatic" than the core processes of everyday verbal expression (Joanette, et al., 1988).

As suggested earlier, RHDs and mildly aphasic patients may score similarly on clinical tests but probably for different reasons. Myers (1986) argued that unusual language behavior with RHD is explained by impairments of attention, perception, and organizational skills. So, let us turn to the primary cognitive impairments caused by right hemisphere stroke.

AWARENESS OF DEFICITS

Justice Douglas' insistence on continuing his Supreme Court duties indicates either a lack of awareness or a denial of disability. McGlynn and Schacter (1989) distinguished among phenomena associated with unawareness. The term **anosognosia** refers to a lack of awareness or recognition of disease or disability. Clinicians have used other terms such as *lack of insight* or *imperception of disease.* In general, patients are unable to become aware of a neurological dysfunction. On the other hand, **denial of impairment** is a psychological defense mechanism; and a patient who is strictly in denial is considered to be capable of awareness of deficit.

Anosognosia is usually observed as lack of awareness of paralysis. For example, a patient with left hemiplegia makes plans to play golf

(Tompkins, 1995). Unawareness of right hemiplegia by LHDs is rare (Cutting, 1978). McGlynn and Schacter (1989) complained about an excessive reliance on subjective reports in research. Pendley and Ramsberger (1996) created a 6-point scale to measure self-awareness of task performances with respect to self-correction behavior and response to a clinician's questions. They found that RHDs were impaired relative to a normal control group and that self-awareness was not correlated with actual task performance.

VISUOSPATIAL FUNCTIONS

Oliver Sacks' (1985) "man who mistook his wife for a hat" was a music teacher with signs of RHD. When describing pictures, Dr. P saw "only details, which he spotted like blips on a radar screen…He had no sense whatever of a landscape or scene" (p. 9). When imagining a stroll through a familiar part of town, he mentioned buildings on his right but not on his left. He approached familiar faces as if they were "abstract puzzles or tests." Sacks sensed that he "faced me with his ears." He saw faces when there were none, as "he might pat the heads of water-hydrants and parking-meters, taking these to be the heads of children" (p. 7). When Dr. P. decided that the examination was over, he looked around for his hat and tugged his wife's head.

Neuropsychological assessment with the WAIS commonly shows a pattern that is reversed relative to aphasia (see Chapter 3). That is, someone with RHD is likely to have a discrepancy score in which the Performance IQ, requiring visuospatial recognition and reasoning skills, is lowered relative to the Verbal IQ (Hom and Reitan, 1990).

Visuospatial Attention

Another patient was a woman who was "only half made-up, the left side of her face absurdly void of lipstick and rouge" (Sacks, 1985, p. 74). Neglect of one-half of space is caused by damage in the parietotemporal region. It is more frequent and/or obvious after RHD, so that **left neglect** is more common than right neglect. Patients with posterior RHD bump into things on their left, leave food on the left side of the plate, dress only the right side, and draw only the right side of an object. Later in this section, we shall take a look at the role of left neglect in wheelchair-related accidents.

Clinical detection of left neglect includes a **crossing out test** of marking lines through circles scattered about a page. A person with left neglect crosses out circles on the right, ignoring the circles on the left. Severity of neglect is measured by the number of omissions. With lines scattered about a page, called the **line cancellation test,** Plourde and others (1993) showed that some RHDs have either severe neglect and others have no or very mild neglect with very few in between. Most subjects with LHD exhibited no or mild neglect.

In a **line bisection test,** a patient is asked to mark the center of a horizontal line. Someone with left neglect marks to the right of midline. Patients with severe neglect perform this task differently from those with mild neglect. Patients with mild neglect vary their mark slightly as line length and position vary, but those with severe neglect mark the line at a fixed distance from the right end (Koyama, Ishiai, Seki, and Nakayama, 1997).

Manipulation of visuospatial attention is demonstrated with a *cued line-bisection test* in which some lines have letters at the right end, others have letters at the left end, and other lines have letters at both ends (Harvey, Milner, and Roberts, 1995). Patients are instructed to name the letter-cues, called "anchors," and then bisect a line in the middle as accurately as possible. There is a bias toward the cued end, even for people without neglect. Harvey was interested in the effect of these cues for patients who already have a tendency to bisect to the right. Unilateral left cues decreased the extent of rightward error as if "dragging" attention leftward. Unilateral right cues did not increase the rightward error. This study provides a hint as to how patients with RHD are trained to compensate for left neglect.

Anosognosia for hemiplegia could be construed as being a symptom of left neglect. However, neglect and anosognosia do not necessarily occur together, and many patients with neglect are aware of their problem (McGlynn and Schacter, 1989). A double dissociation between left neglect and anosognosia for paralysis was demonstrated among 97 patients with RHD (Bisiach, Vallar, Perani, Papagno, and Berti, 1986). Thirty-two of these patients had little or no neglect to account for substantial anosognosia, whereas four patients ignored the left side of the body but were fully aware of motor impairment.

Neglect is thought to be a disorder of selective or focused attention and, thus, is often called *hemi-inattention.* Focusing attention is managed by "special-purpose" attentional systems in specific functional systems. That is, we have a spatial attention mechanism and an auditory attention mechanism. The visual attention mechanism is like a spotlight with an adjustable beam.

Posner discovered that *covert attention* or the cognitive spotlight is impaired, rather than overt shifts of eye movement (Posner, Walker, Friedrich, and Rafal, 1984, 1987). In Posner's theory, there are three stages in shifting covert attention: (1) disengagement from a current focus, (2) moving attention to a target, and (3) engagement of the target. A right parietal lesion prohibits disengagement from a current focus in the right visual field. Visual cues are thought to facilitate disengagement, permitting movement of the internal spotlight to information in the left field (see Arguin and Bub, 1993).

A sense for the internal spotlight was provided by Bisiach and others (1981) in Milan, Italy. In the clinic they asked patients with RHD to imagine the familiar Piazza del Duomo, a large square commanded at one end by a 600-year-old cathedral. Asked to report buildings on each side, patients could report buildings on the right but not on the left. Intact stored structural description of the neglected buildings was exhibited when the patients imagined the piazza facing the opposite direction. Now, the previously neglected buildings were reported from the right-side, whereas the previously reported buildings were ignored.

There are other theories of neglect that are slightly different (Halligan and Marshall, 1994). The proposals indicate that spatial attention is multifaceted; "one should view the distribution of attention over space as the result of a variety of neuronal subsystems that are called into action depending on the cognitive operation undertaken by the subject" (Cubelli, Nichelli, Bonito, De Tanti, and Inzaghi, 1991, p. 155). An indication that spatial attention is a special system occurs with American Sign Language. One RHD patient "correctly uses the left side of signing space to represent syntactic relations, despite her neglect of left hemispace in non-language tasks" (Klima, et al., 1988, p. 323). We shall return to sign language later in the chapter.

Let us return now to the study of wheelchair-related accidents. RHDs with or without clinically diagnosed neglect drove through a wheelchair obstacle course in the courtyard of a rehabilitation center. Obstacles were folding chairs on either side of corridors, and errors were recorded as direct hits or sideswipes. Both groups sideswiped more chairs on the left than the right, and subjects with obvious neglect made more direct hits than those without obvious neglect. All RHDs also made more errors than LHDs who had to steer mainly with the nondominant hand. Some RHDs were taught to scan the course before starting and while driving. The training reduced their direct hits but not their sideswipes (Webster, Cottam, Gouvier, Blanton, Beissel, and Wofford, 1988).

A speech-language pathologist should watch out for the influence of neglect when evaluating language. The role of neglect in reading will be discussed later. However, neglect can affect any test requiring the scanning of a visual array. Word comprehension errors disappeared for many RHDs when investigators controlled for neglect of the left side of picture displays (Gainotti, et al., 1983). The clinician can arrange pictures vertically to the right side or can verbally cue a patient to shift gaze leftward.

Both left hemianopia (see Chapter 2) and left neglect interfere with processing stimuli in the left hemispace. The former is a sensory impairment affecting the ability to see the left of center. These patients are aware of the problem and on their own try to compensate with eye movement. Left neglect, on the other hand, is an attentional impairment. "Patients fail to report stimuli in the neglected area, not because they cannot see them, but because they do not *notice* them" (Myers, 1999, p. 30). These patients are often unaware of the problem and have to be prompted to compensate.

One method for distinguishing a left field-cut from left neglect is to have the patient direct gaze to the left (putting formerly left objects into the center or right field) and then to the right. If an apparent field-cut disappears upon shifting gaze back to the right, then the problem is neglect. However, if the patient still cannot report objects in the left field, then the disorder is hemianopia which "moves with the eyes" (Myers, 1999).

Face Recognition

Like the man who mistook his wife for a hat, bilateral or right parietal lesions can cause a problem with people recognition. Recognizing people is important for maintaining interpersonal relationships and for conducting cogent conversations. Clinical investigation focuses on recognition of faces, which is analyzed in a fashion similar to the recognition of objects (Chapter 6). The ability to process facial features also has significance for recognizing a person's emotional state, which is discussed later.

Difficulties with face recognition parallel problems with objects. As with apperceptive visual agnosia, patients with RHD can have a perceptual disorder that appears as a deficit for recognizing *unfamiliar* faces, that is, new faces or strangers as opposed to family and famous people. Face matching tests show that perceptual difficulty occurs when photographs display the same face in different angles and lighting conditions (Benton, Hamsher, Varney, and Spreen, 1983).

An impairment of *familiar* face recognition, called **prosopagnosia,** is usually caused by bilateral occipito-temporal lesions (Bauer and Rubens, 1985). Failure to name familiar faces has been termed "prosopanomia" (Carney and Temple, 1993). When shown pictures of famous people, patients know they are looking at a face and can identify age, gender, and facial expression but cannot say who people are. Yet, they are able to use voices, clothing, and behavior to recognize acquaintances in a room. Only a few cases with unilateral posterior RHD have been reported (e.g., DeRenzi, 1986; Whiteley and Warrington, 1977).

In face recognition, the facial percept activates a stored recognition unit of someone's appearance (e.g., "She's familiar"). Many patients, who do not exhibit explicit recognition of familiar faces by naming them, still possess implicit or "unconscious" recognition. This covert recognition is detected with electrodermal response and other methods (for review, see Bruyer, 1991). The use of cues to recognize people indicates that patients retain "person identity nodes" in a semantic network (Bruce and Young, 1986). Schweinberger's (1995) priming study mentioned earlier suggests, however, that people with RHD can have difficulty in automatically activating identity nodes with respect to famous faces, whereas activation is normal when presented famous names.

Schweich and Bruyer (1993) examined nine cases of prosopagnosia more thoroughly with a clinical test battery organized according to a model of face recognition proposed by Bruce and Young (1986). Table 8.2 shows some of the subtests in this battery. The investigators found that prosopagnosia is not a homogeneous disorder and can result from damage to different levels of the recognition process. Based on a high-speed short-term recognition task, Schweinberger and others (1992) concluded that group data can be misleading. Some patients with RHD are not impaired in face recognition. Regarding those who are impaired, the problem can be due to misperception or a reduced buffer search speed that might affect performance on recognition tasks.

Visuospatial Orientation

Persons with RHD suddenly find it difficult to find their way around, especially in the unfamiliar maze of hospital corridors. With **topographic disorientation,** a patient fails to orient to the immediate environment such as the hospital. The patient also has difficulty reading maps, remembering familiar routes, and learning new ones

TABLE 8.2 Schweich and Bruyer's (1993) face recognition battery with subtests related to a model of face recognition.

COMPONENT OF MODEL	DEFINITION	SUBTEST
visual analysis	sensory registration of a stimulus	• choose a particular face from choices differing slightly according to facial features
percept	mental representation of stimulus	• copy a drawing of a human face
recognition unit	match pecept to stored structural description	• classify pictures as faces or other objects • select correct face given the person's name
semantic memory	activate person identity nodes	• classify unknown faces according to gender and age • give information about occupation and country of a pictured famous person

(Myers, 1986). This disorder can be attributed to an inability to recognize landmarks, but it also occurs when object recognition is preserved (Ellis and Young, 1988). With **geographic disorientation** a patient relates to immediate surroundings but fails to conceive of general location, claiming to be in China or Africa when actually in Ohio (Fisher, 1982).

The appearance of disorientation occurs with "false memories" in which a patient asserts the existence of two or more places with the same attributes but only one of them exists in reality. Patterson and Mack (1985) reported a case with RHD who described several hospitals in the area where he lived that were similar to his rehabilitation hospital. One was a "floating hospital." It is as if a real place is duplicated in the patient's mind. The problem is known as *reduplicative paramnesia.*

Visuospatial Expression

Impairments of visuospatial motor functions, such as drawing or building something, are called **constructional apraxia.** The most common clinical test is a drawing task. Copying figures is preferred over drawing on command, because the former is less influenced by cultural variations. As noted earlier, RHDs have lower scores than LHDs on the shape copying subtest of the PICA. In other tests, a patient may be asked to draw a clock, house, or flower. Clinical neuropsychologists may present a Picasso-like abstraction called the Rey-Osterrieth figure to be copied. The block design subtest of the WAIS is also used as a test of constructional skill.

First let us consider motor impairments that might interfere with constructional abilities. Anteriorly damaged RHDs are likely to have left hemiparesis, but the unimpaired right side is usually preferred for writing and drawing. Also, limb apraxia is relatively rare with RHD. Estimates vary from no patients with this disorder (DeRenzi, et al., 1969) to 27 percent (Duffy and Duffy, 1989), whereas 68 percent of LHDs may be impaired. This variation is probably due to inconsistent criteria for diagnosing impairment of praxis. Regardless of criteria, we can say that RHDs are less likely than LHDs to have praxic interference with visuospatial skills.

Early comparisons of RHDs and LHDs showed the opposite hemispheric asymmetry regarding constructional apraxia. There was a higher prevalence of constructional apraxia in RHDs than LHDs (e.g., Arrigoni and DeRenzi, 1964). In a more recent study of drawing objects from memory, RHDs had lower recognizability scores than LHDs (Grossman, 1988). In other studies, the two groups turned out to be similar regarding the presence of drawing defiency, with a 30 to 40 percent prevalence in each group (e.g., Arena and Gainotti, 1978; Carlesimo, et al., 1993). Patients with copying deficit have particular difficulty with three-dimensional figures such as a cube (Griffiths, Cook, and Newcombe, 1988).

RHDs and LHDs differ in qualitative features of their drawing deficits. For example, RHDs neglect the left side of a figure and are more likely to have poor spatial relationships among parts. LHDs draw more deliberately, overly simplify drawings, and preserve spatial relationships among parts (Gainotti, and Tiacci, 1970). In drawing a person, RHDs are disorganized and embellish with extraneous detail (Swindell, et al., 1988). Gardner (1982) described RHDs' artistry as "fragmented and disconnected drawing, whose parts, while often recognizable, do not flow or fit together into an organized whole" (pp. 322–323). In general, parietal RHDs draw details incoherently, whereas parietal LHDs omit details in a coherent structure.

Constructional apraxia appears to be caused by different underlying mechanisms. Carlesimo and others (1993) tried to find factors that are strongly related to the drawing performances. For LHDs, the hand used for drawing was the most important factor, and patients drawing with their left hand were the most impaired in this group. For RHDs, visual perception and spatial manipulation appeared to be strong factors.

What is the effect of RHD on the use of American Sign Language, especially the spatially configured syntactic component? In one study, three RH-damaged signers were impaired in comprehension of syntax but not other components of the language. However, they were "flawless" in production of syntactic and other features of ASL (Poizner, et al., 1987). Better production than comprehension is one of those exceptions to the typical pattern for aphasia (see Figure 1.1), which indicates that the comprehension problem was due to something other than language disorder. Problems with visuospatial perception may interfere with comprehension of ASL. Otherwise, like hearing individuals, RH-damage spares fundamental aspects of the use of a language.

Mental Imagery

Deficient visuospatial imagery may underly some of the problems just described. We already know that neglect may involve ignoring the left side of a mental image. Imagery is a "quasi-pictorial" representation that could be either percepts held temporarily in a visuospatial buffer or structural descriptions of objects or scenes activated in long-term memory. After evaluating drawing on command, Grossman (1988) suspected that image-generation is deficient in RHDs and some LHDs.

Let us return to the apperceptive agnosia discussed in Chapter 6. Difficulty matching objects in unusual views indicates that RHDs have difficulty with object-centered or 3-D percepts (see Table 6.1). This problem was thought to point to a failure to execute **mental rotation** for stimulus encoding (Layman and Greene, 1988). Mental rotation is a moving representational process by which we "turn objects around" in our heads (Shepard and Metzler, 1971; Corballis, 1997).

One clinical test of mental rotation is the *Flags Test* by Thurstone and Jeffrey (see Morton and Morris, 1995). A line drawing of a test flag is displayed, and the patient has to judge which of six other flags are rotations of the test flag. Another task is the *Manikin Test* in which male figures are shown upright or upside-down, facing to or away from the viewer (Ratcliff, 1979). The patient has to decide which hand is holding a ball. Case MG with a left parieto-occipital hematoma was impaired with tests of mental rotation but was unimpaired for tests of visuospatial working memory (Morton and Morris, 1995).

Can someone who uses ASL be impaired for comprehending signs that require mental rotation? Most locative statements are produced in the point-of-view of the signer so that a viewer must make a 180-degree rotation to comprehend the spatial relationship conveyed. Some locatives, however, are presented in the point-of-view of the viewer, therefore, not requiring mental rotation.

Patient AM had a right parietal lesion and a pronounced difficulty matching furniture arrangements when one of the arrangements was rotated. This deficit is typical of visuospatial impairment with RHD. However, AM retained an ability to comprehend locative signs that required mental rotation, indicating that linguistic use of space is a different process from nonverbal spatial operations (Emmorey, Hickok, and Klima, 1996).

AUDITORY-VOCAL MODALITIES

A patient may have an impaired ability to recognize sounds despite adequate hearing, called **auditory agnosia.** This term may be used to refer specifically to deficient recognition of nonverbal or environmental sounds such as water pouring or a door squeaking (specifically known as auditory sound agnosia or nonverbal auditory agnosia). RH-damaged individuals are generally normal in recognition of common sounds (Faglioni, Spinnler, and Vignolo, 1969; Spinnler and Vignolo, 1966). Like visual object agnosia, agnosia for environmental sounds usually occurs with bilateral damage, this time in the temporal lobe (Bauer and Rubens, 1985).

Persons with severe aphasia may have normal nonverbal sound recognition or have a severe auditory agnosia along with the language comprehension deficit (Faglioni, et al., 1969; Varney, 1980). Difficulties may be related to verbal mediation. Riege and others (1980) found that aphasic patients with impaired word comprehension were normal in recognizing sounds that would be difficult to label (i.e., bird calls). Auditory agnosia does not seem to be connected to language dysfunction. When it occurs in aphasic persons, it is a distinct disorder that is an "accident of location" of lesion.

What about music or melody processing? Sidtis and Volpe (1988) detected that RHDs were impaired in pitch pattern perception but not speech perception, whereas aphasic subjects had difficulty with speech but not tones. A problem with music after an RH-stroke, called **amusia,** is focused on melody rather than lyrics. In one study, LH-damage caused more problems in recognizing music with familiar lyrics than RH-damage. However, RHDs did worse than LHDs in recognizing music without commonly known lyrics such as "Hail to the Chief" (Gardner, Silverman, Denes, et al., 1977). This study indicated that familiar lyrics are encoded when listening to melodies, a mental skill that helps RHDs but hinders LHDs.

Processing music is a complex matter with components and grammar not unlike language processing (e.g., Handel, 1989). A comparison of RHDs and LHDs indicated that pitch processing is more susceptible to RH-damage and, to a lesser degree, rhythm processing is more susceptible to LH-damage (Shapiro, Grossman, and Gardner, 1981). Imitation of rhythm tapping is part of the Boston Exam for aphasia.

Prior, Kinsella, and Giese (1990) compared RHDs and LHDs with respect to a small battery of music tests. The tests included perception of pitch and rhythm variation in familiar and unfamiliar tunes, as well as production tasks involving imitated tapping and singing familiar and unfamiliar songs. Results were mixed, as comprehensive impairments occurred with LHD and RHD. Both groups were impaired in imitative tapping and singing familiar tunes. LHDs were more impaired than RHDs in rhythm perception and singing unfamiliar melodies.

The **Seashore Rhythm Test** (SRT) is incorporated in the Halstead-Reitan battery (see Chapter 3). It requires patients to discriminate between pairs of musical beats. In clinical circles, it was believed that this test is sensitive to unilateral RH-damage. However, two studies have shown that LH and RH-damaged groups do not differ with the SRT (Karzmark, Heaton, Lehman, and Crouch, 1985; Sherer, Parsons, Nixon, and Adams, 1991). RHDs do appear to have more difficulty than LHDs on the less frequently used **Seashore Tonal Memory Test** (STM), in which patients are asked to discriminate between pairs of three-to five-note melodies (Karzmark, et al., 1985).

The right temporal lobe seems to be responsible for storing and activating familiar melodies. When neurosurgeons used tiny electrodes to stimulate this region, the patients reported hearing an orchestra or a choir (Penfield and Perot, 1963). Sacks (1985) described an elderly woman with a right temporal infarction. In the early months after her stroke, she woke up to hearing familiar songs even though she was nearly deaf and no radio was on. She would ask "Is the radio in my head?" Sacks called this a "musical epilepsy."

Peretz (1993) reported on GL who had a surgically repaired aneurysm on the right side without consequence but then another one on the left side a year later causing Wernicke's aphasia and *atonalia.* GL could not recognize familiar music and did not enjoy it anymore. This patient did not have a sweeping impairment of music processing, as determined by several tests that Peretz conducted. GL recognized melodic contour and intervals, and the disorder was isolated to accessing tonal knowledge.

The French composer Maurice Ravel was also stricken by Wernicke's aphasia. He continued to recognize melodies, but was no longer able to compose. He could not read notes or perform from a score (Gardner, 1982). Although individuals with aphasia can have a music processing impairment, generally people with aphasia retain purely musical competencies; whereas RH-damage causes problems with melodies while retaining the ability to deal with symbolic codes (Botez, Botez, and Aube, 1980).

What about the sound of a person's voice? People with prosopagnosia, caused by bilateral occipitotemporal lesions, can recognize familiar people from their voices. Two tasks have been used to study *speaker recognition* in brain-damaged people. One is a discrimination test in which patients were asked to tell if two voices were the same or different. The other task involved recognizing famous voices (Van Lancker, Kreiman, and Cummings, 1989). Impairment of discrimination or recognition was called **phonagnosia.** Temporal lobe damage in either hemisphere caused voice discrimination deficit. Impaired recognition of famous voices was associated with right parietal lobe damage. Even globally aphasic persons were able to recognize the sound of Johnny Carson or John F. Kennedy.

EMOTION

The neurology of emotion is a complex interaction of systems. It is a feeling in the gut of limbic and autonomic nervous systems and is a message recognized in cognitive cortex. Both hemispheres have been shown to contribute to emotional qualities of behavior, but the RH is dominant (Silberman and Weingartner, 1986). Persons with RHD may display a flat affect or indifference that often accompanies left neglect (Gainotti, 1972). Based on measures of skin response, heart rate, and respiration, RHDs demonstrated **hypoarousal** to tactile stimulation (Heilman, Schwartz, and Watson, 1978) and emotional pictures (Morrow, Vrtunski, Kim, and Boller, 1981).

For cognitive testing, patients are usually examined for recognition of primary emotional expressions in faces, such as happiness, sadness, and anger. RHDs have been found to have difficulty recognizing and remembering facial expressions and recognizing the emotional significance of pictured situations (Cicone, Wapner, and Gardner, 1980; Dekosky, Heilman, Bowers, and Valenstein, 1980; Weddell, 1989). Dissociation of autonomic and cognitive systems was indicated when hypoarousal did not necessarily co-occur with deficient recognition of facial emotion (Zoccolotti, Scabini, and Violani, 1982).

A fairly thorough study of recognition was conducted by Peper and Irle (1997) in Germany. First, they examined "categorical decoding" of primary emotional concepts. Groups of brain-damaged subjects decided if two pictured facial emotions were the same or different, chose the name for a facial emotion, and selected a picture named by the examiner. Then, "dimensional decoding" was tested with respect to intensity of an expression and the positivity or negativity of expressions, called the *valence* of an emotion. From two pictures, subjects had to choose the one that was like a target facial expression according to one of these dimensions. Among the groups studied, patients with right temporal and parietal lesions were uniquely impaired in discrimination, conceptualization, and intensity decoding.

With respect to expression of feeling, Gainotti (1972) described some patients with RHD as having a flat affect, perhaps, indicative of hypoarousal. Facial reactions of RHDs were inaccurate in response to pictures of familiar people, pleasant and unpleasant scenes, and unusual photographic effects (Buck and Duffy, 1980). The expression of emotions appears to be unrelated to recognition of emotion (Borod, Koff, Perlman-Lorch, and Nicholas, 1986). Blonder and others (1993) compared RHDs and LHDs during interviews along with their spouses in their homes. Facial expressions were recorded on videotape. The RHDs demonstrated less facial expressivity than the LHDs, particularly with respect to smiles and laughter.

RHD and LHD transform mood differently with respect to valence. RHDs tend to joke and laugh excessively, a change in a "positive" direction. Aphasic LHDs can be depressive and may cry excessively (Gainotti, 1972). In one study, depression was greatest with anterior LHD. Some RHDs react to cartoons with excessive hilarity, and others are unresponsive (Gardner, Ling, Flamm, and Silverman, 1975). Posterior RHDs may be more depressed than anterior RHDs who can be "unduly cheerful" and apathetic about their disorders (Robinson, Kubos, Starr, Rao, and Price, 1984). Prevailing mood may be related to awareness of deficit.

SECONDARY LANGUAGE DEFICITS

People with RHD exhibit difficulties in language behavior that are extensions of primary cognitive disorders. Left neglect intrudes on reading, and flat emotion can be detected in speech as well as facial expression.

Attention and Reading

"A ROSE is a ROSE or a NOSE" (Patterson and Wilson, 1990). Some people with RHD misread the beginning of words (Riddoch, Humphreys, Cleton, and Ferry, 1990). Other patients omit or misread words on the left side of a page. Some patients have both types of problems (Ellis, Flude, and Young, 1987; Young, Newcombe, and Ellis, 1991). Misreading the left side of words or the left side of a page are symptoms of **neglect dyslexia,** one of the peripheral dyslexias mentioned in Chapter 6. Rare cases of right neglect dyslexia with LH-damage have been reported (e.g., Warrington, 1991).

One test is to present words that can still be words when the first letter is omitted or substituted (e.g, *blight*). Case VB understood targets according to the errors (e.g., *blight* as "light"), indicating that the impairment was in an early point in the process, such as perception or recognition. Of the errors, 66 percent were clear left-side errors, usually substitutions of the first one or two letters irrespective of word-length (e.g., "slain" for *train,* "pillow" for *yellow*). A patient may have many more errors reading orthographically legal nonwords than real words (Arguin and Bub, 1997).

Are words in the neglected space processed at an automatic level? This question was addressed with a priming task in which the prime was a pictured object (e.g., a bat) presented 400 msec before a semantically related target (e.g., *ball*) (McGlinchey-Berroth, Milberg, Verfaellie, Alexander, and Kilduff, 1993). A twist in this study was that the prime was shown in either the left or right visual field. To avoid stimulus-biased attentional adjustments, a nonsense drawing was always presented in the other field. Four patients with left neglect displayed normal semantic priming with primes presented to either field. Thus, neglect was thought to be a disruption of controlled or intentional processing.

What is the effect of left neglect on "reading" American Sign Language? Patient JH was partially deaf since birth and learned ASL in a residential school for the deaf. He was working for an aircraft manufacturer when he suffered a stroke in his right hemisphere. Corina, Kritchevsky, and Bellugi (1996) compared his lateralized sign identification with object recognition. His recognition of objects was strongly affected by neglect, but recognition of signs was not affected. This dissociation is another demonstration that the visuospatial modality per se is not as significant functionally as the system underlying use of the modality. For JH, the intact left hemisphere's linguistic system appears to have overridden the visual attention deficit.

Emotion and Prosody

Along with facial expression, we express our emotions through the intonation or prosody of our speech. Is the disorder of hypoarousal manifested in the sound of a patient's voice? Does the cognitive impairment of recognition occur with auditory input as well as in the look on others' faces? Furthermore, can emotional and linguistic prosody be dissociated by focal brain damage?

A disorder called **aprosodia** has been diagnosed in RHDs. Like classifying aphasias, Ross (1981) proposed that there are receptive and expressive forms of this deficit associated with posterior and anterior lesions, respectively. Some patients speak in a flat intonational contour or monotone (Tucker, et al., 1977; Ross and Mesulam, 1979). Some patients are deficient in identifying emotional tone in mundane sentences, detected in tasks requiring pointing to a happy, sad, or angry face (Heilman, Bowers, Speedie, and Coslett, 1984; Schlanger, Schlanger, and Gerstman, 1976; Tucker, Watson, and Heilman, 1977).

Cancelliere and Kertesz (1990) pursued the notion of clinical syndromes. They gave a test of receptive and expressive affective prosody to 46 patients with left or right lesions, and they concocted a classification based on ranges of test scores. It included a Broca's aprosodia (i.e., expression more impaired than comprehension), a Wernicke's aprosodia (i.e., severe deficit of comprehension), and conduction aprosodia (i.e., repetition more impaired than expression). Patterns of deficit were found to be unrelated to site of lesion. The so-called Wernicke subjects could not be associated with a lesion in the temporal lobe opposite Wernicke's area in the LH. The aphasia model was a device to depict patterns and does not appear to have been pursued seriously since this report.

Tompkins and Flowers (1987) studied the recognition of emotion in statements with a prior context. Intoned sentences with neutral content were placed at the end of paragraphs. The paragraph was congruent or incongruent with the prosodic pattern, and patients with RHD had to choose a label for the conveyed emotion. Deficits were small but statistically significant, and RHDs were helped by context. Effects were attributed to a retained automatic integrative capacity, whereas previously observed impairments were attributed to demands of strategic processing. Yet, Tomkins and Flowers utilized a slow task, so that the factor of automaticity needs to be examined further.

Linguistic prosody includes stress and juncture markers of meaning and sentence structure. A few investigators have pursued the question of whether affective and linguistic prosody can be dissociated. Some studies indicated that RH-damage spares linguistic prosody in receptive and expressive tasks. RHDs comprehended lexical stress normally (e.g., *blackboard, black board*), and most had no problem producing lexical stress (Behrens, 1988; Emmorey, 1987). They produced contrastive stress when answering "Who did what" questions. Others could read aloud declarative sentence contours (Cooper, Soares, Nicol, Michelow, and Goloskie, 1984).

Other researchers found problems with linguistic prosody. Using a reading task, Shapiro and Danly (1985) concluded that RHDs have deficits in producing sentence contours as well as affective prosody. Bryan (1989) found RHDs, especially with parietal lesions, who were impaired in comprehending and producing lexical stress (e.g., *con*vict, con*vict*) and discriminating and recognizing sentence contours. Shapiro and Danly's study stirred closer scrutiny and some debate (e.g., Ryalls, 1986). Behrens (1989) studied a wider variety of sentence contours with a different task (i.e., story completion). Her RHDs were deficient for producing declaratives and yes-no questions but had no problem with imperatives and Wh-questions. A deficit for syntactic contours may only be partial.

There have been few studies that comprehensively compare linguistic and affective prosody with both RHDs and LHDs. In an investigation of comprehension, Pell and Baum (1997) found neither group to have a deficit for emotional prosody. LHDs had a problem with linguistic cues. Also, acoustic analysis showed that RHDs and LHDs utilized duration, fundamental frequency, and amplitude to produce affective and linguistic cues (Baum and Pell, 1997). These researchers could not support previous claims that impairments in comprehending or producing affective tone are common features of RHD.

SPEAKER MEANING

From the previous review, we may predict that people with RHD will have difficulties dealing with elements of external context in communicative situations. Some patients ignore half of extrapersonal space. A few do not recognize objects, familiar people, or music in the background. Some misjudge their location in the world. A few may not recognize the emotion or mood in a speaker's voice or face. These problems are important for the natural use of language, because a speaker's meaning depends on the relationship between an utterance and its context (see Chapter 7).

Interpreting Situations

People with RHD have difficulty recognizing emotion or humor in a pictured scene, whereas aphasic patients do not have this problem (Cicone, et al., 1980; Gardner, et. al., 1975). In one study, patients were asked to group pictures according to a theme or "gist" such as despair or love (Myers, Linebaugh, and Mackisack-Morin, 1985). Some themes, such as hugging, were considered to be explicit. Other themes were implicit, such as love. Unlike aphasic subjects, RHDs had more difficulty sorting according to implicit themes than explicit themes. This pattern indicated that RHDs have a problem with inferring the nature of situations when it is not concrete or obvious.

Another indication of impaired situational inference came from a content analysis of descriptions of the Cookie Theft picture. Myers (1979) looked for "literal" content (e.g., a woman) and "interpretive" concepts (e.g., "She is the mother"). RHDs produced fewer interpretive concepts than normal. When cartoon sequences were used to elicit stories, RHDs omitted inferences that fill in transitions between pictures (Joanette, et al., 1986).

Purdy, Belanger, and Liles (1993) examined the ability of RHDs to draw inferences from a short animated film about a real-life situation. Patients were asked two types of questions. One type was thought to depend partly on general world knowledge, and the other type of question was thought to rely mainly on information in the film. The investigators were particularly interested in testing a belief that people with RHD have a special difficulty in using world knowledge to infer from a situation. In the study, although the patients were more accurate for knowledge-based questions, they did significantly worse than normal controls in answering both types of questions.

Another element of a communicative situation, of course, is the other participant in a conversation. Chapter 7 noted that the exchange of messages relies on a principle of cooperation in which participants try to distinguish between old and new information. The ability to do this depends on estimating the other participant's knowledge of a topic. This may be problematic if a speaker fails to recognize who the listener is. In her book on RHD, Connie Tompkins (1995) cited observations of a difficulty in taking the point-of-view of a listener, especially in being sensitive to the other person's needs.

However, Tompkins (1995) also warned that we could go overboard in anticipating that people with RHD will be insensitive to situations. Stemmer, Giroux, and Joanette (1994) examined the ability to produce direct requests (e.g., "Turn down the radio") and indirect requests (e.g., "I can't concentrate") when presented with contexts calling for one type or the other. RHDs were sensitive to context in that they did not produce direct commands in situations in which an indirect request was appropriate.

Metaphor Comprehension

In addition to indirect speech acts, metaphor is a pragmatic convention used for studying comprehension of a speaker-meaning that differs from literal content. Again, inference is presumed to be necessary. Idiomatic phrases like "bury the hatchet" or "shoot the bull" may come to mind as examples. While such phrases are commonly used in research and pragmatic assessment, they are called *idioms* because they are so common that nonliteral interpretation is likely to be the first meaning that comes to mind in any context. They are different from more creative utterance, such as "The troops marched on" in the context of a room full of unruly children.

The study of metaphor comprehension began with presentation of phrases like *heavy heart* and *colorful music* (Winner and Gardner, 1977). Aphasic subjects chose nonliteral meanings more often than literal meanings and scoffed at absurd literal options. RHDs often exhibited the opposite pattern. They could paraphrase intent of the phrases but still chose pictured literal meanings more often than aphasic subjects (Winner and Gardner, 1977). In another study, idioms were more difficult to comprehend than novel sentences, whereas LHDs again displayed the opposite pattern (Van Lanker and Kempler, 1987).

Clinical researchers have also examined connotative or suggestive meaning. When choosing the most similar pair of words in a triad (e.g., *loving-hateful-warm*), RHDs relied on denotation (e.g., *loving-hateful*) more than connotation (e.g., *loving-warm*). In contrast, aphasic LHDs relied on connotation more than denotation. Normal controls used both meaning components (Brownell, Potter, Michelow, and Gardner, 1984). Later, Brownell wondered if this is a fundamental semantic problem (Brownell, Simpson, Bihrle, Potter, and Gardner, 1990). He compared performance with his connotation triads and a similar semantic task. RHDs were still more impaired in the connotation task, whereas LHDs were equally impaired in both tasks.

Following up Brownell's first study of word-triads, Tompkins (1990) wondered if metaphoric interpretation varies as a function of automatic and effortful levels of processing. She employed a semantic priming task in which a lexical decision target (e.g., *sharp*) was preceded by a metaphoric prime (e.g., *smart*), literal prime (e.g., *dull*), or an unrelated prime (e.g., *warm*). Unlike the dissociations found by Brownell, both related primes facilitated target recognition for RHDs and LHDs. Tompkins argued that the divergence from Brownell's findings was related to his use of a strategic task. RHDs were able to access nonliteral meaning automatically. Impairment lies in controlled operations for choosing pictures or giving definitions.

Again, Tompkins warned of overgeneralization from a few studies. She found that RHDs understand idioms when presented in a sentence context, despite difficulties when asked to define or explain the same metaphors (Tompkins, Boada, and McGarry, 1992). When presented indirect requests, RHDs strangely preferred literal over nonliteral response in one study (Foldi, 1987); but Tompkins (1995) cited other research showing that RHDs can be sensitive to polite requests. As we shall see in the next chapter regarding closed head injury, RHD is not one monolithic syndrome. Inconsistencies are bound to fall out from just a few studies with different experimental procedures. The upside is that the studies show us what to look for in evaluating people with RH-stroke.

DISCOURSE

With their clinical test of discourse comprehension (see Chapter 7), Nicholas and Brookshire (1995) found that RHDs recalled main ideas better than details and explicit information better than implied information. However, aphasic patients and normal controls had the same pattern of ability, indicating that this strategy of assessment may not detect differences between brain damaged groups. This section presents other approaches to the examination of discourse comprehension.

Brownell (1988) contrasted RHDs with aphasic persons according to a simple but powerful framework. He suggested that "aphasic patients often appear to understand more of a conversation or story than one would expect given their impairments with words and sentences, and RHD patients appear to understand less than one would expect given their intact linguistic skills" (p. 249). Early characterizations of RHDs were that they "miss the point" of proverbs and narratives and tend to "wander from the point" when telling a story.

Comprehension

Two investigations focused on inferring relations between propositions. McDonald and Wales (1986) presented items involving spatial (*1a*) and nonspatial (*1b*) inferences.

(1a) The bird is in the cage.
The cage is under the table.
TEST: The bird is under the table.

(1b) The woman held the little girl's hand.
Her daughter was only 3 years old.
TEST: The woman held her daughter's hand.

After hearing the two statements and engaging in a brief distractor task, subjects were tested as to whether they had heard a statement before. RHDs matched normal controls by recognizing true inferences as often as true facts (e.g., *The cage is under the table*).

Another study exposed a deficit. Subjects made true-false judgments about sentence pairs (*2*).

(2) Barbara became too bored to finish the history book.
She had already spent five years writing it.
TRUE-FALSE TEST: Barbara became bored writing a history book.

RHDs made more errors with inferences than with factual statements, indicating a deficiency in combining information between sentences (Brownell, Potter, Bihrle, and Gardner, 1986).

Jokes were among the first devices used to study the detection of coherence in stories. A conclusion becomes a punch line because of surprise relative to expectations in the body of a joke and its coherence relative to a theme (Brownell, Michel, Powelson, and Gardner, 1983). After hearing the body of a joke, subjects selected a conclusion from choices containing a punch line, a suprising nonsequitur, and two coherent conclusions (e.g., *3*). When RHDs fail to choose the punch lines, do they err in favor of surprise or coherence?

(3) BODY: The neighborhood borrower approached Mr. Smith on Sunday afternoon and asked if Mr. Smith would be using his lawnmower. "Yes, I am," Smith answered warily. The neighborhood borrower then replied:
CORRECT: "Fine, then you won't be needing your golf clubs. I'll just borrow them."
SURPRISE: "You know, the grass is greener on the other side."
NEUTRAL COHERENCE: "Do you think I could use it when you're done?"
SAD COHERENCE: "Gee, if I only had enough money I could buy my own."

Asked to pick the funny conclusion, RHDs chose the punch line 60 percent of the time. Normal controls got the joke 81 percent of the time. Therefore, RHDs were deficient but not devoid of a sense of humor. In their errors, they chose surprise over coherence. Later, this study was expanded by using cartoons and adding a humorless story condition, and the results were similar (Bihrle, Brownell, Powelson, and Gardner, 1986). Both studies were considered to indicate that RHDs have a problem with the coherence feature of a narrative.

Another paradigm is to present a few sentences portraying a situation, called a vignette, and then conclude the vignette with a target statement that, to be understood, requires integration with the vignette. Targets have been indirect requests or sarcasm. In one study, short vignettes ended with a conventional indirect request (e.g., "Can you...?") or a request worded to favor literal interpretation (e.g., "Are you able to...?") (Weylman, Brownell, Roman, and Gardner, 1989). Both vignettes established situations in which the most appropriate response was to indirect meaning, so that the study would examine use of linguistic context. RHDs were impaired relative to normal controls but still could use context to comprehend an indirect message.

RHDs also answered questions about vignettes that ended with one person praising or deriding another about a good or poor performance (e.g., golfing) (Kaplan, Brownell, Jacobs, and Gardner, 1990). Subjects were given information about whether the characters liked or disliked each other. The closing comment could be interpreted literally or sarcastically (e.g., *You sure are a good golfer*). RHDs were accurate when conclusions were literally true. Yet, when conclusions were literally false, RHDs had difficulty detecting sarcasm based on the characters' relationship. Patients thought a sarcastic positive statement makes a person feel better, indicating a reduced sensitivity to beliefs and desires of others (i.e., taking another person's point-of-view).

Tompkins and others (1994) looked upon the sporting acceptance of sarcasm as requiring revision of an initial interpretation, and they wondered if this heightened demand on processing is related to working memory capacity. To understand this notion of inference revision, let us examine two versions of a short story presented to subjects:

(4a) Nan invited her new neighbor, Mark, to a party.
He told hilarious stories and everyone enjoyed listening.
Nan's husband said to her, "Good decision. He's really fun to have around."

(4b) Nan invited her new neighbor, Mark, to a party.
He told boring stories and no one enjoyed listening.
Nan's husband said to her, "Good decision. He's really fun to have around."

Story *4a* was congruent in that the second and third sentences convey a positive mood, whereas *4b* was incongruent in that the second and third sentences are inconsistent with respect to mood. Yet, the incongruent story is coherent when the husband's comment is interpreted as sarcasm (thus, requiring revision of an initial interpretation).

Rounding out the experiment, Tompkins presented a simpler story in a third condition. Comprehension was tested with yes-no questions after each story, and working memory capacity was also measured. Results showed that incongruent-sarcasm was more difficult to comprehend than the other stories for all groups. For RHDs, working memory had its highest correlation with the incongruent condition. The investigators concluded that inference revision is especially strenuous for people with RHD.

A few studies addressed sensitivity to overall structure of a discourse. RHDs had difficulty arranging sentences into a story (Delis, Wapner, Gardner, and Moses, 1983) and sequencing frames of cartoons (Huber and Gleber, 1982). In one study, the crucial thematic statement for a story was put at its usual position at the beginning or at an unusual position at the end. Subjects were tested for recalling main ideas (Hough, 1990). For normal controls, there was no effect of delaying the theme. However, RHDs scored much better when the theme was early than when the theme was delayed. Hough decided that these subjects were "unable to utilize the macrostructure as an organizer in apprehending the paragraph" (p. 271). Another possibility is that RHDs recognize common macrostructure, and exceptions create hardships for processing narration.

Discourse Production

Eisenson (1962) characterized extended verbal expression with RHD as "empty." This characterization was supported by content analyses that demonstrated reduced informativeness of description or narration (Joanette, Goulet, Ska, and Nespoulous, 1986; Trupe and Hillis, 1985). Trupe and Hillis found some patients to be verbose, whereas others exhibited a paucity of utterance.

As indicated in Chapter 7, the assessment of discourse production has two key elements, namely, the method of eliciting a sample and the method of analysis. We can elicit discourse without analyzing the features that make it coherent. The study of discourse with RHD has been quite varied. Characteristics of the research are compared to the study of closed head injury in the next chapter (see Table 9.9). In the study of RHD, picture-elicitation has been used more often than spontaneous conditions. Narrative has been the most frequently studied type of discourse, and information or content analysis has been used more than cohesion or macrostructural analyses (Davis, O'Neil-Pirozzi, and Coon, 1997).

Trupe and Hillis (1985) found some RHDs were overly literal and focused on detail in picture description. The following example is a description of the Boston Exam's Cookie Theft picture:

> *"Well, it's on 8½ x 11 inch paper overall covered by plastic. Looks like it may have been done with drawing pens and India ink on white paper. It's less than 20 pound paper. Else you wouldn't have used black to keep it from shining through. I see window and curtain somebody has pulled back and hospital-type curtains exposing a window and utensils on table, pan or a pot, curtains drawn back with strings tied. Kitchen curtains, no particular design on them. A valance at the top of the curtains with an ordinary angular design. The rest of the curtains only called curtains because of their placement and overall lack of color. There's evidence that the paper was punched for a three ring binder before it was made. The room seems to be filled with air since the curtains have a billowing effect" (p. 94); reprinted by permission of the publisher, BRK).*

As indicated earlier, RHDs have been said to wander from the point or theme when telling stories. In several studies, autobiographical stories and story-retelling included event-sequence errors, confabulations, digressions, and embellishments (Gardner, et al., 1983; Myers, 1979; Rivers and Love, 1980; Trupe and Hillis, 1985). RHDs varied widely in script production; some were tangential, and others terminated too soon (Roman, Brownell, Potter, Seibold, and Gardner, 1987). Patients were compared with normal controls in telling a story from a short video, and they were deficient in cohesion and number of episodes told to a naive listener (Uryase, Duffy, and Liles, 1991). On the other hand, Bloom and others (1995) found that RHDs were not deficient in telling stories with respect to completeness, logic, and whether they had a beginning, middle, and end.

Aware of some of the early research on storytelling, a group of neuropsychologists decided to try out a different scoring system for the Logical Memory subtest of the *Wechsler Memory Scale* (see Table 9.6) in which a patient is asked to recall two short stories (Webster, Godlewski, Hanley, and Sowa, 1992). The system consisted of scores for recalling essential thematic information and nonessential details and for producing intrusion errors. RHDs recalled a normal number of essential propositions but recalled fewer details and produced significantly more idiosyncratic intrusions than controls and LHDs, similar to behavior on Glosser and Goodglass' word-association test cited early in this chapter.

Indications of possible difficulties come from a study that included telling a story from a cartoon (Davis, et al., 1997). The cartoon, called the Flower Pot story, shows a man walking his dog when a falling flower pot hits him on the head. He gets angry and storms into the building where the pot came from. After rapping on a door, a female culprit appears. She is nice to his dog, and he tips his cap without mentioning the bump on his head (Huber and Gleber, 1982; also Snow, et al., 1995). Here are a couple of versions from individuals with RHD:

> *"It looks like the man is out walking his pet dog, and it looks kinda like he's lost, and he's looking for help. So he goes banging on one of the doors, and a lady opens her door, and out runs her pet. Looks like he's asking her for directions, and she gives 'em to him."*

> *"The first one it looks like he's returning home with a stray dog. He takes him in. The third one. Fourth one, he's banging on the door. Fifth one,*

he's giving the dog a bone. Sixth one, he seem to be pleased with him. And the dog is taking off with his bone."

The first one is a good story with a theme, characters, motivated events, and related resolution. Yet, it is the wrong story with an incorrect detail about the pet. The second version is also the wrong story and has inaccurate details and less logical coherence than the first story.

Davis was concerned that subjects might have had problems with interpretation of visual stimuli. Subjects were more accurate when retelling a story told to them. Myers and Brookshire (1994) compared visual and inferential complexity of pictures, and found that complexity had little influence on information content. Bloom and others (1993) presented picture sequences that had an emotional theme (i.e., a pet gets hit by a car), a visuospatial theme (i.e., moving a box from a chair), or a procedural/neutral theme (i.e., how to fry an egg). Instead of measuring content, they looked for certain pragmatic features of the stories (e.g., topic maintenance, conciseness). Emotional content impaired RHDs' discourse and seemed to facilitate aphasic discourse.

The general point is that our picture of RHDs' discourse may depend on our choice of methods of elicitation and analysis. We should be hesitant about forming a diagnostic opinion from one task or one story.

CLINICAL ASSESSMENT

A few guides are available to help the clinician assess the unique communicative difficulties that might occur for some people with RHD. One is the *Rehabilitation Institute of Chicago Evaluation of Communication Problems in Right Hemisphere Dysfunction* or RICE (Burns, Halper, and Mogil, 1985). This evaluation covers general behavior patterns, visual scanning and tracking, writing, pragmatic communication, and metaphorical language. General behavior includes orientation examined in an interview. Writing is an opportunity to look for neglect dyslexia and linguistic problems with sentences. Pragmatic communication is profiled with very general rating scales for intonation, gesture, a few conversational skills, and narrative abilities. Metaphoric language is examined by asking a patient to explain proverbs and idioms (e.g., *Look before you leap*).

There are a couple of other devices. One is *The Right Hemisphere Language Battery* first reported in an article by Bryan (1988). The test controls for visual perceptual deficits in assessing lexical-semantic comprehension, metaphor appreciation in listening and reading, verbal humor appreciation, comprehension of inferred meaning, production of emphatic stress, and conversational discourse. Another test is the *Mini Inventory of Right Brain Injury* (Pimental and Kingsbury, 1989). This brief screening includes some tests for primary impairments, affective language behavior, and pragmatic language such as humor and metaphor. Tompkins (1995) also recommends the measures and tests of functional communication reviewed here in Chapter 7.

MARTIN EXETER'S RIGHT HEMISPHERE

Martin Exeter was fully aware of his impairments. During the first few weeks, he was restricted to getting around in a wheelchair. He wondered if he would ever be able to play golf with his son Peter, again, although progressing from the wheelchair to a walker and then to a cane were happy accomplishments. They helped Peter to feel better, too. After a few months, his grades started to return to where they were.

The often reserved professor was surprised and delighted that he could still carry a tune, and words came out better when he sang a favorite song. This became a warm-up exercise in therapy every now and then, although he could tell that his first clinician was self-conscious about her own singing. He had never thought his drawing was very good, but sometimes a simple sketch came in handy when a referent was not being communicated precisely enough through speech. His first clinician was also self-conscious about her own drawing. She would have him practice but seldom did it herself.

Martin had no trouble expressing his feelings. In fact, Jackie remarked that she could read his emotions much better than before his stroke. She had to depend even more on what his face said. However, she was startled by sharp cursing that thankfully did not happen too often. For Martin, it was frustrating to be unable to do such simple things like walking and talking. For a while, it made him angry. Then, he became depressed and did not want to see his friends. Toward the end of his month in the Pocumtuck Rehabilitation Unit, he would hide from visitors.

SUMMARY AND CONCLUSIONS

The chapter began with the speech-language pathologist's point-of-view with respect to traditional assessment of language. These tests were constructed with aphasia in mind, and so people with RHD do fairly well with them. The chapter also came close to completing the landscape of cognitive signs of neurological impairment (Table 8.3). The primary impairments of RHD involve visuospatial and auditory processing. We should not expect that every person with RHD will have all of these disorders. The research just tells us what is possible, especially when revealed by the clinical neuropsychologist's evaluation.

In its contrast to LH-dysfunction, RHD sheds some light on the nature of aphasia and communication. We have a better idea of the resources remaining relatively intact in aphasic individuals. Also, we see what happens to communicative ability without language disorder, and what can happen to language behavior without language disorder.

The growing literature on verbal behavior with RHD is filled with contradictions. Some researchers find deficits in recognizing emotional or linguistic prosody, whereas others do not find these deficits. Some find RHDs who are sensitive to situations, whereas others find RHDs who are

TABLE 8.3 A selection of disorders and their usual site of lesion.

HEMISPHERE	SITE	IMPAIRED FUNCTION	DYSFUNCTION
Left	Frontal, Broca's area	Speech programming	Apraxia of speech
	Perisylvian	Language	Aphasia
	Parietal	Calculation	Acalculia
		Drawing	Constructional apraxia (details)
Right	Temporal	Melody recognition	Amusia
	Parietotemporal	Visuospatial attention	Left neglect Neglect dyslexia
	Parietal	Orientation	Topographic & geographic disorientation
		Spatial construction	Constructional apraxia (structure)
		Speaker recognition	Phonagnosia
	Parieto-occipital	Object-centered perception	Apperceptive visual agnosia
Bilateral	Frontal motor area	Execution of speech	Dysarthria
	Temporal	Sound recognition	Auditory agnosia
	Occipital	Object recogntion	Associative visual agnosia
	Occipitotemporal	Face recognition	Prosopagnosia

not. Some find RHDs who cannot tell a coherent story, whereas others find RHDs who can.

This is a relatively young field of study. Subject selection has been rather broad, and just about anyone with RH-damage seems to be fair game. Studies of aphasia, on the other hand, inherently consist of LHDs with a more circumscribed location of lesion. Also, a wide variety of methods have been based on common sense, neuropsychological assessment traditions, and precedents in the study of aphasia. Only a few have been modeled after the study of visuospatial and music processing, emotion, and discourse in independent sciences.

CHAPTER 9

TRAUMATIC BRAIN INJURY AND RELATED SYNDROMES

"It was kind of a freak accident. I was on a motorcycle and I didn't have my helmet buckled. I just put it on, you know, and didn't buckle it. I was comin' down the road, and there's like an island in the road, you know, there was an island with two telephone poles in the middle, and I bounced off both those poles. Bounced off and flew forty feet through the air and lost my helmet in the meantime. And my brains were leaking out on the ground, and then I got to the hospital, and I was in a coma for four months. I was supposed to croak but I didn't. I fooled them all."

Traumatic brain injury impairs cognitive functions that have a wide reach. These general cognitive systems include attention, memory, and a resource management capacity called the executive system. After 18 years of examining 2,500 head injured cases, Hagen (1981) sorted them into three general diagnostic categories:

- residual cognitive impairment without language dysfunction
- disorganized language secondary to cognitive impairments
- predominant language-specific disorder, or aphasia

These possibilities indicate that the speech-language pathologist has an important role in the evaluation of persons with head injury. It can cause aphasia or, like right hemisphere dysfunction, can cause language difficulties that are expressions of other cognitive impairments. The clinician's job is to figure out which is which.

HEAD TRAUMA

Traumatic brain injury is the most common cause of death under age 38 in the United States. The most typical head injured person is male, single, of lower socioeconomic status, and high school educated or less (Anderson and McLaurin, 1980; Cooper, 1982). More than half are caused by motor vehicle accidents (MVAs). Falls are the next major cause. The most common contributing factor is alcohol use, and most injuries occur in summer or fall. In one study, 12 percent of head injuries were precipitated by interpersonal violence, and most of these were self-inflicted or stemmed from domestic problems (Rimel and Jane, 1983).

If the human skull is placed on the ground and weight is slowly piled on, it can support three tons (Rolak, 1993). Nevertheless, violent forces can damage the skull, and the brain can be damaged without harm to the skull. Head injuries have been broadly classified according to whether the skull is displaced, meninges are torn, or cortex is violated. A common approach is to distinguish **open** (i.e., penetrating) from **closed** (i.e., nonpenetrating) head injuries. Mechanisms of injury are quite variable (Table 9.1).

Large samples of war-related open head injuries revealed a great deal about cerebral dysfunction. Small caliber weapons provided Luria (1970b) with "cleanly punched out" lesions to study. Investigations followed World War I (Goldstein, 1942), World War II (Luria, 1966; Newcombe, 1969; Russell and Espir, 1961), and the

TABLE 9.1 Classification of head traumas (Brookshire, 1997).

TYPE	DEFINITION	SUBTYPE	DESCRIPTION	CAUSES
open	skull fragments penetrate brain tissue	high velocity	projectiles perforate or pierce the skull, bringing hair and skin with them	gunshots explosions
		low velocity	concentrated blunt trauma causing skull fracture rather than perforation	blows to head MVAs
closed	foreign substances do not penetrate brain tissue	acceleration	unrestrained head struck by moving object or moving head strikes stationary object	blows to head falls MVAs
		nonacceleration	fixed head struck by moving object	blows to head

Vietnam war (Mohr, Weiss, Caveness, Dillon, Kistler, Meirowsky, and Rish, 1980). High-velocity injuries from modern weapons can be quite devastating, causing extensive *laceration* (i.e., tearing) of brain tissue. Low-velocity traumas are like closed head injuries, except for the laceration of brain tissue when skull fracture is severe.

Most of this chapter is devoted to **closed head injury** (CHI) because it is a common form of trauma in a civilian population and its consequences are unique compared to dysfunctions presented in previous chapters. Table 9.1 distinguishes acceleration and nonacceleration injuries. The latter are usually much less severe than acceleration traumas. Nonacceleration causes *contusion* (i.e., bruising) of the brain's surface at the point of impact, called impression trauma.

The **primary effects** of acceleration traumas occur at the moment of impact. Brookshire (1997) detailed two types of forces. Linear acceleration causes both contusion at the point of impact (i.e., *coup* injury), and contusion opposite the point of impact (i.e., *contrecoup* injury). Angular acceleration, on the other hand, creates more twisting forces on the brain and usually produces more severe injuries.

In either case, violent movement against the sharp bony floor of the skull damages the "orbital" underside of the **prefrontal area** (see Figure 1.3) and the **anterior temporal lobes.** Neuropsychologists identify particular cognitive deficits or "syndromes" with damage to each of these regions. Because the lateral walls and roof of the skull are smooth, laceration is uncommon in the superior frontal lobes and the parietal and occipital lobes. In addition, twisting or stretching forces cause **diffuse axonal injury** (DAI). This stretching (or "shearing") of white fiber tracts within the cerebrum and brain stem occurs more with high speed traffic accidents than with blows or falls.

The brain's responses to such trauma are called **secondary effects.** Accumulation of fluid (i.e., edema) over the first few hours causes swelling and intracranial pressure. Because of laceration of blood vessels, a variety of hemorrhages can occur. Reduced pulmonary output can reduce blood flow to the brain, causing some ischemic damage. Widespread embolism can occur within hours. Sometimes secondary effects are dominant, such as when a person is conscious for a while before lapsing into unconsciousness.

THE TRAUMA UNIT

When a hospital is notified that a trauma patient is on the way, the beepers of the Trauma Team are activated simultaneously for a trauma code. All members not occupied with patient responsibilities proceed immediately to the booth in the emer-

DRI

gency room for trauma patients. The Trauma Surgery Attending Physician is the team leader. The team includes the Senior Trauma Surgery Resident, Resuscitator, Airway Manager, Procedure Residents, Primary Nurse, Nurse Assistant, and X-Ray Technician.

On the Resuscitator's count of three, the team and paramedics transfer the patient from a transport litter to a gurney. The Nurse Assistant removes the patient's clothing and obtains vital signs. The Resuscitator directs the team to establish an airway and an access to intravenous fluids. The oropharynx and nasopharynx are suctioned for blood, secretions, and foreign matter. When the patient is stabilized, the Senior Resident confers with the Team Leader and Resuscitator regarding an evaluation plan, which includes a CT scan. An unstabilized patient is taken immediately to an operating room. Depending on the nature of trauma, the surgeon evacuates subdural hematomas and/or repairs the skull and removes foreign matter.

A patient may be classified as a "talker" or "nontalker" in the emergency room. A nontalker is assessed for state of arousal. Pupils are checked for size and reaction to light. A thumb pressed by an eyebrow might elicit a motor response. Is respiration abnormal? Does eye gaze respond to commands? The aroused or talking patient is questioned for awareness of surroundings.

Around 25 percent of head injured people are nontalkers at hospital admission (Rimel and Jane, 1983). Loss of consciousness, or **coma,** is usually attributed to diffuse axonal injury. Acute care decisions are based partly on depth of coma, which is commonly assessed with the *Glasgow Coma Scale* (GCS) (Jennett and Teasdale, 1981). Ratings are obtained for eye opening, motor response, and verbal behavior. The maximum "coma score" is 15. Depth and duration of coma are indicators of severity of injury (Table 9.2). A critical decision path for multiple trauma patients may specify that a medically stable patient with a GCS less than 12 should get a CT scan before surgery.

The conscious patient exhibits a temporary period of diminished awareness called **post-traumatic amnesia** (PTA). The patient cannot remember events occurring before and after the accident. PTA is temporary and usually lasts much longer than the duration of coma. With the *Galveston Orientation and Amnesia Test* (GOAT), a patient is asked about current location, time, and date, and about recollections before and after injury (Levin, O'Donnell, and Grossman, 1979). In subject descriptions for research publications, duration of PTA is often added to information about coma to indicate severity of brain injury.

TABLE 9.2 Bases for estimating severity of traumatic brain injury.

	GCS SCORE	DURATION OF COMA
mild	13–15	less than 20 minutes
moderate	9–12	
severe	8 or less	more than 24 hours

Hannay and Levin, 1989; Jennett and Teasdale, 1981.

Mild head injury or **postconcussive syndrome** is diagnosed when there is loss of consciousness for 20 minutes or less, a GCS score of 13 or better upon admission, no known structural damage to the skull or brain, a hospital stay of no more than 48 hours, and a relatively brief period of PTA (Binder, 1986; Parasuraman, Mutter, and Malloy, 1991).

CLINICAL NEUROPSYCHOLOGY

Because of its important role in assessing the effects of traumatic brain injury, let us become more familiar with *clinical* neuropsychology. It is a specialized area of practice in clinical psychology and, thus, is different from *cognitive* neuropsychology. Initially, psychologists applied tests used for the evaluation of neurologically intact populations to the assessment of neurologically impaired populations. Then from "its parent disciplines of neurology and psychology," neuropsychology began to "develop an identity of its own in the 1940's" (Lezak, 1983). A chronology of neuropsychological assessment and its origins is shown in Table 9.3.

TABLE 9.3 Chronology of the development of clinical neuropsychological test batteries, from the early period of applying tests constructed for normal children and adults to a more recent period of tests intended for neurologically impaired populations (Lezak, 1983).

	ASSESSMENT	DESCRIPTION	REFERENCE
1900s	Stanford-Binet Intelligence Scale	Terman's revision of the first intelligence test (in France) at Stanford University; some use with brain damaged patients	Terman and Merrill (1937)
1930s	Weisenburg & McBride	first comparison of aphasic patients to normals with standardized tests	Weisenburg and McBride (1935)
1940s	Wechsler-Bellevue Scale	developed at Bellevue Hospital in New York City; used in hospitals during World War II	
	Armed services test batteries	screening of newly enlisted personnel; origin of some neuropsychological tests	see Lezak (1983)
1950s	Wechsler Adult Intelligence Scale (WAIS)	refinement of Weschler-Bellevue Scale; became the core neuropsychological test	Wechsler (1955)
1970s	Halstead-Reitan Neuropsychological Test Battery	6–7 hours of tests, including the WAIS; standardized for neuropsychological evaluation	Reitan and Wolfson (1985)
	Mini-Mental State Exam (MMSE)	brief standardized screening evaluation	Folstein, Folstein, and McHugh (1975)
1980s	WAIS-R	revision of WAIS	Wechsler (1981)
	Rancho Los Amigos Scale	rates general level of cognitive function	Hagen (1981)
	Luria-Nebraska Neuropsychological Battery	controversial standardization of Luria's informal clinical tests	Golden, Hammeke, and Purisch, (1980)
1990s	BROCAS SCAN	bedside screening taking 20–30 minutes; sensitive to mild impairment	Neppe and others (1992)

Unofficial guidelines for training have been published (Bornstein, 1988a, 1988b). A clinical neuropsychologist should be licensed or certified as a psychologist in the state where he or she practices. The American Board of Professional Psychology (ABPP) certifies clinical psychologists and recognizes specialty certification by the American Board of Professional Neuropsychology (ABPN) established in 1981. The credential is called a *diplomat in clinical neuropsychology.*

Because the ABPN was formed relatively recently, many competent neuropsychologists are not credentialed.

Qualifications is one issue addressed by Stern (1995) in an article advising attorneys on how to conduct a direct examination of a neuropsychologist in a trial. For example, someone with traumatic brain injury may be seeking compensation from a defendant (a test for faking memory deficit is presented later in this chapter). Stern explained that the neuropsychologist compares test findings to the patient's academic, vocational, medical, and psychiatric records to estimate the effect of injury on cognition and personality and on social and emotional behavior. State jurisdictions vary as to whether a neuropsychologist is allowed to render opinions regarding the status of the brain and its relationship to function. However, many states do permit a clinical neuropsychologist to discuss, for example, the function of the frontal lobe, how it can be injured, and what the residual impairments are likely to be.

A complete neurospychological evaluation can be done during the period of PTA, but the examiner expects random changes in pattern of deficit upon repeated testing. As indicated in Chapter 10, functional recovery can be quite rapid so that by two years postinjury the individual can attain a near average IQ on the WAIS (see Table 3.1). The **Digit Symbol subtest,** requiring concentration and speed, continues to reveal difficulties. In one study, the only significant impairment was with this subtest (Table 9.4). A much larger sample of 263 cases of CHI had a mean Full Scale IQ of 83.00 with a Verbal IQ of 85.79 and a Performance IQ of 81.28. The Digit Symbol subtest was a low 5.26 (Cullum and Bilger, 1986).

A general rating of cognitive impairment and behavioral characteristics has widespread use. It is called the **Rancho Los Amigos** scale or RLA scale (Table 9.5). Experimental subjects are often described or selected according to levels in the RLA scale. A subject may have had severe head injury but, at the time of study, have a relatively mild overall dysfunction of RLA level VI.

TABLE 9.4 Comparison of 20 CHIs and 20 matched controls on selected subtests of the WAIS-R. The CHIs had severe injuries at least 18 months prior to testing.

		CHI	CONTROLS
Full Scale IQ		95.60	102.80
Verbal	Arithmetic	9.10	9.90
	Similarities	9.35	10.30
	Digit Span	9.40	11.35
	Vocabulary	8.40	10.25
Performance	Digit Symbol	7.80	12.05
	Block Design	10.20	11.40

Schmitter-Edgecombe, Marks, Fahy, and Long, 1992.

ATTENTION

Table 4.3 introduced the levels and functions of attention. Cortical arousal to any environmental stimulus depends on the reticular activating system in the brain stem (see Figure 1.3), and damage to this system is thought to cause the comatose state (Trexler and Zappala, 1988). Once a patient is aroused or conscious, levels of awareness vary from stupor (or "obtundation") to alertness. An alert patient can still be distractible, or can have difficulty focusing attention.

Selective or focused attention is thought to be managed by connections between the thalamus and prefrontal cortex, called the *thalamofrontal gating system* (Trexler and Zappala, 1988). These structures are vulnerable to the forces of CHI. Ponsford and Kinsella (1992) studied a group with severe CHI just one to three months postinjury. The researchers presented several color naming tasks. One consisted of printed names of colors in different colors, so that the word *red* might be printed in blue. This is called the Stroop interference task. The color name could be a distraction when the task is to name the color of the print (i.e., *blue*). CHIs were slower but as accurate as controls, indicating that focused attention was intact in the Stroop task. Sustained attention was

TABLE 9.5 Rancho Los Amigos Scale of cognitive-behavioral function (Hagen, 1981). Only a few characteristics of each level are shown, rendering this summary insufficient for using the RLA.

LEVEL	GENERAL RESPONSE	DEFINITION SUMMARY
I	No response	unresponsive to all stimuli
II	Generalized	nonpurposeful, inconsistent, or gross response to stimuli; may have delayed response to pain
III	Localized response	responses related to stimuli but inconsistent. responds to some commands
IV	Confused-agitated	bizarre behavior, incoherent utterance, short attention span, uncooperative
V	Confused-inappropriate, nonagitated	follows simple commands, affected by complexity of task, better attention span, has difficulty learning new things
VI	Confused-appropriate	remote memory returning, recent memory still deficient, some goal-direction
VII	Automatic-appropriate	oriented in familiar situations, improved but shallow recall of recent activities, lacks insight and judgment
VIII	Purposeful-appropriate	capable of new learning, remote and recent memory good, poor stress tolerance; supervision not needed

examined in the same study. Subjects watched lights go on and off and pressed a button whenever a target light appeared. Again, CHIs were slower but not less accurate than controls and performance did not deteriorate over the time of the task.

Nevertheless, a common complaint is a struggle with concentration. Documenting such complaints with mild head injury has been particularly difficult. When a victim is seeking damages, a defense attorney makes sure that a jury hears the phrase "mild head injury" over and over (Stern, 1995). Parasuraman and others (1991) studied sustained attention one month after injury in a group with mild CHIs. The investigators presented a series of digits, and subjects simply had to press a button whenever a target digit appeared. There was no deficit with clear stimuli, but a deficit appeared when stimuli were obscured to make them more difficult to encode. Compared to Ponsford's study, it appears that reduction of vigilance depends on the task. Parasuraman concluded that the findings "join a growing body of evidence that mild CHI can lead to measurable deficits in cognitive functioning" (p. 789).

PERCEPTION AND RECOGNITION

Studies of CHI indicate that, at least during the first year postinjury, patients can have difficulties with visual perception or what investigators may call "stimulus encoding" (Shum, McFarland, Bain, and Humphreys, 1990). Visual matching and other visuospatial tasks in test batteries can be especially problematic (Bernstein-Ellis, Wertz, Dronkers, and Milton, 1985; Luzzatti, Willmes, Taricco, Colombo, and Chiesa, 1989). The encoding impairment is likely to disappear over time.

Face perception and recognition were studied according to a stage-theory similar to Table 8.2 (Parry, Young, Saul, and Moss, 1991). Three tasks were administered, and each was thought to address a different component of the recognition process. The researchers wanted to determine if different disorders could be identified in a group with severe CHIs. The group was impaired overall in comparison to a control group. Four of 15 patients had distinctive disorders: one on facial expression recognition (i.e., perception), one on unfamiliar face matching (i.e., perception), and two on familiar face recognition (i.e., access to recognition unit). The results indicate that some patients with CHI have specific face processing problems.

Years after his injury, case PH remained unable to copy shapes and recognize familiar people (Young and De Haan, 1988). He was still able to recognize people by their voices or clothing, indicative of intact semantic memory. The instructive thing about PH was that he could not identify people when asked to judge whether faces were familiar, but he matched familiar faces faster than unfamiliar faces. The latter finding suggested that a "covert" level of recognition was preserved.

MEMORY

A common tool is the **Wechsler Memory Scale** (WMS) which contains seven subtests (Table 9.6). The sum of subtest scores is called the Memory Quotient (MQ). Performance on the WMS is not necessarily related to overall intelligence. A case whose frontal lobe was penetrated by a billiard cue was impaired on this memory test but had a Full Scale IQ of 123 (Kapur, 1994). The MQ has been criticized for promoting the idea that memory is a unidimensional function and for representing memory as an odd variety of cognitive functions (Lezak, 1983). Also, the test is heavily weighted on verbal abilities and immediate memory skills.

Traditional clinical tests of memory have an unclear relationship to theories of memory. Our survey of the study of aphasia has given us some idea of the distinction between working memory and long-term memory. By now we should also be sensitive to the corresponding distinction between process and the stable storage of knowledge. Processes, constrained by working memory, make contact with knowledge in long-term memory. These processes are involved in the *acquisition* of new information and the *activation* of old or stored information whenever it is needed for a task. Basic investigation of CHI has been sensitive to these and other distinctions in what we now know is a multidimensional memory system.

Short-Term and Working Memory

The Digit Span subtest of the WAIS has exposed a deficiency of short-term buffer capacity in patients with CHI (see Table 9.4). A patient can be left with only an STM deficit six months after injury (Van der Linden, Coyette, and Seron, (1992). Duration of short-term retention can be studied with a **continuous recognition memory task.** For example, a series of drawings may be presented and some are repeated. As each drawing appears, a subject reports if the drawing is "new" or "old" (i.e., like one seen before). In a study of adolescents with CHI, Hannay and Levin (1989) found that short-term recognition memory varied as a function of severity of injury. Those with mild head injuries performed like normal controls, whereas moderately and severely injured subjects were impaired.

TABLE 9.6 Subtests of the Wechsler Memory Scale (Wechsler, 1945).

SUBTEST	DESCRIPTION
I. Personal and current information	asks for age, birthdate, and current and recent public officials
II. Orientation	questions about time and place
III. Mental control	say alphabet, count by fours
IV. Logical memory	immediate retelling of two short stories
V. Digit span	forward and backward, slight difference from WAIS subtest
VI. Visual reproduction	immediate recall of three designs
VII. Associate learning	recall of related and unrelated word-pairs

Another method for testing duration of retention in STM consists of placing a few seconds between a subspan series of digits and the recall test. Also, a subject is asked to count backwards during the interval in order to minimize rehearsal of the list. One version of this paradigm is the *Portland Digit Recognition Test,* which has been used to determine if financial incentives influence the measurement of cognitive deficit in mildly head injured people (Binder, 1993). A group seeking compensation was compared to a group not seeking compensation. CHI was caused by falls, motor vehicle accidents, and timber cutting or sawmill accidents. The no-compensation group was superior to the compensation-seeking group, which is consistent with the possibility that the compensation-seeking group was exaggerating memory deficits or malingering (also, Trueblood and Schmidt, 1993).

Many studies, including the studies of attention mentioned earlier, have led to identifying "mental slowness" or **slow information processing** as a fundamental consequence of head injury. Pronounced deficit in the Digit Symbol subtest of the WAIS is a clinical indication of this problem. Sternberg's (1975) classic *short-term memory scanning* procedure provides a more precise picture of processing speed and style. In Chapter 7, the scanning process was implicated in the hunt for a pronoun's antecedent in the short-term buffer (i.e., Bill or Mary).

The Sternberg task is a short-term recognition test in which response time is measured. A short series of digits (i.e., within memory span) is presented, followed immediately by a test digit. Subjects indicate if the test digit was in the preceding list. Researchers vary the length of the digit-series in order to determine scanning speed and type of search (i.e., terminating at recognition or exhaustive no matter when the match is found). The task was given to severe CHIs who were at least 18 months postinjury (Schmitter-Edgecombe, et al., 1992). Again, the subjects with CHI were slower than controls, but they scanned exhaustively and made matching decisions like the controls.

Long-Term Memory

Amnesia involves previously acquired memories that reside in long-term memory. The disorder is not related to overall intelligence. In one study, mildly and severely amnesic subjects did not differ in Full Scale IQ on the WAIS (Schacter and Graf, 1986). Head injured patients experience two types of difficulty:

- **retrograde amnesia** involves forgetting memories acquired *before* injury (e.g., "remote memory")
- **anterograde amnesia** involves forgetting memories acquired *after* injury (e.g., "recent memory")

Severity of retrograde amnesia increases as the memory gap extends further into the past. Any experiment or clinical assessment must delve into memories acquired prior to injury. Depending on a patient's age, an interview may explore recollections from contemporary life, early adulthood, and childhood (e.g., Van der Linden, Bredart, Depoorter, and Coyette, 1996). Memory for impersonal world events might be quizzed with questions organized according to periods of time (e.g., Beatty, Salmon, Bernstein, and Butters, 1987; Warrington and Sanders, 1971). During recovery, the amnesic gap shrinks toward the time of injury. A mild gap comprises 30 minutes prior to injury and is usually long-lasting.

Compared to retrograde amnesia, anterograde amnesia is more prominent and resilient after a patient regains consciousness. The patient does not remember meeting hospital personnel and does not remember what happened in therapy. Thus, cognitive rehabilitation is affected by the duration of post-traumatic amnesia. PTA is said to end when a patient "remembers today what happened yesterday and does not begin each day with a blank mind" (Jennett and Teasdale, 1981, p. 89). Because anterograde amnesia involves information acquired after the injury, investigations have commonly consisted of new learning procedures.

Can the nature of these amnesias be pinpointed with respect to features of the memory system? Are retrograde and anterograde amnesias different cognitive disorders? Two main issues have been considered. One is whether people with CHI have a characteristic difficulty with one type of information storage, such as semantic or episodic memory (review Chapter 1). The other question pertains to whether the impairment is a disappearance of information from long-term storage or is a disruption of processes that make contact with preserved long-term storage.

Several cases have been presented to address the question of whether memory deficit is specific to one type of information. Gene, who suffered a severe head injury in a motorcycle accident, was one of these cases (Schacter, 1996). He could not recall day-to-day events and could not remember specific events from any period in his life. He could not recall motorcycle trips with his friends or a train derailment near his home. Yet, he could remember facts such as the floor plan of his childhood home and names of friends and schools. He could discuss the nature of his work prior to injury but could not recall events that had occurred while on the job. He could tell how to change a tire but could not recall ever having changed one. The deficit was with episodic memory, not semantic memory.

Conway and Rubin (1993) proposed a hierarchical organization of **autobiographical knowledge.** The highest level consists of *lifetime periods* that are measured in years or decades such as the high school years or a period of living in one place. For example, patient PS retained memory only for his service in World War II (Hodges and McCarthy, 1993). The middle of the hierarchy contains *general events* that are extended episodes measured in days, weeks, or months, such as a vacation or a practicum experience. The bottom of the hierarchy is the store of *specific events* measured in seconds, minutes, or hours. Based on the study of Gene and other cases, Schacter (1996) suspected that event-specific knowledge is episodic and more general levels of autobiographical knowledge are recorded in semantic memory.

AC, a 38-year-old teacher with a master's degree, was found unconscious in the street and remained in a coma for three months (Van der Linden, et al., 1996). After regaining consciousness, he was given an interview that distinguished between *personal semantic memory* of facts, such as where he had lived and names of school teachers, and *autobiographical incidents* about specific events. AC could remember semantic information indicating that he "knows who he is," but he could not remember specific events from any of the periods tested. He recalled people who were famous before his injury and facts learned afterward such as names of therapists and location of the rehabilitation center. Like Gene, AC's episodic memory was impaired in some way, and semantic memory at least had not been erased.

Assuming pre-traumatic memories were acquired normally, then retrograde amnesia can be either a destruction of stored memories or a retrieval problem. The spontaneous gradual return of remote memories is indicative of preserved storage and a damaged retrieval mechanism. By itself, however, this does not account for the retrieval of memories of the distant past better than memories of the more recent past (Squire, 1987).

Anterograde amnesia has been studied with tasks requiring the recall of recently presented information. In a paired-associate learning task, a list of unassociated word-pairs is presented for a subject to study (e.g., WINDOW-REASON). Then, recall or learning is tested two ways. An **explicit test** consists of presenting the first word of a pair (e.g., WINDOW-) to see if the pair is remembered. A subject is aware that memory is being tested. Prior to the explicit test, the subject is also given a word-stem completion task that can be done without prior exposure to the list (e.g., REA___). Performance on this test could be affected by priming or, namely, by the facilitating effect of prior experience. By seeing if the subject completes stems from the list more accurately or faster than stems not in the list, this turns out to be an **implicit test** of list learning (Schacter and Graf, 1986).

The terminology for this distinction varies (Table 9.7). However, results are fairly consistent. Schacter and Graf (1986) found impairment with

TABLE 9.7 Different terminology for two levels of the memory test. The terms tend to identify different aspects of the same thing.

LEVELS OF RECALL TEST				DEFINITION
automatic	covert	implicit	incidental	without awareness that prior learning or memory is being tested; "unconscious"
effortful	overt	explicit	intentional	with awareness that prior learning or memory is being tested; "conscious"

Levin, Goldstein, High, and Williams, 1988; Schacter and Graf, 1986; Young and De Haan, 1988; Vakil, Blachstein, and Hoofien, 1991.

explicit testing but not with implicit testing. Implict recall also indicates that new information can be acquired and retained for a while. The impairment lies in effortful retrieval processes. Yet, there is also the stimulus encoding problem mainly in the first year postinjury and the problem with distractibility. Both can make it difficult to acquire new information (Freedman and Cermak, 1986).

Amnesic Syndromes

Amnesia has many causes but has some consistent characteristics. Anterograde and retrograde forms typically co-occur in one patient. Also, explicit memory is impaired whereas implicit memory is spared. Besides trauma, amnesia is caused by temporary loss of oxygen (anoxia), ruptured anterior communicating artery aneurysm, Alzheimer's disease, and herpes encephalitis (see Table 2.3). Researchers often group these etiologies together in studies of the amnesic syndrome (e.g., Schacter, Harbluk, and McLachlan, 1984). However, individuals have been particularly informative regarding content and organization of the knowledge store as well as regarding the neurology of memory.

HM became an historic case in neuropsychology after the surgical removal of structures deep within the medial portion of both temporal lobes (Milner, Corkin, and Teuber, 1968). One of these structures was the hippocampus. Two years later, HM scored a Full Scale IQ of 112 on the WAIS. However, he did not recognize hospital staff that he saw regularly and forgot when he had recently eaten a meal. Besides his anterograde amnesia, HM also had retrograde amnesia for events several years prior to his operation. HM is thought to have provided the first direct evidence that the medial temporal lobe, the hippocampus in particular, plays an important part in memory.

Schacter (1996) wrote of two rounds of golf with Frederick who was in the early stage of Alzheimer's disease. It was a test. One round was on a familiar course, and the other on an unfamiliar course. Frederick could still play golf, indicative of retention of procedural memory. He retained perfect use of golf vocabulary, considered to be indicative of semantic memory. He also followed the "rules" by choosing the right club, knowing who putts first, and evaluating slopes on the green before putting. However, he would forget the shots he had just hit. He could not find his ball after being the first to drive off the tee, that is, when there was a delay between hitting the ball and looking for it. After the round was over, unlike most golfers in the clubhouse, he could not remember a single shot from the round. Frederick had a specific problem with episodic memory.

Similar problems specific to episodic memory have been reported in patients with herpes encephalitis (see Table 2.3). SS could not recall episodes from any time in his life (Cermak and O'Conner, 1983). Like Gene, he could recall lifetime periods and general events, which Schacter believed to be stored in semantic memory. Herpes encephalitis, however, can have the opposite result when damage is concentrated in the anterior temporal lobes. There is a comprehensive failure to recall from semantic memory but a retained ability to remember specific episodes (DeRenzi, Liotti, and Nichelli, 1987).

Sometimes a patient remembers what someone said but cannot remember who said it, which is called **source amnesia.** In one study, two people acted as sources of information in a cued recall task. The two experimenters alternated in asking and answering questions about famous people (e.g., What job did Bob Hope's father have? *fireman*). A few items later, subjects were asked the question again and were asked to provide the answer and state who asked the particular question. A mixed group of amnesic subjects were unable to recall that either of the experimenters was the source of information, a problem not exhibited by normal controls (Schacter, et al., 1984).

Functional Memory

Do laboratory tests predict everyday memory? This question was posed by Sunderland, Harris, and Baddeley (1983) in a comparison between self-reports of everyday memory and a variety of experimental and clinical tests (e.g., continuous recognition, story recall, and paired-associate learning). Also, a group about three months after injury was compared to a group between two and eight years postinjury. Patients and their relatives filled out questionnaires for rating the frequency of occurrence of memory errors over the previous few weeks. They also took home booklets that contained checklists regarding the same 35 items for indicating whether the memory failure occurred each day for seven days.

The 35 items in the questionnaires and checklists were selected according to five categories. Here are some examples that might inform any work with a patient's memory:

Speech

- Forgetting the names of friends or relatives or calling them by the wrong names.
- Forgetting something you were told a few minutes ago. Perhaps something your wife or a friend has just said.
- Forgetting to tell somebody something important. Perhaps forgetting to pass on a message or remind someone of something.
- Repeating a story or joke you have already told.

Reading and Writing

- Forgetting what the sentence you have just read was about and having to re-read it.
- Unable to follow the thread of a story. Lose track of what it is about.

Faces and Places

- Forgetting where you have put something. Losing things around the house.
- Failing to recognize television characters or other famous people by sight.
- Getting lost or turning in the wrong direction on a journey or walk you have often been on.

Actions

- Forgetting to do some routine thing which you would normally do once or twice in a day.
- Starting to do something, then forgetting what it was you wanted to do. Maybe saying, "What am I doing?"

Learning New Things

- Unable to remember the name of someone you met for the first time recently.
- Forgetting to keep an appointment.

Sunderland and his colleagues found that the relatives' questionnaire correlated with 6 of 14 test performances for the long-term head injured group but not for the recently injured group. The patients' questionnaire did not correlate with any of the laboratory tests. The results reflect the instability of memory in the first few months after injury and indicate that formal tests may not be predictive of everyday memory, at least, in the way that everyday memory was assessed in this study.

Sense of Self

In the journal *Aphasiology,* Brumfitt (1993) led a discussion of the effect of aphasia on a person's identity or "sense of self" (see Chapter 12). This question is also relevant regarding the impact of amnesia on an individual's sense for who he or she is. Patients like AC, the teacher who was found unconscious on the street, can recall facts about themselves stored in semantic memory and, thus, retain a fundamental personal identity. They just cannot remember specific events.

A severe retrograde amnesia can have devastating consequences. Schacter (1996) commented on the aftermath of Gene's motorcycle accident: "A life without any episodic memory is psychologically barren...Nothing much happens in Gene's mind or in his life. He has few friends and lives quietly at home with his parents...he thinks little about the future. It does not occur to him to make plans..." (pp. 149–150). Another patient could not remember most of what happened in his life prior to a bilateral thalamic stroke, but he could remember details about his service in the navy during World War II nearly 50 years before (Hodges and McCarthy, 1993). In fact, his identity became so attached to that period that he came to believe that he was still in active service and would have to return to his ship soon.

EXECUTIVE FUNCTIONS

"Action disorganization" is caused by an impairment of the central executive component of working memory (Baddeley, 1986). Shallice (1988) called it a Supervisory Attentional System (SAS). Although a central executive is occasionally associated with any aspect of working memory (e.g., Van der Linden, et al., 1992), it usually refers to the management of resources in dual-tasks and in the performance of multiple actions. Tasks used to assessed the executive appear to be related to success at work.

The general assumption is that simple routine or highly skilled actions are carried out quickly and efficiently in the automatic processing mode. The executive system, on the other hand, is thought to be invoked intentionally for novel or difficult actions or when errors occur in routine actions. It regulates attentional resources to reach a goal. Let us assume that a goal is to get to work. According to Duncan (1986), executive function starts with *goal lists* such as taking a shower, getting dressed, and eating breakfast before going to work. An *action-list* is the mental operations and overt actions engaged in meeting these goals. *Self-monitoring* or means-ends analysis compares current states and goal states, ensuring that goals are being met.

Impaired executive control produces what is known as **dysexecutive syndrome.** Executive control applies to any information-processing domain, and the syndrome should be manifested in a wide variety of tasks. The **Wisconsin Card Sorting Test** (WCST) (Grant and Berg, 1948) is often used to test executive function. It is said to test abilities to identify abstract categories and shift cognitive set. The WCST contains 64 cards depicting one to four colored shapes. Patients must determine a sorting strategy according to a criterion that an examiner has in mind (e.g., color or shape) and that is deduced from the examiner's feedback (i.e., "right" or "wrong"). Once a patient uses one criterion consistently, the examiner changes the criterion.

In one study, CHIs exhibited fewer sorts and more perseverative errors than normal controls on the WCST (Gansler, Covall, McGrath, and Oscar-Berman, 1996). In general, patients have difficulty shifting response sets and evaluating their performance.

The **Tinker Toy Test** was developed to assess executive function (Lezak, 1982). A patient is presented with 50 assorted Tinker Toys and is instructed to "make whatever you want." Fifty persons with CHI were given this test at least 24 months after receiving medical clearance to return to work (Bayless, Varney, and Roberts, 1989). Half of the group, however, had not returned to work, and the other 25 had been employed for at least six months or had returned to their previous employment. All but one who had returned to work scored normally, but nearly half of those who did not return to work scored below the worst control subject. Thus, the Tinker Toy Test may have some prognostic value for returning to work.

FRONTAL LOBE SYNDROMES

The pre-frontal area is another region of the brain commonly damaged in CHI (see Figure 1.3). Prefrontal damage causes changes in intellectual skills and personality (Benson and Stuss, 1986). This is a vast region, however, prompting Kertesz (1994) to advise that frontal lobe syndromes vary greatly according to type of pathology and size and location of lesion. He added that "no such entity as a single frontal lobe syndrome or frontal lobe disease exists, although this terminology is used frequently" (p. 569). Problems associated with frontal lobe damage are attention disorder, executive dysfunction, amnesia, and personality disorder.

One frequently studied pathology is the hemorrhagic rupture of an **anterior communicating artery aneurysm** (ACAA or ACoA, or AACA for "aneurysm of the anterior communicating artery"). In addition to variation in the acronym, descriptions of this "syndrome" have been quite variable because of inconsistencies in procedures, use of control groups, and time post onset of the study (DeLuca, 1992).

Godefroy and Rousseaux (1996) were interested in processes underlying increased distractibility with ACAA. They found patients to be deficient in focused and divided attention. However, other patients were not specially impaired in tests of attention and concentration relative to a group with intracranial hemorrhages, indicating that attention disorder may not be unique to ACAA (DeLuca, 1992).

Disorders of memory and executive control are thought to combine as a *dysexecutive memory impairment* in cases of ACAA (Parkin, Yeomans, and Bindschaendler, 1994). The problematic pattern of deficit occurs as intact recognition memory but impaired recall on tasks equated for difficulty. Recognition is a way of testing memory or learning without requiring retrieval (i.e., "Did you see this before?"), whereas recall tasks require explicit retrieval of information. Scrutiny of recall tasks indicated patients have difficulty implementing retrieval strategies, which is considered to be one job of the executive system.

The Wisconsin Card Sorting Test has been thought to be particularly sensitive to frontal lobe damage. Patients with ACAA have performed poorly (DeLuca, 1992). However, in another study, subjects with focal frontal lesions did not perform differently from a nonfrontal group. Some subjects with extensive frontal damage scored well, and researchers suggested that the test cannot be used alone as an index of frontal lobe damage (Anderson, Damasio, Jones, and Tranel, 1991; also, Ahola, Vilkki, and Servo, 1996).

Damage to the frontal lobes can produce dramatic behavioral changes that vary according to size and location of lesion (e.g., Crowe, 1992). Damage to the forward convexity is known to cause *apathetic syndrome*. Medial frontal damage tends to cause *akinetic syndrome* or lack of initiative. Gene, the motorcyclist, had these arousal disorders. He became less outgoing and less active than he was before the accident. Orbitofrontal damage (inferior frontal), which is common with CHI, makes it difficult to control impulses. This difficulty is known as *disinhibition syndrome* or "behavior disorder." A patient may engage in outrageous displays including sexual inappropriateness and running away or "elopement."

The **Minnesota Multiphasic Personality Inventory** (MMPI) is part of the Halstead-Reitan battery and is the most widely used objective personality measure (Hathaway and McKinley, 1951). It is a 566-item true-false questionnaire requiring sixth grade reading skills. Answers contribute to four *validity scales* (i.e., test-taking competency) and 10 *clinical scales.* Interpretation of the clinical scales is based on a pattern of scores that can be related to normal control subjects and diagnostic groups of psychiatric patients. Neuropsychologists are careful to avoid blind psychiatric interpretation without taking medical conditions into consideration.

INSIGHT AND EMOTION

Patients are often unaware of their behavior or personality changes, an anosognosia that is linked to frontal lobe damage (McGlynn and Schacter, 1989). While family members become stressed by a patient's anxiety and bad temper, the patient denies such disturbances. Persons with CHI also may not complain of physical disabilities. Neuropsychologists say that patients have a **posttraumatic insight disorder** that is observed as an underreporting of the severity of impairments.

Several studies show that patients with mild or severe head trauma often underestimate memory impairments (McGlynn and Schacter, 1989). They realize their memory is worse but are not aware of the severity of deficit. Family members feel that the memory impairment is more serious than the patient does (e.g., Van der Linden, et al., 1996). Patients with more left hemisphere damage are more likely to report memory problems than patients with more right hemisphere damage. A patient might admit to a slight memory problem upon questioning but still insist that returning to work is a realistic goal. Some training of compensatory strategies may be accompanied by an increase of self-awareness in the training tasks, but this more realistic estimate of deficit sometimes does not carry over to the work setting.

Investigators found that, at six months postinjury, CHI patients continued to underreport severity of deficits. Other patients with CHI demonstrated greater insight at one year and two-to-three years postinjury (Godfrey, Partridge, Knight, and Bishara, 1993). However, improved insight was accompanied by increased emotional dysfunction. Depression and anxiety were found to be less in the first six months postinjury than later, and these problems peak between seven and 12 months after injury (Lezak and O'Brien, 1988). The delayed onset of depression may be the result of a gradually increasing awareness of impairments. In general, patients may be difficult to engage in rehabilitation during the first year because of unrealistic treatment goals, while a later challenge is the negative reaction to an emerging understanding of impairment.

Neuropsychologists have tried to document the life-altering effects of disability. Stambrook and others (1991) administered self-report questionnaires to obtain perspectives of patients and their spouses. One questionnaire addressed emotional, psychological, and physical problems. Another measured extent of emotional distress. A third questionnaire measured social and free-time activities and negative social behaviors. Stambrook compared CHIs and a group with spinal cord injury. Moderately impaired CHIs and spinal cord injured patients were equivalent on all measures. Severely impaired CHIs were distinctive in being more bewildered, depressed, and hostile than the other groups. Wives rated the severe CHIs as being more belligerent, helpless, and withdrawn than the others.

LANGUAGE

At the beginning of this chapter, Hagen (1981) was cited for suggesting that CHI in some cases causes cognitive disorders without language problems and in other cases causes aphasia or language problems that are secondary to cognitive disorders. Wertz (1985) referred to the secondary deficits as "language of confusion" (e.g., McDonald, 1993). Let us begin our examination of language with results of clinical tests.

Clinical Tests and Diagnosis

What proportion of CHIs have aphasia? Heilman, Safran, and Geschwind (1971) administered an unspecified aphasia examination to 750 patients with CHI and concluded that only two percent had aphasia (also, Schwartz-Cowley and Stepanik, 1989). Fifty patients were studied elsewhere, and they had minimal deficits on language tests except for 40 percent who had naming difficulties (Levin, Grossman, and Kelly, 1976). Among Heilman's 13 diagnosed with aphasia, nine had anomic aphasia and four had Wernicke's aphasia. Hartley and Levin (1990) said that acute CHIs can display language behavior similar to Wernicke's aphasia, which evolves to anomic-like aphasia as orientation improves.

Sarno, Buonaguro, and Levita (1987) examined 25 CHIs nearly four months after injury with four tasks from a standard aphasia battery. The tests consisted of naming, sentence repetition, word fluency, and the Token Test of sentence comprehension. The patients were impaired in all tasks to levels found in stroke-related aphasia. Sarno decided that they had found "parallel aphasias which characterized both CHI and CVA aphasic patients" (p. 336). Earlier, Sarno (1980) had concluded that 32 percent of a head injured group had aphasia whereas others had a "subclinical aphasia" with no apparent deficit in conversation but still an impairment in word fluency.

Thirty severe CHIs received an Italian translation of a German test for aphasia plus some more naming tasks and tests of other cognitive functions (Luzzatti, et al., 1989). Sixteen subjects had unilateral lesions according to CT scan. On the aphasia test, CHIs scored in the range for mild language deficit. Of 18 subjects classified as aphasic, 11 were diagnosed as having Broca's aphasia according to test criteria. However, presence of dysarthria influenced classification of six of these nonfluent cases.

Porch identified three **bilateral signs** with respect to performance on the PICA: (1) a visual-auditory reversal with either auditory subtests higher than the visual object matching subtests, (2) high verbal ability near levels of receptive modalities, and (3) unusually low copying in subtests. To examine the validity of this diagnostic aid, Bernstein-Ellis and others (1985) gave the PICA to 15 cases of traumatic brain injury. The patients had deficits in all areas of language function, but statistical analysis showed a unique pattern. Visual matching was worse and writing sentences was better for patients with TBI than for those with stroke-related aphasia. Yet, the bilateral signs did not distinguish traumatic injury. Ten of the head injured patients showed one sign, five showed two signs, and none displayed all three.

These studies indicate that some patients with CHI exhibit deficits on language tests. The studies also leave an impression that clinical investigators differ with respect to diagnosing these deficits as aphasia. However, even if everyone agrees on what aphasia is, findings are going to differ when one sample size is 750 and another is 25. One sample may have more predominantly unilateral lesions than another. Yet, there is an impression that "language of confusion" has been diagnosed as aphasia or, at least, as "subclinical" aphasia. Holland (1982) did not mince words: "if the language problems seen in closed head injured patients don't look like aphasia, sound like aphasia, act like aphasia, feel, smell or taste like aphasia, then they aren't aphasia" (p. 345).

A debate over diagnosis of aphasia has implications for treatment. Sarno and others (1987) concluded that "the traditional language rehabilitation approaches implemented with CVA aphasic patients are appropriate for the management of aphasia in CHI patients as well" (p. 336). On the other hand, Holland (1982) stated that CHI patients "will not be terribly responsive to the traditional methods by which we have come to treat aphasia" (p. 345). This apparent disagreement dissolves if we agree that CHI is not a homogeneous neurological condition and is similarly diverse in its consequences. It is possible that CHI patients with secondary language deficits may not be responsive to traditional aphasia methods, whereas CHI patients with aphasias caused by more focal insults may be responsive to these methods.

Language Comprehension

The experimental study of language comprehension with CHI is a barren landscape compared to the study of aphasia caused by stroke. To examine lexical contact with semantic memory, Haut and others (1991) presented a unique priming task in which subjects made rapid judgments about whether a second word is a member of the semantic category of the first word. The subjects with CHI were primed, indicating that semantic organization was preserved both before and after one year postonset. However, the patients were also slow. This result is consistent with Schacter's clinical observation of preserved semantic memory (while access to episodic memory is impaired) and is consistent with the robust finding that CHI reduces the speed of information processing in working memory.

A few persons with CHI have been featured in cognitive neuropsychological studies of word-reading disorders (see Chapter 6). Seven of them are summarized in Table 9.8. We can see that there is no single CHI-related reading disorder, although the peripheral dyslexias caused by attention disorders should not be surprising. Case GG, who had a hematoma drained from the right hemisphere, is striking for his "lower neglect dyslexia." He had the usual left neglect dyslexia; but, when words were arranged vertically, he misread the final letters of words arranged top-down and the initial letters of words arranged bottom-up (Nichelli, Venneri, Pentore, and Cubelli, 1993). The disorder was located roughly at a peripheral level of stimulus representation.

Patients with CHI were compared with patients with stroke-related aphasia on Caplan's Thematic Role Battery introduced in Chapter 4 (Butler-Hinz, Caplan, and Waters, 1990). The battery tests "final interpretation" of various canonical and noncanonical sentence structures and employs the enactment strategy of manipulating toy animals. Pattern of difficulty among sentence-

TABLE 9.8 Summary of word-reading disorders caused by CHI. Four of the seven would be classified as peripheral dyslexias (see Chapter 6).

CASE	CAUSE	READING DISORDER	DESCRIPTION	REFERENCE
MA	motor vehicle accident	pure alexia, letter-by-letter reader	nonaphasic; evidence of impairment extending beyond reading	Sekuler and Behrmann (1996)
HT	motorcycle accident	letter-by-letter reader	had mixed aphasia; impairment differing from others' word-length effect; attention deficit	Price and Humphreys (1992)
JB	struck by motorcyclist	neglect dyslexia	with normal language, main complaint was reading problem; misread left side of words; related to attention deficit	Riddoch, Humphreys, Cleton, and Ferry (1990)
GG	fall from a scaffolding	neglect dyslexia	left neglect dyslexia, but also lower neglect for words presented on a vertical axis	Nichelli, Venneri, Pentore, and Cubelli (1993)
MP	struck by motor vehicle	surface dyslexia	fluent speech with paraphasias; regularity effect in reading and writing; impaired activation of whole-word units in single orthographic lexicon	Behrmann and Bub (1992)
DE	motorcycle accident	deep dyslexia	Broca's aphasia; difficulty reading function words & abstract words; deficit in recognizing silly sentences	Patterson (1979)
RL	motor vehicle accident	deep dyslexia	agrammatic speech with neologisms; semantic paralexias & concreteness effect; spontaneous recovery of primary semantic route	Klein, Behrmann, and Doctor (1994)

types was similar between groups. However, French-speaking clinical groups differed in that the stroke-group had more severe impairment than the CHI-group; but English-speaking clinical groups did not differ in severity of deficit. The French stroke-group was more impaired than the other three groups, attributed mainly to the small size of each group. The similarity of pattern led the investigators to conclude that LH-stroke and CHI cause qualitatively similar sentence comprehension impairments.

One lesson of Chapter 5 was that we should delay conclusions about the nature of disorder until we have a body of on-line research that taps into ongoing sentence processing. Tyler (1985) reported some unusual on-line studies of DE who, at age 16, was involved in a motorcycle accident and apparently had a secondary occlusion in the left internal carotid artery. There was no evidence of RH-damage. A few years before, he was involved in some studies of dyslexia (e.g., Patterson, 1979). Apparently DE's main disorder looked, sounded, and acted like aphasia, as his Boston Exam indicated that he was "a typical Broca's agrammatic patient." Tyler began her studies around 13 years after the accident.

With the word-monitoring procedure, Tyler (1985) initially examined "global" capabilities without a clear relationship to a particular comprehension mechanism. DE was handed a word on a card (e.g., *church*) and was instructed to press a button as soon as he heard it. Tyler presented normal sentences (*1a*), anomalous sentences that retained syntactic form (*1b*), and scrambled utterances without syntactic or semantic sense (*1c*).

(1a) Everyone was outraged when they heard. Apparently, in the middle of the night some thieves broke into the *church* and stole a golden crucifix.

(1b) Everyone was exposed when they ate. Apparently, at the distance of the wind some ants pushed around the *church* and forced a new item.

(1c) They everyone when outraged heard was. Of middle apparently the some of the into the broke night in thieves *church* and crucifix stole a golden.

In such studies of linguistic violations, the normal processor slows down in the vicinity of errors. DE's response also slowed down as semantic sense and syntactic form were stripped away. He was unlike normals, however, by not responding with increasing speed as the location of target words was changed from left to right in anomalous sentences like *1b.* Tyler diagnosed this absence of word-position effect as an impairment in detecting the syntactic structure of these sentences.

A second word-monitoring experiment was more focused, as Tyler examined sensitivity to violations of verb-argument relations. The target-word was placed in either a correct context (*2a*), a selection violation after verbs that take a direct object (*2b*), or a strict subcategorization violation after verbs that do not take a direct object (*2c*).

(2a) The crowd was waiting eagerly. The young man grabbed the *guitar* and...[one more clause].

(2b) The crowd was waiting eagerly. The young man drank the *guitar* and...[one more clause].

(2c) The crowd was waiting eagerly. The young man slept the *guitar* and...[one more clause].

Slowed response in the vicinity of verb-argument violations indicated that DE was sensitive to verb-argument structure. The longest response was for subcategorization violation (*2c*). Tyler suggested that DE retained this lexically-driven capacity, so that difficulties with anomalous sentences in the first experiment had to be because of a problem with some other aspect of syntax.

Later, Tyler (1989) focused on anomalous sentences to see if DE could detect phrase-level structural violations (called "local" violations). A baseline condition contained a target-word in a normal phrase (*3a*). Then, word-order violations were placed in the same location as in *3b.*

(3a) An orange dream was loudly watching the house during smelling lights because within these signs /a slow *kitchen*/ snored with crashing leaves.

(3b) An orange dream was loudly watching the house during smelling lights because within these signs /slow very *kitchen*/ snored with crashing leaves.

Tyler also located the target-word early or late in the sentence; and, again, DE did not have the normal position effect (replicating the result in 1985). He also had the normal pattern of slowing down when there was a local structural violation late in the sentence. This result along with his verb-argument ability led Tyler to conclude that DE could assign structure at a local level and was, in fact, dependent on this level of syntactic processing.

Language Production

When CHI causes linguistic impairments, "anomia is the primary linguistic deficit reported" (Hartley and Levin, 1990, p. 356). Boles (1997) found that patients with traumatic brain injury and Alzheimer's disease make more visual misperception errors than stroke patients with aphasia (e.g., *can* for *drum*). In discussing misnaming, Holland (1982) argued that impaired language behavior need not be indicative of aphasia. Errors with CHI may be perceptually-based or confabulatory and, thus, may be produced by visual agnosias discussed in Chapter 6.

As with the RHD, deficit is most frequently evident in word fluency tasks. Several investigators studied CHI with a letter-fluency task (e.g., Gruen, Frankle, and Schwartz, 1990; Wertz, et al., 1986). Lohman and others (1989) found that the number of words produced per letter increased as RLA cognitive level increased from V to VII (see Table 9.5). These investigators also found substantial reductions in words produced for nine categories such as clothes, furniture, and birds. Typicality of words was unusual for only two categories, which is again consistent with the retention of fairly good semantic organization.

Another component of the Halstead-Reitan battery is the **Thurstone Word Fluency Test** developed in 1938 (see Pendleton, Heaton, Lehman, and Hulihand, 1982). In this short test, a patient is asked to produce words to a couple of letters; but the main difference from other tests is that the response is in writing. Pendleton's research team administered the test to several neurologically impaired groups, comparing effects of localized and diffuse lesions. They found that letter-fluency is disrupted by any type or location of damage. Frontal and left-hemisphere damage produced more difficulty, but the test did not discriminate frontal and diffuse lesions.

Crowe (1992) wanted to see if the different frontal lobe syndromes mentioned earlier behave differently on the FAS letter-fluency test. All groups had reduced levels of response, despite the impaired impulse control of the orbitofrontal group (mainly CHIs). The CHIs produced more uninhibited responding, such as random neologisms, than a medially damaged group consisting of a variety of neuropathologies.

Word-finding deficits may translate into information deficiencies in discourse. Ehrlich (1988) elicited picture descriptions from severe CHIs at various times post onset. A standard content analysis showed no difference from normal controls in syllables per minute and number of content units produced. However, the clinical group produced fewer content units per minute.

Glosser and Deser (1991) studied interviews with nine patients at RLA Levels V to VII. The CHIs produced paraphasias but did not produce more indefinite or generic words than normal controls. The patients made some syntactic errors and had some grammatical omissions but spoke at a normal level of syntactic complexity.

DISCOURSE

Holland (1982) suggested that "it is in the area of language pragmatics that aphasia and head injured language most vividly contrast" (p. 347). We may suspect that anterograde amnesia and either apathy or disinhibition would affect interpersonal interactions. Retrograde amnesia and dysexecutive syndrome may influence story-telling.

"Conversational problems may take the form of rambling talk that moves unpredictably from topic to topic, lack of social initiation, or lack of inhibition which may result in language that is inappropriate or offensive" (Gobble, Dunson, Szekeres, and Cornwall, 1987, p. 369).

Nicholas and Brookshire (1995) commented on the dearth of research on discourse comprehension with CHI. They gave their *Discourse Comprehension Test* to a group with traumatic brain injury and, as noted in Chapter 7, these patients performed similarly to RHDs and aphasic patients. If there is a special influence of attention deficit or other primary impairments on this level of language comprehension, asking about main ideas and details in stories does not seem to tap into it.

A few investigators, such as Carl Coelho (1995) at the University of Connecticut, have specialized in the study of CHI. Others have specialized in the study of RHD (Chapter 8). As a result, research has had broadly differing styles according to the discourse elicited and the analysis employed (Table 9.9). The study of CHI has relied less on pictures to elicit discourse and has utilized more cohesion analysis and less information analysis. A standard comprehensive strategy for assessing discourse production across clinical groups has not yet materialized. However, a broad multi-task approach was recently initiated by Snow, Douglas, and Ponsford (1995).

Microstructure

In an unpublished dissertation, Wyckoff reported that CHIs produced a deficient number of cohesive ties and had an additional problem with accuracy when telling stories (cited in Mentis and Prutting, 1987). Hartley and Levin (1990) analyzed Wyckoff's data and decided that it contained three general profiles:

- confused discourse soon after injury, containing frequent inaccuracies, repetitions, and revisions
- cohesive discourse that is accurate but sometimes wordy or inefficient
- impoverished discourse with short utterances, little cohesion, and limited content

Published studies contain different conclusions. For example, Mentis and Prutting (1987) assessed cohesion for three patients at or above RLA Level VII. Subjects made high scores on a test for aphasia, and syntax was judged to be preserved. Subjects engaged in 10 minutes of conversation with a familiar partner, described their work or rehabilitation program, and produced routines (e.g., how to play a sport or bake a cake). The subjects used fewer cohesive ties than normal controls for description and routines. Glosser and Deser (1991) found nine CHIs to be unimpaired in referential cohesion. Glosser and Deser studied lower levels of function (V-VII), limited discourse to

TABLE 9.9 Characteristics of discourse research through 1994 in 13 studies of CHI and 21 studies of RHD. Some totals are over 100% because investigators often used more than one procedure (Davis, et al., 1997).

	N	DISCOURSE TYPE	STIMULUS/TASK	ANALYSIS
CHI	13	8% description 38% narration 46% conversation	62% spontaneous 38% picture elicitation	23% information, content 54% cohesion 31% macroanalysis 31% conversational
RHD	21	33% description 57% narration 14% conversation	29% spontaneous 52% picture elicitation	48% information, content 14% cohesion 29% macroanalysis 10% conversational

interviews, and looked for ties only within the preceding three "verbalizations."

Liles, Coelho, Duffy, and Zalagens (1989) compared elicitation procedures with four CHIs at RLA Level V and above. Two stories were elicited with pictured stimuli. One story was told after viewing a 19-frame filmstrip. The other story was told about a Norman Rockwell painting that remained in view during narration. Two CHIs were deficient in cohesion, and all CHIs presented cohesive styles that differed according to condition. While viewing the Rockwell painting, CHIs decreased pronoun reference and increased lexical cohesion relative to telling stories from memory. The diminished cohesion was attributed to the requirement of translating a static representation into a dynamic series of events.

Macrostructure

Liles and others (1989) studied completeness of narrative structure with respect to the presence of an initiating event, actions, and a consequence marking the attainment of goal. Three of four subjects produced no complete episodes for telling a story from a Rockwell painting. The report did not say whether CHIs deviated from story structure in any particular way.

Two other studies compared levels of discourse. Glosser and Deser (1991) studied thematic coherence by judging topic maintenance through an entire discourse. CHIs were distinctly impaired, contrary to their good cohesion and sentence form. Deficit was described as being greater for "global" coherence than for "local" cohesion. In a study by Coelho, Liles, and Duffy (1991), two patients with CHI displayed opposite patterns of ability. One had poor cohesion but good story structure. The other had poor story structure but good cohesion.

Two patients at the RLA Level VII told the Flower Pot story quite differently (see Chapter 8). One gave the following fairly accurate version:

(4) "Looks like the guy got hit on the head with a flower pot, and he's probably swearing or something. He's gonna go up and paste the guy one. He's banging on the door, and the woman goes up, 'Oh, nice doggie.' And he's all sucked in. And he's showin her the bump on his head. She gave the dog a bone."

Technically, *the woman* has no antecedent in the narration as an instance of signaling lexical coreference. Also, the order of the last two events is reversed. However, this is a rather picky analysis of a fairly good story compared with another patient when telling the story from memory:

(5) "The apartment of the Mrs. Jones or Mr. Jones each waving his cane up her, cause he was watering the plants and fell out the window."

Snow, Douglas, and Ponsford (1997) were concerned about the selection of control groups or norms for the diagnosis of deficit. For example, should *4* be considered to be deficient? In Snow's study, 26 TBIs were compared to two groups. One was a slightly older group of orthopedic patients who were similar demographically to the head injured group. The other control was a somewhat younger group of university students considered to be demographically dissimilar from the clinical group. The TBI group differed from the students but not from the orthopedic group in productivity and content measures. The TBI group differed from both control groups with respect to a pragmatic measure (e.g., topic maintenance, situational appropriateness).

Thus, with some measures, identification of "deficit" depends on our frame of reference. Sociolinguistic variations need to be explored more before we settle on a normative basis for diagnosing discourse disorders.

Conversation

As indicated in Table 9.9, conversational interactions have been investigated much more frequently with CHIs than RHDs. Some of these interactions are bolstered by a series of planned questions, which Snow, Douglas, and Ponsford (1995) called "semi-structured conversation." In general, the studies give us more ideas on how to assess functional communication. Some clues about what to look for come from the test of everyday memory presented earlier in the chapter. Head injured patients are asked if they forget things they were just told or forget what they had just said, perhaps, repeating a recent story or joke.

Coelho and his colleagues (1993) compared five mildly aphasic patients with five CHIs at the highest RLA level in conversations on topics of the patients' choosing. Both clinical groups had difficulties initiating and sustaining conversation, and it was difficult to discern differences between them. Their communication partners had to assume more communicative burden than in control interactions between two neurologically intact partners (e.g., topic and turn initiation). The CHIs were described as especially subdued or requiring prompting to talk.

In New Zealand, psychologists examined interactions with a significant other and an opposite-sex stranger (Marsh and Knight, 1991). CHIs were more than 18 months postinjury. These clinical subjects and significant others engaged in problem-solving tasks requiring them to reach a consensus. Interaction with the stranger was conducted in the guise of a social break in which the stranger took a seat next to the patient and asked, "How has everything been going this morning?" The interactions were evaluated with the *Behaviorally Referenced Rating System of Intermediate Social Skills* (BRISS) developed by Wallander and others (1985). In the problem-solving interactions, verbal communication was hampered by word-finding problems, lack of coherence, and the use of inappropriate expressions. With the opposite-sex partners, CHIs were passive and appeared disinterested.

In Sydney, Australia, Skye McDonald investigated the pragmatic sensitivities of two cases who had been in motor vehicle accidents. She was especially interested in the influence of the disinhibition syndrome associated with frontal lobe damage. As indicated earlier in this chapter, the syndrome includes disorganization and poor impulse control or self-regulation.

In one study, McDonald (1993) isolated a component of conversation by having the two patients explain how to play a game to a naïve listener who was blindfolded. She wanted to examine the ability to meet the informational needs of a listener, and she developed ratings based on Grice's maxims of conversation (see Chapter 7). For example, the maxim of quantity states that a speaker will say no more or less than is required. Scales classified whether there was too much or too little repetitiveness and detail. Both subjects were disorganized and ineffective in the task. One was repetitive, and the other had too little detail. Cohesion was not a problem, but statements were irrelevant or badly sequenced, making instructions very confusing.

McDonald and van Sommers (1993) focused on the use of polite indirect requests. They presented various situations verbally and asked the two subjects how they would respond (e.g., asking a stranger for the time, asking to borrow a car, hinting that you want to leave a dinner party). The subjects appeared to appreciate the situations but had difficulty formulating requests indirectly. Attempts at indirect requests ended up being more impulsively direct than those of control subjects. The investigators concluded that "impaired problem-solving ability and poor behavioural control also disrupt normal social communication skills" (p. 313). Later, they had similar findings with a group of 15 patients mostly with CHI (McDonald and Pearce, 1998).

SUMMARY AND CONCLUSIONS

Cases with closed head injury can be quite different from cases with stroke. The condition of the damaged brain is quite different. Cognitive impairments can also be quite different. Furthermore, the needs of a younger population with CHI differ from an older population with stroke. CHI has direct impact on parents, brothers, and sisters, whereas stroke has direct impact on spouses and children.

Young people with CHI have deficits of attention, episodic memory, learning new information, and behavioral organization. Sometimes their personalities seem to change as they become irritable or impulsive. Some seem to be unconcerned or unmotivated. On the other hand, older adults with stroke can concentrate for long periods, remember their past, absorb new information, and structure their daily routines. They tend to maintain their pre-stroke personalities and have normal reactions to sudden disability. Many are highly motivated to improve their language abilities. Thus, CHI presents a special challenge for rehabilitative teamwork among neuropsychologists, psychologists, and speech-language pathologists.

Except for the cases in which a focal trauma causes a nearly classic aphasia, a striking difference between the effects of stroke and CHI is the level of residual or chronic language ability. People with CHI are likely to be able to retrieve words and formulate fluent sentences. Many have such mild and subtle impairments that they seem ready to return to school or work. Upon returning, some succeed but many fail because of demands that exceed their concentration or patience. Their communicative difficulties appear in the organization of discourse and in pragmatic aspects of conversation related to primary cognitive impairments.

Chapter 10

RECOVERY AND PROGNOSIS

"Marty talks for a living," Jackie Exeter thought during those first few days in the hospital when she realized Martin was safe but unable to muster more than a few words. They would have to cancel his speech in Brussels. A more important concern was that Martin talked for fun. Talking was a major part of who he was and who they were together and what they did with their friends. "Would he talk again?" "How long would it be before they would have a normal conversation?"

Besides the Exeters, payment providers have a stake in what can be expected from recovery. In this chapter, we shall explore the facts obtained from behavioral measurement in clinical research. A great deal of the information pertains to the factors that enable clinicians to make general predictions about amount of recovery and its eventual outcome. Most of the chapter is about recovery from stroke. Traumatic brain injury is discussed near the end. What happens in a patient's head, neurologically or cognitively, is a matter of speculation; and the possibilities are explored at the end of the chapter.

STROKE AND FUNCTIONAL OUTCOMES

Martin's early disorientation along with aphasia made it appear as if his entire brain was impaired. Chapter 2 explained why structurally intact regions far from the site of infarction are dysfunctional during the acute period. Rapid early improvements are the result of a subsiding diaschisis. Lifting the cloud of global confusion reveals the *sparing* of regions of the brain rather than recovery from infarction per se (Laurence and Stein, 1978).

As Martin entered the period of living with infarction, he also improved in remaining areas of impairment. It is characteristic of stroke that most patients improve regardless of whether they enter rehabilitation. This is called **spontaneous recovery.** A general impression of recovery was obtained in a longitudinal study of 92 patients with ischemic stroke (Skilbeck, Wade, Hewer, and Wood, 1983). The investigators followed functions of daily living with the Barthel Index (see Chapter 7) for two-to-three years postonset. They measured statistically significant progress during the first three months post onset. Between three and six months, improvement occurred but was not significant, and no change was measured after six months.

Health care professionals and payment providers want to know the **functional outcome** of services provided in the hospital. "Outcome" is a term that is currently used to refer broadly to the benefits of medical and clinical treatments (Mariner, 1994). Desired results are specified according to objectives, and preserving life is the desired outcome of emergency diagnosis and treatment of stroke. For long-term rehabilitation, "outcome measurement" has become the means of documenting whether functional therapeutic objectives are being attained.

One outcome indicator is a patient's discharge destination. Physicians would like to predict whether a stroke-patient will eventually be discharged to home (a good outcome) or long-term institutionalized care (a poor outcome). In one study, 172 patients were examined initially during the first two weeks after onset (Henley, Pettit, Todd-Pokropek, and Tupper, 1985).

Researchers recorded information about medical history and obtained CT scans, measures of sensory and motor functions, a rating of activities of daily living, and a couple of measures of cognitive functions. CT scan data were not predictive of discharge outcome. Predictors of independent living included attentiveness, cooperation during testing, and high scores on motor-sensory and cognitive evaluations.

The *Functional Independence Measure* (see Chapter 7) has become a common measure of functional outcome in trauma-related rehabilitation programs as well as stroke-related programs (Cook, Smith, and Truman, 1994). The FIM has also been evaluated for its predictive value. When administered six days after admission to an acute care hospital, the FIM is helpful in predicting discharge to home, a rehabilitation center, or a nursing home (Mauthe, Haaf, Hayn, and Krall, 1996). When the scales are given upon admission to a rehabilitation center, around two months after stroke, the severity level of the full-scale is suggestive of outcome after 60 days of therapy (Oczkowski and Barreca, 1993). The FIM is also predictive of "burden of care" at home, measured according to the minutes of assistance per day provided by a caregiver (Granger, Cotter, Hamilton, and Fiedler, 1993).

MEASURING RECOVERY OF LANGUAGE

Recovery of language has been documented in a variety of circumstances, including studies in which untreated patients were compared to treated patients. We find information about spontaneous recovery in this research. In one study, "patients were prevented from attending therapy by extraneous factors, such as family or transportation problems, but were willing to come back once again to the unit after six months or more in order to take the second examination" (Basso, Capitani, and Vignolo, 1979, p. 191). Elsewhere, "inclusion of a no speech therapy group was considered ethically acceptable because there was considered to be reasonable doubt whether the speech therapy service available to these patients was effective" (Lendrem and Lincoln, 1985, p. 744).

We may measure either **clinical improvement** in tasks used for clinical assessment or **functional improvement** in solving communicative problems of daily living. It has been suggested that "improvement which is not reflected in the patient's daily life is not improvement in fact" (Sarno, Sarno, and Levita, 1971, p. 74). Most investigators have measured clinical language behavior with the *Porch Index of Communicative Ability* (e.g., Lendrem and Lincoln, 1985) or the *Western Aphasia Battery* (e.g, Kertesz and McCabe, 1977; Pashek and Holland, 1988).

It would be good to remind ourselves of the scores associated with these tests (see Chapter 3). The following sections introduce the fundamental components of recovery. Most data is from clinical measures taken from patients in rehabilitation programs, but studies of spontaneous recovery are given special mention. The reader will discover that *variability* is a central theme. It would be inappropriate to rely on any single study to support one opinion or another about recovery from aphasia.

Proportion of Patients that Improve

What is the likelihood that language ability improves at all after stroke? In early studies, only about 50 percent of patients made recognizable improvement according to general rating scales or vaguely reported testing methods (Basso, Capitani, and Vignolo, 1979; Godfrey and Douglass, 1959; Marks, Taylor, and Rusk, 1957). Then, according to PICA measurement, 90 percent of untreated patients were found to improve over the first 10 weeks postonset (Lendrem and Lincoln, 1985). The proportion dropped to 79 percent between 10 and 22 weeks. Thus, standardized and reliable measurement has painted a more hopeful picture than cautious clinical judgments.

Amount

Reliable measurement enables us to quantify progress instead of relying on subjective judgment. Amount of improvement is determined by subtracting an earlier test score (i.e., pre-test) from a later score (i.e., post-test). The result is a "difference-score" or "change-score." Change scores have been reported for a variety of intervals between the first and second test.

In studies of recovery, *initial scores* have been obtained at different times postonset. Sarno and Levita (1971) obtained functional ratings on 28 patients at bedside within two days postonset, when some had "a total lack of responsiveness and, quite probably, total absence of consciousness" (p. 177). Other investigators obtained a few initial scores between four and nineteen days postonset (Bamber, 1980; Hanson and Cicciarelli, 1978). In another study, the first test was conducted at discharge from acute care with a median stay of 20 days (Holland, Greenhouse, Fromm, and Swindell, 1989). When the initial score is obtained early in the acute phase, the change-score will include the fading of diaschisis.

Researchers often prefer to wait until the medical condition stabilizes and pattern of language deficit is apparent before giving the first comprehensive test. Therefore, the first score may be obtained around one month after onset (e.g., Deal and Deal, 1978; Wertz, Collins, Weiss, et al., 1981), sometimes depending on the time of admission to a rehabilitation center (Pickersgill and Lincoln, 1983).

In studies of spontaneous recovery, the *final score* may not always be obtained at the point of maximum recovery. Investigators tend to give the final test at three or four months postonset, thus, possibly not detecting all the progress that might have been made (e.g., Kertesz and McCabe, 1977). Lendrem and Lincoln (1985) re-tested at 6-week intervals beginning at 10 weeks postonset and concluding at around eight months. Deal and Deal (1978) reported on progress for an interval of one to 12 months.

In studies of patients in rehabilitation, the final test is often given around one year postonset (e.g., Wertz, et al., 1981). Also, change-scores may be based on final scores at termination of treatment (Deal and Deal, 1978) or *peak scores* achieved before treatment is terminated (Bamber, 1980; Hanson and Cicciarelli, 1978). Thus, investigators have reported end-points tied to slightly different clinical circumstances, such as a decision to end treatment as opposed to the continuation of treatment.

The most consistent fact arising out of this inconsistent research is that aphasic patients are widely variable in amount of recovery. This is a central clinical problem, making prediction seem to be impossible. In one study of mostly untreated subjects, the WAB's Aphasia Quotient (AQ) progressed an average of 16.64 percentage points (Kertesz and McCabe, 1977). Yet, one subgroup improved 5.16 points; and another, 36.80 points. The PICA has yielded ranges of spontaneous progress of 0.34 to 2.72 (Deal and Deal, 1978) and –0.49 to 5.18 overall response level points (Lendrem and Lincoln, 1985). Therefore, a group mean is not indicative of individual progress.

Treated aphasic patients display similar variability. Three small-sample studies had remarkable agreement in average amount of change measured with the PICA over the first year postonset (Table 10.1). Just looking at change scores, we may be tempted to inform the Exeters that Martin is likely to improve around 3.30 points in the first year. Unfortunately, we cannot promise this improvement for anyone. A treated aphasic

TABLE 10.1 Amount and Variability of Change in PICA Overall Scores in Three Studies of Mixed Aphasic Groups.

	N	INITIAL	FINAL	CHANGE	RANGE
Hanson and Cicciarelli (1978)	13	9.48	12.72	3.24	0.98–4.29
Deal and Deal (1978)	17	9.14	12.52	3.38	0.51–7.16
Bamber (1980)	13	8.40	11.65	3.25	0.10–6.18

client may improve between 0.10 to 7.16 response level points.

A final comment has to do with how we interpret a change-score. Researchers speak of "significant progress" with respect to an objective statistical analysis. In Lendrem and Lincoln's (1985) repeated administrations of the PICA, spontaneous progress did not become statistically significant until five months postonset. Some clinical researchers distinguish between *statistical significance* and *clinical significance* of recovery data. With a large experimental group, a small change-score may be statistically significant; but it may not represent a meaningful change in a patient's life. For an individual patient, a small change may be clinically significant depending on what it represents functionally (e.g., progress in answering yes-no questions amidst a battery of tests).

Final Outcome

What will an aphasic person be like at the end of recovery? The aforementioned final or peak scores are a numerical indication of level of language ability that can be attained around a year after stroke. In research, the end of recovery is usually demonstrated with a series of measures showing a **plateau** of slightly variable scores. These scores indicate that the final linguistic outcome usually falls short of normal function.

In their study of spontaneous recovery over four months postonset, Kertesz and McCabe (1977) reported that one-fifth of 93 subjects attained levels above the cut-off AQ of 93.8 on the WAB. Twenty percent of this group had hemorrhages and traumatic injuries. Later, Kertesz (1985) categorized outcomes of mostly untreated patients with AQs taken at an average of two years postonset. He placed 27 percent in the excellent category (75–100 AQ); 24 percent were good (50–75); 24 percent were fair (25–50); and 25 percent ended up in the poor category (0–25).

The final scores in Table 10.1 are indicative of average PICA overall outcomes for thromboembolic patients in treatment until a year postonset. However, outcomes ranged from 8.69 to 14.88 across the three studies. Thus, many were far from a neurologically intact group that scored between 13.40 and 14.99 overall (Duffy, et al., 1976). About one-third of the aphasic subjects represented by the table reached into the "normal" range. The highest levels after a year were auditory comprehension and word repetition, which were around or above 14.50. Verbal subtests averaged 12.52, while describing the function of objects lagged behind at 10.87 (Hanson and Cicciarelli, 1978).

Aphasic patients do not return to normal function, because the loss of brain cells is permanent. These cells do not grow back. This difficult reality restrains recovery. To the extent that "recovery" implies a cure, there is an uneasiness over the use of this term. Some clinicians prefer to speak of "progress" or "improvement," instead of recovery. The Exeters probably did not want to overhear us quibbling over terminology. In this chapter, all three terms are used somewhat interchangeably because "recovery" has a common usage with a mutual understanding of the constraints upon it.

Saying that a patient might improve 3.30 points or end up with a 12.00 on the PICA does not say much about the *quality of life* that can be achieved. Schuell and her colleagues (1964) documented the number of patients that returned to school, entered vocational training, or re-entered employment. In her youngest group with "simple aphasia," 14 percent entered school or vocational training while 19 percent resumed employment. In a group with a diagnosis similar to Broca's aphasia, 33 percent entered vocational training and 27 percent found employment. Schuell explained that the less impaired aphasic clients had more difficulty accepting employment that was less demanding than their previous jobs. The more successful group seemed more determined to improve and to adjust realistically to deficit. Among the most impaired groups, no one entered vocational training or became employed.

Rate

Although final outcome varies, we may still wonder how long it takes to get there. Payment providers are particularly interested in the length of time that progress can be expected. It is one thing to say that a patient may improve 3.30 points, and it is another thing to say that it will take four months or four years. Our information comes from research that has regularly employed certain time-frames, namely, from onset to 3 months, 3 to 6 months, 6 to 12 months, and beyond 12 months. Most data comes from the first twelve months.

The distinction between final and peak test scores is worth reconsidering with respect to investigations that address rate of recovery. A final score may be based on a decision to terminate treatment that was independent of what actually happened in recovery per se. A peak may be reached any time along a plateau, sometimes after recovery has ceased. Thus, a final score may underestimate and a peak score may overestimate the time that recovery stops.

In the study by Skilbeck and others (1983), the Barthel Index was supplemented with Sarno's FCP to measure recovery of communicative skills by subjects with LHD. Significant progress occurred across the first three months with gradual but nonsignificant improvement thereafter, extending beyond the 6-month plateau recorded with the Barthel Index. The researchers had the impression that no improvement occurred after one year.

One of the most consistent findings is that progress is more rapid in the first two or three months postonset than in any period thereafter. This recovery curve is illustrated in Figure 10.1. Lendrem and Lincoln (1985) found statistically significant progress between 4 and 22 weeks (1 to 5.5 months). A comparison of 10 weeks to 34 weeks yielded change that was not significant. The shape of this curve applies to both spontaneous recovery and progress during rehabilitation. For one group of aphasic patients receiving language treatment until 11 months postonset, 65 percent of their progress occurred within the first four months (Wertz, et al., 1981).

Duration of spontaneous recovery has been an important consideration with respect to determining the efficacy of treatment. For patients in a rehabilitation program, clinicians are tempted to conclude that progress can be attributed to a treatment when the improvement is observed after spontaneous recovery is assumed to have run its course. Since a study by Butfield and Zangwill (1946), the belief has been that spontaneous recovery lasts around six months, so that it is safe to say that any progress afterward is caused by therapeutic intervention. However, this belief has been difficult to substantiate because of the reluctance to withhold treatment for more than three or four months postonset.

Kertesz and McCabe (1977) discovered spontaneous progress after six months. Wernicke's aphasia showed substantial gains between six and twelve months. Also, recovery in terms of overall function may mask progress that continues for specific functions (e.g., Hagen, 1973). With statistical analysis of change-scores, the magnitude of difference is a function of the interval between measures. An amount of progress achieved in three months may be achieved again over the next eighteen months.

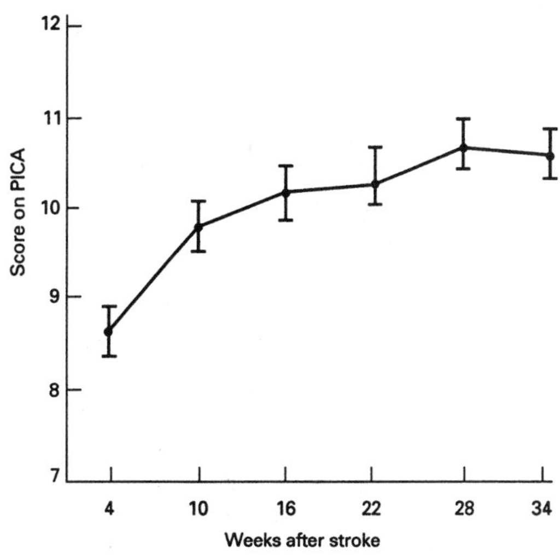

FIGURE 10.1 Progression of means and standard errors for overall PICA response levels by 41 patients.

Reprinted by permission from Lendrem, W. & Lincoln, N. B., Spontaneous recovery of language in patients with aphasia between 4 and 34 weeks after stroke. *Journal of Neurology, Neurosurgery, and Psychiatry,* 48, 1985, p. 747. British Medical Association, publisher.

Rate of recovery is also highly variable among individual patients. In studies of treated patients, one took over seven months to improve 4.01 points overall on the PICA, whereas another took about eight months to improve only 0.98 points (Bamber, 1980; Hanson and Cicciarelli, 1978). Also, duration of recovery may be quite different between patients improving the same amount. Two patients improved almost 3.00 points but took about four and nineteen months to do so. Two others, who improved 4.84 and 5.22 points, took 7.7 and 30.4 months, respectively.

Substantial progress has been found in some cases receiving treatment well beyond the first year (e.g., Broida, 1977; Sands, Sarno, and Shankweiler, 1969). A group of 35 patients with infarcts, hemorrhages, and one trauma were given the PICA at 3, 6, 12, 24, 36, and 55 months postonset (Hanson, Metter, and Riege, 1989). These patients were receiving varied amounts of individual treatment until 24 months and mostly group treatment after 24 months. Many patients showed steady and substantial improvement in the overall score until 24 months. After this point, patients either held steady or declined. Those that declined tended to have the mildest aphasias, and contributing factors included declining health and depression.

Pattern

An overall measure is less informative than attending to specific communicative functions. An overall measure may also be misleading. A patient may progress substantially in one function while regressing in another, but this result would balance out in an overall score. Just as a subject-group mean may not reflect individual scores, a patient's overall change-score may not be indicative of individual test or skill changes. Most comparisons in the research have been between auditory comprehension and oral expression. Auditory scores on the PICA end up being better than the verbal scores, reflecting their relationship at the beginning.

Spontaneous recovery for the four months postonset was differentiated according to eight subtests of the WAB (Lomas and Kertesz, 1978). The observations included two auditory comprehension tasks, one repetition test, and five expressive tasks mainly requiring word retrieval. The investigators concluded that comprehension fares better than verbal expression in early spontaneous recovery. Auditory comprehension has had a better outlook for treated patients, as well (Basso, et al., 1979; Kenin and Swisher, 1972; Prins, Snow, and Wagenaar, 1978).

Following recovery to its peak with the PICA, Hanson and Cicciarelli (1978) found a different pattern. Verbal functions improved more than auditory functions. However, auditory functions reached their peaks sooner than expressive functions (i.e., around 5.5 months vs. over 8 months). Amount of progress in auditory functions may be smaller, because this initially less impaired function reaches a test's ceiling. Standard tests may keep us from observing further progress. Also, when a patient is followed long enough, verbal expression may overtake auditory functions in amount of progress but not in the final outcome.

Another approach to following the changing pattern of aphasia is through the WAB's filter of syndrome diagnosis. Kertesz and McCabe (1977) recorded "transformation from one clinically distinct group to another as defined by the subscores on subsequent examinations" (p. 15). Thirty-three percent ended up with a syndrome that differed from the initial diagnosis. "Broca's, conduction, and Wernicke's aphasics usually become anomic aphasics when recovery reaches a plateau" (Kertesz, 1979, p. 99).

In Pashek and Holland's (1988) study, evolution of aphasia took two paths. One was a rapid day-to-day fluctuation, sometimes back and forth between syndromes during acute hospitalization. The other path was gradual over weeks or months. Fluent aphasias rarely evolved to nonfluent aphasias.

In a retrospective study, researchers found records of patients who had at least two WABs within the first two months poststroke (McDermott, Horner, and DeLong, 1996). Those who changed syndromes progressed a significantly greater amount than those who did not change syndromes, indicating that good recovery pushes a patient through different patterns of impairment.

APPROACHES TO PROGNOSIS

The documentation of amount, rate, and final outcome of recovery demonstrated that it is nearly impossible to predict the long-range future based on an early and general diagnosis of aphasia. We must identify more specific factors that are related in some way to whether a patient does or does not get much better.

Porch, Collins, Wertz, and Friden (1980) identified three strategies of prediction:

- **behavioral profile approach** which involves "evaluating the aphasic patient with a variety of listening, reading, speaking, and writing tasks; constructing a profile of his performance; and comparing this profile with the change made by previous patients with a similar profile" (p. 313);
- **statistical prediction** or the use of early test scores to predict subsequent test scores, perhaps, with a mathematical formula;
- **prognostic variable approach** in which we compare "a patient's biographical, medical, and behavioral characteristics against how these variables are believed to influence change in aphasia" (p. 312).

The behavioral profile approach, employed by Schuell and others (1964), is not used often except for the extent to which initial syndrome diagnosis is known to imply a pattern of recovery. The goal of statistical prediction is implied in any attempt to relate an initial test score to later scores, such as studies of the FIM (e.g., Oczkowski and Barreca, 1993). This goal was thought to have been achieved with the PICA for aphasic patients (e.g., Porch, 1981; Wertz, Deal, and Deal, 1980). The most common clinical strategy, however, is the prognostic variable approach.

Rational use of prognostic variables depends on a body of investigations into factors that are thought to be predictive of recovery. A "real factor," such as size of lesion, is one that has a direct influence on the recovery process. Other factors, such as the timing of initial test, may be useful predictors but do not influence recovery per se.

Prognostic indicators fall into two other broad categories (Table 10.2). *Endogenous factors* are attributes that a patient brings to rehabilitation. The clinician can do nothing about many of these factors (e.g., size of lesion, age). *Exogenous factors* are external to patients and are often a function of clinical decisions or circumstances. Timing of initial evaluation is a predictor that depends on when treatment is initiated or when a referral is made.

We try as soon as possible to predict whether a patient's prospects are at least favorable or unfavorable. First, we gather pertinent information regarding medical history, neurological diagnosis, and initial test results. The collective impact of the factors is estimated, and prediction is framed in general terms. So far, we are not able to compute a numerical prediction without the risk of being misleading. Perhaps, the most striking development in the past 15 years has been the investigation of brain imaging for providing concrete clues to a patient's future. What we know about the main factors is presented in the following sections.

TABLE 10.2 Many of the factors studied as to whether they have a relationship to recovery from stroke.

ENDOGENOUS		EXOGENOUS
Neurological	*Functional*	
size of lesion	severity of deficit	timing of initial test language treatment
site of lesion	syndrome	
age	motivation	
gender		
race		
handedness		

TYPE OF STROKE

The gradual recovery described so far is mainly characteristic of thromboembolic cases. Hemorrhage is likely to have different outcomes because the hematoma "displaces the fibre bundles without completely destroying them" (Basso, 1992, p. 340). Hemorrhage appears to produce alternating periods of progress and plateau; and recovery may not begin for months following a small intracerebral hemorrhage (Rubens, 1977a). In Kertesz and McCabe's (1977) study of spontaneous recovery, some patients with hemorrhage had large and rapid recovery, whereas others had little or no recovery.

Two other studies showed better recovery with hemorrhage than ischemic stroke. Holland and others (1989) gave the WAB at discharge and at one and two months postdischarge. Type of stroke had a moderate influence on progress during this period, with hemorrhage being more favorable than infarction. Basso (1992) reported on a comparison of 46 patients with intracerebral hemorrhage and 101 patients with infarctions. These patients were examined less than six months postonset and then 6 months later. More patients with hemorrhage had substantial recovery. The most significant progress occurred in reading and writing.

Nagata and others (1986) studied neurological factors in recovery, especially by measuring cerebral blood flow during a period beginning at two-to-four weeks postonset and concluding at least three months after onset. In a group with infarction, blood flow gradually improved and was correlated with recovery. Among patients with hemorrhage, blood flow was highly variable and was not related to recovery. Their explanation pointed to the instability of compression by a hematoma on adjacent brain tissue.

SEVERITY OF IMPAIRMENT

For infarction, **severity of brain damage** need no longer be estimated from behavioral examination. CT scans permit a physician to look at the damage relatively soon after a stroke. The hope has been that characteristics of the lesion would provide a concrete aid in predicting a patient's linguistic outcome. In general, larger lesions are related to less recovery, which is most evident when comparing very large and very small lesions (Goldenberg and Spatt, 1994; Kertesz, Harlock, and Coates, 1979; Knopman, Selnes, Niccum, and Rubens, 1984; Mazzoni, Vista, Pardossi, Avila, Bianchi, and Moretti, 1992).

Naeser and her colleagues (1998) examined 12 aphasic patients one year and then 5 to 12 years poststroke. They found that lesion borders had expanded over this period of time. The reason for this slight but statistically significant increase in lesion size is not understood. The possibilities include degeneration of adjacent cells, a hypoperfusion creating the appearance of degeneration, or problems in other small arteries (although no patient had been diagnosed with a second stroke). Curiously, Naeser also found significant progress in naming and phrase length in patients with nonfluent speech. Evidently the gradual expansion of lesion borders had no negative effect on the patients' language behavior.

Speech-language pathologists suspect that **severity of dysfunction** can be predictive of recovery. The general belief has been that "there is a negative correlation between severity of aphasia in the early recovery period and the amount of improvement which occurs during the recovery process whether or not speech therapy is given" (Sands, et al., 1969, p. 204). That is, the more severe the impairment before one month postonset, the smaller the change-score. However, there are some exceptions around the edges of this generalization.

In a couple of studies, initial severity of overall language impairment around one month after onset was unexpectedly correlated in a positive direction with amount of recovery by patients with thromboembolic stroke (Bamber, 1980; Hanson and Cicciarelli, 1978). That is, patients with the most severe disorders tended to change the most. However, the lowest initial PICA overall scores in both studies were 5.85 and 6.63. Inclusion of more severely impaired patients may have left a different impression. Also, aphasic subjects with mild impairment had small amounts of recovery because of the ceiling effect built into the test.

The value of severity of deficit as a predictor may depend on when the first test is administered. Wallesch, Bak, and Schulte-Mönting (1992) found the first two weeks to be an unstable platform from which to predict recovery. Severely impaired patients were unpredictable, which was one reason for delaying a prognosis for Martin Exeter until the end of the acute period. On the other hand, Mazzoni and others (1992) found that distinguishing severe from moderate impairment at 15 days postonset was related to spontaneous recovery over the subsequent six month period. It is possible that the platform begins to become more stable at the end of the first two weeks.

Lomas and Kertesz (1978) studied spontaneous recovery with 31 aphasic subjects divided into four groups based on initial levels of comprehension and verbal fluency. These groups were tested within one month postonset and were re-tested two and one-half to four months later. Relative amounts of progress are shown in Figure 10.2. The low-fluency/high-comprehending group made the most progress. The low-fluency/low-comprehending (i.e., "global aphasia") made the least progress. The two high-fluency groups (i.e., "posterior aphasias") made moderate amounts of progress. Pattern of improvement varied among these groups. Patients with low comprehension improved mainly in receptive functions, whereas those with high comprehension improved receptively and expressively. No group improved in word fluency in the early months postonset.

Initial severity of auditory comprehension deficit appears to be a factor. In a study by Gaddie and others (1989), high-comprehending subjects made much more recovery of *expressive* language than low-comprehending subjects. However, initial severity of comprehension deficit may not be predictive of recovery of *comprehension* with severe aphasia. Also, good initial word comprehension is predictive of good recovery in naming (Knopman, et al., 1984).

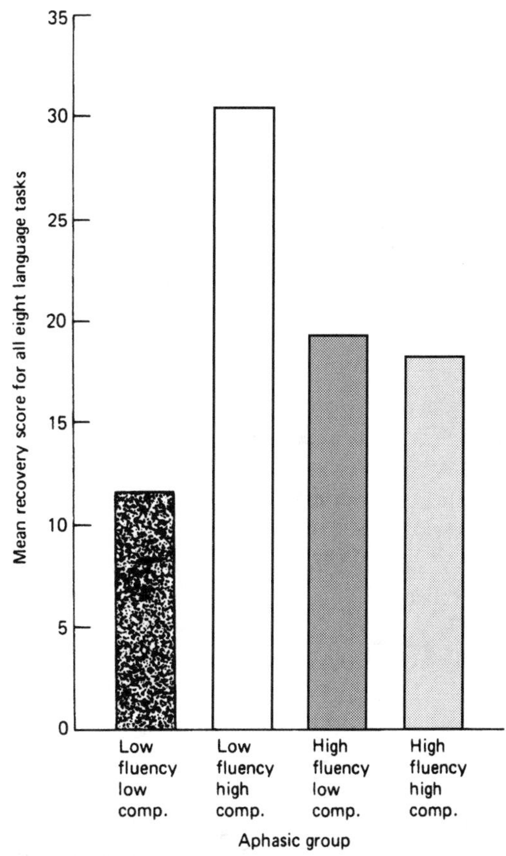

FIGURE 10.2 The overall amount of spontaneous language recovery differs among groups defined according to level of comprehension and fluency. These amounts are from the first four months after onset.

Adapted by permission from Lomas, J., and Kertesz, A., Patterns of spontaneous recovery in aphasic groups: A study of adult stroke patients. *Brain and Language,* 5, 388–401, 1978.

TYPE OF IMPAIRMENT

Site of lesion and type of aphasia are interrelated factors. Syndrome has been studied according to the general distinction between nonfluent and fluent disorders or according to specific syndromes. Investigators have found that size and location of lesion may be prognostic indicators with respect to particular syndromes.

Site of Lesion

Site of lesion in the left hemisphere has a pronounced effect depending on whether it is in the primary language zone around the Sylvian fissure or in the borderline areas encircling the primary language zone. The latter tends to cause transcortical aphasias. Recovery occurred more often in patients with penetrating trauma in marginal zones than in those with perisylvian damage, and several with marginal damage made rapid and complete recovery (Luria, 1970b). Rapid and near-total recovery of transcortical aphasias has been observed by Rubens (1977a) and Kertesz and McCabe (1977).

Deficits caused by **subcortical lesion** recover differently from those caused by cortical stroke. Using SPECT to measure hypoperfusion to other regions of the brain, Vallar and others (1998) found that improvement of blood flow is related to the best recovery. In distinguishing between thalamic and nonthalamic sites of damage (see Chapter 2), we should again be cautious in thinking about aphasic-like symptoms because of the possibility that some of the language deficits are not genuine aphasias.

With thalamic hemorrhage, aphasic symptoms disappeared completely by the end of the second month (Rubens, 1977a). Patients in Kirk and Kertesz' (1994) study were retested with the WAB at 3, 6, and 12 months. Several patients with predominantly thalamic infarcts recovered completely or dramatically by 3 months postonset. One patient with symptoms of Wernicke's aphasia did not improve much, and one with early diagnosis of global aphasia was much improved in comprehension and repetition by the 6-month measure.

Kennedy and Murdoch (1991) assessed four cases with nonthalamic or capsulostriatal hemorrhage at 3, 6, and 12 months postonset. Each case had some aphasic symptoms at 3 months, but two of these cases had AQs above the 93.8 cut-off for language deficit in most of their assessments over time. Regarding cases in Kirk and Kertesz' study, those diagnosed with anomic aphasia either recovered completely by 3 months or were still mildly anomic. Symptoms of global aphasia occurred with lesions extending into white matter posterior to the capsulostriatal region, and symptoms persisted for several months. The investigators concluded that subcortical language deficits generally resolve dramatically over time.

Broad Classification of Dysfunction

Dividing aphasic patients according to dichotomies has produced inconsistent results. Patients with expressive or nonfluent aphasia have been found to make more progress than receptive or fluent aphasias (Butfield and Zangwill, 1946; Godfrey and Douglass, 1959; Marks, et al., 1979; Wertz, Kitselman, and Deal, 1981). In other studies, nonfluent and fluent aphasias did not differ (McDermott, et al., 1996; Prins, Snow, and Wagenaar, 1978; Sarno and Levita, 1979). In the study by Mazzoni and others (1992), however, nonfluent aphasias had less progress in verbal expression and in reading and writing than fluent aphasias. The dichotomy may be too broad for meaningful study of recovery, especially when researchers are so varied in selecting patients in each of these categories. In turn, fluency diagnosis may be too general to be of assistance for prognosis.

Research focuses increasingly on the major syndromes. In Kertesz and McCabe's (1977) study of spontaneous recovery, data within each group represented varying time intervals after onset, and some subjects were followed much longer than others. Starting at a mean AQ of 85.5, anomic aphasia was similar to global aphasia in having the smallest amounts and slowest rates of progress. Lendrem and Lincoln (1985) compared four syndromes with the PICA overall score. Pashek and Holland (1988) followed short conversations throughout acute hospitalization; and then, starting at one-month, the WAB was administered regularly until 7–12 months poststroke.

Global or Severe Aphasia

We are especially concerned about prospects for patients with chronically global or severe aphasia. Holland, Swindell, and Forbes (1985) followed patients who presented with global aphasia upon admission to the hospital. Short conversations were recorded daily during acute care, and the WAB was given at regular intervals until a year poststroke. Some cases evolved to other forms of aphasia by the time of acute hospital discharge, whereas others remained globally aphasic for months. A sign of whether a patient might remain globally aphasic was whether verbal expression changed rapidly in the conversations. Those with chronic global aphasia exhibited minimal or no change during hospitalization.

In Kertesz and McCabe's study of patients who were not receiving language treatment, global aphasias changed by an average AQ of 5.16 in contrast to a nearly 37-point improvement by nonfluents with Broca's aphasia. When 13 patients with global aphasia were diagnosed within the first 30 days, four remained global and seven evolved to Broca's aphasia within the next two or three months (McDermott, et al., 1996).

Pockets of progress in specific functions can occur. During early spontaneous recovery, low-comprehending patients improved in comprehension but not expression (Lomas and Kertesz, 1978). Within one year postonset, seven severely impaired patients receiving treatment made significant gains in auditory language comprehension and gesturing; and most of this progress occurred between six and twelve months postonset (Sarno and Levita, 1981).

Size and site of lesion can vary. Using CT scans, Ferro (1992) found five types of lesion that caused global aphasia in the first month poststroke:

- Type 1: large middle cerebral artery infarction encompassing anterior and posterior regions
- Type 2: anterior infarction with variable damage to underlying deep nuclei and white fiber tracts
- Type 3: subcortical infarction
- Type 4: parietal infarction involving supramarginal and angular gyri
- Type 5: simultaneous infarctions in frontal and temporoparietal regions

Based on a comprehensive aphasia battery, the subcortical group (Type 3) had the best prognosis. Some cases with circumscribed anterior (Type 2) or subcortical lesions (Type 3) "recovered completely" after six months (see also Kirk and Kertesz, 1994). Good progress could be characterized as improving to a Broca's or transcortical aphasia, which is consistent with Kertesz and McCabe's observation of global aphasia. Prognosis was very poor, however, for patients with large Type 1 infarctions.

Naeser (1994) reported on her team's retrospective study of global aphasia in which the first clinical test was given between one and four months poststroke, and a second test was given over a year later. She separated cases into two groups. In one group, cases had a cortical and subcortical lesion across frontal, parietal, and temporal lobes. The other group was the same except for an absence of damage to Wernicke's area. This group had a significantly greater recovery of word comprehension, but there were no differences between the groups in measures of language production.

Brookshire's (1997) review of early studies of global aphasia led him to conclude that "the presence of global aphasia at 1 month post onset is an ominous prognostic sign" (p. 247). However, preliminary research indicates that progress is possible in some cases. The problem lies in identifying the cases that are mostly likely to improve. Positive indicators are lesions that are mainly subcortical, the absence of damage to Wernicke's area in the temporal lobe, and probably a corresponding early improvement in auditory comprehension.

Wernicke's Aphasia

Wernicke's aphasia is also a severe impairment but with fluent verbal production. These patients displayed a bimodal distribution of recovery in Kertsz and McCabe's study. Some improved little. Others improved by at least 20 AQ points. Four of 13 ended up in the anomic category according to WAB profiling. Patients with higher initial test scores and less jargon did better than others. Lendrem and Lincoln found that Wernicke subjects had poorer outcomes at eight months than the other syndromes. Frequently flat lines of recovery are displayed in Figure 10.3.

Kertesz and others (1993) wanted to determine if lesion size and location would be predictive of recovery in 22 cases of Wernicke's aphasia diagnosed between 14 and 45 days poststroke. Patients were grouped according to whether they had good, moderate, or poor recovery after one year. Poor recovery was related to damage extending beyond Wernicke's area to the supramarginal and angular gyri bordering the parietal lobe. Good recovery to high AQ scores was associated with small lesions sparing much of the superior and middle temporal gyri.

Naeser (1994) reported results of a similar strategy in which patients with Wernicke's aphasia were classified at six months as having good or poor recovery. Differing from Kertesz, Naeser could not find a relationship between recovery and damage to the parietal lobe. However, there was a distinct relationship to the amount of damage to Wernicke's area. All patients with good recovery had damage in half or less than half of Wernicke's area, whereas all poorly recovered cases had larger lesions.

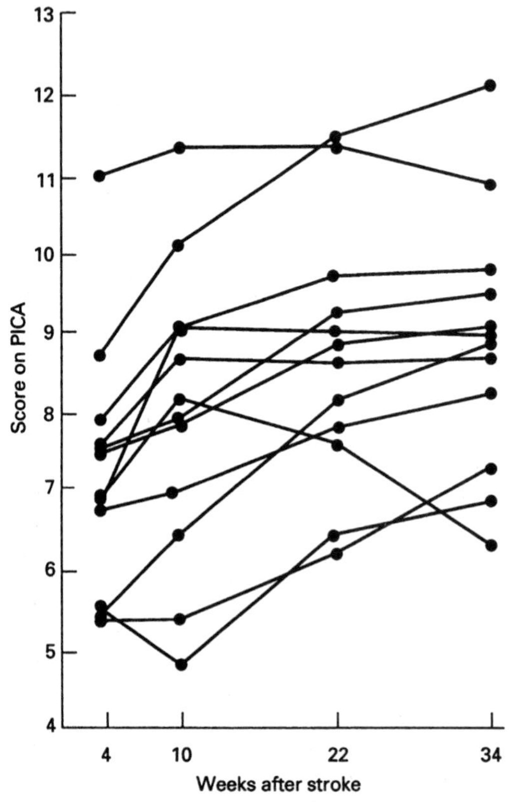

FIGURE 10.3 Spontaneous recovery of persons with Wernicke's aphasia.

Reprinted by permission from Lendrem, W. & Lincoln, N. B., Spontaneous recovery of language in patients with aphasia between 4 and 34 weeks after stroke. *Journal of Neurology, Neurosurgery, and Psychiatry,* 48, 1985, p. 746. British Medical Association, publisher.

Broca's Aphasia

In Kertesz and McCabe's study, four patients with Broca's aphasia had spontaneous improvement averaging 36.8 AQ points. Compared to the others, this syndrome had the greatest amount of recovery and had varied outcomes of fair, good, and excellent. Figure 10.4 shows the variability of PICA overall scores over eight months postonset. With respect to early evolution, patients with Broca's aphasia either remain in the same category or progress to a milder more fluent form (McDermott, et al., 1996).

Naeser (1994) reported on a comparison between a small group with Broca's aphasia and others with more severe expressive deficit of either no speech or mainly stereotyped words or phrases. No single lesion site could discriminate between these groups. However, cases with

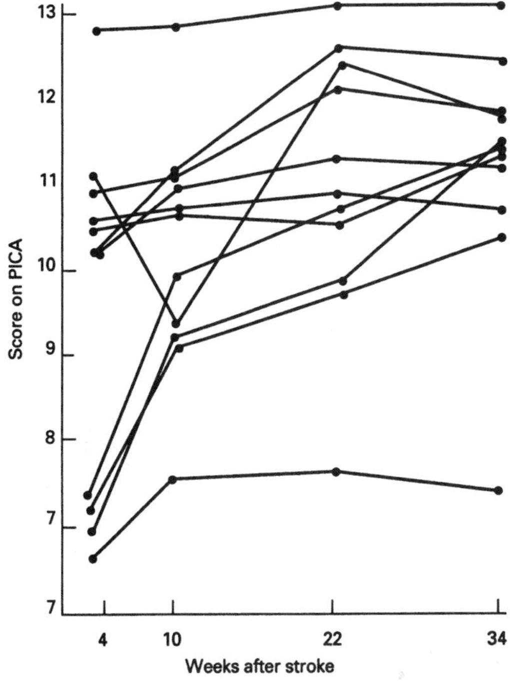

FIGURE 10.4 Spontaneous recovery of persons with Broca's aphasia.

Reprinted by permission from Lendrem, W. & Lincoln, N. B., Spontaneous recovery of language in patients with aphasia between 4 and 34 weeks after stroke. *Journal of Neurology, Neurosurgery, and Psychiatry,* 48, 1985, p. 745. British Medical Association, publisher.

Broca's aphasia had less damage in two subcortical areas.

Conduction Aphasia

Conduction aphasia has been judged to be between Broca's and anomic aphasias in overall severity of language impairment. Patients seem to remain in a milder form of conduction aphasia or follow the fluent route to anomic aphasia, sometimes within the first three months (McDermott, et al., 1996; Pashek and Holland, 1988). In Kertesz and McCabe's (1977) study, conduction aphasia had an amount of recovery comparable to Broca's aphasia and reached nearly maximum AQs in some cases. Most anomic, conduction, and transcortical aphasias had excellent outcomes; and many rose above 93.8 for the AQ.

One case was followed by Gandour and others (1991) for six months after onset. BH developed conduction aphasia after a second stroke. He could follow simple commands and produced fluent utterances with occasional paraphasias. However, when asked to repeat *No ifs, ands or buts,* he said "sucklent incadiblems." BH evolved from a "reproduction" form of conduction aphasia (i.e., reading aloud as impaired as repetition) to a "repetition" form (i.e., reading aloud resolved). Chronic short-term memory impairment was indicated by improvement in Part V of the Token Test but not in Parts III and IV. Phonemic paraphasias were rare one month poststroke and were nonexistent five months later.

OTHER FACTORS

Several other factors have been studied extensively or have been suspected to be prognostic based on common sense or theories of functional organization of the brain.

Age at Onset

Chronological age per se may be more of a predictor than a real factor. Kimmel (1974) wrote that "when we find age changes or age differences, it is important to keep in mind that these findings only point to changes that occur with age but do not indicate the possible causes of these changes" (p. 33; see Tompkins, Jackson, and Schulz, 1990). Growing older is accompanied by changes in biological function, susceptibility to disease, and cognitive and social changes.

The experimental support for a patient's age as predictor has been mixed. Correlations between age and recovery were not significant in several studies (e.g., Basso, et al., 1979; Keenan and Brassell, 1974; Kertesz and McCabe, 1977; Sarno, 1981; Sarno and Levita, 1970). Yet, Sands and others (1969) called age "the most potent variable influencing recovery," because five subjects making the most change averaged 47 years of age and five making the least change averaged 61 years. Holland and others (1989) found age to be a strong predictor over two or three months postonset. McDermott and others (1996) found patients younger than 65 making more progress than patients above 65. A similar result occurred with respect to age 70 (Pashek and Holland, 1988).

In sum, Pashek and Holland warned that age by itself is a precarious predictor, and older patients may differ according to whether they have dementia and other pathologies. Basso (1992) concluded that age "is not a very important factor in recovery." We may contemplate age as a favorable or unfavorable indicator with respect to extremes, especially when youthful middle age or older adulthood is accompanied by medical or motivational conditions that create a positive or negative climate for therapeutic success.

Gender

Gender is considered because of the possibility that men and women differ in distribution of cognitive functions between the hemispheres (e.g., Moir and Jessel, 1991). The suspicion has been that verbal and nonverbal capacities are more evenly distributed in women, whereas men have the more familiar asymmetric division of labor. However, a great deal of data supporting this idea is indirect, based on comparisons between verbal and nonverbal tasks thought to be related to one hemisphere or the other. If the difference is true, women should have a more favorable prognosis because the RH already has more linguistic capability. This issue has been difficult to address because of the amount of research done in male-dominated veterans' hospitals.

Gender was found not to be a factor in several studies (e.g., Kertesz and McCabe, 1977; Lendrem and Lincoln, 1985; Sarno, Buonaguro, and Levita, 1985; Sarno and Levita, 1971). However, it was a factor in the predicted direction in a few other studies. In a study of nearly 400 patients, females did improve more than males in spoken language but not auditory comprehension (Basso, Capitani, and Moraschini, 1982). In cases of severe aphasia, women had more improvement than men in auditory comprehension (Pizzamiglio, Mammucari, and Razzano, 1985). More research needs to be done before we can trust this factor.

Handedness

Handedness or overall *laterality* of motor functions are commonly assessed by clinical neuropsychologists. For reasons similar to gender, handedness could be a clue to recovery because of evidence that left-handed people have more bilateral representation of language in the brain than right-handers (Springer and Deutsch, 1998). However, these differences apply to half of left-handers at the most. The factor is of particular interest with respect to right- and left-handed people getting aphasia after damage to the left hemisphere.

Data on this question is scarce, partly because left-handers are relatively rare and because of the tendency to study only right-handers. In a study of traumatic injuries, Luria (1970b) found an effect of familial left-handedness in right-handers. That is, pure right-handers without family history of left-handedness did not recover as quickly. Basso and her colleagues (1990) found that non-right-handed patients with stroke-related aphasias did not differ from right-handed patients. Borod, Carper, and Naeser (1990) followed the progress of left-handed patients and found patterns of change that were similar to right-handers.

Race

Race was considered in Holland and others' (1989) multivariate analysis of spontaneous recovery up to three months postonset, and they found that it did not matter. Wertz, Auther, and Ross (1997) compared African-Americans and Caucasians across the course of a 44-week treatment study that began a month poststroke. Progress was measured with the PICA, Token Test, and a word fluency task. The two clinical groups did not differ in initial severity and in amount and rate of improvement of auditory and oral language skills over 10 months.

Time of Initial Test

The recovery curve (see Figure 10.1) tells us that amount of recovery depends on when we initially test a patient after stroke. We can expect a smaller amount of improvement the later a patient is referred. Pickersgill and Lincoln (1983) measured overall progress of 1.01 points with the PICA over an eight week period, much less than the change-scores in Table 10.1. However, patients were tested initially at an average of five months postonset at the time of admission to a rehabilitation program.

Yet, the timing of first test within the first two months is probably unrelated to change measured over a year, as indicated in Bamber's (1980) study and in an analysis of data reported by Hanson and Cicciarelli (1978). Thus, starting treatment anytime within two-months is not likely to be related to subsequent progress, but a program started much later is likely to be accompanied by less improvement.

Additional Considerations

There are other factors that make sense but have not been studied much. In one study, *history of previous stroke* did not matter with respect to progress over the first three months (Holland, et al., 1989). *Length of hospital stay* was a moderate predictor, as 20 days or less was more favorable than 21 or more days. Like age, this is one of those indicators tied to more direct or "real" influences such as the reasons for a short stay (e.g., smaller infarct, less severe deficit, good medical condition).

Other possible factors include *education,* which may have more influence on response to therapy than on recovery per se. *Motivation* can be related to more concrete circumstances, such as good health and a realistic goal of returning to work. Tompkins and others (1990) complained that investigators continue to examine the same old variables with the same old measures. They recommended that researchers consider the influence of auditory processing, personality and attitude with available scales, and social support system.

A more exotic possibility is that *morphological asymmetry* or a person's brain size can affect recovery. Burke and his colleagues (1993) reviewed some previous work indicating that globally aphasic patients with a *right* hemisphere larger than the left recovered better than patients without this asymmetry of brain structure. Others found no relationship between structural asymmetries and recovery. Burke's team decided to do their own study and reviewed medical charts at the Albuquerque VA Medical Center from 1976 to 1986. They came up with a different result.

Burke's team compared the relative size of each hemisphere on CT scans to PICA overall scores recorded initially at one month poststroke and at one-month intervals until a year poststroke. Posterior width asymmetry favoring the left was associated with a faster rate of recovery and higher outcome at one year than right posterior asymmetry or equal hemisphere size. This so-called "occipital asymmetry" included portions of Wernicke's area and the temporoparietal boundary. Their conclusion was that a larger posterior *left* hemisphere hemisphere is a more efficient language processor and provides more intact brain for facilitating recovery. More research probably needs to be done before neurologists routinely measure brain size as a clue to prognosis.

BILINGUAL RECOVERY

Does a bilingual person recover languages differently? Exceptions to the equivalent recovery of two languages have long been associated with the "rules" of Ribot and Pitres (see Chapter 6). The rules indicated that any difference would have something to do with which language is the native tongue and/or which is the most familiar language.

- *rule of Ribot* ("primacy rule"): the first learned or native language recovers first

- *rule of Pitres:* the most frequently used language recovers first

Obler and Albert's (1977) review of the literature indicated that Pitres' rule describes recovery more often than Ribot's rule. That is, the most recently used language recovers faster more often than the other languages. In the published reports, the degree to which this pattern occurred depended somewhat on age. Patients over 60 were less likely to recover the most recent language than younger patients. This pattern was also more likely to be followed in multilingual than bilingual persons. The reliability of this characterization is confounded by definition of "most frequent/familiar language," partly because functional bilinguals use two languages depending on the situation.

Paradis (1977) got a different impression from his review of 138 cases of bilingual aphasia reported in the literature. He found many possibilities (Table 10.3). Contrary to the previous emphasis on differential recovery, nearly half the cases improved according to a **synergistic** pattern in which progress in one language is accompanied by comparable progress in the other language. Subsequently, Paradis and others (1982) described another category. In *alternate antagonism* (or "seesaw recovery"), "for given periods of time, the patients could speak only one language, and the available language would alternate for consecutive periods" (p. 56). A critical suspicion regarding reports over the past century is that clinicians may be more inclined to report differences between languages or that journals may be more inclined to publish them.

TRAUMATIC BRAIN INJURY

The major problem in studying recovery after traumatic brain injury is that there is great variability in type and severity of brain pathology (Prigatano, 1987). Aphasia is not often transparent, and other cognitive disorders may be a primary concern. Parameters of recovery are often related to functional considerations such as psychosocial status and vocational adjustment and are recorded with broad rating scales. Contrary to the common measurement of language, investigators rely on undefined descriptors such as "mild, moderate, and severe" to characterize dysfunction and improvement.

Recovery

Table 10.4 shows four general phases in recovery from closed head injury (CHI). Cripe (1987) associated treatment strategies with each phase. Outcome is often represented in terms of whether

TABLE 10.3 Patterns of recovery between languages in bilinguals (Paradis, 1977).

PATTERN	DEFINITION	PERCENTAGE
synergistic (parallel)	two languages progress at the same rate and were similarly impaired at the beginning; nearly identical recovery curves	41
synergistic (differential)	two languages improve at the same rate but were impaired to different degrees at the start; curves separate but parallel	8
selective	one language improves but the other does not improve	27
successive	one language recovers after another; one seems dormant while another is progressing, and the dormant language starts improving weeks or months later	6
antagonistic	one language progresses but the other regresses	4
mixed	two systematically intermingled languages	?

TABLE 10.4 Phases in recovery from closed head injury (Cripe, 1987).

PHASE	DESCRIPTION	TREATMENT ORIENTATION
coma	loss of consciousness lasting hours to months	
post-traumatic amnesia (PTA)	beginning when consciousness is regained and ending when a patient can remember day-to-day events	assistance with attention and orientation; complex cognition is avoided
rapid recovery	significant progress over three to six months depending on severity	focus on basic skills; minimize unrealistic expectations
long-term plateau	persisting residual deficits; progress is painstakingly slow	emphasis on adjusting to disabilities

a patient has returned to independent functioning or previous employment.

In all severe head injuries, PTA exceeds one day. Conclusion of this phase may be recognized when a patient begins to remember conversations a few hours earlier. In more than 90 percent of cases, PTA lasts more than a week; and more than four weeks in 60 percent (Jennett and Teasdale, 1981). The longer this period lasts, the more difficult it is to recognize exactly when it ends; and identification of the end of PTA can be one or two weeks off.

In a study of cognitive recovery, groups with CHI were evaluated at different periods postonset (Bond, 1975, cited in Prigitano, 1987). Most improvement in Full Scale IQ with the WAIS occurred in the first six months after injury. Progress was slower thereafter until two years postonset. In a longitudinal study, Lezak (1979) found significant improvement of memory extending to 6-to-12 months postonset but no significant change thereafter.

Patients with CHI have been observed to recover language to a functional level by four months postonset (Groher, 1977) and to normal levels on an aphasia battery by six months (Levin, Grossman, Sarwar, and Meyers, 1981). Persistent deficit was associated with persistent hematomas in the left hemisphere. After reviewing studies, Levin (1981) found "an overall trend of improvement that may eventuate in restoration of language or specific defects ('subclinical' language disorder) in naming or word finding in about two-thirds of the patients who are acutely aphasic" (p. 441). Adolescents with CHI still had deficits of verbal expression one year after onset (Campbell and Dollaghan, 1990).

Luzzatti and his colleagues (1989) followed 18 patients with several language and neuropsychological tests. The time periods were highly variable. The first test was given at a median of five months postinjury and the second from 4 to 36 months postinjury. Progress was more evident in an aphasia battery and a categorical word-fluency task than in supplemental neuropsychological measures. Findings were probably influenced by the early recovery that was not observed and ceiling effects with certain tests.

Prognosis

Type of head injury was explored by Luria (1970b), who found that progress differed depending on whether head wounds were nonpenetrating (closed) or penetrating (open). Most cases of penetrating injury to language areas (93%) continued to be clinically aphasic after two months postonset. However, 63 percent of nonpenetrating injuries to language areas remained aphasic (meaning that more recovered). An extreme difference of sample size weakens the impact of this comparison, but data on damage to marginal language areas also showed that nonpenetrating injury had a higher frequency of "total recovery." This study is suggestive of the rapid and large recovery that sets CHI apart from more focal lesions.

Severity of injury is probably a factor. Patients with only diffuse swelling have a better level of recovery than those with additional diffuse axonal injury (Uzell, Dolinskas, Wiser, and Langfitt, 1987). Severity of injury is usually estimated by duration of coma and/or PTA. "Most mild injuries...show substantial recovery and are often back to work within 3 to 6 months postinjury," noted Prigatano (1987, p. 603). "Patients with moderate injuries...and severe injuries...are quite *variable* in their recovery course."

Prigatano (1987) cited a study by Bond that focused on **PTA duration** as a predictor. When PTA was under 3 weeks, IQ improved from 94 to 100 in six months. When PTA was 4–6 weeks, IQ improved from around 80 to 92 in six months and reached 100 after 12 months postonset. When PTA was 8–11 weeks, a pattern of recovery was also evident. The verbal scale improved faster than the performance scale over the first 6 months. Afterward, the performance scale progressed slowly until two years postonset. In general, PTA under 7 weeks is accompanied by the early rapid recovery associated with CHI. If PTA is longer than 12 weeks, progress is not promising.

EXPLAINING RECOVERY

One of Julianna Exeter's friends told her, "I heard that the right side of the brain takes over or that you can teach the right side to talk."

The survey of prognostic factors included neurological conditions that might contribute to recovery from stroke, such as the relative size of one hemisphere or the size of lesion. Now, we consider changes in the brain that may occur after a stroke and that may allow recovery to occur. Two general types of changes are considered. One is the structural repair of damaged regions, and the other is a compensatory contribution from structurally intact regions such as the right hemisphere.

Early in this chapter, it was stated that cortical cells do not grow back. However, neuroscientists have not given up on exploring the possibility that there can be some **repair** of the damage or a restoration of the damaged region. *Spontaneous regeneration* of damaged nerves was demonstrated in animals in the 1930s and 40s by Weiss and Sperry (Rose, 1989). Sperry cut the optic nerve of salamanders. The nerve regenerated, and sight was restored. The optic nerve in mammals, however, does not regenerate.

Other theories of recovery are based on the global notion of the brain's *plasticity* or flexibility. A child's brain is maximally flexible as it is continually learning new things. Plasticity in an adult brain is also indicated by new learning. However, does the adult brain make adjustments subsequent to stroke? According to **functional substitution,** a structurally intact area assists in or takes over an impaired function. Like the comforting thought from Julianna Exeter's friend, the right hemisphere (RH) may take over language functions to such a degree that it becomes a substitute for the damaged left hemisphere (LH). This used to be called the "spare tire" theory.

There can be some subtle variations in substitution. One is whether new RH involvement in language processing could happen spontaneously or as a result of therapy. After damage to the motor cortex on one side in adult rats, increased dendritic arborization has been shown to occur nearby and in the opposite hemisphere. Also, the nervous system in animals has been shown to be responsive to environmental stimulation. Rearing animals in the dark reduced protein synthesis in the visual cortex, and exposing these animals to the light resulted in increased protein synthesis in geniculate bodies and cortex. Detector cells in the visual cortices of adult cats varied as a function of the type of visual environment in which the cats were reared (Keefe, 1995; Rose, 1989).

Another dimension of substitution pertains to whether the RH (or any intact region) had a capacity for the impaired language function before the stroke. *Spontaneous substitution* would indicate that language skills already existed in the substituting region. A demonstration of this in normal adults would contribute to this theory of recovery. *Therapeutic substitution,* on the other hand, would be indicated if the RH became more involved because of language therapy. This would suggest that the RH did not have an important role in the rehabilitated function before the stroke. For a long time, these were handy logical possibilities. Then researchers started to look for a basis for believing, at least, that the role of the RH changes after stroke.

One group of studies relied on indirect "observation" of brain function with techniques for studying functional asymmetry (Moore, 1989). Presenting stimuli simultaneously to each ear, called dichotic listening, is one of these techniques. Normally there is a right-ear advantage (REA) in response to verbal stimuli, which is considered to be indicative of the expected LH role in verbal processing. Curiously, various studies have shown a left-ear advantage (LEA) in aphasic people. This LEA has been interpreted as the RH taking a greater role in language function. Niccum and Speaks (1991) suggested that other factors could account for the results, but Moore and Papanicolaou (1992) countered by noting that there is other evidence converging on an increased role of the RH.

Now, scientists can observe brain function more directly after stroke with neuroimaging techniques. In Italy, Cappa and his colleagues (1997) obtained PET scans from eight aphasic patients two weeks after stroke. In the acute stage, there was diminished metabolism in both hemispheres, indicative of diaschisis. Then, metabolism increased significantly in both sides of the brain for all subjects six months later. Moreover, changes in Token Test comprehension and spoken naming were correlated more with specific changes in the right hemisphere than in the left.

Besides substitution, a logical possibility is some sort of **reorganization** which suggests that an aphasic person accomplishes a functional goal in a new way. An area of the brain does not change; instead, spared areas not normally involved in a function are recruited for the performance of a task. Luria (1970b) called it *intersystemic reorganization.* Such response to damage is often thought to be encouraged by rehabilitation rather than being something that happens spontaneously.

Investigators may speak of the formation of "new pathways." No new association tracts are sprouted. The idea is like taking another existing route to work because a bridge has collapsed on the most efficient route. This type of adjustment is often proposed in cognitive terms with respect to CN-models presented in Chapters 4 and 6. For example, Carlomagno and Parlato (1989) described treatment of writing that supposedly detours a collapsed graphemic route to production, possibly by way of a semantic or phonological "lexical relay."

In Germany, Hans Karbe and his colleagues (1998) believe that they found physiological evidence of left brain reorganization associated mainly with improvement in Token Test scores. PET scans were obtained three-to-four weeks after stroke and then over a year later for seven severely aphasic patients. Metabolism was measured while patients did a word repetition task. As a presumed compensatory response one month after stroke, areas of both hemispheres were activated that are not normally active for the repetition task. The best language recovery over the following year was related to restored metabolism in the left superior temporal lobe, not increased metabolism in the RH. The investigators concluded that "left hemispheric structural reorganization is significantly more effective than the right hemispheric compensation" (p. 227).

MARTIN EXETER'S RECOVERY

Martin Exeter was progressing more rapidly than many persons with aphasia (Table 10.5). His improvement in comprehension accuracy in the first two months was important for conversation. He could answer questions about what he was trying to convey, and he could detect when he was misunderstood. In the first few months, he was having a hard time managing his frustration. Just naming a picture never felt particularly "good." He would humor the therapist with a smile, but it was not

TABLE 10.5 Some "progress notes" concerning Martin Exeter's functional progress.

TIME POST ONSET	LANGUAGE	FUNCTIONAL SKILLS	LISTENER'S BURDEN
2 months	sporadic comprehension pretends to read newspaper word-finding delays agrammatic phrases	gets basic ideas across supplements with gesture depressed and reclusive	lots of yes-no questions anxiety over impatience Jackie speaks for Martin sometimes
6 months	mildly agrammatic sentences more fluent but still slow reads headlines & first paragraphs writes short phrases	gets most ideas across sense of humor returning avoids work-related topics invites friends to house	fewer questions Jackie more patient close friends adjusting
12 months	slow but nearly complete sentences reads newspaper articles slowly	practices with computer pursues social situations cannot follow conversations	minimal burden for dinner conversation
18 months	aphasia not apparent to strangers Martin senses word-finding problems reads professional articles slowly writes with computer very slowly	friendly debates too fast to get the fine points thinks about returning to work	patient with his misinterpretations balancing encouragement with reality

what he was used to thinking of as an accomplishment.

Over time, word-finding quickened and grammatical morphemes filled gaps. His verbal production became generally more fluent. His therapist would report that he seemed more like someone with anomic aphasia than Broca's aphasia. By 18 months after his stroke, Martin was nearly his former self in everyday conversations with family and friends.

In two years, it was difficult for a stranger to tell that Martin had a language disorder. However, he could tell that his processing system was imperfect. He remained quiet in social gatherings, because his friends talked too fast and took turns too quickly. His confidence was still shaken. He was slow finding words about obscure or complex topics. Even with these difficulties, he was beginning to contemplate a return to teaching. The stroke did not destroy his memory of the issues he had wanted to debate with students and colleagues. Yet, reading journals was laborious, and writing a couple of sentences usually took an hour.

SUMMARY AND CONCLUSIONS

Important decisions about services are based on notions of recovery. Recovery is greatest and swiftest during the first two or three months postonset and slows down until six months after onset. Some believe that language does not improve after six months or a year. However, recovery has been demonstrated in some patients up to one year and, in a relatively few patients, beyond one year. The problem with these observations is their variability. We need to have a way of managing a caseload based on an ability to predict who is likely to progress the most in the least amount of time.

The referring physician is interested in our opinion about prospects for recovering language, especially if the patient is provided language treatment. We want to be sure that the physician and family are also thinking about recovery of communication, which, as indicated in Chapter 12, involves more than language per se. We also make a point of documenting recovery of language comprehension as well as verbal expression, considering that physicians often focus only on speech.

Like the physician, we shy away from prediction during the first week after onset. We are more willing to make a general prediction later in the first month. Our prognosis pertains to the likelihood that a patient can benefit substantially from treatment. This is close to a binary decision, namely, either a patient can benefit from treatment or treatment is not likely to help. Of course, the physician's opinion regarding type, size, and site of lesion is important. Our job is to document initial severity of deficit and follow a patient's early spontaneous progress. A focal infarction preserving the comprehension area along with some early spontaneous progress are all fairly positive signs.

Although this chapter presented recovery by patients in rehabilitation programs, it avoided discussing treatment as an exogenous factor. Evidence for the effects of treatment remains to be considered in the following chapters.

Chapter 11

PRINCIPLES OF LANGUAGE RESTORATION

With respect to the three levels of medical conditions set forth by the World Health Organization (see Table 1.6), this chapter focuses on treating language *impairment.* The next chapter deals with *disability* and *handicap.* These two chapters should be applicable to all degrees and types of aphasia, whereas the final chapter contains procedures directed at specific impairments.

When treatment is oriented to impairment, the initial goal is to repair or restore damaged cognitive processes. For someone with aphasia, this means trying to fix damaged psycholinguistic processes. For someone with closed head injury, it is likely also to mean trying to fix damaged systems of attention or memory.

REHABILITATION SETTINGS

A speech-language pathologist came to Martin Exeter's bedside in the Stroke Unit and quickly evaluated his language abilities and oral motor function (including swallowing). She recommended some communicative strategies for him and his family, and offered encouragement to everyone.

Martin's rehabilitation went through four phases. He was transferred from the Stroke Unit to the Rehabilitation Unit of Pocumtuck Medical Center where he received subacute inpatient therapy for about a month, following the recommendations in his initial clinical report (see Figure 3.5). Then, he began the chronic phase by returning to the Rehabilitation Unit as an outpatient for about three months. He took a "vacation" from therapy for a couple of months, until he heard about a university-based program in another state. After three months at the university, he returned home and began his own regimen of daily language exercises. Thinking about returning to work, he sought help at the speech-language clinic in his own university. The variety of rehabilitation settings is summarized in Table 11.1.

Post-stroke care has become the responsibility of a **rehabilitation team.** Besides a speech-language pathologist, the team minimally includes a physical therapist, occupational therapist, and social worker.

- *Physical therapy:* to improve strength and range-of-motion of large muscle groups. The therapist's concerns include ambulation and transfers between bed and wheelchair.
- *Occupational therapy:* self-care, work, and play activities. The therapist is particularly concerned with manipulation of utensils for grooming, eating, and other self-care tasks.
- *Social services:* for psychological, residential, and vocational needs.

Reasons for more integrated teamwork in recent years include the sharing of reimbursement resources and the widespread use of general outcome scales such as the FIM (see Chapter 7). In many rehabilitation centers, team members meet regularly so that, for example, language treatment can be coordinated with occupational therapy.

TREATING AN IMPAIRMENT

The activities of language treatment are similar to research and assessment. In research and assessment, tasks are designed for observing failures and successes. In treatment, some of the same tasks are carefully chosen for eliciting a patient's best

TABLE 11.1 Rehabilitation settings including common estimates of length of stay as inpatient or length of therapy.

SETTING	TYPE OF CARE	NOTES	LENGTH OF THERAPY
acute care hospital	in-patient acute	ensure survival discharge when medically stable	less than 7 days
rehabilitation hosptal	in-patient postacute or subacute	often in acute care facility therapy as soon as possible short-term treatment	less than 4 weeks
rehabilitation center	out-patient chronic	independent facility long-term rehabilitation	weeks or months
home health care	residential chronic	patient's home Home Health Agency (HHA)	weeks or months
nursing home	residential chronic	skilled nursing facility (SNF) private practice contracts	weeks or months

performances. Brookshire, Nicholas, and others (1978) studied 40 videotaped treatment sessions conducted in various regions of the United States. The clinicians did basically the same thing when administering treatment. That is, all therapy tasks contained the following components:

- clinician's stimulus
- patient's response
- clinician's feedback

Any treatment task consists of the clinician's stimulus and the expected response. When working on comprehension, the stimulus is a word or sentence. The response tends to be nonverbal so that production difficulties do not distract from comprehending (e.g., pointing to a picture). When working on production, the minimal stimulus may be a picture of an object, and the patient is asked to make a verbal response. Table 11.2 shows some basic tasks for some general objectives.

We are now interested in improving rather than just observing a patient's response. We help the patient by modifying or supplementing a stimulus or by providing informative feedback. For example, in a comprehension task, we may simplify a linguistic stimulus to improve the response. For a naming task, we may supplement a picture with hints about an object's name.

Nearly all of the methods of aphasia therapy conform to one of two fundamental approaches to structuring and administering these tasks. One approach is *behavior modification* which appears widely throughout education and rehabilitation fields. A stimulation or *stimulation-facilitation* approach is more specific to aphasia treatment. The ensuing discussions point out some of their

TABLE 11.2 Some basic tasks in treatment of aphasia.

TO IMPROVE:	CLINICIAN'S STIMULUS	PATIENT'S RESPONSE
auditory comprehension	Says a sentence while showing three pictures	Points to one of the pictures
reading comprehension	Shows a sentence while showing three pictures	Points to one of the pictures
spoken word-finding	Shows a picture of a common object	Says name of the object
written word-finding	Shows a picture of a common object	Writes name of the object

differences with respect to assumptions about the nature of aphasia, targets of treatment, method for obtaining a correct response, the therapeutic mechanism in a task, the number of items in a task, and the clinician's response to a patient's error.

BEHAVIOR MODIFICATION

Behavior modification is derived from learning theory. It has been said that it is used because clinicians make an assumption that aphasia is a loss (or erasure) of linguistic knowledge. Because this assumption is usually erroneous, other clinicians have argued that behavioral therapies are invalid or inappropriate for aphasia (e.g., Sullivan and Brookshire, 1989). Yet, a strict behaviorist would deny any interest in the nature of aphasia. The goal is simply to change behavior, and its hidden causes are irrelevant.

Among the types of behavior modification technique, **operant conditioning** has been preferred for modifying volitional behavior. A patient responds to a stimulus and is rewarded after an adequate response. Operant treatment for aphasia was common in the 1960s (e.g., Brookshire, 1967; Holland and Harris, 1968). It then faded from clinical aphasiology for a while and reappeared in the early 1980s in conjunction with single-subject experimental designs in efficacy research (see Chapter 13).

The Task

The first step in planning this type of therapy is to select a behavior to be treated. The **target behavior** is often quite specific such as yes-no responses to questions, production of the auxiliary *is,* or production of certain social phrases. We may start with a task that elicited responses during initial assessment. The response need not have been produced at a high rate of success.

Because behavioral treatments are geared to specific responses, there may be a tendency to *treat-to-the-test.* In this approach, "the clinician identifies tests in which a patient's performance is deficient and constructs treatment tasks that mimic the content and structure of those tests" (Brookshire, 1997, p. 248). For example, a naming task in treatment is likely to be quite similar to the naming task in assessment. Holland and Sonderman (1974) devised a task similar to the Token Test for treating auditory comprehension.

If a response does not come through simple presentation of a stimulus, a clinician often uses a procedure called **modeling** by instructing a patient to imitate a specific response. In Thompson and McReynolds' (1986) treatment of sentence production, the clinician "sequentially modeled the first two words of the target response then the remaining words of the target response, instructing the subject to repeat each portion as it was modeled" (p. 198). Responses sometimes appear to be forced (Sullivan and Brookshire, 1989).

Behavioral methods have entailed the training of specific sets of responses to a small set of stimuli. Thompson and Kearns (1981) trained the production of 10 names to 10 pictures until a patient reached a criterion of success. That is, the same items were elicited repeatedly. Kearns and Salmon (1984) trained the auxiliary *is* in 10 specific sentences. A small number of specific items is especially common when working with a severe impairment.

Feedback

In operant training, "consequences of the behavior serve to control the frequency of its occurrence" (Mowrer, 1982, p. 204). Reinforcement should increase the frequency of a desired behavior, and negative feedback (or "punishment") should decrease the frequency of errors or undesirable behavior. Clinicians usually employ verbal praise such as "good" or "nice job," called **incentive feedback** (Brookshire, 1997). Kearns and Salmon (1984) presented redeemable coupons and tokens after correct responses. A *reinforcement schedule* is a rate at which an accurate response is rewarded. In continuous reinforcement, each correct response is rewarded. In intermittent reinforcement, only some correct responses are rewarded (e.g., Thompson and Byrne, 1984).

A clinician's response to a patient's inadequate response distinguishes operant conditioning from stimulation-facilitation methods. In operant conditioning, errors may be "consequated" by verbal punishment. Tonkovich and Loverso (1982) administered a "verbal reproof" such as *No, that wasn't right.* Thompson and Byrne (1984) simply said *No, not quite.* A computer may be programmed to emit a "cheerful sound" after a correct response and a "negative tune" after an error (Scott and Byng, 1989).

Another option is **information feedback** (Brookshire, 1997). That is, we point out the degree to which a response approximated the instructed expectation (e.g., "It's not a complete sentence" or "Close, but you should have put 'was' in front of the verb"). Brookshire recommended information feedback for self-motivated clients who are unaware of the target or the relationship between the target and an inadequate response. Simple positive feedback after correct responses may be considered to be informative.

COGNITIVE STIMULATION

Stimulation-facilitation originated in the clinical work of Hildred Schuell. Her contemporaries followed her lead (e.g., Darley, 1982; Eisenson, 1984), and she continued to influence prominent clinicians such as Brookshire (1997), Duffy (1994), and Shewan and Bandur (1986). The term "cognitive" is added to the notion of stimulation in order to indicate the approach's reliance on an understanding of the nature of aphasia. Clinicians give more thought to treatment of comprehension and formulation processes.

Theoretical Targets of Treatment

Schuell stated that "what you do about aphasia depends on what you think aphasia is" (Sies, 1974, p. 138). Brookshire (1997) has elaborated: "Most clinicians and investigators agree that aphasia is not a loss of language (either vocabulary or rules) but is the result of impairments in processes necessary for comprehending, formulating, and producing spoken and written language" (p. 249). Current "diagnostically based" or "theory-driven" treatments are consistent with the broad assumptions underlying stimuluation.

Brookshire advocated a *treat underlying processes approach* which steers clinicians away from replicating tests and toward cognitive processes assumed to be responsible for impaired performances. Treating a process should lead us away from targeting specific stimuli and responses and toward targeting general processes or abilities that may underlie a patient's response pattern. In principle, "treating a general process may affect several specific communicative abilities that depend on the process" (Brookshire, 1997, p. 249). For example, when targeting the process of word-finding, a clinician may employ word production tasks not used in assessment, increasing the likelihood of improving divergent abilities and sentence production.

Chapters 4 and 5 presented some psycholinguistic processes such as lexical access and syntactic parsing, but these processes are not yet well-understood with respect to aphasia. Current clinical practice tends to target general processing systems such as comprehension. When therapy is said to target comprehension, a clinician is speaking of a mental process, not a behavior. A behavior consists of pointing to pictures in response to spoken sentences, and one of Brookshire's points was that the comprehension system is built to deal with a variety of stimulus-response relationships.

Accurate Response

We start therapy with what a patient can already do, which is demonstrated directly or indirectly in initial testing. That is, we rely on tasks that produce a high frequency of accurate responses without training. This is known as the **success principle.** Brookshire (1997) wrote that "a good general rule is to keep patient performance at 60% to 80% immediate correct responses during the beginning of a given task" (p. 225). Starting at 80 percent accuracy or higher is possible when including slow responses.

Following the success principle ensures that a patient is practicing normal processing. Repeated failure, in effect, is the practice of an ineffective or aberrant cognitive process. Also, errors beget errors. Brookshire (1972) discovered that erroneous naming on one trial increased the likelihood of error on the next trial. Brookshire and Nicholas (1978) found that three or four consecutive errors reduced the chance of subsequent correct response to almost nil. When a patient starts making 30% or more errors, we adjust the task to make it easier, or we switch to a different task in which normal processing is resumed.

Schuell said that "I do not teach aphasic patients words. I stimulate language processes and they begin to function. Words come out that I never used" (Sies, 1974, p. 138). In the stimulation approach, the antecedent event is the driving force behind improving responses, as opposed to the consequent event in behavioral therapy. Darley (1982) suggested maximizing the "arousal power" of a stimulus, and Duffy (1994) recommended that stimulation be strong enough to elicit a response without forcing it. Rosenbek and his colleagues (1989) wrote that "our feeling that good clinicians can—by their stimulus selection, ordering, and presentation—elicit responses from all but the most severe or sullen patients, causes us to emphasize antecedent over consequent events" (p. 137).

Schuell added that "I am going to depend largely on auditory stimulation, because I think language is most dependent on this perceptual system" (Sies, 1974, p. 139). Another reason for relying on the auditory modality is that it is the least impaired of the language modalities. Schuell believed in bombarding a patient with stimulation and requiring many successful responses, making therapy quite different from the other hours in a patient's day.

Number of Items

Shewan and Bandur (1986) put stimulation techniques together in a package called Language Oriented Treatment (LOT). "In LOT the same stimuli are not used over and over again... different stimuli at a comparable level of difficulty are presented to elicit responses" (p. 13). A patient could say "car" in response to "You buy a ___," "You wreck a ___," and "You fix a ___." Conversely, more than one response may be acceptable for one stimulus (e.g., You drive a *car, Ford, bus* and so on).

The key is that the particular words or sentences presented or produced do not matter as long as the targeted process is being exercised. In fact, it may be advantageous to vary item content, because progress may be more likely to generalize to untreated stimulus-response content that depends on the same process (Thompson, 1989). In the jargon of behavioral modification, this principle is known as "training sufficient exemplars."

Feedback upon Error

Restimulation is the alternative to verbal reproof after a patient makes an error. Brookshire (1997) noted that "many clinicians tend to avoid negative feedback, perhaps because they do not wish to discourage their patients" (p. 230). Schuell and others (1964) stated that "the objective is to get the language processes working, not to teach the patient that whatever he says is wrong" (p. 342). According to this philosophy, the stimulus was probably not adequate if a patient fails to respond, and *we stimulate the patient again* instead of correcting errors (also, Duffy, 1994).

There should be little need for restimulation, when stimulation is planned to be powerful enough to elicit a good response most of the time. When the occasional inadequate response does occur, we first say "let's try it again" and then repeat the initial stimulus. If simple repetition does not work, we repeat the stimulus supplemented with cues such as the first sound in a naming task. However, if a patient exhibits frustration and starts making errors at a frequency of more than 30 percent, then we modify the task so that the stimulus is more powerful. That is, the restimulation becomes the antecedent event for the modified task.

Brookshire (1997) suggested that "incentive feedback does not play an important part of treatment of most brain-damaged adults" (p. 229). Most patients are self-motivated. Many know their target and are aware of the difference between their response and their target. Information feedback is often used in biofeedback techniques for motor speech disorders, when patients are trying to achieve subtle pitch or intensity changes. For most aphasic patients, Brookshire preferred **general encouragement** that is not necessarily contingent on adequacy of response (e.g., "You're doing fine," "You're doing much better today").

In sum, clinicians have taken different approaches to the treatment of aphasia. These differences are illustrated in behavioral and stimulation methods. The main contrasts are summarized in Table 11.3.

PROGRAMMED STIMULATION

How does treatment progress over time? Principles of programmed learning keep stimulation treatment on a track defined by a goal. Treatment changes across sessions because a patient changes. Stable treatment is a sign of a stable patient. LaPointe (1985) referred to the overall approach as programmed stimulation (see Table 11.4).

The terminal behavior specifies an intermediate goal of a treatment plan (e.g., *to produce complete sentences*). The plan for progressing toward the goal is called a "program." Multiple goals may be established, suggesting that a plan consists of multiple programs such as one for comprehension and one for production. A clinician documents goals but usually does not write out a complete program for each goal. Manuals for aphasia therapeutics provide sample steps in progression from initial to terminal behaviors. Experienced clinicians are able to follow fundamental principles in keeping treatment on a goal-directed track without having to document each step.

Historically, long-term treatment of aphasia has been a series of little victories. Principles of programmed learning state that moving from an initial behavior to a terminal behavior requires small steps. The idea is that if the next step is similar to the current step, then capacities shown in the current step should transfer readily to the next step. The same processes are being used in each

TABLE 11.3 Comparison of cognitive stimulation and operant conditioning in carrying out a treatment task.

COMPARISON	COGNITIVE STIMULATION	OPERANT CONDITIONING
Theoretical assumptions	Belief that aphasia involves impaired cognitive processes and preserved linguistic knowledge	No assumptions about the nature of aphasia
Targets of treatment	Treatment of cognitive or psycholinguistic processes	Treatment of particular behaviors in relation to environmental events
Obtaining an accurate response	Behaviors naturally elicited by a stimulus most of the time	Modeling when responses are not forthcoming naturally
Therapeutic mechanism	Power of a stimulus to elicit a response repeatedly	Behavior changed through consequences or the clinician's feedback
Number of items in a task	Large number of different stimulus items that may vary from session to session	Restricted number of stimulus items repeated across sessions
Feedback upon error	Restimulation	Punishment

TABLE 11.4 Programming terminology applied to stimulation treatment.

TERM	DEFINITION	EXAMPLE
initial behavior	starting point of a treatment plan	names actor in picture of simple event
terminal behavior	end point of a treatment plan	complete statement of simple event
program	steps from initial behavior to terminal behavior	(1) names actor (2) names action (3) produces actor & action (4) produces the complete statement
response criterion	basis for going from one step to the next	each step is 90% accurate before changing response instruction

step, and the next step should present an easily surmountable new obstacle.

A small step is created by changing only one variable in the current task. These variables exist mainly in the clinician's stimulus and client's response. We may make a stimulus sentence slightly more complex, or we may increase the length of verbal response that we instruct a patient to produce. One approach to stimulus adjustment is called **fading,** in which we gradually remove supportive cues so that the stimulus becomes more like what would occur in real life.

Formal programs usually include a somewhat flexible response criterion as the basis for moving to the next step. In Shewan and Bandur's (1986) LOT, a 70 percent criterion was frequently recommended. A patient had to achieve this level of accuracy on consecutive blocks of 10 trials before we could assume that processing is sufficient for handling the next level of difficulty. Brookshire (1997) suggested a 90 to 95 percent criterion, especially because a task should start at a 70 to 80 percent level.

With managed care, the elements of Table 11.4 might be modified in at least two ways. The terminal behavior is more likely to be functional, such as requesting an item at a grocery rather than just producing a particular linguistic form. Second, a step of progression is more likely to represent changes in multiple variables rather than just one at a time. Many patients skip steps successfully, anyway; and small steps may be quite inefficient for cases that show bursts of improved processing. For example, once a patient starts producing verbs regularly, other elements of a sentence may naturally follow without specific treatment. It may be more useful, in this case, to shift stimulus conditions to real-life communicative problems or settings.

WORD-FINDING

One of the main goals in Martin Exeter's early language treatment was to improve word-finding efficiency. This was not unusual, because every patient has some kind of word-finding problem. Technique usually revolves around the object-naming task. A week after his stroke, Martin named common objects promptly and without help around 50 percent of the time. The therapist found that a "hint" or cue would raise his word-finding to about 80 percent. Therefore, this is where treatment began. The goal was for him to be naming at 80 percent without hints in a couple of weeks.

Cue Responsiveness

> *If an aphasic cannot bring forth an intended response himself, it is sometimes possible to lead him to do so by eliciting a response first in a more automatic way and then in more and more voluntary ways by gradually withdrawing the facilitations incorporated in the stimuli. This passage from more automatic to more voluntary constitutes the core of rehabilitation (Basso, et al., 1979, p. 192).*

We use cues to elicit words automatically or without training. Several studies have been done to determine the arousal power of cues for aphasic patients. Naming cues fit into two broad categories (Table 11.5). Semantic cues provide information about the target-word's meaning, and the most frequently studied version is a carrier phrase conveying superordinate, functional, or locational information (e.g., "It's a sport"). A purely semantic cue provides no intentional information about the target-word's form. Cognitively speaking, semantic cues may be said to activate an area in semantic memory. A lexical or phonological cue provides information about a word. It is usually the first sound or syllable (e.g., "It starts with /b/"). It gives no additional information about meaning. Cognitively speaking, lexical cues point to a form in the mental lexicon. Either type of cue is more effective in eliciting names than a picture alone (Stimley and Noll, 1991).

In the research, cues have been presented either prior to showing an object, called *prestimulation* (Pease and Goodglass, 1978; Stimley and Noll, 1991), or they have been presented as restimulation after naming difficulty or naming error (Li and Williams, 1990; Kohn and Goodglass, 1985; Love and Webb, 1977). Generally, cues are more effective as the severity of naming deficit decreases. A phonological cue is more effective than semantic cues and other lexical cues such as a printed or rhyming word. In one study, phonemic cues elicited names about 50 percent of the time, and semantic cues were effective around 30 percent of the time (Li and Williams, 1989).

Some exceptions have been observed. The greater power of phonemic cues applied to nouns but not to verbs. For an action naming task, phonemic and semantic cues were equally effective around 40 percent of the time (Li and Williams, 1990). Semantic cues were more effective for verbs than for nouns.

Phonemic cue superiority is slightly more pronounced for Broca's aphasia relative to aphasia in general (Table 11.6). Some investigators left the impression that phonemic cues are especially useful for cases of Broca's aphasia that have the most difficulty in naming (Bruce and Howard, 1988; Love and Webb, 1977). Regarding the fluent aphasias, cues were more effective for conduction aphasia than the other fluent syndromes. Cues have been least productive for Wernicke's aphasia.

Self-Cueing

If an aphasic person can identify the first letter of a word in a tip-of-the-tongue (TOT) state and retrieves words when a clinician provides the first sound, then maybe the patient can generate his or her own cues to facilitate retrieval. This would

TABLE 11.5 Common cues used to facilitate spoken object-naming. Carrier phrases create syntactic probabilities that may be helpful.

SEMANTIC CUES	EXAMPLE	LEXICAL CUES	EXAMPLE
Definition	"It uses ink and you write with it."	Phoneme (first sound/syllable)	"puh"
Function	"You use it for writing."	Rhyming word	"It's not ten; it's a ___."
Semantic associates	"Pencil," "ink" "It's like a pencil."	Spelling	"p-e-n"
		Printed word	PEN
Carrier phrase	"A ball-point ___." You write with it. It's a ___."	Modeling	"pen"
Location	"You find it on a desk."		

TABLE 11.6 Percentages of naming to phonemic lexical cues and carrier phrase-semantic cues in prestimulation cueing of difficult items (Pease and Goodglass, 1978) and restimulation cueing among groups equated for severity of naming deficit (Li and Williams, 1989, 1990).

	APHASIA		BROCA		WERNICKE		CONDUCTION		ANOMIC	
	Phon	*Sem*	*Phon*	*Sem*	*Phon*	*Sem*	*Phon*	*Sem*	*Phon*	*Sem*
Prestimulation			54	20	42	11			72	38
Restimulation	48	31	55	28	41	22	62	41	34	36
Restimulation	45	29	52	25	38	19	59	39	32	35

make the patient more independent of the clinician. It sounds like a good idea. It was reported first by Berman and Peele (1967). They described training a patient to write the first letter, sound it out, and generate his own carrier phrase; but they did not submit the program to experimental scrutiny.

Bruce and Howard (1988) studied possiblities with 20 persons who had Broca's aphasia, only half having been helped by clinician-generated phonemic cues. These researchers figured that the patients should be able to point to the first letter of a word that cannot be retrieved, sound out (or recode) the letter, and use the sound as a cue. Yet, only six patients could identify first letters upon failing to name objects. None retrieved words upon identifying the first letter. Only two could sound out letters, and none displayed all three abilities. Attempts to train the recoding skill were laborious. Thus, the reports of compensatory self-cueing have been discouraging so far.

Theory-Driven Naming Therapy

Some clinicians have applied theory-driven research to the study of treatment. Byng (1994) stated the fundamental premise: "any treatment that can address the language deficit in aphasia must begin with a theory about the nature of the deficit" (p. 266). This premise goes back to Schuell's admonition that what we do about aphasia depends on what we think aphasia is. The modern version of this notion is more specific in that treatment is designed to either target an impaired process or escort the language system around the impairment as a compensatory strategy (see Chapter 13 for more examples). Let us become familiar with this approach through its application to naming.

The model of object-naming (see Figure 4.2) is a frame of reference for establishing objectives and explaining results of a therapy procedure. The arousal power of cues is considered to be evidence that aphasic impairment lies in lexical retrieval instead of being a loss of lexical storage (Howard, Patterson, Franklin, Orchard-Lisle, and Morton, 1985a). Phonological cues are superior to semantic cues possibly because the stimulus-object already activates semantic memory through the object recognition capacity of most aphasic persons. Thus, semantic cues may be redundant; and the aphasic person, who knows what he or she wants to say, still needs help for accessing or retrieving the word. One thought has been that a stroke raises the thresholds for lexical activation and that form-related cues lower the threshold or raise the activation level.

Treatments have been designed to repair the semantic system (Nickels and Best, 1996b), the phonological output lexicon (Bastiaanse, Bosje, and Franssen, 1996; Miceli, Amitrano, Capasso, and Caramazza, 1996), or the route between semantic and lexical systems (Marshall, Pound, White-Thomson, and Pring, 1990). In considering these studies, we should keep in mind that most of them involve the administration of treatment several months after onset rather than when treatment is usually provided in the health care system. The therapies are classified as two general types, namely, phonological (or lexical) treatment and semantic treatment.

Howard and his colleagues (1985a) administered a **phonological treatment** to determine the therapeutic value of lexical cues. Eight patients were given a package of word repetition, rhyme judgment, and rhyming cues. Phonemic cueing was superior to no cueing for one session; but, after a 30-minute interval "filled with general chat and a cup of coffee," trained names were retrieved no better than before treatment and no better than names that were not cued. Later, a similar treatment without rhyming cues was given to 12 patients for four days across one week or eight days across two weeks (Howard, et al., 1985b). Six weeks later the superiority of treated items faded. Howard's studies raised a question as to whether only a few sessions of lexical cueing is sufficient to restore the retrieval process for lasting use.

Raymer and others (1993) administered a phonological treatment to patients with Broca's aphasia. Detailed analysis indicated that one patient's disorder was squarely in the phonological output lexicon, whereas the other three had a "lexical-semantic impairment." Each patient received the same naming procedure consisting of three levels of restimulation. Upon a patient's failure to name an object, the clinician tried a rhyming cue, then the initial phoneme, and then the word itself for repetition. The therapy was given for 15-to-20 sessions. Some cases improved in the naming of untreated items and in word production on tasks not used in therapy (i.e., reading aloud and written naming). There was no clear relationship between treatment effects and diagnosis.

Semantic treatments steer a patient toward activating concepts associated with words. The unique feature is that patients are not required to produce a word during the therapy, as if the semantic system is to be exercised in isolation of word-finding. That is, activation of the semantic system precedes lexical access in Figure 4.2. One version of semantic treatment centers around word comprehension. This *picture-word matching* technique may be supplemented with a semantic judgment task. Progress in naming, especially regarding untreated items, has been mixed (Nickels and Best, 1996b) if not somewhat disappointing (Pring, Hamilton, Harwood, and Macbride, 1993).

Another version of semantic therapy is called *semantic feature analysis,* in which the object in a naming task is accompanied by various cues. An object is placed in the center of a "feature analysis chart" containing cues to various types of conceptual associations (e.g., "is used for ___," "has ___," "reminds me of ___"). A patient is asked to complete the phrases and write answers in boxes surrounding the object. Boyle and Coelho (1995) tried this procedure with a patient diagnosed with Broca's aphasia. Naming treated and untreated items improved, but spontaneous speech did not get better. Lowell, Beeson, and Holland (1995) tried this procedure for three cases with fluent aphasias, and two of the subjects improved in naming.

Phonological and semantic treatments were compared in a couple of studies. One comparison showed the two procedures to be equally effective but with limited generalization (Howard, et al., 1985b). Le Dorze and others (1994) alternated two versions of semantic therapy, one involving word forms and the other without word forms, with a single patient. Naming improved for items drawn from the procedure involving words but not for items drawn from the other procedure, indicating that including words in a semantic task is important.

In sum, the logic underlying theory-driven treatments is compelling, but the few studies so far have exposed some inconsistencies that make it difficult to understand how a theory of naming is to be applied. For example, patients with Broca's aphasia have received either phonological or semantic therapies. This could mean that a diagnosis of Broca's aphasia is too vague for selecting word-finding treatments or that investigators are uncertain as to how a treatment is to be selected once a diagnosis is made. Conversely, patients with different aphasias have been getting the same treatment, suggesting that different syndromes have the same naming disorder (which has been shown to be possible). Limited generalization beyond the therapy can be attributed to the small amount of treatment studied in some instances and to the fact that experimental treatments have usually been given 10 or more months postonset.

MEASUREMENT AND GENERALIZATION

The health care system demands that clinicians document whether a patient is getting better. We can take three approaches to measuring progress during a period of treatment:

- charting performance of treatment tasks
- repeating a standardized test (e.g., "pre-post test")
- regular probing with specific goal-related tasks that are independent of treatment

Probably the least time-consuming approach is to measure performance in the task(s) used as treatment. The practice of setting criteria for changing tasks indicates that clinicians measure performance in treatment activities (e.g., LaPointe, 1985). A change of 70 to 95 percent accuracy would indicate that a patient is improving (as well as becoming successful with increasingly difficult tasks). Graduate students are often required to measure treatment as part of their clinical training.

Measuring the treatment, however, presents conflicts between some principles of treatment and the need for reliability of a progress measure. One conflict is between starting treatment at a high rate of accuracy (e.g., 80%) and starting measurement at a low baseline for showing clear change (e.g., 20%). Another conflict is between a flexible responsiveness to patients in therapy and the consistency required for reliable measurement.

The conflict between flexibility and consistency can be resolved by employing separate tasks for conducting treatment and measuring progress. Treatment can be flexible and at a high rate of success, and measurement can be consistent and can begin at a relative low level. One implication of this separation is that the task used for measurement is likely to differ from the task used as treatment.

This fortuitous difference provides an opportunity to measure generalization (Kearns, 1989). Clinical researchers commonly distinguish acquisition and generalization. **Acquisition** refers to a new behavior appearing consistently during a training activity. In terms of learning theory, a patient is said to have acquired the behavior. Yet, our goal is that a patient use a new behavior beyond the therapeutic task. **Generalization** refers to progress in "something else," either in other conditions or with untrained responses. Studies of treatment often contain measures of both acquisition and generalization.

The types of generalization consist of stimulus and response generalization, and maintenance (Table 11.7). The importance of stimulus generalization has been known for a long time. For example, the last step of Taylor and Marks' (1959) classic naming program was the use of their core

TABLE 11.7 The three types of generalization.

TYPE	DEFINITION	TREATMENT	TRANSFER
stimulus	trained response to stimuli that differ from treatment	yes-no to a list of questions	yes-no to other questions at home
response	untrained response to the stimuli used in treatment	says "car" to picture of a Toyota	says "Toyota" to same picture
maintenance	trained stimulus-response pairs after completion of treatment	says 10 food names in 60 seconds	same outcome six months later

vocabulary in "everyday life without the help of a picture, a word card, or a therapist" (p. 16). In addition, response generalization should occur with improvement in a general process such as word-finding. As Schuell stated, words start coming out that she never used in therapy.

Stimulus and/or response generalization can be observed with what researchers call a **generalization probe.** A probe takes a few minutes to administer and is usually given at the end of a session, sometimes called a post-session probe. Post-session probes are given daily, on alternate days, or once per week. Reliability is maximized by using at least 10 items and, of course, by administering the task the same way each time.

A systematic approach to probing is illustrated with *matrix training.* One example comes from a study of gesture training (Tonkovich and Loverso, 1982). The basic idea was to train a few signed agent-object messages with the hope of improved gesture production in 25 additional combinations not trained (Figure 11.1). Edges of the matrix defined training items (T). Other items (I) were for assessing transfer a short distance from training (i.e., untrained combinations of trained verbs and nouns). Pairs outside the matrix (E) were for assessing transfer a greater distance from training (i.e., both elements not trained). All subjects improved with untreated gestures. Three of four subjects reached the level of 100 per cent accuracy achieved in acquisition of the seven treated pairs (also, Oleyar, Doyle, Keefe, and Goldstein, 1991).

A treatment activity and a generalization probe are linked by a goal. The treatment is the means to achieving the goal. The generalization probe tells us whether we are meeting the goal. Because a treatment is a means to an end, goals and measures pertain to behaviors that differ from the treatment. For example, a treatment may consist of imitation tasks, but our goal is *not* to make a patient a better imitator. Instead, our goal may be to improve spontaneous verbalization. We can document progress toward meeting this goal by

	MILK	COKE	TEA	COFFEE	JUICE	WATER	BEER	WINE
SPILL	SPILL MILK T	SPILL COKE T	SPILL TEA T	SPILL COFFEE T	SPILL JUICE E	SPILL WATER E	SPILL BEER E	SPILL WINE E
DRINK	DRINK MILK T	DRINK COKE I	DRINK TEA I	DRINK COFFEE I	DRINK JUICE E	DRINK WATER E	DRINK BEER E	DRINK WINE E
BUY	BUY MILK T	BUY COKE I	BUY TEA I	BUY COFFEE I	BUY JUICE E	BUY WATER E	BUY BEER E	BUY WINE E
POUR	POUR MILK T	POUR COKE I	POUR TEA I	POUR COFFEE I	POUR JUICE E	POUR WATER E	POUR BEER E	POUR WINE E

T = Training Items (7)
I = Intramatrix Generalization Items (9)
E = Extramatrix Generalization (16)

FIGURE 11.1 A matrix of verb + object pairs for training gesture and sign combinations. (T) = items trained, (I) = generalization items within the training matrix, and (E) = generalization items outside the training matrix.

Reprinted by permission from Tonkovich, J. & Loverso, F., A training matrix approach for gestural acquisition by the agrammatic patient. In R. H. Brookshire (Ed.), *Clinical aphasia conference proceedings.* Minneapolis: BRK, 1982, p. 284.

measuring spontaneous verbalization, not by measuring the imitation used as the therapy. Another example is shown in Table 11.8.

COMPUTER-ASSISTED TREATMENT

"Teaching machines" were part of the wave of programmed instruction in the 1960s. These devices provided automated presentation of stimulus "frames" and feedback upon response (e.g., Holland, 1970; Sarno, Silverman, and Sands, 1970). The machines were quickly reviled by Wepman (1968) as being a "devil's box" coming between a therapist and a patient. Now, computers are a ubiquitious fixture in clinics as well as patients' homes.

We have become familiar with the essential role of computers in studying the automatic processes of language comprehension and production. For about 20 years, Richard Katz (1995) has been showing us how computers can supplement standard treatment (also, Crerar, Ellis, and Dean, 1996). Companies such as *Parrot Software* have developed sophisticated programs for work on reading comprehension, semantic categorization, visual attention, short-term memory, and reasoning. Thus, tasks are available for cognitive impairments associated with CHI and RHD. The software is capable of providing hints to correct response and data on performance over time, including how often the patient requested hints.

Let us consider a commercial naming program in which a photo of an object appears, and the patient is to type the name. If the patient needs help, the clinician or patient can use the mouse to click on one of three types of cues (i.e., first letter, brief description, carrier phrase). However, here is where we might become concerned about the computer. A gorgeous banana split appears on the screen. A patient types out "fudge." The computer says this is incorrect. The patient might just as well have typed "mars." Because of such glitches, the clinician usually runs through a program before leaving a patient to run it alone. Fortunately, many aphasic patients will chuckle over the computer's aphasia and just move on to the next stimulus.

Deloche and others (1993) administered a computer-assisted written naming program to two patients who had suffered hemorrhages. The patients were moderate-to-mildly impaired, one diagnosed with conduction aphasia. Priming was part of the therapy, in that a form-related or semantic cue was shown simultaneously with a picture to be named in some conditions. The two patients maintained improvements one year after therapy not only in written naming but also in untrained spoken naming and handwriting.

GROUP TREATMENT

A great deal of treatment during and after World War II was conducted with patients in groups (Huber, 1946; Sheehan, 1946; Wepman, 1951). The large number of patients in military hospitals made groups necessary, but it also came to be viewed as a valuable supplement with its own dynamics that do not occur in individual treatment. Most clinicians do not utilize groups as a substitute for individual treatment.

Because groups can be constituted for different purposes, there is no single entity for which the label "group therapy" suffices. When someone reports that group therapy was conducted, we can assume only that it involved two or more clients. Kearns (1994) and Brookshire (1997) have

TABLE 11.8 The relationship of a treatment and a measure to a goal.

BEHAVIORAL GOAL	TREATMENT PROCEDURE	GENERALIZATION PROBE
improve naming from baseline of 40% to 80%	sentence completion at 90% accuracy	simple naming using words not practiced in treatment

reviewed different approaches. Generally, groups are formed for the following purposes:

- *treatment* of cognitive and psycholinguistic impairments
- *maintenance* of communicative gains achieved in prior treatment programs
- *transition* from a treatment program to real-life (i.e., community reintegration)
- *support* for patients and/or families while the patient is undergoing other treatment programs

Multiple purposes can be operative for a single group, such as the support that patients provide each other as they work on cognitive or communicative treatment goals. Groups for any purpose may include family members or volunteers used in ways reported in the next chapter on functional rehabilitation.

EFFICACY OF STANDARD APHASIA TREATMENT

A speech-language pathologist is required minimally to document whether a patient is progressing during the period of treatment. Because managed care also encourages that treatment be attempted as soon as possible, it is often provided during the period of maximum spontaneous recovery in the context of a rehabilitation team. In these circumstances, we cannot determine whether language therapy is the cause of progress. This section presents some studies that have addressed whether language treatment makes a difference in a patient's recovery (see also, Holland, Fromm, DeRuyter, and Stein, 1996). It is important information for clinicians looking to establish or preserve a treatment program.

The Meaning of Efficacy

Bloom and Fischer (1982) wrote of the "three eff's" of accountability in clinical practice. *Effort* is documented as the number of patient-visits and the length of a visit. *Efficiency* is a measure of effort with respect to time (e.g., visits per day). However, working hard and efficiently does not guarantee the third "eff" or *efficacy,* which is the effect of a treatment on recovery of language skills.

Some clinicians have brought the notion of functional improvement to bear on an additional distinction between efficacy and *effectiveness,* the latter referring to whether treatment causes a change in functional abilities or in daily life (e.g., Brookshire, 1994). This fine-tuning of our wording appears to have some inconsistency, as Robey and Dalebout (1998) distinguished between the benefit of "treatment delivered under ideal conditions" as efficacy and "treatment delivered under routine conditions" as effectiveness (p. 1227).

A generalization probe per se does not provide evidence for efficacy or effectiveness of treatment, because other factors could account for progress any time postonset (e.g., neurological changes, medications, living environment, other activities). Demonstration of a cause-effect relationship has obligatory and optional components. The obligatory component is to control for other factors that could be present while treatment is being administered. The optional component lies in the type of progress measurement chosen, namely, the extent to which treatment causes generalization beyond the treatment.

Large Group Studies

Because of the difficulties in conducting large-scale comparisons of treated and untreated groups, only a few such studies have been reported. For an ideal examination of efficacy, the only difference between the groups should be that one is receiving a treatment and the other is not receiving a treatment.

The largest efficacy study in terms of number of subjects was carried out in Italy (Basso, Capitani, and Vignolo, 1979). Most subjects had aphasia caused by stroke. The researchers used the size of treated and untreated groups to maximize their similarity. Subjects entered the no-treatment group, because they "were prevented from attending therapy for extraneous factors, such as family or transportation problems" (p. 191). It took 30 years to complete the study; but the comparability of groups was still weakened by the nonrandom selection. Not being able to attend therapy may have made the untreated subjects differ from treated subjects in other respects, such as communicative environment or motivation to get better. Yet, the groups were similar in educational and socioeconomic levels, and in distribution of types of aphasia, etiology, and gender.

The treated and untreated groups were subdivided according to the time postonset that treatment was initiated. Some subjects received treatment less than two months after onset. Others began treatment between two and six months postonset; and other subjects did not start treatment until after six months. The dependent variable was the percentage of subjects making a substantial improvement of at least two points relative to a five-point scale. Main results are summarized in Table 11.9. At each period, the proportion of subjects making such progress was higher in the treated group. Percentages were lower but the differences between groups were still pronounced after six months. The study showed that treated subjects are more likely to make substantial improvement than untreated subjects, but the study did not indicate relative amounts of progress with respect to measures that were developed long after this major undertaking had begun.

In Canada, Shewan and Kertesz (1984) compared three treated groups with an untreated group "who did not wish or who were unable to receive treatment" (p. 277). The groups ranged from 23 to 28 subjects with ischemic or hemorrhagic strokes. The therapies consisted of language-oriented treatment (LOT), stimulation-facilitation therapy, and an unstructured support therapy provided mainly by nurses. LOT was a decision-making process for treatment developed by Shewan (Shewan and Bandur, 1986), and stimulation therapy was associated with Schuell's methods (Duffy, 1994). Few details about differences between procedures were reported. Treated subjects received three hours of treatment per week for a year.

Progress was measured with the WAB's LQ and CQ and with the ACTS at regular intervals beginning within the first month and then at 3, 6, and 12 months postonset. With an analysis of covariance for the "last LQ," treatments together produced a better outcome than choosing not to have treatment. Both treatments by speech-language pathologists had a better outcome than no-treatment, whereas the unstructured group did not differ significantly from no-treatment. There was no difference between LOT and stimulation therapy. The treatment effect occurred mainly in the 6-to-12 month period postonset.

Poeck, Huber, and Willmes (1989) followed the progress of 68 treated aphasic patients with the *Aachen Aphasia Test* in Germany. The treated subjects were compared with the spontaneous recovery of 92 subjects in 17 departments of neurology where aphasia treatment was not available at

TABLE 11.9 Percentage of substantially improved subjects in each of six groups (Basso, et al., 1979). Groups were defined as treated or untreated and whether treatment was initiated within 2 months, 2–6 months, or after 6 months postonset.

	TIME POST ONSET		
	< 2 months	*2–6 months*	*> 6 months*
Auditory Comprehension			
Treated (N = 107)	88	65	50
Untreated (N = 86)	50	48	16
Oral Expression			
Treated (N = 162)	59	39	29
Untreated (N = 119)	33	9	4

the time. Treatment was said to be similar to Shewan's LOT, but it was three times the amount. It was given in five 60-minute individual sessions and four 60-minute group sessions per week. Treatment periods lasted six-to-eight weeks. The treated group was divided into an early group receiving treatment between one and four months postonset and a late group treated between four and 12 months postonset. For some in the late group, treatment occurred beyond the final measurement of spontaneous recovery. A "chronic" group started after 12 months.

The progress of each treated subject was computed by correcting for spontaneous recovery. That is, treatment effects were determined by "subtracting" the control group's spontaneous recovery from the progress that occurred. With these corrections, significant treatment effects occurred for 78 percent of the early group and 46 percent of the late group. Poeck and his colleagues thought that these estimates were low because of the strictness of the correction. No correction was made for the chronic group; but 68 percent showed significant improvement, which should be of interest to those who believe that progress cannot occur after the first year.

Treatment Comparisons

In the United States, a massive project was undertaken to compare individual treatment with group treatment (Wertz, Collins, Weiss, et al., 1981). Several VA Medical Centers participated in a fastidious effort to match treatment groups according to several criteria and assign subjects randomly to each group. For over three years over one thousand patients were screeened, and 67 met the criteria. Eight hours of treatment per week was started at one month postonset. Each group received treatment for 11 weeks or until about four months postonset. Due to attrition, a total of 34 subjects were followed for 44 weeks or until about a year postonset.

The only difference between treatments was that individual treatment had greater progress in the PICA overall score than group treatment. Otherwise, both methods were similar in being accompanied by significant progress. The only suggestion of treatment efficacy per se was a common one. That is, significant improvement occurred after six months, the point at which spontaneous recovery is believed to have ceased.

The next report from the cooperative study addressed a comparison between two other categories of treatment (Wertz, Weiss, Aten, et al., 1986). One type was treatment in the clinic by a speech-language pathologist. The other was a home-based treatment by a volunteer who had received six-to-ten hours of training. The treatments began about seven weeks after onset. Eight-to-ten hours per week were devoted to the treatments for 12 weeks. Comparisons to periods of no-treatment were introduced partly by using these groups as their own controls. That is, treatment was followed by 12 weeks without treatment. Yet, because the spontaneous recovery curve biases this design to favor the period of treatment, a deferred-treatment group was added. This group, beginning about eight weeks postonset, had 12 weeks without treatment followed by 12 weeks of clinic-treatment.

The progress made by the clinic-treatment group was significantly greater than that made by the deferred-treatment group over the first 12 week period. The home-treatment group was between these groups, not differing significantly from either one. The three groups did not differ from each other at the end of the 24 week study period or about eight months postonset, indicating that delaying treatment for a while does not matter ultimately.

A summary of the major group studies is shown in Table 11.10.

Small Group Comparisons

Several studies with smaller groups and/or less experimental control have been reported. Wepman (1951) found that 68 aphasic patients, whose treatment had begun at least six months postonset, improved in grade level from 3.8 to 9.1. Fourteen cases reported by Broida (1977), where treatment was started at least 12 months postonset, improved an average of 10 overall percentile points

TABLE 11.10 Characteristics of the large studies of treatment efficacy.

INVESTIGATORS	LOCATION	GROUP COMPARISON	INITIATION (POST ONSET)	INTENSITY AND DURATION
Vignolo and Basso	Italy	stimulation no treatment	within 2 months 2–6 months after 6 months	
Shewan and Kertesz	Canada	language-oriented stimulation unstructured support no treatment	1 month	3 hours/week 52 weeks
Poeck, Huber and Willmes	Germany	language-oriented no treatment	1 month 4 months	9 hours/week 6–8 weeks
Wertz and many others	USA	individual group	1 month	8 hours/week 44 weeks
Wertz and many others	USA	professional volunteer	7 weeks	8–10 hours/week 12 weeks

on the PICA. Three patients improved as much as 19 and 22 points. Hagen (1973) compared treated and untreated groups in a study that "commenced when all subjects were discharged from the physical rehabilitation program six months post-onset" (p. 456). The treated group had substantial progress in language functions for which the untreated group had no improvement. Other investigators have found impressive progress in patients whose treatment was not started until four to seven months after onset (Butfield and Zangwill, 1946; Deal and Deal, 1978).

Holland (1980b) bumped into some data pertaining to treatment efficacy during standardization of the CADL. Twenty-eight subjects were retested at intervals varying from eight to 15 months, and the first test was given no sooner than four months postonset. Many patients improved in their test scores. Thirteen receiving treatment had significantly more improvement than the 15 who did not receive treatment. The groups turned out to be comparable in several prognostic factors. This "post hoc" study had its weaknesses; but if Holland had not known the basic principles of designing efficacy research, then she would not have recognized her accidental study.

Studies Showing No Effect

Two group studies indicated that treatment has little effect. A study by Sarno, Silverman, and Sands (1970) has been trotted out in support of opinions that aphasia therapy is of little value. Their comparison of treated and untreated groups consisted of patients who were severely impaired at 27-to-41 months postonset. Therefore, the study was restricted to a particular group with a poor prognosis and to a period after stroke when treatment is not usually provided.

Another study stirred some controversy. Lincoln and her colleagues (1984) tried to randomly assign patients to treated and untreated groups. From a pool of 327 at six weeks postonset, patients were assigned to one of the two groups. The treated group was to receive two hours of therapy per week for 24 weeks for a total of 48 hours of treatment. There was no difference between groups at the end of the study period, over eight months postonset.

Several speech-language pathologists published a letter in *Asha* magazine expressing serious reservations about Lincoln's study (Wertz, Deal, Holland, Kurtzke, and Weiss, 1986). For example, there were no criteria to ensure that patients had aphasia. There was no evidence that subject assignment produced matched groups, a possibility weakened by 134 drop outs over four weeks before the study began. After the study began, about 74 percent of the treated subjects dropped out at some point. The two hours of therapy per week were considered to be "minimal" for most clinics, and only a few subjects actually received the full 48 hours of therapy. The letter concluded that "when one does not treat patients who may or may not be aphasic, those patients do not improve" (p. 31).

Robey's Meta-Analysis

At the University of Virginia, Randall Robey (1998) has analyzed group studies of efficacy with a technique called meta-analysis. It is "a mathematical means for synthesizing independent research findings scattered throughout a body of literature" (p. 173). In a tutorial, Robey and Dalebout (1998) advised that "science requires converging evidence from all independent experiments as the basis for a compelling conclusion" (p. 1227). They suggested that "thoughtful reviews of salient literature" are insufficient for this purpose. A meta-analysis of independent experiments determines the *weight of scientific evidence* bearing on a research hypothesis.

Robey's first report dealt with 21 studies and addressed general questions about efficacy. The study showed that recovery of treated patients was nearly twice the recovery of untreated patients when treatment was begun during the acute period. There was a smaller effect favoring treated subjects when treatment was started after the acute period. The requirements of meta-analysis dictated that more studies had to be found to address more specific questions about amount and type of treatment.

A more recent analysis included 55 studies, and Robey (1998) replicated the results of the smaller study. Focusing on amount of treatment, the strongest effects occurred for moderate amounts started in the acute or post-acute periods (i.e., 2–3 hours/week) in comparison to low (i.e., less than 1.5 hours/week) and high amounts (i.e., more than 5 hours/week). In an attempt to compare types of treatment, Robey noted that the most frequently reported type was "not specified," and most specified types were not studied often enough to meet statistical requirements for comparison. Regarding severity of aphasia, it was especially telling that no study examined mild aphasia explicitly. Severe and moderate aphasia had strong treatment effects in the acute stage.

Limitations of Group Efficacy Research

Robey (1998) concluded that the group investigations substantiate the value of standard treatments for aphasic people in general. Few studies have been replicated and, "as a result, many outcomes are singular observations and practically independent of all others" (p. 183). For more specific information, the research has shown mainly that intensive individual treatment does not differ greatly from intensive group treatment (Wertz, et al., 1981) and that two similar language treatments administered by a speech-language pathologist are equally effective with respect to clinical tests of language ability (Shewan and Kertesz, 1984).

Group studies have high hurdles to overcome. The main challenge lies in establishing a no-treatment control group that is comparable to a treated group. Self-selected groups (i.e., according to subject choice, not random assignment) run the risk that "the characteristics causing a subject to be assigned to a no-treatment group may also affect how they perform on the measures used to assess the effects of treatment" (Brookshire, 1994, p. 7). In addition, the treatments studied may not be typical of current clinical practice. Robey (1998) was concerned about the failure to report information. For example, "an ambiguous or absent description of a treatment protocol under test is a troubling matter" (p. 183).

Robey concluded that the basic issue regarding treatment efficacy has been settled and that resources should now be directed toward answering more specific questions. He suggested that future studies establish a criterion for meaningful or beneficial change. Clinicians have turned to single-case experimental designs as one means of answering the more specific questions (see Chapter 13), and a recent meta-analysis indicated that treatment effects are large in the published studies (Robey, Schultz, Crawford, and Sinner, 1999).

MANAGED CARE

The health care system in the United States is driven by the desire to provide maximum benefit at minimal cost. Health care professions have provided input to this system with information about the amount and type of services needed to achieve maximum benefits.

Where the government pays for health care, rehabilitative services can extend for a longer period than what is most likely to occur in the United States. In Belgium, the duration of "legally reimbursed" therapy "does not exceed 2 years" (Seron and de Partz, 1993). At the Brussels Neuropsychological Rehabilitation Unit, an initial evaluation often takes one to two months and consists of the cognitive neuropsychological "case study" approach described in previous chapters. We should keep this perspective in mind as we examine some of the innovative programs that appear to have room to develop in Canada and other countries (see Chapter 12).

Reimbursement

Managed care has transformed reimbursement for medical and rehabilitative services in the United States. We have become familiar with the **health maintenance organization** (HMO), which is a private insurance plan that contracts with a medical group or groups to provide a full range of health care services to enrollees who pay a fixed monthly fee. A medical group tends to be a **preferred provider organization** (PPO), which is a network of health professionals approved by an HMO to provide services to plan members at a discount. One early development was the use of **diagnosis-related groups** (DRGs) as a basis for reimbursement. DRGs is a classification of hosptial in-patients with implications for likely utilization of resources. Table 11.11 presents basic terminology regarding reimbursement.

Medicare is an insurance program provided by the United States government for persons over age 65. The program consists of two parts.

- **Part A** provides necessary inpatient medical services within the first 90 days in a hosptial and first 100 days in a skilled nursing facility (SNF). Reimbursement is guided by DRGs. Now a hospital receives a single payment per-patient.
- **Part B** pays for subsequent physician-prescribed services in a hosptial, clinic, or at home. A clinician submits a short certification form to the physician, noting planned visits per week and an anticipated maximum duration of treatment. Certification also requires a brief statement of short-term goals that are within a patient's immediate grasp and long-term goals for the duration requested.

The Balanced Budget Act of 1997 changed Medicare reimbursement dramatically. For Part B, the significant change was the introduction of

TABLE 11.11 Terminology for reimbursement in managed care.

TERM	DEFINITION
co-payment	additional fee for a service paid by insurance plan members
prospective payment system (PPS)	payment determined before provision of services, rather than the former *retrospective payment* following services
fee-for-service	payment for each service provided (discouraged in managed care)
capitation (CAP)	payment per-person; fixed monthly payment for all medical care of an individual (encouraged in managed care)

an annual $1500 cap on services per patient. One cap is to be shared by speech-language pathology and physical therapy, while occupational therapy has its own $1500 cap. The cap applies to inpatient rehabilitation, rehabilitation centers, and home health agencies. It does not apply to outpatient clinics in hospitals. Of course, this situation may be temporary because of ongoing campaigns to remove caps and restore funding.

A new "clinically driven" prospective payment system (PPS) is being implemented in SNFs, according to Susan Boswell for the *ASHA Leader*. Reimbursement is computed based on a series of steps:

- Minimum Data Set (MDS): assessments by 5, 14, and 30 days post admission; every 30 days thereafter
- Resource Utilization Group (RUG): from MDS, patients classified according to intensity of therapy needed
- Payment Per Patient Day: conversion of RUG categories into per diem payment rate
- Resident Assessment Protocols (RAP): added assessment by day 5 or 14 as the basis for treatment plan

The amount that a SNF is reimbursed depends mainly on a patient's RUG category. A patient may be classified for a low intensity of rehabilitation or an "ultra high" level of intensity (Davolt, 1998).

Influence on Aphasia Treatment

Clinical objectives have become increasingly reimbursement-driven. Inpatient care in the acute and subacute phases consists of a combination of language restoration and compensatory procedures to facilitate communication as soon as possible (Boyle, 1994). Regarding subsequent outpatient settings, Elman (1994) noted that "it is not unusual to receive a treatment authorization for only six language therapy sessions to rehabilitate someone with aphasia" (p. 10). This restriction may or may not come after the patient has received language treatment at an inpatient facility.

Any limitation on number of sessions forces speech-language pathologist to be maximally efficient. Initial evaluation is relatively brief (e.g., 30 minutes), with more evaluation being integrated into treatment as "diagnostic therapy." For treatment, the following adjustments are made to the traditional practice of focusing on direct language stimulation for a long period of time:

- making direct language treatment as functional as possible
- instituting compensatory communicative strategies quickly
- training the family or volunteers to conduct language treatment at a patient's home
- involving trained volunteers to facilitate communication in real-life settings

These adjustments are the principal topics of the next chapter. For now, let us consider one of these practices as it has been employed for the goal of restoring as much language function as possible.

Several investigators have explored the value of volunteers for providing language stimulation. The VA cooperative study indicated that a trained spouse or friend can conduct effective treatment at home (Marshall, Wertz, Weiss, et al., 1989). Other studies found no difference in progress when treatment was provided by professionals and volunteers (David, Enderby, and Bainton, 1982; Meikle, Wechsler, Tupper, Benenson, Butler, Mulhall, and Stern, 1979; Quinteros, Williams, White, and Pickering, 1984). Professionals performed all evaluations and trained the volunteers, indicating that volunteers may be helpful when they are under the direction of a speech-language pathologist.

Ethical Practice

The Code of Ethics of the American Speech-Language-Hearing Association addresses the following:

- providing services with the appropriate clinical certifications
- maintaining adequate records of professional services

- engaging in any form of dishonest practice or misrepresentation of services or outcomes

Minimal documentation includes the basis for diagnosis and ongoing records of treatment objectives, procedures, and measures of progress. Possible misrepresentation includes diagnosis of a nonaphasic cognitive impairment as aphasia, prediction of recovery for a patient with progressive disease, and documentation of progress when there has been no progress.

Beauchamp and Childress (1994) help us identify fundamental ethical issues, based on a construct developed in the 1970s by a national commission for the protection of human subjects (also, Strand, 1995). Conflicts can arise between three legitimate considerations identified in Table 11.12. Regarding patients' autonomy, they have "a common law right to choose what care they will or will not accept" (Mariner, 1994, p. 43). A corollary to the clinician's beneficence or desire to "do good" is the need to prevent harm, called *nonmaleficence.* Third, there is society's need for justice or fairness in distribution of services given limited resources. Conflicts can be minimized by conducting a clinical practice with integrity and by following ASLHA's code of ethics.

PATIENT-ORIENTED DECISIONS

This section reviews common decisions regarding the goal of restoring language functions. We shall see how some of the basic principles in this chapter were applied in the subacute (or post-acute) phase of Martin Exeter's language rehabilitation. As indicated before, he was referred to the Rehabilitation Unit from the Stroke Unit providing acute care. The clinician followed the stimulation approach in which "treatment focuses on reactivating or restimulating language processes, rather than on teaching specific responses" (Brookshire, 1997, p. 249).

Patient Selection

The decision to provide inpatient language treatment is based on the likelihood that treatment will be beneficial in conjunction with the patient's ability to pay. The likelihood of beneficial treatment is related to many factors such as motivation and health as well as severity of language impairment. Ability to pay includes whether the patient has insurance or is eligible for Medicare. Medicare has a history of approving some trial treatment for any patient. Whether a clinic receives

TABLE 11.12 Framework for discussing ethical issues and conflicts.

COMPONENT	DEFINITION	POTENTIAL CONFLICT
patient's autonomy	or "respect for persons"; the right of an individual for self-determination	*patient vs. clinician:* a patient does not want therapy that a clinician thinks is needed
professional's beneficence	the desire to contribute to another person's welfare and protect another from harm	*clinician vs. patient:* a clinician prescribes a communication board that a family member refuses to acknowledge
social justice	fairness in distribution of services given limited resources (third-party considerations)	*clinician vs. third-party:* a speech-language pathologist prescribes care that a third-party is unwilling to pay for
		third-party vs. clinician: a third-party pays for services that are inappropriate or unnecessary

continued payment for improving patients depends partly on judicious selection of patients.

Martin had several factors going for him. He had suffered a focal infarction with some immediate spontaneous recovery. He was relatively young at age 55 and in good health besides his stroke. He was oriented to his surroundings and quite aware of his deficits. He was highly motivated and had a supportive family willing to participate in treatment.

Let us consider some of factors that might work against a decision to recommend a full treatment program:

- an aphasic patient may be unlikely to improve due to etiology, such as a progressive neuropathology.
- aphasia may be too severe to warrant the expense of individualized linguistic therapeutics that, so far, have been shown to have little effect on communicative ability.
- an aphasic person may have too many complicating conditions; for example, a patient may be too sick to muster the energy or desire for the effort that language therapy entails; also, a patient may have a dementia or psychological problems that would interfere with typical language therapy.
- mildly impaired patients may not need therapy considering their circumstances and motivation; however, others with subtle disorders have linguistically demanding lives, and work on the slightest impairment may have dramatic consequences for them.

When to Begin

Martin's treatment began around a week after his stroke. There have been differing opinions regarding the best time to begin individualized treatment. Wepman (1972) worried about adverse psychological reaction to intensive therapy during the acute (and subacute) period and recommended delaying language treatment until the chronic aphasic impairment becomes evident. He argued that a clinician should provide only "a supportive psychological role" during the emotionally delicate acute phase. On the other hand, Eisenson (1984) insisted that language therapy begin "as soon as the patient is able to take notice of what is going on and is able to cooperate in the effort" (p. 180). A neurologist agreed and wrote, "I believe that the therapy should be as intensive as the general medical situation will allow" (Rubens, 1977b, p. 1).

Some research addresses the question of whether starting time makes a difference in the efficacy of treatment. We know that a patient often makes much greater progress during the first two or three months than the next three months. An argument can be made that treatment is most effective while the brain is adjusting during the period of spontaneous recovery. In Robey's (1998) meta-analysis of 55 studies, treatment was found to be effective when started in the acute period (i.e., under 3 months postonset), post-acute period (i.e., 3–12 months), and chronic period (i.e., 12 months or later). The magnitude of effect decreased over time, leading Robey to conclude that "aphasic individuals should receive treatment as early in their recoveries as is possible" (p. 181).

Goals and Task Selection

Because Martin had a variety of interests, the subacute treatment was designed to improve all modalities. The clinician worked on auditory comprehension and verbal expression to enhance his independence in conversation. Reading and writing were also targeted because of Martin's vocational needs for these skills. He also enjoyed reading and writing. The following goals were established, based partly on initial test performance (see Figure 3.5):

- *improve paragraph comprehension from 5/12 to 10/12*
- *increase number of words and phrase-length in conversation about family and work*
- *improve sentence-level reading*
- *increase written naming from 2/10 to 7/10*

Treatment was established to be consistent with objectives but also to be conducted at a level that was likely to be successful. The clinician also considered semantic content that would be functional and interesting. Martin's wife extended two of the exercises by administering tasks at home. The initial lesson plan is sketched in Table 11.13.

The Treatment Session

Each session has a beginning, middle, and end. Brookshire (1997) divided a session into five segments shown in Table 11.14. For an hour session, a clinician may plan to begin with a warm-up period and conduct three or four tasks to take 40 minutes. In Martin's sessions, the clinician usually had time to work in three of the four major areas of the plan. As a result, each session was a little different from the previous one. Occasionally the "cool-down" period was used for generalization probes.

A speech-language pathologist also plans to be flexible. In addition to bringing prepared materials, the clinician is likely to have blank cards and a pen for creating new materials when a surprise topic arises or when a sudden shift in stimulus difficulty is needed. If a patient is having a "bad day," the clinician may shift treatment to a lower level.

On some days a patient may just want to talk, and a clinician may want to be sympathetic to the patient's desire. However, the clinician has to make a judgment as to whether listening for a while is necessary for achieving successful stimulation on that day. The patient may need to vent, which should clear the air to resume treatment. In general, the clinician needs to manage valuable treatment time by gently steering the patient into planned activities.

SUMMARY AND CONCLUSIONS

Treatment for aphasic impairment begins with an assessment to determine a patient's language problems and areas in which stimulation may address these problems. An impairment is translated into a goal. For example, if a patient is impaired in word-finding, then a goal is to improve word-finding. A behavioral version of this goal would be to increase number of accurate spoken naming responses to pictured objects (keeping in mind that other tasks can be used to exercise word-finding). During assessment, a clinician may learn that word-finding can be stimulated with a cue or by imitation. This is where treatment of word-finding might begin.

TABLE 11.13 Martin Exeter's first treatment plan.

BEHAVIORAL GOAL	TREATMENT PROCEDURE	GENERALIZATION PROBE
improve discourse comprehension from 5/12 to 10/12	clinician reads aloud short paragraphs from newspapers, and Martin answers questions about them; homework includes newspaper reading with Jackie	BDAE paragragph comprehension task
increase number of words and phrase-length in conversation	speed naming drill; repetition drill for phrases of increasing length	word counts and phrase-length measure from regular conversations
improve sentence-level reading	clinician types sentences for verification about family and current events	clinical sentence reading test
increase written naming from 2/10 to 7/10	write names of family members from photos; phonemic cues provided initially; homework includes spelling correction and sentence completion	written naming of common objects

TABLE 11.14 Brookshire's (1997) segments of a treatment session.

SEGMENT	DESCRIPTION
hello	• conversation about what has happened since previous session
accommodation	• short warm-up period of easy or error-free tasks
work	• heart of session focused on treatment objectives
cool-down	• positive conclusion with easy or error-free tasks
goodbye	• conversation about the session and plans for next session

Tasks are chosen to stimulate the impaired process at a high level of response accuracy. A somewhat different task may be chosen to measure whether a general objective is being met and especially for measuring generalization from the treatment. For example, treatment may be a naming task in which stimuli are supplemented with various cues and fast responses are reinforced. The measurement may be a simple naming task without cues and feedback to see if the patient is improving in naming without therapeutic assistance. In general, a treatment should be open to flexible reaction to a patient's success and demeanor, whereas a generalization probe is inflexibly controlled to be reliable.

Meta-analyses of the studies of treatment efficacy indicate that there is sufficient investigation for us to conclude that language treatment makes a difference for aphasic patients. One warning is that the treatments examined in large group studies have been atypical with respect to the managed care environment in which patients receive less treatment than the subjects received in these investigations. One positive finding is that treatment can help aphasic individuals beyond 6 months postonset (e.g., Basso, et al., 1979; Shewan and Kertesz, 1984) and even beyond the first year (e.g., Broida, 1977; Poeck, et al., 1989). There is very little solid empirical support for the occasionally stated opinion that language treatment cannot make a difference for someone with aphasia.

Managed care has put limits on the amount of treatment. Currently we have no evidence to suggest that less treatment is less effective. Moreover, managed care has not forced a change in the fundamental principles that we follow in administering language treatment. Current therapy may actually be different from many of the formally studied therapies, partly because current therapy may be more functional. We consider functional modifications of treatment in the next chapter.

CHAPTER 12

FUNCTIONAL THERAPEUTICS AND OUTCOMES

This chapter examines therapeutics aimed at disability and handicap. Demands of the health care system for functional outcomes in a short period of time have motivated a functional approach to treatment of language disorders. Repairing linguistic impairment may address communicative disability only partially. We employ several strategies to improve communication, and they generally stem from the following goals:

- maximize use of residual linguistic capacities
- develop augmentative or alternative modes of communication
- maximize psychological and emotional adjustment to language impairment
- improve the role of partners and settings in facilitating communication

With respect to treatment at the level of handicap, many clinicians advocate that we have a role in helping the patient and family to recover as much of their former communicative life as possible. In a rehabilitation center, this role is coordinated through regular meetings of the rehabilitation team. This orientation has been expressed often in the literature by clinical aphasiologists in Europe, Canada, and universities in the United States. Changes in family roles and communicative dynamics are likely to have implications for generalization of a professional clinician's treatment. Reciprocally, success in linguistic and communicative treatment may encourage positive family adjustments.

However, other speech-language pathologists define and carry out their functions more narrowly. These clinicians may be working on a contract basis, traveling to multiple skilled nursing facilities. Thus, they spend relatively little time in any one location. They focus on direct speech and language stimulation, and they have little opportunity to coordinate with other members of the rehabilitation team and with members of a resident's family. These clinicians may approve of parts of this chapter, and then they do the best they can.

BRIDGING THE CLINICAL-FUNCTIONAL GAP

Jeffrey Metter (1986), a neurologist, wrote a letter to *Asha* magazine in which he referred to a paradox between documentation of a patient's improvement in clinical tasks and his observation of no progress when conversing with the patient. The clinician observed acquisition, but Metter did not observe generalization. This distinction between clinical progress and functional progress has frustrated many clinicians. Long before managed care, we wanted to figure out ways to transfer progress in clinical tasks to a patient's daily life.

At least, we want to see the progress in a treatment generalize to different materials used in the same activity. However, simple stimulus and response generalization has been limited with some of the treatments presented in Chapters 11 and 13. A study of naming therapy by Thompson and Kearns (1981) produced good news and bad news. The good news was that treatment had an effect on behavior. The bad news was that progress with a small list of words used in therapy was not transferring to very similar lists of words not being used in therapy. It seemed that the treatment used in the study would have to be applied to every word the patient might use in daily life.

One reason for Metter's observation may be extreme differences between the standard treatment setting and real-life communicative situations. Clinical settings contain minimal distraction. Patients interact with supportive people who know what aphasia is. Following principles advocated in Chapter 11, repetitive drills are designed to undercut deficits and stimulate success. On the other hand, real-life presents a rough road of communicative potholes for someone with language impairment. This difference might be called the "clinical-functional gap."

Looking across the gap, Busch (1993) recommended three broad functional goals that would be acceptable to Medicare:

- The patient will communicate basic physical needs and emotional status.
- The patient will engage in social communicative interactions with immediate family or friends.
- The patient will carry out communicative interactions in the community.

These goals are oriented to stimulus generalization. That is, we want to see a patient produce formally trained key phrases whenever a physical need arises. We want to see a patient produce behaviors in the presence of family that had been practiced with a clinician.

It has been said that clinicians would "train and hope" that clinical progress would transfer to a client's daily life (Thompson, 1989). Hope can be replaced by a bridge across the clinical-functional gap. In principle, the bridge can be built by **programming for generalization.** The steps of this programming are forged by changing stimulus conditions and response expectations in the direction of modeling real-life communicative problems. For this transition, we have used group therapies or have introduced tasks that seem important to a patient's daily life (e.g., Aten, 1986). However, Brookshire (1997) suggested that "many do not pursue generalization in a systematic way" (p. 235).

Closing the gap systematically is accomplished by bringing attributes of natural situations into the clinic and by moving the patient somewhat gradually into situations outside of the clinic. This approach has also been applied to rehabilitation for head injury: "For those who are making the transition to a home setting, guidelines establishing routines for spontaneous real-life situations should be developed and implemented prior to returning to independent living" (Starch and Falltrick, 1990, p. 28). In the words of Simmons-Mackie and Damico (1997), we make clinical conditions more "authentic."

Especially for severely impaired patients, it may be valuable to begin with standard direct procedures, focusing on a specific process in a situation free of anxiety and distraction. A patient may need to become comfortable with an awkward nonverbal strategy before trying it outside the clinic. Later, the clinic can become more natural by encouraging the patient to deal with communicative failures. For example, a mid-stage of treatment for people with CHI involves increasing "frustration tolerance" (Ylvisaker and Szekeres, 1986).

In general, functional programming involves making adjustments in **contextual variables** as well as linguistic variables. Table 12.1 is organized according to hypothetical steps for closing the clinical-functional gap (e.g., Bellaire, Georges, and Thompson, 1991). In reality, however, Table 12.1 is more of a menu of options for functional treatment, rather than a literal sequence of steps. The number of sessions allotted under managed care in the United States may not permit us to proceed according to the logic of stepwise programming. Treatment may move down the list quickly or may skip options by involving family members and entering real-life settings after a few sessions. Later, this chapter presents various ways in which this work has been done.

FUNCTIONAL STIMULATION

Our patients still want to improve the operation of impaired language processes. Maintaining this traditional objective, standard treatment exercises can be more functional than might have been

TABLE 12.1 Contextual variables to consider in generalization training.

STAGE OF TREATMENT	CONTEXTUAL VARIABLE	EXAMPLES
Direct training	world knowledge	name photos of family members
	environment (props)	read phone book sports box scores
Generalization training	form of interaction	conversational interaction
	purpose	role-play phoning family member buying plane ticket
	people	interactive activity with spouse volunteer
	setting (at clinic)	role-play shopping with props or in a hospital store
	setting (at home)	shop at grocery in neighborhood

indicated in Chapter 11. We may think of it as "functional repair."

Functional repair begins with the goal of maximizing the likelihood of stimulus and response generalization. That is, if a patient is failing to progress with stimuli and responses not specifically exercised in treatment, then no progress will be seen in Dr. Metter's office or at a patient's home. Brookshire's principle of aiming treatment at a process rather than a specific word or sentence is an essential first step in creating conditions that can achieve some degree of generalization. If word-finding is genuinely improved, then the use of language should be better in a number of circumstances and with a wide variety of words.

In her review of generalization research, Thompson (1989) concluded that four features of treatment should maximize the possibility of transfer:

- a sufficient number of training responses
- a sufficient number of training conditions
- activities that incorporate aspects of the generalization environment
- strategies for mediating generalization

In the single-subject experiments that did not show much generalization, treatment tended to have the behavioral orientation of drilling a small sample of language with one task.

Brookshire (1997) collapsed Thompson's suggestions under the notion of **training sufficient exemplars.** For one thing, this means training a wide variety of words within a semantic category. Instead of naming five foods, a patient practices naming 20 or 30 foods. It also means training a behavior in a variety of stimulus conditions; and, according to this principle, flexibility extends to participants in an interaction and settings in a rehabilitation center. Behaviorally oriented clinicians began to present varied stimuli to elicit a particular response and accept varied responses to a particular stimulus as a strategy of "loose training" (see RET in Chapter 13).

Once we loosen our stimulation activities, we enhance functionality by molding semantic content according to a patient's world and interests. Standard or commercial materials are constructed to be familiar or appropriate for the greatest number of people. Their functionality stems from being objects and events that are common in the activities of daily living. Yet, content may also be selected to be personally relevant. What does the patient like to talk about? We can conduct "contextual inventories" to find out the unique content of a patient's life (Simmons-Mackie and Damico, 1996).

Personally relevant content is often chosen the first day of treatment. Wallace and Canter (1985) compared personal and nonpersonal content for severely aphasic persons. Personal content was defined as items pertaining to self and the immediate environment. The comparison was made for auditory comprehension (e.g., *Is your birthday in December?* vs. *Is Christmas in December?*), reading comprehension, repetition of nouns, and naming object-drawings (e.g., *television* vs. *chicken*). The investigators found that personally relevant material was easier to understand than nonpersonal content.

Our contextual inventories should also reveal activities that are common in a patient's daily life. Then, we may do a **functional analysis** of targeted situations (e.g., restaurant, airport, bridge club, sporting events). What are the basic language functions used in these situations? A situation may require some reading, some talking, or some writing. Rather than stimulating reading or writing according to a general program, stimulation could be planned to correspond to the linguistic level, semantic content, and purpose of an everyday situation or a situation that is personally relevant to the patient (e.g., Parr, 1992, 1996). Reading the phone book or street signs is functional. Reading playing cards or the box scores may be interesting. In general, we should let the patient, not a clinician's comfort, motivate the content and activity of treatment.

COMPENSATORY BEHAVIORS

Nonverbal modalities can be supplements to fragmentary or vague speaking or alternatives for patients with intractable expressive impairment. Severity of aphasia motivates us to attempt training alternative modes directly following principles of elicitation and programming applied to verbal behavior. Many modes and systems have been tried (Kraat, 1990; Silverman, 1989), sometimes with patients whose aphasia was questionable but who still needed a mode of communication.

Communication Boards

Communication boards are often introduced early for patients with severe motor speech disorders, especially for those without linguistic or other cognitive deficits. The boards provide a means of communicating until speech or writing become functional. With minimal language impairment, words and phrases can be used freely without pictures or symbols. Pointing to letters provides flexibility for forming any word or phrase, but it is much slower. Some clinicians, however, delay use of communication boards because of a belief that they decrease motivation to speak.

Severely aphasic patients may rely more on pictures for basic needs that cannot be readily expressed by pointing or natural gesturing (Collins, 1986). Severely nonfluent patients may have enough comprehension for pointing to words. Patients with more severe comprehension deficits require some training in the use of simple printed material. In the Netherlands, Visch-Brink and others (1993) train patients to use a "Language Pocket Book," which consists of word lists and pictures organized by category or situation. Part of the training includes work on conceptualization such as sorting words into functional categories. Any patient along with frequent communication partners may need some practice in the functional use of boards or notebooks.

Bellaire and others (1991) studied acquisition and generalization of communication board use for two patients with Broca's aphasia. The boards contained 15 line drawings of items for a coffee hour, such as social greetings, requesting food, and providing personal information. Individual treatment involved responding to requests from a clinician. Generalization training began with role-playing coffee hour situations in individual sessions, and, in the next phase, the clinician accompanied the patient to the social hour. The patients acquired requests and personal information responses but did not readily generalize use of the boards to the social setting. Instead, patients relied on vocalization or head nods that had been used before training. The investigators suggested that communication boards may be more useful for individualized content that cannot be easily expressed through natural gesturing.

Pointing behavior is a valuable communicative tool, and some real-life settings may be more communicatively accessible than others. Menus are communication boards. For ordering in a restaurant, one need only read and point to an item on the menu. Some menus have many pictures of the food. Major stores have catalogues. At home, a patient can tear out pages as a shopping list and use them for asking about the location of a product. Bus stations and travel agencies have brochures. Functional analysis of a situation includes identifying compensatory materials and strategies that are accessible in the situation.

Gesturing and Drawing

As indicated in Chapter 7, many aphasic persons retain a capacity for gesture and drawing, whereas others are impaired. Use of these modes for communication depends on their intelligibility when they are impaired and a patient's willingness to use them. Patients with Broca's aphasia may spontaneously use more gesture than usual. Those with Wernicke's aphasia gesture the way they talk and may require some training if they are to clarify some of their spontaneous gestures (Le May, et al., 1988; Smith, 1987).

Training has been designed for pantomimic gesture (e.g., Coelho and Duffy, 1990). **Visual Action Therapy** (VAT) takes a patient through several steps involving object manipulation to train the use of pantominic gestures (Helm-Estabrooks, Fitzpatrick, and Barresi, 1982). The program begins with matching tasks for perception and recognition of objects and proceeds to gesturing of function with the object in hand and then without the object.

If a pantomime is to replace speech as a communicative mode, it should be reasonably intelligible. Flowers and Wyse (1985) examined intelligibility of pantomimes produced by normal adults who used only their nonpreferred hand. A receiver, familiar to the sender, wrote the name of an object that was demonstrated. Subjects' gesturing was highly variable, with a 46 to 91 percent level of transparency to receivers outside of a natural situation. Like playing charades, clear pantomiming does not come naturally; but the forced-choice method probably functions like a natural situation that narrows the possible meanings. In data available for the Duffys' referential abilities test, four normal subjects were 97 percent accurate (Duffy, et al., 1984).

Drawing may be attempted long postonset after traditional language treatments prove to be unsuccessful (e.g. Rao, 1995). There have been a few reports of training (Lyon, 1995a). Morgan and Helm-Estabrooks (1987) instituted "Back to the Drawing Board" with two cases of nonfluent aphasia who copied cartoons of increasing complexity. Lyon and Sims (1989) trained "expressively restricted" patients with a wide range of overall severity of aphasia. For three months, the patients were given a cued training program. Then, transfer to communicative use was encouraged with an interactive procedure. The patients improved as a group. Holland (1995) tried to teach drawing to patients with Broca's, Wernicke's, and conduction aphasia. She encouraged self-motivated used of natural drawing abilities; but, blaming her own poor drawing skills, Holland concluded that her attempts were "notably unsuccessful."

Gestural Codes

At one time, Amer-Ind Code was enticing because it is descriptive of referents and can be used with one hand (Skelly, 1979). The iconicity of Amer-Ind and American Sign Language (ASL) has been examined according to their transparency, namely, the extent to which someone unfamiliar with the code can guess a gesture's meaning. Amer-Ind was 54 percent guessable, and ASL was 10 to 30 percent guessable (Daniloff, Lloyd, and Fristoe, 1983). From reports on training patients to use Amer-Ind, Skelly (1979) concluded that "there was almost universal dissatisfaction expressed concerning transfer from the cued retrieval/replicative stage to self-initiated use" (p. 40).

Coelho and Duffy (1987) studied acquisition of 23 Amer-Ind signs and 14 fabricated signs. Their training method had steps for imitation, recognition, and "naming" with each gesture. The goal for the study was to develop an ability to name referents. Generalization was measured with respect to naming untrained pictures with trained gestures. The ability to acquire these signs was negligible for patients below the 35th percentile on the PICA. Those above this level increased their ability to acquire and generalize signs as a linear function of severity of aphasia.

Later, Coelho (1990) attempted training selected Amer-Ind and ASL signs. Two of his four patients were below the 35th percentile. Stages of treatment led to varying the agent (i.e., *man, woman*) with two verbs (i.e., *cook, eat*) and eight objects (e.g., *tomato, fish, egg*). Coelho concluded that "the production of sign combinations from previously acquired single signs does not occur spontaneously—that is, without training—and that even with training, at least within the context of the present experiment, the maintenance effect is weak" (p. 399). Later in the chapter, Coelho's programmed generalization to natural settings will be presented.

Blissymbols, a system of pictograms, was presented to four patients with global aphasia (Johannsen-Hornbach, Cegla, Mager, Schempp, and Wallesch, 1985). Two patients interacted with the clinician using these symbols, and one of these patients used the system on a limited basis living with his mother. Another patient progressed enough in speaking so that Blissymbols became unnecessary (also, Funnell and Allport, 1989). Koul and Lloyd (1998) compared symbol learning by patients with "moderate global" aphasia and RHD. The training involved pointing to choices of Blissymbols in response to a spoken name. Aphasic patients were equivalent to normal controls in learning the associated pairs, whereas the RHDs recognized fewer symbols. The potential for using pictured symbols with severe aphasia is explored further in the next chapter.

Patients with traumatic brain injury have been trained in pantomimic gesture and Blissymbols (e.g, Coelho, 1987). Clinicians have reported acquisition of abilities in clinical tasks but have not reported convincing transfer to real-life communication (Kraat, 1990).

Purdy, Duffy, and Coelho (1994) trained 15 nonfluent patients in responding with a communication board and gestural symbols. They found that the patients did not use as many gestures in a structured conversation task as they used in direct training, and patients continued to prefer verbal over nonverbal response. Nevertheless, the investigators were particularly interested in whether the patients would spontaneously switch to one modality when an attempt with another modality failed. Patients switched modalities only 39 percent of the time, but they were successful in conveying messages 73 percent of the time when they did switch.

Contrary to the belief that gesturing inhibits speaking, gesturing may draw out verbalization when other methods fail. In one study, a gesture was paired with naming, but naming was better with gesture for nonfluent subjects, not fluent subjects (Hanlon, Brown, and Gerstman, 1990). Rosenbek and his colleagues (1989) stated that "our assumption is that verbal expression can be improved by the appropriate pairing of performances or with the systematic use of unique sensory inputs" (p. 218). The first step of training is to teach gesture recognition. The next step involves modeling a gesture and word for imitation. If a patient should spontaneously start talking while gesturing, it is likely that the patient can benefit from other treatments for language production. The challenge is to maintain the verbal response after the gesture is faded.

Adaptive Language Strategies

There is more than one way to convey a meaning or message linguistically. In principle, when an aphasic person has difficulty constructing one linguistic form to convey an idea, another linguistic form might be attempted to convey the same general idea. Positive symptoms are indicative of spared language skills that can serve as adaptive mechanisms for conveying a message. Holland (1978) argued that it is okay for a patient to be "in the ball park, rather than pitching a verbal no-hitter."

Residual language capacities are most evident in anomic and Broca's aphasias. Patients with either type of aphasia tend to make adjustments automatically without intervention. Someone with anomic aphasia uses sentence production ability to produce circumlocutions around words that cannot be found at the moment. People with agrammatic aphasia access semantic and lexical stores to produce structurally simplified versions of an idea. Thus, saying "girl tall and boy short" is pretty close to saying that the girl is taller than the boy. The clinician's job is to reinforce meaningful circumlocution and simplification. The clinician avoids inhibiting communication by forcing a patient to shut down crucial subsystems of language production.

INTERACTIVE THERAPIES

One step toward natural communicative conditions is to modify clinical interaction to conform to the structure of conversation. For aphasic patients, a clinician does not have to train conversational structure per se. Instead, a more natural interactive structure is an opportunity to apply communicative modalities and strategies that have been practiced in direct training. Also, patients may increase confidence in their communicative abilities in a more natural interaction. Conversation is a collaboration between partners. A patient may come to realize that he or she does not have the sole responsibility for the success of communication (see Figure 1.2).

PACE

Interaction can be modified from the basic naming task to incorporate the features of face-to-face conversation. One strategy for doing this is called **Promoting Aphasics' Communicative Effectiveness** (Davis and Wilcox, 1985). Procedures follow four principles representing special features of conversation (Table 12.2). Any one principle may be applied in adjusting traditional tasks, but the four principles together make the interaction like conversation. PACE still is an artificial interaction which, in a progression from clinical to functional activities, falls short of real conversation.

TABLE 12.2 The four principles and essential procedures of Promoting Aphasics' Communicative Effectiveness (Davis and Wilcox, 1985).

PACE
1. **The clinician and patient exchange new information.** Instead of having a picture of an object or event (called the message) in simultaneous view of the clinician and patient, a stack of message-stimuli is placed face down to keep messages from the view of a message receiver. A client selects a card and attempts to convey the message on the card. The *Brussels modification* is to place a screen about eight inches or 20 centimeters high between the patient and clinician, and the message receiver chooses the message from options (Clerebaut, Coyette, Feyereisen, and Seron, 1984).
2. **The clinician and patient participate equally as senders and receivers of messages.** This principle puts the turn-taking feature of conversation into the interaction. The clinician and client simply alternate in drawing a card and sending messages.
3. **The patient has a free choice as to the communicative modes used to convey a message.** Contrary to training one modality such as gesture or drawing, the patient is left to choose the mode that is used for any message. We do not tell a client to perform in a particular way.
4. **The clinician's feedback as a receiver is based on the patient's success in conveying the message.** The new information condition should make this inevitable for both participants. Our feedback should let the client know if he or she got the idea across. If we already know the message, we should respond as if we did not know.

In the new information condition, a message sender need only convey what is necessary to get the idea across. Message-stimuli can be pictures of objects or events or anything else a clinician wants to try. Turn-taking takes us out of a directive role and places us on equal footing with the patient. Our turns as sender are opportunities for modeling communicative behaviors that a patient is capable of using but may not be choosing. We may use direct instruction to train a communicative modality such as gesture or drawing, but in PACE we allow a client to choose modalities. Modeling shows that gesture is a reasonable option for getting the idea across.

Also, the patient can practice a few skills that are unique to conversation. One is responsiveness to a listener's attempts to interpret what the patient is trying to convey. Another skill is responsiveness to communicative failure and the use of repair or revision in trying to get a message across.

Investigators either have used PACE and compared progress in different functions or have compared PACE with another procedure with respect to the same functions. After PACE therapy for eight patients, communicative abilities improved but not language skills according to standard language tests (Carlomagno, Losanno, Emanuelli, and Casadio, 1991). For a patient with conduction aphasia, PACE was compared with traditional stimulation for improving naming, and more progress in naming was shown during the PACE phases of treatment (Li, Kitselman, Dusatko, and Spinelli, 1988). Avent and others (1995) compared a sentence stimulation technique with a "PACE-like" procedure emphasizing nonspeech modes of picture description. Results were mixed among three aphasic patients, with one favoring the "nonverbal treatment," one favoring the "verbal treatment," and the other showing no difference.

Other studies dealt with the responsiveness of patients to a clinician's modeling. Glindemann and others (1991) examined the influence of modeling names or descriptions. Patients with mild aphasia were more likely than others to switch between names and descriptions as a function of what the clinician does as sender. Greitemann and Wolf (1991) found that modeling can have an influence across verbal and gestural modalities and that the use of speech does not necessarily disappear as gesture increases. Glindemann and Springer (1995) were unimpressed with the modeling function for severe aphasia and for training compensatory communicative behavior. They recommended systematic stepwise training for this purpose. However, modeling was intended primarily to help a patient become comfortable about choosing trained modalities, and Glindemann and Springer viewed PACE as an "enrichment" of traditional treatment that motivates patients to use all available communicative options.

Scripted Dialogues

Conversational coaching was developed by Holland (1991) who provides a patient with a short script written slightly too difficult for the patient to produce. The patient should be able to read aloud simple sentences, but a script may also be created with few words and a few pictures. The script incorporates communicative strategies that had been trained or suggested more directly. These strategies include "conversational management," such as asking a listener to slow down, to be discussed later in the chapter. The approach is another "bridging framework to initiate transfer of strategy use to patient-generated conversation" (p. 204).

First, the patient and clinician practice by following the script. The patient reads the script one sentence at a time. The clinician's job is to evaluate communicative effectiveness and suggest ways of conveying the information differently. The patient then may practice with another listener, often a family member. The clinician reminds the patient of strategies and sometimes coaches the listener (e.g., "If you don't understand, it's probably better to ask him to say it another way"). This activity is videotaped, and the participants get together to view and discuss it. The entire procedure may be repeated with a stranger as the listener.

Supported Conversation

In 1979 the wife of an aphasic person recognized a need for a program after discharge from therapy, and so she founded The Aphasia Centre-North York in Toronto (Kagan and Gailey, 1993). This community-based program is now named for her and is called the Pat Arato Aphasia Centre. Other community-based programs in Canada and elsewhere have been reported (e.g., Hoen, Thelander, and Worsley, 1997). In Australia, Hersh (1998) established a Talkback Group modeled after the Arato Centre. The Group provides free ongoing social interaction after patients are discharged from formal rehabilitation.

A normal atmosphere is fostered at the Arato Centre by referring to aphasic participants as "members" instead of patients or clients. The program has two phases. A 12-week introductory program is for educating members and their families, improving communication, and providing psychological support. Then a 16-week program offers conversation groups, music therapy, art classes, family/caregiver groups, and other options. Volunteers, such as students interested in a rehabilitation career, serve as conversation partners.

The communication intervention is called **supported conversation for adults with aphasia** (SCA), with a focus on severe language impairment (Kagan, 1998). SCA is based on the premise that working on the skills necessary for conversation, such as a PACE activity, is not the same as actually having an adult conversation. There are a couple other key assumptions:

- access to conversation is denied aphasic people because of a perceived lack of competence
- competence is revealed by a "communication ramp" (i.e., skilled partner) to conversation opportunities

Volunteers at the Arato Centre are trained in a workshop that includes an instructional video, role-playing, work with a group of members with severe aphasia, and an apprenticeship with experienced volunteers.

Table 12.3 contains reported characteristics of supported conversation. Kagan (1998) claimed that emphasis on "natural-sounding conversation ...differentiates the SCA approach from other similar-sounding approaches" (p. 820), although Kagan did identify these other approaches. Within

TABLE 12.3 Reported characteristics of supported conversation with severe aphasia (Kagan, 1998).

FEATURE	DETAIL
acknowledgment of competence	reinforce a member's capacities
	sound natural and adult
revealing competence	ensure that a member comprehends
	ensure that a member has a response mode
	verify a member's communicative attempt
simultaneous use of techniques	create natural flow and timing of modalities

this interactive atmosphere, aphasic members practice communicating by any means. Particular attention is given to an extensive manual of pictographs used to identify conversational topics and support getting a message across.

Holland (1998) was concerned that some clinicians are uncomfortable conversing with aphasic patients, and she detected a bias against conversation as a therapeutic medium. She asked "what relegates conversation to some sort of sleazy, shady, unreimbursable Neverland that must...follow the real goods—the therapy" (p. 845)? Chapter 7 indicated that conversation is often studied by interviewing patients. Thus, some clinicians who think they are engaged in real conversation are really engaged in something else. Holland (1998) stated that "interview models" emphasize a receiver function over a participant function, and she provided examples of the difference from a chat about "my most embarrassing moment" (p. 846):

- interview model: "Today we are going to talk about the most embarrassing thing that ever happened to us. Why not begin, Joe?"
- conversation: "You're not gonna believe what happened to me yesterday...Can you top this?'

PARTNERS AND SETTINGS

We also introduce an aphasic person's world into the therapeutic process. One goal is to extend generalization of clinical progress to natural circumstances. In this section, family members are discussed not with respect to doing traditional stimulation but, instead, with respect to their role in communicative interactions.

Role-Playing in the Clinic

Role-playing provides an opportunity to induce the use of varied speech acts such as advising, warning, and arguing. A situation is created in which conflict is likely. The clinician and patient proceed to disagree over what to have for dinner or over how much to spend for a vacation.

Family members can be a part of many settings; but other partners, such as a waitperson in a restaurant, are an integral part of a particular setting. Like people, settings influence language behavior in the extent to which they are familiar and demanding of the language processor. Driving a car involves reading simple signs quickly. After standing in line at the bank, we are expected to take care of business quickly.

One step before entering these settings is to recreate them in the clinic. Hospitals have cafeterias and shops. The occupational therapy department is likely to have a model living environment. The hospital may have a driving simulator. A few hospitals have a fairly expensive simulated world called "Easy Street Environments" (Simmons, 1989). They are replicas of common settings such as bank, grocery, restaurant, store, and a city street with a bus and a car.

Schlanger and Schlanger (1970) divided "simulated life situations" into nonstress situations such as planning a picnic and stressful situations such as going out to dinner. The stress situations could be pleasant (e.g., going out to dinner) or unpleasant (e.g., dealing with an emergency). In these activities, the client plays a role that would normally be assumed in these circumstances. For various situations, the clinician and patient begin to anticipate communicative problems and work together to figure out how a functional goal could be achieved with the patient's communicative resources.

A relatively minor shift in simple role-playing occurs when the clinician assumes the role of other persons in a communicative situation (e.g., a cab driver, a telephone operator, the minister, a waitperson in a restaurant). One characteristic of people in the community is their lack of knowledge of aphasia. By pretending to be ignorant of aphasia, the clinician can learn about the communicative failures that the patient is likely to face. Then, strategies for dealing with these failures can be developed.

In training two nonfluent patients to use symbolic gestures, Coelho (1991) first provided direct treatment in producing a gesture to a picture of a food item and then had the patient practice in Easy Street's restaurant. The clinician played the role of waiter, asking questions such as "What kind of sandwich would you like?" Probes for generalization included real waitresses asking similar questions in an actual restaurant. One patient generalized use of gestures to the natural setting, but a more severely impaired patient did not.

Hopper and Holland (1998) contrasted such **situation-specific training** with approaches, such as PACE, which are applicable to any situation. The investigators felt that managed care has moved treatment toward activities that establish functional independence in real-life tasks. They reported training two patients with Broca's aphasia to communicate over the phone in emergencies at home. Treatment consisted of the following three steps:

- describe a pictured emergency situation
- if the description was incorrect, answer *wh*-questions about components of the situation
- with the picture present, role-play the scenerio with the clinician asking "What is your emergency?"

Six pictured emergencies were trained, and four other pictures were used for a generalization probe. The patients improved over 10 sessions in responding to treated and untreated scenerios. Of course, success in communicating over the phone in a real emergency must be determined from interviews with family members.

Partners in the Clinic

Most of the previously cited approaches involve the clinician as communicative partner, but a patient's real-life partners can play a role in promoting generalization by coming into the clinic (e.g., Armstrong, 1993; Le Dorze, et al., 1993). Clinicians have found that PACE is a relatively easy activity for a spouse to slip into (e.g., Davis and Wilcox, 1986; Visch-Brink, et al., 1993). Familiar and unfamiliar listeners are an important part of Holland's (1991) Conversational Coaching.

Community Reintegration

Before going to a nearby restaurant with a group of clients, a woman with severe Broca's aphasia worked in a clinic on pointing to items on a menu as a means of ordering for herself. She pretended to order while a clinician gave her feedback. When the client got to the restaurant, she was stymied because the waitress was at the other end of the table listening for orders. While role playing might have anticipated the need to motion for the waitress to come over, there is no guarantee that role playing and other clinical activities will anticipate everything that happens in the real thing.

After training gestures for food items, Coelho (1991) concluded that "although the 'Easy Street' setting was useful as an intermediate step, it should not be used in place of true natural settings...There appear to be certain aspects of real-world settings that cannot be simulated, for example, conversations stopping, persons staring, waitresses' embarrassment, all as the aphasic individual struggles to communicate, and these need to be overcome by the aphasic patient for true generalization to occur" (p. 217).

How might resumption of activities be facilitated, especially when clinicians do not have time to accompany patients outside a rehabilitation center? Lyon (1992) established **Communication Partners** in which an adult volunteer from a patient's community "serves as the vehicle with which activities of the patient's choice are introduced, either at home or in the community where they naturally occur" (Lyon, Cariski, Keisler, Rosenbek, Levine, Kumpula, Ryff, Coyne, and Blanc, 1997, p. 694).

The program has two phases. The first occurs in the clinic for six weeks. Supervised by a speech-language pathologist, the volunteer and client become comfortable with each other in a variety of plausible situations. The volunteer practices several communicative strategies such as the following (Lyon, et al., 1997, pp. 705–706):

- Listen for a general theme rather than specific words.
- If a spoken message is not clear, encourage use of gestures.
- If the message is still not clear, encourage the client to draw.
- Draw your best guess as to what the client is trying to say.
- Verify what you think you know every 1 or 2 minutes.

The second phase of Communication Partners is 14 weeks and consists of outside activities. In the first of two weekly sessions, the clinician assists in reviewing the previous week's activity and planning the next activity to be carried out as the week's second session. The second session involves the aphasic client and the volunteer partner and is conducted in the home or at a community site. Types of activities include a favorite from the past (e.g., gardening, card playing, grocery shopping), an activity considered but never tried before (e.g., learning computer skills), and volunteering in the community (e.g., visiting a day-care center).

For some older and severely impaired aphasic individuals, their community is the nursing home in which they live temporarily or permanently. A nursing home may contain a skilled nursing facility (SNF), which is very much like a hospital ward. The SNF may provide rehabilitation with the hope that the resident can become independent enough to return home eventually. The nursing home may also contain an independent living area for people without serious medical and physical problems. Opportunities for social integration are more readily available. Instead of a restaurant, there is a cafeteria. Partly through the efficient use of in-service education, a speech-language pathologist can help the staff reinforce communicative skills being trained in individual sessions.

CHANGING COMMUNICATIVE CONTEXTS

This section shifts emphasis from putting a patient in communicative contexts to changing them. It was indicated before that an aphasic individual is not solely responsible for the success of communication. We should observe patients and family members conversing to identify areas in which the family member can make adjustments. The PACE procedure is a controlled interaction in which problematic speaking and listening behaviors might be more apparent.

One investigation showed that aphasic people comprehend better when their spouses make adjustments in their utterances (Linebaugh, Margulies, and Mackisack-Morin, 1984). These adjustments included increased pauses and redundancy in describing pictures. Simmons and others (1987) found that training spouses to modify their behavior led to a reduction of interruptions of their aphasic partners.

The patient may utilize strategies of **conversational management.** For example, someone with mild aphasia may not be able to process conversation at its normal rate. The aphasic person starts to get lost and is too embarrassed to say so. However, instead of allowing others to restrict his or her ability to comprehend and respond, the patient can ask people to reduce their rate of speech or repeat every now and then. Holland (1991) called these "comprehension strategies," and they included asking others to simplify or elaborate their messages.

Let us suppose a mildly impaired patient is going through a divorce and must deal with a future ex-spouse and a lawyer over the phone. In the clinic, we can play the roles of these persons so that the patient can practice asking the spouse or the lawyer to explain slowly, to repeat, or to be available if a question should come up after hanging up the phone. If the spouse and lawyer cannot agree to these conditions, then perhaps the conversation should be at another time. This situation can make an interesting script in Conversational Coaching. This dress-rehearsal may strengthen confidence and the likelihood that the patient will use these strategies outside the clinic.

Lubinski (1981) wrote about **environmental language intervention.** A "communicatively impaired environment" has the following characteristics: (1) strict rules governing communication, (2) few places for a private conversation, (3) a staff that devalues communication between residents and between residents and staff, (4) many residents with multiple problems including dementias, and (5) physical conditions that reduce communicative efficiency such as linear or distant seating and poor lighting and acoustics. Clinicians should employ their diplomatic and persuasive skills to effect modifications of these conditions (Lubinski, 1988). New and remodeled nursing homes include spaces for private meetings with family and friends, attractive areas for social gatherings, and seating in the dining room that facilitates face-to-face interaction.

PSYCHOSOCIAL ADJUSTMENT

Psychosocial adjustment should have a bearing on success of interpersonal communication and, thus, on meeting goals of rehabilitation (Parr, 1994). Communication disorder changes daily life and presents a challenge to maintaining a satisfying lifestyle (Herrmann, 1997; Herrmann, Johannsen-Horbach, and Wallesch, 1993b; Letourneau, 1993). This section addresses the beliefs and emotions held by clinicians and family members as well as those held by the patient.

Clinician Characteristics

Martin Exeter's language and outlook became much improved over the first six months, and he became curious about whether he could teach again. However, memories of his rehabilitation were tarnished by an experience with one clinician. He worked with her briefly during the three-month treatment at a university in another state. One day the clinician told him that he would never get his memory back. The prediction lodged in Martin's mind as "you'll never teach again."

Rehabilitation is supported by the relationship between a clinician and a client. Rapport and trust contribute to the therapeutic process. In discussing these factors, Cyr-Stafford (1993) suggested that "the serene attitude of the knowledgeable professional who is familiar with these situations is reassuring to the person with aphasia" (p. 108). Our technical skills are not enough for a therapeutic relationship to flourish. If a patient is uncomfortable with a clinician, the patient quits. Our "people skills" are supportive of language rehabilitation.

Wulf (1979) commented on her first contact with her therapist with a "radiant smile": "And this was the first miracle speech therapy wrought for me. No word was needed—it was the magic of a look—an instantaneous rapport partly because my innermost messenger had told me that it would be that way" (p. 50). **Unconditional positive regard** creates a positive climate for therapeutic change. The influential clinical psychologist Carl Rogers (1961) defined it as "an outgoing positive feeling without reservations, without evaluations" (p. 62). Depression, frustration, and anger are allowed in the clinical setting without reservation or evaluation by the clinician.

Yet, studies have shown that patients and their families are likely to express more optimism than speech-language pathologists (e.g., Herrmann and Wallesch, 1989). An aphasic adult detects body language and prosody conveying negative attitudes. Sacks (1986) stated that "one cannot lie to an aphasic person." In a survey by Skelly (1975), patients "cited numerous subtle signs of impatience from those around them which were deeply discouraging—audible sighs, tightening of the mouth muscles, shoulder and eye movements, and drumming fingers" (p. 1141). A few clinicians may confuse aloofness with professionalism and exude a coolness that intimidates family members.

Wulf (1979) also wrote that a speech-language pathologist's rare talent is "being able to hop on anybody's wavelength and stay there until the aphasic has learned how to climb the unending tortuous crag facing him" (p. 50). In a survey of clients who evaluated attributes of a good clinician, "empathetic-genuineness" ranked second to technical skill (Haynes and Oratio, 1978). **Empathy** is a capacity to sense the feelings and personal meanings that another person is experiencing at each moment. We cannot walk in an aphasic person's shoes, but we can convey that we understand the problems created by brain damage.

Experienced clinicians are familiar with the soothing of frustration that comes with statements like "I know, you know what you want to say but just can't think of the words to say it." A speech-language pathologist may be the first person to convey this understanding. A patient discovers someone who knows that he or she is not stupid and believes there is someone in the hospital who can help with the exasperation of trying to talk. A client is inclined to accept the rigors of clinical advice when he or she knows that the helper understands the problem.

Rogers (1951) advised that "it is the counselor's function to assume, in so far as he is able, the internal frame of reference of the client...to lay aside all perceptions from the external frame of reference while doing so, and to communicate something of this empathic understanding to the client" (p. 29). An external frame of reference includes stereotypic conceptions according to gender, age, race, or religion. Ageism, for example, may entail a fear of the elderly that interferes with addressing a client as an individual (Davis and Holland, 1981). Prospective clinical aphasiologists should evaluate their attitudes regarding these attributes so that they can keep them out of clinical interactions and can attain unconditional positive regard and empathy for their patients.

A third clinician characteristic is **patience.** A family member, accustomed to a certain pace of conversation or feeling compelled to help a loved one, may jump in quickly when a patient is slow to respond. An experienced clinician, on the other hand, knows that the goal is to increase the patient's independence and allows some time for generating a response. Family members, who are used to quick cures of diseases, may become distressed over the relatively slow rate of progress that is common with stroke-related dysfunction. An experienced clinician knows that progress moves in small steps and takes some time.

Patient Adjustment

In the first three-to-six months postonset, a patient receives treatment in a climate of psychological adjustment. Martin seemed to go through some phases in coping with the sudden loss of verbal skills, motor function, and functional independence. The grief response has been a model for stages of psychological adjustment to sudden language dysfunction. Tanner and Gerstenberger's (1988) four stages were denial, frustration, depression, and acceptance. Whether aphasic patients actually go through this sequence has not been clearly established. These and other reactions contribute to the handicap caused by communicative disability (Le Dorze and Brassard, 1995).

In Chapter 8 on RHD, **denial** of impairment was introduced as being a psychological defense mechanism in contrast to absence of awareness of deficit. Not all patients deny their aphasia, but, for some, it may be a patient's premorbid coping style, and it "allows patients to borrow time while they come to terms with reality" (Sarno, 1993, p. 325).

Martin struggled with **depression** or discouragement, which is common after a stroke. Depression is more common with good comprehension and nonfluent aphasia than with other types of aphasia (Starkstein and Robinson, 1988). Physicians have advised that depression may not be just a stage of coping that a patient passes through. Herrmann, Johannsen-Horbach, and Wallesch (1993a) suggested that it is likely to be an unavoidable neurochemical consequence of stroke. The spectrum of post-stroke depression includes *emotional lability* which is sudden laughter or crying for no apparent reason. Treatment of severe depression or pathological crying has included antidepressant medication (Andersen, 1997).

Because Martin could no longer teach, write, argue with his daughter Julianna, or play golf with his son Peter, he began to wonder if aphasia was attacking his personal identity. He would say "I want to be me again." Brumfitt (1993) argued that motor and communicative disabilities batter a person's **sense of self.** Holland and Beeson (1993) supported this concern, adding that "as clinicians, we will be involved with individuals and family members as they mourn the insult to the prestroke identity, and as they make adjustments to the sense of self" (p. 581). Fundamental to an aphasic person's identity is his or her adulthood. Caring family members may start to treat the patient like a child, especially with respect to communicative style.

Van Eeckhout (1993) worked with patients who were artists or talented artistically. The aim was not "to spark creativity in persons with aphasia, but, rather, to revive the persons' former personality" (p. 89). One patient regained enough drawing ability with the left hand to take a job as illustrator. Another patient had Wernicke's aphasia but retained the ability to play any melody on the organ. Through continued revelation of this retained skill, the patient regained self-confidence and wrote 32 compositions since his stroke. A third patient, who was a singer and poet, received music therapy as the primary mode of communicative stimulation. Part of his therapy involved composing songs about aphasia.

Martin was fortunate that his colleagues visited often in the hospital. Later, they enthusiastically accepted Jackie's invitations to the house. As he progressed, he would stop in at the department on campus occasionally. He fought off ideas that his busy colleagues were ignoring him intentionally at times. After all, they were busy. Nevertheless, Sarno (1993) reported that **social isolation** is the most frequently cited consequence of aphasia in surveys of aphasic patients and that 70 percent believe that people avoid them because of their aphasia. Programs mentioned previously, such as Communication Partners or the Arato Centre in Toronto, were designed to relieve social isolation.

Le Dorze and Brassard (1995) interviewed patients and family members. Aphasic patients cited some of the following changes in their lives:

- interpersonal relationships: disruption of family relations, friction with spouse, loss of authority over children, fewer contacts with brothers and sisters, anxiety in meeting strangers.
- autonomy: loss of employment, physical dependency, feeling of powerlessness.

A patient may quickly exhibit **unproductive coping mechanisms** as a shield from impairment (Eisenson, 1984). In interviews with 20 aphasic patients, Parr (1994) found that they employed a variety of ways of dealing with their disabilities. One patient was resigned to his impairments but pursued an active life. His relationship with his wife improved during his rehabilitation. Another patient, however, responded to his condition with "angry fatalism." He was unwilling to discuss many things about his condition, including possibilities for functional progress through rehabilitation. Patients below age 65 were more likely than older patients to take action and control in their situation.

Family Adjustment

Immediately following a stroke, the family is likely to be overwhelmed with the sense that they nearly lost a husband, wife, father, or mother. Suddenly a hospitalized life partner appears to be vulnerable to the slightest encroachment, and a skittish spouse wants to protect him or her 24 hours a day. The devoted spouse may return home only overnight, sleeping partly dressed in case there is a call from the hospital. Spousal adjustment hopefully follows a path from selflessness to a renewed sense of self, a path that may parallel the patient's progress.

Martin's family had to make changes in their lives. Jackie went through phases similar to Martin's. She was sometimes angry, sometimes depressed. Some early coping mechanisms were understandable but unproductive. Aphasia is a family problem, turning family dynamics upside down (Rollin, 1984). A spouse becomes annoyed with a patient's swearing, feels heightened responsibilities, becomes increasingly fatigued, and drops some favorite activities to attend to the patient (Labourel and Martin, 1993; Le Dorze and Brassard, 1995; Ponzio and Degiovani, 1993).

A patient's inability to carry out customary roles causes family members to assume new roles. Regarding traditional roles of marriage partners, a male patient may no longer be able to provide income, sign the checks, and park the car. Dalhberg noted the following: "Since I'd grown up in middle-class America, I was used to taking care of 'masculine' details. I signed into hotels, picked up the bags, gave taxi directions, and ordered in restaurants." His wife added: "I looked forward to the time Clay would be able to do the managing again. It wasn't the physical exertion I minded as much as the loss of my female enjoyment of being 'taken care of'" (Dahlberg and Jaffe, 1977, p. 52).

Porter and Dabul (1977) applied transactional analysis (TA) to helping spouses understand the situation and return to a balance. A spouse has to respond to shifts in Adult, Parent, and Child ego states by the patient. "He acts like a child." In the aphasic person, the Adult state is often weakened and turned into the dependent state of the Child. "He just sits around all day and watches TV." Childlike ego involvement dominates as impulsiveness and a continual attention to "me, me, me." The Parent state diminishes with an inability to conform to social acceptability. Other patients may exaggerate the Parent by becoming overly protective of the spouse, constantly monitoring his or her activities. We may begin to imagine the toll this takes on a spouse and children living at home. A spouse, in turn, can become overly protective of a patient.

Julianna had been notified only that her father had suffered a stroke. It did not take long for Martin to figure out that she was considering leaving school to be with him and help out at home. She was afraid he was going to die, and so she hovered over him and pampered him as if he were an infant. He tried to assure her with his ability to squeeze a rubber ball, and he did not want to feel guilty about interfering with her life. She felt better after having a chance to see his early progress, and she returned to school the next semester. Later, they would communicate regularly through e-mail, which became part of Martin's self-imposed rehabilitation.

Peter was having a difficult time adjusting. He was living at home and could sense his mother's frustrations, although she tried to make everything seem normal. Maybe that made it harder than it already was for him to talk about it. Everyone was feeling his or her way. Peter had to help out more around the house, doing some of the repairs and yardwork that he and his father used to do together. His life was changing and he did not like it, but he would not say anything for fear of appearing to be selfish.

Zraick and Boone (1991) found that spouses develop different attitudes toward their aphasic spouse than "control spouses." The investigators used an attitude assessment technique called Q-methodology in which spouses sorted and ranked 70 attributes according to what was most and least representative of the aphasic person. In general, spouses had more negative attitudes than controls, indicating that spouses' attitudes had changed after onset. The most prevalent perceived characteristics of the impaired spouse were *demanding* and *temperamental* in contrast to *mature* and *kind* for controls. Least prevalent characteristics for the clinical group included *sexy, mature,* and *intelligent.* Spouses of nonfluent patients had more negative attitudes than spouses of fluent patients, which, in part, could have been due to the more frequent presence of hemiplegia in the nonfluent group.

Jackie's sense of loss did not last long, once she realized that Martin was safe and could communicate in some ways. Others had real tragedies to deal with. She felt she still had a partner and realized that it would be better for both of them if she cultivated those feelings and showed them often. She did not have to learn to park the car or pay the bills. She and Martin had tried to balance or share roles. She knew about the finances and did not have to scramble to figure them out.

Jackie also tried to find out as much information as she could about stroke and aphasia. She read several pamphlets and books such as Strokes: What Families Should Know *(Shimberg, 1990) and* Living with Stroke *(Senelick, Rossi, and Dougherty, 1994). She did* Yahoo *searches on the internet and found information in sites for medical schools and professional associations. She shared some of the information with Julianna and Peter. She brought print-outs to Martin's clinicians. She also found information on therapy procedures that were promoted as being promising. Because Martin was a professor, Jackie knew to ask if the data at a Website was peer-reviewed. Over time she learned that she did not have to anticipate every need, and she and Martin became equals again.*

Probably the best source of support was a group of family members and aphasic people that met once a month at Martin's hospital. Jackie met wives who had been through the same experience. They shared stories. They laughed. Each meeting had a social time and a formal presentation either by a professional or by a member of the group. She and Martin would go together. He was inspired by seeing others like him talk before the group about a family vacation or a particular problem. ***Support groups*** *often have one of the follow sponsors:*

- The **American Heart Association** sponsors "Stroke Clubs" that include persons with varied problems (Sanders, Hamby, and Nelson, 1984).
- The **National Aphasia Association,** founded by Martha Taylor Sarno at Rusk Institute of Rehabilitation Medicine in New York City, is promoting community awareness and encouraging the creation of similar support groups specifically for aphasic persons and their families.

- The **National Head Injury Foundation** and its state organizations have provided legislative advocacy and have sponsored local survivor groups.

Also, European countries have formed Aphasia Associations for families (e.g., Wahrborg and Borenstein, 1989, 1990). Many programs are reported in the literature (Hoen, Thelander, and Worsley; 1997; Hubert and Degiovani, 1993; Mogil, Bloom, Gray, and Lefkowitz, 1978; Rice, Paull, and Muller, 1987; Webster and Newhoff, 1981).

DOCUMENTING FUNCTIONAL OUTCOME

Unless a clinical procedure (e.g., using a phone) is identical to a functional objective (e.g., to improve using the phone), the functional outcome of a treatment is documented with a generalization probe or a report from a family member that the patient is doing something new. As indicated in Table 11.8, a generalization probe is a measure of progress toward an objective. It is not a measure of performance in a treatment. For example, if a goal is "to carry out communicative interactions in the community," then we document observations of communicative interactions in the community.

According to Busch (1993), clinicians should document "significant functional change" in patient performance for Medicare. The meaning of "significant" can be unclear. Citing the official guidelines, Busch said that it refers to "a generally measurable and substantial increase in the patient's present level of communication" compared to the level of communication when treatment began. The requirement was not intended to refer to a percentage of improvement on a specific language task.

Holland (1998) suggested that while "third-party intermediaries like to see numbers...they have never told us what to count" (p. 846). She added that, besides our "professional obsession with counting linguistic units," we can count "sociolinguistic units of conversation, such as ideas encoded, topics maintained...repairs completed, messages transmitted and so forth" (p. 846).

A fairly straightforward approach to documenting social change is to compare what a patient can do before and after therapy. Before therapy, the clinician records specific activities that a patient has discontinued due to stroke or other brain injury. After therapy, the clinician records which of these activities the patient now pursues. For example, a patient may have stopped working after a stroke but, after therapy, has returned to work. Lyon recorded specific activities that were initiated during treatment and then were continued after treatment concluded. These activities included grocery shopping, attending a Stroke Club, maintaining a bank account, participating on a church committee, volunteering at a day-car center, and so on (Lyon, et al., 1997).

Social validation is a component of single subject experiments. It pertains to whether progress reaches "the demands of the social community of which the client is a part" (Kazdin, 1982). Thompson and Byrne (1984) used a probe called a *novel social dyad* to observe production of trained social conventions. The dyad was a five-minute conversation in a "comfortable, nontreatment room" with an unfamiliar person (i.e., undergraduate students). The clinicians also gave the probe to two normal adults as a standard for interpreting peak levels of progress reached by aphasic patients. The wide range of scores exhibited by the controls exposed a problem with interpretation of natural progress: "we really don't know what patients are supposed to do when they go out into the real world because we don't always know what non-brain-damaged people do" (p. 142).

Sarno (1993) urged that we look into using **quality of life** measures. In a study of functional progress over a five-month period, Lyon and his colleagues (1997) found no progress with respect to the Boston Exam and the CADL. However, significant change was detected with two non-standard questionnaires related to goals of the treatment. One measure was a "Communication Readiness and Use Index" that questioned a client's comfort, confidence, and skills when conversing with family members or strangers. The other was a "Psychological Well-Being Index" re-

TABLE 12.4 Reminder of functional treatment methods, differentiating between those conducted in the clinic and those conducted outside the clinic.

IN-CLINIC		OUTSIDE-CLINIC
Direct Stimulation	*Interactive*	
Personalized stimulation	PACE	Communication Partners
Functional task stimulation	Conversational Coaching	Conversational management
Communication boards	Supported Conversation	Environmental intervention
Gesturing & drawing	Role-playing	

garding life satisfaction and general comfort with self and others.

Hoen and others (1997) used the *Psychological Well-Being Scale* (Ryff, 1989) to evaluate their community-based rehabilitation program. This scale presents many statements addressing autonomy, environmental mastery, personal growth, positive relations with others, purpose in life, and self-acceptance. Patients are asked to strongly agree or strongly disagree on a six-point scale. The clinical investigators created a condensed version by selecting the easiest statements for aphasic persons to understand.

An essential characteristic of functional outcome is that it should represent a real and meaningful change in a patient's life. This is what Dr. Metter was looking for. There can be a perception of dishonesty in advertising the effects of a language treatment program with a picture naming score without evidence of change at home. Scherzer (1992) argued that "only successful results will convince politicians that long-term rehabilitation is worth investing in. Therefore, we have to be very careful and absolutely honest in our statements, not exaggerating good results and not venturing out with over-optimistic predictions" (pp. 102–103).

SUMMARY AND CONCLUSIONS

Communicative treatment for aphasia is aimed at helping a patient maximize the capacity to comprehend and convey messages through any means. Functionality comes with the use of communicative capacity in real-life situations. The contexts interacting with the language system are internal and external to a patient. The internal contexts roughly consist of the patient's world knowledge, belief system, and emotional state. The external contexts consist of settings and other people. These contexts suggest a menu of variables that clinicians consider in providing a functional or pragmatic treatment program. Table 12.4 is a reminder of approaches surveyed in this chapter.

A great deal of functional or pragmatic treatment does not repair damaged language processes or teach something new. Instead, it reduces fear. We walk patients to the end of the diving board and ask them to "look down." It increases confidence in the use of retained capacities or of processes repaired as a result of stimulation. For severely impaired patients, a clinician's job is to determine communicative capacities and then maximize confidence in and opportunities for their accepted use.

CHAPTER 13

TARGETING SPECIFIC DISORDERS

This final chapter presents refinements of treatment and explorations that may be predictive of the future in aphasia rehabilitation. Many of the procedures are experimental in that they were provided in controlled conditions (e.g., without other therapies). Rather than thinking of therapy as being for aphasia in general, we will be thinking about therapy for specific symptoms or for diagnoses of specific cognitive impairments. Although the focus is on syndromes, the chapter progresses roughly from the word-level to discourse and text.

In concluding with the discourse-level, the chapter reaches the final stages of Martin Exeter's rehabilitation. Over a couple of years, his communicative skills and self-confidence improved to a point where he was considering a return to some of his professional activities. He missed lecturing. However, he was not sure of his understanding of difficult concepts or his ability to follow his own train of thought, as well as still being uncertain about his swiftness in retrieving psycholinguistic terminology. These concerns contributed to the late-stage goals of his treatment.

STUDYING INDIVIDUAL CASES

The future of aphasia treatment may be scouted in studies of individual cases. In the clinic, a speech-language pathologist's minimal obligation is to measure and document a patient's progress during a period of treatment. Proving the cause of a patient's progress, on the other hand, requires a control of variables that is difficult to achieve in the usual clinical circumstance. About all a clinician can do is interpret progress occurring after six months as caused by something other than spontaneous recovery, but attributing this progress to treatment is still not a sure thing.

Single-case experimental designs provide clinical investigators with a means of controlling variables in order to determine cause-effect relationships. Unlike group studies of efficacy, single-case studies enable a researcher to explore nuances of specific treatment procedures. Although clinicians have been encouraged to employ these designs while providing treatment, an adequate study usually requires external funding to pay for the time involved. Nevertheless, a general knowledge of these designs should help a speech-language pathologist be a better consumer of treatment products that are purported to be efficacious.

A single-case experiment differs from a **case study.** The former institutes control of variables, whereas the latter is primarily descriptive of a patient's history and treatment. A case study may include measures taken before and after a treatment; but, without controls, conclusions about the cause of any change must be considered to be without foundation. Like any experiment, a single-subject design consists of two components:

- manipulation of an independent variable or treatment
- a measure of a dependent variable related to a goal of treatment

A subject is said to serve as his or her own control. That is, a comparison between the presence and absence of a treatment is performed with one subject, rather than one subject (or group) receiving treatment and another subject (or group) not receiving treatment.

The strategies of single-case experimentation have been detailed in several books (e.g., Barlow and Hersen, 1984; Kazdin, 1982; McReynolds and

Kearns, 1983), tutorials (Kearns, 1986; McReynolds and Thompson, 1986; Willmes, 1990, 1995), and critical reviews (e.g., Fukkink, 1996). These strategies are summarized in Table 13.1. Single-case and group designs have given us different perspectives. Group designs have viewed treatment over the first year postonset, but single-case designs have often been applied years following onset.

One type of experiment consists of alternating phases of no-treatment (i.e., baseline) and treatment. The minimal ABA design is common (e.g., "test-treat-test"). Although some have put forth the claim that this design can establish efficacy (e.g., Behrmann and Byng, 1992), it is not enough to nail down causation, especially when the A-phase is a single test. However, a more complete ABAB design may not be in the best interest of a client, because the most demanding experiment requires that a patient's performance be "reversed" in the second A-phase to nail down causation (i.e., a return to initial baseline level). "Careful consideration must be given to the consequences of reverting to baseline for the client and those who are responsible for his or her care" (Kazdin, 1982, p. 124).

In clinical aphasiology, the more frequent strategy is a multiple baseline design. A straightforward example is Thompson and Kearns' (1981) study of a cueing treatment for naming deficit for a patient with anomic aphasia. Figure 13.1 shows that the study was actually a series of ABA designs applied sequentially to four dependent variables, called a "combined-series" design (Fukkink, 1996). The dependent variables were four different lists of words elicited in naming tasks. Two lists were from one semantic category (i.e., A1 and B1), and the other two lists were from another semantic category (i.e., A2 and B2). The cueing treatment was applied to one list and then to the other three in succession. Upward trends occurred only when treatment was instituted. Concluding that the treatment had an effect is based on the small likelihood that the timing of the changes could have been caused by something else.

When comparing treatments given to a single patient, one treatment must follow another. Both alternating treatment designs (ATD) and

TABLE 13.1 Summary of basic single subject experimental designs.

	DESIGN	NOTATION	DESCRIPTION
single treatment effects	pre-post treatment	ABA	bordering a treatment (B) with baselines (A)
	alternating phases	ABAB	alternating periods of baseline (A) and a treatment (B)
	multiple baseline	MB	a single treatment applied sequentially to different behaviors or settings; baselines for each behavior or setting are obtained throughout the study
comparing treatments	alternating treatments	ATD	two treatments given within a single day; repeated in different orders for several days
	cross-over	BCBC	alternating treatment periods (B & C phases); in different sequences for at least two subjects (e.g., BCBC, CBCB)

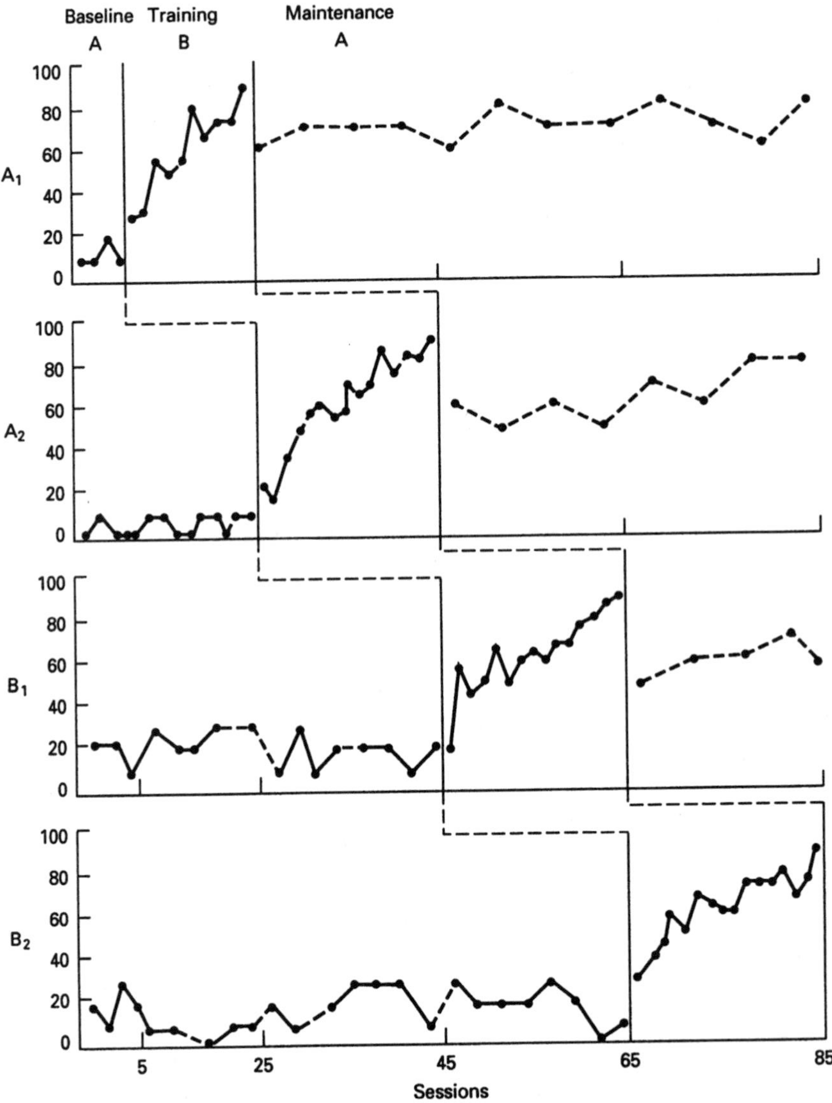

FIGURE 13.1 Probing an anomic patient's progress according to multiple baseline design. Clinicians obtained percent of naming across four sets of words during periods of baseline and treatment.

Reprinted by permission from Thomson, C, K. & Kearns, K. P., an experimental analysis of acquisition, generalization, and maintenance of naming behavior in a patient with anomia. In R. H. Brookshire (Ed.), *Clinical aphasiology conference proceedings.* Minneapolis: BRK, 1981, p. 39.

cross-over designs contain elements intended to control for sequence-effects, namely, the effect that one treatment might have on another that follows.

The ATD is also known as the simultaneous-treatment or concurrent schedule design. As in other designs, it begins with a baseline of the dependent variable. Then, the different treatments are administered on the same day (i.e., "simultaneous" treatments). Each day thereafter, the order of treatments is reversed, and the two daily sequences are randomly alternated across several days. Probes of the dependent variable are obtained for each treatment so that a graph of the treatment phase shows two sets of data (e.g., Avent, et al., 1995).

Cross-over designs have been commonly used in Europe to compare aphasia treatments (e.g., Springer, et al., 1991). For one patient, one treatment phase (B) precedes another treatment phase (C). For another patient, the second treatment (C phase) precedes the first treatment (B phase). A study may stop at this point or continue by alternating phases. With this design, a second subject is necessary to balance sequence effects.

An important component of single-case research is that several data points should be collected across a phase, rather than simply "bordering" each phase with a pre- and post-treatment test. The goal is to determine the *trend* across a phase. A trend could be flat, upward, downward, or random variation. The problem with just two data-points bordering a phase is that they could be derived from random variation and, thus, do not present conclusive evidence regarding how the patient was doing across the phase. The requirement of obtaining sufficient data points is one reason why single-case experiments are difficult to do when a clinician is strapped for time.

GLOBAL APHASIA

In focusing on particular disorders, let us begin with patients who have severe impairment of comprehension and little verbal expression (Collins, 1997; Peach and Rubin, 1994). Following principles of stimulation, direct repair of the language system would begin with the simplest language and the simplest tasks. Following principles of functional treatment, many clinicians try to establish or encourage any means of communication as soon as possible. First, however, we should be sure that a patient has a true global aphasia (see Chapter 2).

Candidacy for Treatment

Robert Marshall (1987) raised eyebrows by asserting that "aphasiologists spend excessive time in the treatment of globally aphasic clients but tend to dismiss the needs of the mildly aphasic person because they are less obvious" (p. 60). Although the accuracy of these assumptions can be questioned (e.g., Parsons, 1987b), the cost effectiveness of treating global aphasia was put on the table for public debate.

More recently, Brookshire (1997) stated that "the presence of global aphasia at one month post-onset is an ominous prognostic sign." He added that "the healing effects of time apparently have little effect on the language capabilities of most patients who remain globally aphasic beyond the immediate post-onset period" (p. 247). He suggested that at least two of the following symptoms indicate that a patient may not have the capacity to become a functional verbal communicator:

- stereotypic utterance along with severely impaired comprehension
- inability to match objects
- unreliable yes-no response to questions
- semantic or neologistic jargon without awareness and self-correction

We should note that these projections pertain to linguistic communicative capacity, not necessarily nonverbal communicative capacity. Even when improvement occurs across a period of treatment, it may have taken months or years to achieve (e.g., Samples and Lane, 1980).

In responding to Marshall's bleak characterization of the recovery data, Edelman (1987) suggested that lack of progress in overall language test scores may hide progress in comprehension and gesturing. Brookshire (1997) stated that a brief period of trial therapy can be indicative of whether a patient can benefit from a full treatment program, but he added that "prolonged treatment to reinstate functional verbal communication for such patients is rarely successful" (p. 248). Nevertheless, he acknowledged that new treatment programs may alter this outlook.

One study indicated that intensity of language treatment can make a difference (Denes, Perazzolo, Piani, and Piccione, 1996). Seventeen patients received treatment of auditory comprehension along with some stimulation of multiple expressive modalities in conversation. Treatment was begun around three months postonset. Nine patients received 60 sessions over a six-month period (2–3/week), and eight patients received 130 sessions over six months (5/week). More patients receiving the more intensive therapy made significant improvement.

Comprehension

Treatment of auditory comprehension can be devised according to a logical application of principles introduced in Chapters 11 and 12:

- set a reasonable functional goal
- start with a task that has a high level of accuracy
- upon meeting a criterion of success, move to a more demanding task
- measure progress toward meeting the goal

Improved comprehension can have far-reaching consequences. A goal of achieving a high level of accuracy in comprehending sentences is functional in the sense that comprehension can facilitate conversational interaction (e.g., answering another's questions). However, because treatment should begin at a level of high accuracy, it may have to begin with a task that is easier than the floor of initial assessment. For example, a word comprehension task may have two pictured choices instead of the six or eight in an aphasia test. To measure progress toward the goal, a brief test of sentence comprehension should be administered regularly. The lesson plan might look something like Table 13.2.

We should have a patient's attention for repetitive drills. In a hospital, a patient may arrive at the clinic tired from physical therapy or in a state of depressed vigilance due to trauma. Alerting signals, such as the patient's name or "Ready?", may be presented before each stimulus. Collins (1986) tried to heighten interest with playing cards in simple matching and sequencing tasks. Awareness, as well as functionality, may be heightened when the task is individualized, as in pointing to pictures of family members.

For word comprehension, several variables can be manipulated to adjust difficulty. The lexical stimulus may be repeated or presented with a printed word. Redundant verbal context might help in identifying an object. Pictures can be varied in semantic relatedness and can be supplemented with printed words. However, despite all of the logical manipulations that could generate a brilliant stepwise program, a patient represented by Table 13.2 should be progressing quickly out of the word-level treatment in order to meet the sentence-level goal. Stimulation should be awak-

TABLE 13.2 A lesson plan for treating auditory comprehension for someone with global aphasia.

GOAL	TREATMENT	GENERALIZATION PROBE
improve functional sentence comprehension from 10% to 70% accuracy	point to pictures (2-choices) given common words and family names	10-item sentence comprehension test, including yes-no biographical questions and functional commands

ening a process. If a patient is not improving over three or four sessions, then it is not likely that much repair of the language system is possible in an affordable amount of time (although there is little published data supporting this suggestion).

At a slightly higher linguistic level, four patients with severe aphasia were trained to follow simple verb-noun commands such as *take glove* and *cover fork* (Oleyar, et al. 1991). The patients had AQ scores from the WAB of 19.4 to 48.8. Treatment consisted of pairing a spoken command with a model of the action. The clinician also gradually increased the time between the command and the model. Two of the four subjects responded favorably to the treatment by improving with trained commands without models and generalizing to untrained commands.

Language Formulation

Sarno and Levita (1979) noted that a few words could make a remarkable difference in someone's life over an inability to produce words. In principle, treatment begins with what a patient can do verbally; and people with global aphasia easily produce verbal stereotypes with no relation to a situation. They can be prodded into counting to ten or singing a song.

Clinicians try to harness whatever utterances are produced spontaneously. If we can get them under our control, then we may help a patient to produce them more appropriately and in greater variety. Helm and Barresi (1980) formalized this common practice in a program called **Voluntary Control of Involuntary Utterances.** It began with presenting the printed form of an utterance just heard. If the utterance was repeated as if read aloud, it was considered to be more volitional. If a different word was produced, a stimulus card was written for that word. No treatment was pursued for any utterance that was difficult to elicit a second time. When reading aloud and repetition elicited responses, an object-picture was presented in a transition to naming tasks. Patients improved in independent testing and were reported to use some of the words appropriately in conversational interaction.

Schonle (1988) reported a treatment called *compound noun stimulation* for chronic global aphasia more than three years postonset. Object-drawings labeled by compound words were presented (e.g., *wheelchair, football*), and the first part of the word was used to cue the second part. The goal was to elicit words. This procedure was compared with a standard naming activity in which simple words were elicited by repetition. Compound naming improved from 0 to 94 percent over four weeks, whereas standard naming improved from 0 to 12 percent. A second treatment phase advanced performance further and only a slight drop occurred five weeks after the end of treatment. Schonle did not address whether word-retrieval in conversation was improved.

Brief trial therapy usually does not produce functional improvement in verbal behavior for patients who have global aphasia at one month postonset. At least, clinicians can determine level of comprehension and ability to communicate nonverbally. It is more common that the clinician's primary role "is to help the family and other caregivers structure the patient's daily life environment to take advantage of the communicative abilities that the patient has retained" (Brookshire, 1997, p. 248).

C-VIC

Speech-language pathologists have been relentless, if not heroic, in seeking a communicative mode for globally impaired patients. This effort includes the use of various shapes as symbols. Patients were trained to comprehend statements, questions, and commands constructed out of such symbols arranged in syntactic order. One team of investigators examined cut-out paper shapes that were also used to give chimpanzees a means of communicating with humans (Glass, Gazzaniga, and Premack, 1973).

Gardner and others (1976) tried a system called **Visual Communication** or VIC. Although aphasic subjects displayed a knowledge of syntactic relations, there was no sign of functional use of the system. However, such unconventional methods indicated that globally aphasic persons may have more language capacity than is usually exposed by aphasia tests (Shelton, Weinrich, McCall, and Cox, 1996).

For a decade, a team of researchers led by Michael Weinrich at the University of Maryland has been developing a computerized version of Visual Communication called C-VIC. The program contains a hierarchically organized picture vocabulary that is displayed as cards on the screen. Verbs are animated to facilitate comprehension. A patient can arrange nouns around verbs without regard to syntax. A sentence looks like a row of picture cards. The clinician makes a statement on one row, and the patient responds on a second row.

Weinrich's research team has used C-VIC mainly to explore the linguistic capacity of persons with global aphasia, and they found that this capacity is heterogeneous. C-VIC is currently limited for use as an augmentative communicative device, partly because learning the system takes up to two years (Shelton, et al., 1996). In other research, Naeser (1994) found no relationship between lesion size and response of severely impaired patients to training with this system. Two patients with severe Broca's aphasia (i.e., good comprehension) were trained to produce basic sentences with varied tense marking with C-VIC. Additionally, their spoken sentence production was improved after the training (Weinrich, McCall, Weber, Thomas, and Thornburg, 1995; Weinrich, Shelton, Cox, and McCall, 1997).

AGRAMMATIC PRODUCTION: EMPIRICAL TREATMENTS

Clinicians have experimented with several methods aimed at increasing the verbal productivity of patients with agrammatism. These methods can be classified according to the distinction between data-driven and theory-driven research introduced at the beginning of Chapter 4. Data-driven or empirically-based therapies are derived mainly from observations of how aphasic persons respond to stimuli. Theory-driven therapies, introduced in Chapter 11 for naming, are a more recent development.

HELPSS

The *Helm Elicited Language Program for Syntax Stimulation* (HELPSS) is intended to increase the syntactic variety and complexity of utterances (Helm-Estabrooks, 1981). It is recommended for agrammatic patients with good comprehension and a mean length of utterance of two-to-five words. Another recommendation is that we measure progress with Cookie Theft picture description (Helm-Estabrooks and Albert, 1991).

The procedure was modeled after a story-completion task used to elicit 14 syntactic forms in a study by Gleason, Goodglass, Green, Ackerman, and Hyde (1975). A hierarchy of structural difficulty was based on results of that study. Pluralized nouns and progressive verbs were among the easiest forms to produce, whereas it was very difficult to add -s for subject-verb agreement and produce the future auxiliary.

The story-completion format elicits 11 types of sentences, and each story is accompanied by a picture. The program also consists of two broad levels for training each type of sentence. In Level A, the target phrase is included in the story so that a patient can repeat. In Level B, the patient is to complete the story with the target phrase. A response criterion of 90 percent accuracy determines movement up the sentence-type hierarchy within each level. A subsequent study showed that the sequence of difficulty was not appropriate for all patients (Salvatore, Trunzo, Holtzapple, and Graham, 1983).

A couple of studies led Helm-Estabrooks and Albert (1991) to conclude that the "efficacy" of HELPSS has been demonstrated. These were mainly pre-post test studies showing progress in sentence production (Helm-Estabrooks, Fitzpatrick, and Barresi, 1981; Helm-Estabrooks and Ramsberger, 1986).

In early single-subject studies, HELPSS caused little stimulus or response generalization (Doyle and Goldstein, 1985; Salvatore, 1985). A similar procedure was applied successively to baselines for production of imperative transitives and intransitives (e.g., *Read a book, Stand up*), declarative transitives and intransitives (e.g., *He fixes cars, She dances*), and Wh-interrogatives (e.g., What is your name?). This multiple baseline study indicated that the procedure can influence production of these sentences because of changes in each baseline that coincided with the sequential introduction of the treatment (Doyle, Goldstein, and Bourgeois, 1987).

A more recent study was focused on measures of generalization with respect to therapies for improving sentence production (Fink, Schwartz, Rochon, Myers, Socolof, and Bluestone, 1995). HELPSS was administered to four nonfluent patients in three sessions per week, and each session ended with a story telling task. The investigators examined the extent to which generalization occurred in circumstances differing from the treatment. One probe consisted of pictures and questions designed to elicit specific types of sentences. Generalization to this probe was observed, but generalization did not occur in a narrative production task.

Behavioral Treatment

In behavioral methods, sentences are elicited through modeling. One technique for lengthening utterances is called **forward chaining** in which a clinician "sequentially modeled the first two words of the target response then the remaining words of the target response, instructing the subject to repeat each portion as it was modeled" (Thompson and McReynolds, 1986, p. 198). **Reverse chaining** involves presenting all but the last word as a "completion task" and, then, eliciting an increasingly longer form by subtracting words from the carrier phrase toward the first word. In the 1980s, these methods were usually reported along with single-subject experimental designs to determine cause-effect relationships between a treatment and generalization probes.

For Kearns and Salmon's (1984) study of two cases of Broca's aphasia, the goal was to increase production of complete sentences containing the auxiliary *is* (e.g., *The boy is drinking*). Treatment consisted of imitative and spontaneous production tasks, and reinforcement was contingent upon complete sentence productions. Results for one subject are seen in Figure 13.2. Beginning with the baseline phase, probes were administered regularly to assess progress with trained and untrained auxiliary productions (upper graph). Generalization to production of a different type of sentence (lower graph) was measured with a probe of untrained copula production (e.g., *The man is a cowboy*).

Efficacy was studied with reversal of training as the second baseline phase (i.e., no training) followed by reinstatement of training. Reversal consisted of two parts. The first part was a kind of "counter-therapy." That is, agrammatic productions of previously untrained copula forms were reinforced, and the clinician ignored complete productions. In the second reversal phase, the same strategy was applied to trained auxiliary forms. After these two reversal phases, auxiliary training was resumed. The basic point was to determine if auxiliary production can be placed under a clinician's control.

The results are seen by following the trend of performance from phase to phase. Performance improved with both trained and untrained forms during the first training period, deteriorated during reversal phases, and improved again when auxiliary-is training was reinstated. Maintenance of progress was seen two and six weeks after termination of treatment. The treatment effect is indicated by the reversal and restoration of performance. Kearns and Salmon reported that generalization to spontaneous production was not achieved.

With four agrammatic subjects, Thompson and McReynolds (1986) compared a "direct-production" approach and an "auditory-visual" approach to training *Wh*-question production (e.g., "What is he drinking?"). The former method was presumed to be a behavioral treatment, and the latter was thought to be characteristic of stimulation methods. The comparison of fundamental approaches hinged on use of single stimulus presentation in direct-production/behavioral treatment and multimodal presentation in auditory-visual/

stimulation (although Table 11.3 indicates that there are other distinctions).

An alternating-treatments design was used to compare procedures. Procedures were alternated each day between morning and afternoon sessions. "To control for possible interaction effects of the two treatments, each treatment was applied to different interrogative constructions" (p. 197). The researchers found that direct-production was more effective for acquisition of trained *Wh*-questions, but the treatment did not generalize to untrained interrogative types.

Response Elaboration Training

Behavioral training of a few specific items was not causing generalization to untrained items. So, the clinicians decided to modify the treatment. One change was called **loose training,** which introduced flexibility in stimuli and in the response to be reinforced (e.g., Thompson and Byrne, 1984). One version is *Response Elaboration Training* (RET) developed by Kevin Kearns. In this procedure, "the clinician shapes and elaborates spontaneously produced client utterances rather than targeting preselected response" (Kearns, 1985, p. 196). Kearns wanted to expand a patient's independence as a communicator by encouraging initiation of responses, and he considered RET's intent to be somewhat similar to PACE therapy (Kearns, 1986b). RET appears to promote generalization and is effective for conduction and anomic aphasia, as well (Yedor, Conlon, and Kearns, 1993).

Table 13.3 shows the steps for one stimulus item (Kearns and Potechin Scher, 1989; Kearns

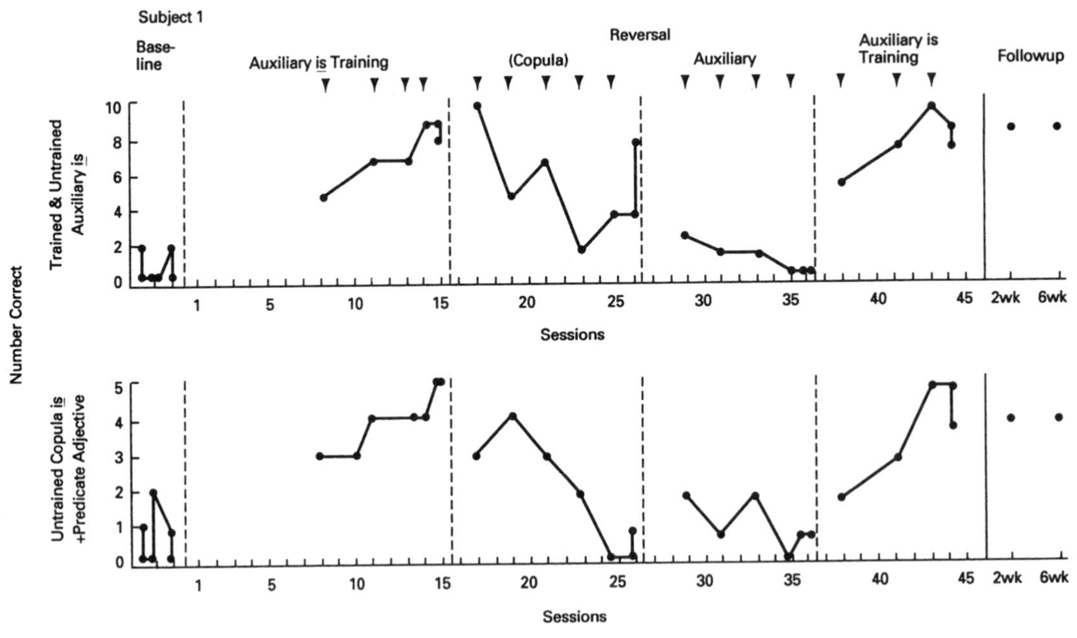

FIGURE 13.2 Results of continuos probes of correct production of trained and untrained auxiliary *is* (top) and untrained copula *is* (bottom) by one agrammatic subject. Arrows at the top mark sessions in which criterion was met for trained items. Improvement occurred for trained and untrained forms during the treatment phases.

Reprinted by permission from Kearns, K. P. & Salmon, S. J., An experimental analysis of auxiliary and copula verb generalization in aphasia. *Journal of Speech and Hearing Disorders,* 49, 1984, p.158. American Speech-Language-Hearing Association, publisher.

and Yedor, 1991). Kearns asked a patient to describe a simple event and then used modeling and shaping to encourage an expanded description. The model in step (2) is an expansion of a patient's initial response (i.e., "Man...sweeping"). In step (3), a *wh*-question stimulates production of additional information. In step (4), the clinician models a combination of the initial response and the subsequent response to the question. The patient practices elaborated imitations. The key is to avoid training a specific target response.

RET was introduced with a patient who had Broca's aphasia (Kearns, 1985, 1986b). Following a multiple baseline design, treatment was initiated for one set of 10 pictures and was delayed for another set. Probes for the untreated sets were taken on alternate days when treatment was not scheduled (Figure 13.3). Treatment of the first set was discontinued so that it would not confound treatment of the second set. A treatment effect is observed in the upward trends of performance beginning with each treatment. The flat baselines indicate that repeated testing by itself had little effect. Some generalization occurred for a third set of pictures but did not occur for the second set before treatment was instituted. Whereas the patient had decreased in his verbal score on the PICA over the six months prior to this treatment, his score improved across this period of treatment.

Cueing-Verb Treatment (CVT)

Once called a "verbing strategy," *cueing-verb treatment* (CVT) was designed to improve production of verbs, which was thought to be a special difficulty for people with agrammatism (see

TABLE 13.3 Steps of *Response Elaboration Training* (RET) for a picture of a man sweeping the floor.

RET STEPS	CLINICIAN'S STIMULUS	PATIENT'S RESPONSE	CLINICIAN'S FEEDBACK
(1) Elicit initial verbal response to picture	line drawing of simple event (man with a broom) "Tell me what's happening in this picture."	"Man...sweeping."	
(2) Reinforce, model & shape initial response			"Great. The man is sweeping."
(3) Wh-cue to elicit elaboration of initial response	"Why is he sweeping?"	"Wife...mad."	
(4) Reinforce, model, and shape the two patient responses combined			"Way to go! The man is sweeping the floor because his wife is mad."
(5) Second model and request repetition	"Try and say the whole thing after me. Say 'The man is sweeping the floor because his wife is mad'."	"Man...sweeping... wife...mad"	"Good job."
(6) After reinforcement, elicit a delayed imitation of the combined response	"Now, try to say it one more time."	"The man... sweeping because his wife...mad."	

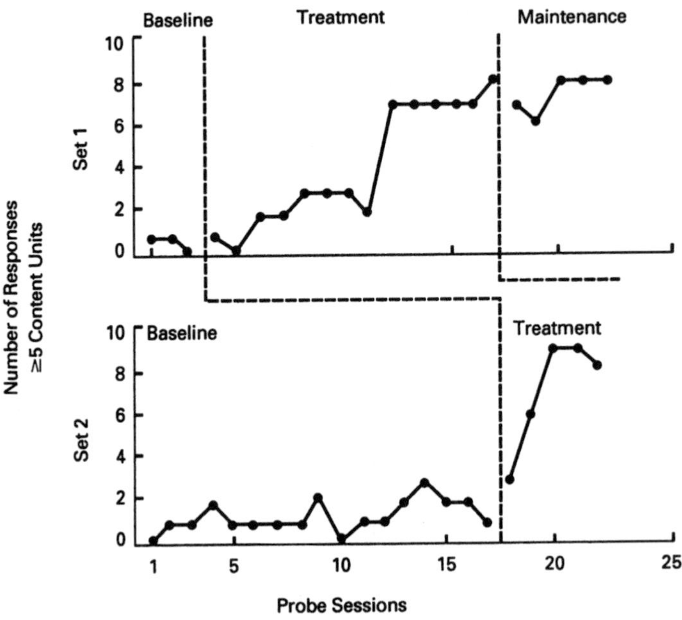

FIGURE 13.3 Continuous probes of responses containing at least five content units for the initially treated set of pictures and the second set for which treatment was delayed. Improvement with a set of pictures was contingent on treatment of that set.

Reprinted by permission from Kearns, K. P., Response elaboration training for patient initiated utterances. In R. H. Brookshire (Ed.), *Clinical aphasiology* (Vol. 15). Minneapolis: BRK, 1985, p. 199.

Chapter 5). Because of the grammatical information encoded with verbs, it was hoped that improved verb-finding would pull noun-phrase arguments along with them (Loverso, Prescott, and Selinger, 1988; Loverso, Selinger, and Prescott, 1979). The procedure has been used with nonfluent and fluent aphasias.

Generally, we present a verb as a pivot-stimulus and then ask who- and what-questions to elicit arguments around the verb. We try to elicit sequences of increasing length. CVT has been administered and reported in different ways since its introduction in 1979 (Table 13.4). The initial version of the program had two levels differing according to the length of sentence to be practiced (Loverso, etal., 1979). Level I was designed to elicit subject-verb sentences. If a patient could not produce SV sentences 60 percent of the time, then backup procedures included copying and repeating the sentence or a comprehension task. Level II was similar except that questions were asked to elicit an SVO sentence.

Selinger and others (1987) decided to modify the procedure for a severely aphasic patient. Three levels were staged from copying sentences, to a comprehension task, and finally to generating a sentence given the verb. A third version was reworded to correspond to more modern linguistic terminology regarding thematic roles (Loverso and Milione, 1992). Also, contrary to the first version, sentence generation followed repeating and pointing. With a computer version of CVT, a degree of efficacy was demonstrated (Loverso, Prescott, Selinger, and Riley, 1989).

TABLE 13.4 The original version and one modification of cueing-verb treatment.

LOVERSO, SELINGER AND PRESCOTT (1979)	LOVERSO AND MILIONE (1992)
I Given the verb, supply a subject	IA Copy/repeat actor+action
IA Given a subject-verb phrase, copy and imitate it	IB Select correct actor from array and repeat/copy actor+action
IB Given the verb, choose a correct subject from an array of four	I Self-generation of actor+action both verbally and graphically
II Given the verb, supply a subject and an object	IIA Copy/repeat actor+action
IIA Given the subject-verb-object, copy and imitate it	IIB Select correct actor from array and repeat/copy actor+action
IIB Given the verb, choose a correct subject from an array of four and choose a correct object from an array of four	II Self-generation of actor+action both verbally and graphically

Other investigators have attempted to train sentence production through the stimulation of verb-retrieval (e.g., Fink, Martin, Schwartz, Saffran, and Myers, 1993). Fink and others (1997) employed a task centered around the verb to be used to complete a story. One example follows (p. 42):

Clinician: Someone *carried* the sofa. It was the mover. Did I say the mover *dropped* the sofa?
Patient: No, he *carried* the sofa.

Agrammatic patients improved across six sessions in the use of trained verbs and verbs that were simply "exposed" during probing. In a case study, verbs were better than nouns for cueing sentence production; and a treatment of verb-finding was accompanied by improved sentence production (Marshall, Pring, and Chiat, 1998).

Melodic Intonation Therapy (MIT)

Melodic Intonation Therapy (MIT) is based on the observation that nonfluent aphasic patients sing better than they talk. It is a carefully crafted program developed at the Boston VA Medical Center by Robert Sparks. The program has been reported in considerable detail and has been around for some time (Sparks, Helm, and Albert, 1974; Sparks and Holland, 1976). Candidates for the procedure are patients with good auditory comprehension and minimal improvement in speech production by more standard clinical procedures.

The essence of MIT is to have a patient "sing" an utterance. Several steps lead a patient into singing language, and then additional steps involve fading artificial melody from the production. Patients have been reported to proceed through the program successfully (Albert, Sparks, and Helm, 1973). Performance in MIT by severely nonfluent patients can be spectacular. However, reports have been elusive regarding response generalization to situations outside the context of the program.

AGRAMMATIC PRODUCTION: THEORY-DRIVEN TREATMENTS

In the 1990s, a few groups of clinical researchers began to report extensively on what they claimed are uniquely theory-driven or "model-guided" treatments for aphasia. Actually, a theoretical basis for treatment is not entirely new in that Schuell thought that therapy should be consistent with what we think aphasia is (see Chapter 11). This position has been rearticulated more recently by clinical researchers such as Sally Byng (1994) in England.

Currently, investigators are exploring the application of more modern and detailed theoretical developments. Treatments are based on a diagnosis of impairment in the cognitive system or, for aphasia, in the psycholinguistic system. When applied to agrammatism, treatments are motivated by a theory of language production. A treatment might repair an impaired process or facilitate the establishment of an alternate route around the crippled process.

Externalization of Schemas

Luria (1970b) may have originated theory-motivated treatments of grammatical difficulties. He believed that agrammatic utterances are the result of difficulty with accessing structural representations. His "externalization of schemas" was intended to raise structural representation to a conscious level of awareness. He would present visual cues to grammatical categories in syntactic order, such as stick-figures of agent, action, recipient. Sometimes three coins or buttons were all that was necessary. While pointing to each cue, patients magically produced a complete utterance. This cueing procedure became the basis for a more elaborate system (Davis, 1973). A patient would practice elicited sentences as the clinician gradually faded the cues.

Diagnostic-Based Treatment

At the University of Maryland, Rita Berndt, Charlotte Mitchum, and Ann Haendiges set up a framework for refurbishing the theoretical influence on treatment of sentence production. They presented a treatment for EA, who had nonfluent aphasia and "problems with phonetic aspects of speech" (i.e., apraxia of speech). This case study represented a "a solution to the problem of where to focus treatment of the sentence production impairment in aphasia" (Mitchum, Haendiges, and Berndt, 1993, p. 71).

The Maryland team contrasted their approach to HELPSS which, they claimed, is "aimed exclusively at the level at which the sentence is spoken" (p. 71). They stated that the alternative is "to direct treatment at the earlier stages of the sentence production process...that presumably precede phonetic implementation" (p. 71). More specifically, Mitchum explored the possibility that EA was impaired in the positional level of Garrett's model of sentence production (see Figure 5.1). Yet, after extensive evaluation of EA, she concluded that she "cannot precisely identify the cause of his failure to construct an adequate sentence" (p. 85). Mitchum could conclude only that some sort of dysfunction exists prior to the selection of output modality (i.e., speech or writing).

The treatment for EA consisted of written naming of actions (i.e., verb production). The speech modality was not stimulated. Mitchum and her colleagues (1993) predicted that "If the impairments...affect processing components that are executed prior to the modality 'split,' ...generalization across modalities should occur even if only one modality of output is practiced" (p. 76). They found that spoken sentence production improved following treatment of written sentence production.

Let us examine this study for a moment. The diagnosis of disorder at a level prior to the motor stage is equivalent to saying that the patient had a language disorder in addition to phonetic problems. The diagnosis had essentially the same specificity as identifying aphasia in contrast to apraxia of speech. Moreover, the cross-modal generalization achieved with the treatment is a common goal in treatments based on Schuell's understanding that aphasia is a central disorder underlying the modalities. Thus, clinical aphasiologists did not need to revolutionize their work, yet. More experimentation needed to be done before we could say that modern theory sharpens our focus relative to traditional clinical practice.

Mapping Therapy

Another application of theory hinged on a more specific diagnosis. Could agrammatic production be caused by a mapping impairment? To put this proposal in perspective, we should review the mapping hypothesis regarding sentence comprehension discussed in Chapter 5. Applied to Garrett's model of production, impairment lies in the transition from the functional level of predicate-argument structure to the positional level of surface ordering and inflectional selection (Schwartz, Saffran, Fink, Myers, and Martin, 1994). Mapping therapy is intended to repair this transitional operation.

Candidates for the procedure usually fit the following profile:

- agrammatic production (usually Broca's aphasia)
- "good" grammaticality judgment ability
- "poor" comprehension of reversible sentences, including more role reversal than lexical errors

These selection criteria indicate that identification of asyntactic comprehension is crucial for diagnosing the basis for expressive agrammatism. Moreover, the theory of mapping in comprehension contributes to the therapeutic approach (i.e., mapping thematic role interpretations onto intact structural representations).

Three research teams have been exploring mapping therapy for improving sentence production (Byng, Nickels, and Black, 1994; Marshall, Pring, and Chiat, 1993; Schwartz, et al., 1994). Byng and Schwartz used the therapy to improve comprehension as well as production. Their slightly different techniques have certain fundamental common features:

- the goal of improving sentence production
- therapy tasks that do not require production (e.g., metalinguistic tasks)
- thematic role cueing similar to Luria's externalization of schemas

Similar to the semantic treatments of naming (see Chapter 11), mapping therapy is thought to stimulate a level of the sentence production process before production actually occurs. Thus, like the naming treatments, producing utterances is not a key feature of mapping therapy. Versions of this method are summarized in Table 13.5.

One difference among mapping methods is that Byng's group built a generalization stage into their therapy. This stage incorporated thematic cues to aid in the production of sentences during a PACE activity. Other versions of mapping have not contained a generalization stage, indicating

TABLE 13.5 Summary of mapping therapies for improving sentence production.

INVESTIGATORS	LOCATION	TREATMENT STEPS	RESEARCH
Sally Byng Lyndsey Nickels Maria Black	Birkbeck College London	patient sorts color coded phrases into sentence; patient describes same action (color cues); PACE therapy (color cues available)	3 cases improved in verb and sentence production
Jane Marshall Tim Pring	City Hospital London	present simple actions on video; ask questions about agent, recipient, and action	spontaneous production did not improve in case studied
Myrna Schwartz Eleanor Saffran Ruth Fink	Moss Rehabilitation Hospital Philadelphia	present printed sentence; ask questions about agent, recipient, and action; patient underlines agent, recipient, and action (pens used as color cues)	6 subjects improved in comprehension and production

that clinicians hoped for a greater jump over the gap between the treatment and more functional sentence production.

Mapping therapy is similar to cueing-verb treatment's emphasis on awareness of thematic roles around a verb. One procedural difference is that CVT involves the direct elicitation of production, whereas mapping therapy emphasizes metalinguistic tasks that do not elicit utterances. In this sense, mapping therapy has been thought to tap into a mental process leading to sentence production.

Movement Therapy

Cynthia Thompson and Lewis Shapiro explored a treatment modeled after a different type of theory, namely, linguistic theory of sentence structure (see Shapiro, 1997). As an account of aphasic impairment, linguistic theory was mentioned in Chapter 5 in association with Caplan's linearity hypothesis and Grodzinsky's trace-deletion hypothesis of altered structural representations that may be computed for comprehension. Linguistic theory is not generally tested in the time-based psycholinguistics laboratory as a model of mental processing. Yet, Thompson and Shapiro spoke of the "mapping" of structural levels in a way that could give linguistic theory a psychological character. Studies of treatment may be a test of the "psychological reality" of linguistic constructs.

The clinical investigators studied the construct of *movement,* which shows how sentence structures are related to each other (Thompson, Shapiro, Ballard, Jacobs, Schneider, and Tait, 1997). For example, a *wh*-question is said to be created from a declarative statement (e.g., *The woman followed the man*) by "moving" the direct object (e.g., *the man*) from its position after the verb to the front of the sentence (e.g., *Who did the woman follow*?). In linguistic terms, a *trace* is left behind in the position vacated by the moved noun-phrase, enabling us to identify *Who* as the direct object. Some type of movement characterizes most questions.

Thompson and Shapiro were interested in whether linguistic theory predicts generalization of treatment effects across baselines defined according to type of *wh*-question. Superficially, we might think that treatment of one type of *wh*-question could generalize to all other *wh*-questions. However, there are two types of movement with respect to *wh*-questions. One type of movement underlies *who* and *what* questions, and the other underlies questions beginning with *when* and *where.* Thompson and Shapiro found that treatment of *who* questions generalized to *what* questions but not to the other type of *wh*-question (Thompson, Shapiro, Tait, Jacobs, and Schneider, 1996). This was an instance in which a theory predicted a clinical outcome that would not necessarily have been predicted without knowledge of the theory.

Another theory-motivated feature of this research was the treatment itself. The treatment contained steps that modeled the linguistic notion of movement (that is, we cannot be sure that movement is a mental process). Using cue-cards with the printed words of a sentence, patients started by repeating and reading a simple sentence such as *The girl hit the boy* (akin to deep structure). The short-term goal was to help agrammatic patients produce *wh*-questions such as *Who did the girl hit*? In early steps, a patient was provided with additional cue-cards including one with *Who* at the end of the first sentence. Subsequent steps included moving the *wh*-cue to the beginning of the sentence. All moves led to a sequence of cues depicting the question (e.g., Thompson and Shapiro, 1994).

ASYNTACTIC COMPREHENSION

Treatment of language comprehension for Broca's aphasia tends to start with sentences. General programs for sentence comprehension have consisted of manipulating length and basic structural characteristics to increase the difficulty of a task. A few clinical investigators have been evaluating treatments that may be appropriate for a cognitive impairment thought to cause asyntactic comprehension.

Externalization of Schemas

As with sentence production, Luria (1970b) attempted to improve sentence comprehension by increasing conscious awareness of syntax. Diagrams which "differ little from those used in common grammar texts" were shown in association with a spoken or printed sentence. The diagrams consisted of stick figures for actors, drawings of actions, and ideograms showing basic spatial relations. For example, *on* was represented as a ball on a plane, and *under* was represented as a ball beneath a plane.

The purpose was "to externalize the meaningful relationships implied by the constructions and compensate for the inner schemata which the patient lacks" (p. 443). Phrases like *mother's daughter* were split into parts so that a patient could analyze structure. Two pictures represented the meaning of each word. A demonstrative was added for cueing the word serving as modifier (e.g., "*this* mother's daughter").

Mapping Therapy

The belief motivating mapping therapy was that asyntactic comprehension is caused by an impairment of the hypothesized mapping mechanism. Patients were assumed to have problems making conscious agent-object order decisions for reversible sentences. As indicated earlier, two research teams employed mapping therapy for improving both comprehension and production (Byng, et al., 1994; Schwartz, et al., 1994).

Byng (1988) found two patients who erred with reversible declarative (e.g., *The man kisses the woman*) and locative sentences (e.g., *The man is beside the woman*). She treated only locatives and measured comprehension of other types of sentences. In a treatment that was similar to Luria's externalization of schemas, comprehension was cued with a "meaning card" showing relations between noun phrases. Colors were also used to cue noun-phrase location in a sentence. One patient's progress in understanding locatives spread to untreated reversible sentence-types, which Byng interpreted as repair of a mapping mechanism that contributes to comprehending all sentences.

The Maryland research team treated EA with another version of mapping therapy (Haendiges, Berndt, and Mitchum, 1996). This patient had a comprehension impairment considered to be more severe than the typical deficit in Broca's aphasia. Treatment consisted of practice with three auditory comprehension tasks. One consisted of sentence-picture verification. Another was a standard picture-choice task. In the third task, EA was instructed not to respond to the clinician's comparison of active and passive versions of one message. In all tasks, the clinician pointed out specific thematic components of a picture (i.e., agent and recipient). Because the patient's progress generalized to some untreated sentences but not others, Haendiges and her colleagues forthrightly concluded that mechanisms besides mapping were probably contributing EA's impairment.

Comments on Theory-Driven Strategies

Most clinicians may agree with Schuell that an appropriate treatment is derived from an understanding of the nature of aphasia. The theoretical basis for stimulation treatment has been that aphasia is thought to be primarily an impairment of processing rather than a loss of linguistic knowledge. The main difference between current theory-driven treatments and the stimulation approach is that the current treatments are intended to address specific processes rather than a vague notion of processing in general. The testing of more specific theories is an ongoing work, and theory-driven treatments should be considered to be part of this unfinished endeavor.

Caramazza (1989) expressed misgivings over the "unfulfilled promise" of theory-motivated treatments that were in their infancy. He suggested, "we need to ask ourselves whether we would have used a different therapeutic strategy had we had a different hypothesis about the functional lesion in the patient" (p. 395). He added that any hypothesis about the nature of deficit "is of limited use in specifying an informed therapeutic strategy because the content of our cognitive theories does not specify the modifications that a damaged system undergoes as a function of the different types of experiences with which a patient may be presented" (p. 393). Holland (1994) echoed this concern over the lack of a theory of therapeutic effects.

The clinical consumer of treatment ideas should ask a couple of questions.

- **Is the treatment really new, or is it a repackaging of an established approach?** For example, Mitchum and others' application of Garrett's production model did not carve out any new ground with respect to diagnosis or treatment. Clinicians may already be doing the theory-driven treatment. Only the rationale may be new. Thompson and Shapiro's linguistic approach led to some treatment procedures that had not been reported before.
- **Has the diagnostic basis for a treatment been validated in basic research?** Chapter 5 indicates that the diagnosis of a mapping disorder, at least, should be considered to be just one of several current explanations of agrammatism. Treatment studies might include comparisons between therapies that follow from alternative explanations of a symptom pattern (e.g., a "parsing therapy" vs. mapping therapy). Meanwhile, clinical investigators should do a better job of presenting their work in the context of alternative theories or explanations.

We may also be tempted to challenge theory-driven treatments regarding their efficacy. However, this would be a rather selective application of a common challenge. All treatments should be scrutinized for efficacy, and a harsh demand for efficacy in the early stages of a particular investigation risks inhibiting the discovery of new methods.

WERNICKE'S APHASIA

Wernicke's aphasia presents some unique problems for rehabilitation such as a poor "therapeutic set" (Sparks, 1978). With a lack of awareness of deficit, the patient does not appear to comprehend the reason for being in the clinic. Our expectations soon after onset should be uncertain, because some patients recover a great deal of language ability whereas others do not progress very much. Early progress in treatment may be an indication of likely overall progress. Brookshire's (1997) ominous prognostic signs for global aphasia included symptoms of Wernicke's aphasia such as severe comprehension deficit and extensive jargon without awareness of the disorder.

Auditory Comprehension

Treatment of comprehension is the first step in dealing with this type of aphasia. People with frank Wernicke's aphasia are terrible repeaters, so that direct stimulation of production through modeling is generally unsuccessful. In a sense, we cannot enter treatment of formulation through the front door. Comprehension training doubles as a means of improving functional communication and as a means of setting up skills that can be used to gain control over expression.

The first goal is to establish a therapeutic set or, namely, consistent response to a clinician's stimulation. We may have to begin with simple modeling of a clinician pointing to a picture. The patient may be trained to point to a picture of an object in response to an environmental sound. When the patient gets the idea of listening and pointing, we begin to use words as stimuli with appropriate referents for response. Family names and photos may be used. Numbers may be readily recognized with response cards showing simple quantities. Once reliable responding is established, we sneak simple levels of word comprehension into the treatment.

Press for speech can interfere with auditory processing. We should direct attention to listening by inhibiting this tendency to talk excessively. Whitney suggested a "stop strategy" in contrast to a "go strategy" for Broca's aphasia (cited in Holland, 1977). The idea was to keep the person with Wernicke's aphasia from talking during comprehension training. An alerting signal such as a raised hand is often all that is needed to remind the patient to stop talking when the task is to listen. As comprehension improves, we look for improved recognition of jargon.

Mitchum and her colleagues (1995) saw a need to provide mapping therapy for ML, a case who had moderate Wernicke's aphasia and who had been studied previously with other treatments. Auditory stimulation was about the same as the treatment given to EA, except that the active and passive sentence comparison was not included. Progress generalized to auditory sentences with untreated verbs and to reading sentences. Progress did not generalize to understanding longer sentences or to sentence production.

Jargon

Self-monitoring is considered to be important for getting control over unwieldy verbal expression. Jane Marshall and her colleagues in London studied four patients with a dissociation between comprehension and self-monitoring. That is, comprehension ability was good, but the patients still could not recognize their own jargon. The patients appeared to have an impairment of feedback processes (Marshall, Robson, Pring, and Chiat, 1998). Further evaluation showed that the patients could recognize neologisms when repeating words but not when naming, suggesting that the feedback problem arises when accessing semantics.

This semantically related problem led Marshall to try a semantic therapy program for naming. The treatment consisted of comprehension tasks involving associating printed words with pictures, and it was carried out for six sessions plus homework assignments. The investigators were disappointed that the patients made no progress in naming, but the patients improved in recognizing neologisms for treated items but not for untreated items. In all, the treatment did not have a dramatic effect on the feedback mechanism.

We may have to see if repetition appears spontaneously during comprehension drills before trying intentional repetition to elicit meaningful speech. Exactly how this happens and how often it happens does not appear to have been studied systematically. Patients may get to the point where we can use standard methods of modeling, chaining, and so on. When volitional repetition begins, we can build a program for eliciting language. However, this may take months beyond the number of sessions allotted under managed care. Special funding may be needed to explore thoroughly the effects that language stimulation can have on jargonaphasia.

CONDUCTION APHASIA

Treatment studies of conduction aphasia are about as rare as studies of Wernicke's aphasia. The discovery that sentence comprehension problems are similar to those in Broca's aphasia indicates that comprehension training may be similar. In fact, tasks for making syntactic judgments and arranging words into sentences were embedded in a program to treat phonemic paraphasias (Cubelli, Foresti, and Consolini, 1988). Kearns' RET program has also been helpful for people with conduction aphasia (Yedor, et al., 1993). For targeting the definitive problems of conduction aphasia, investigators have focused on repetition or phonemic paraphasias.

A pair of studies was devoted to improving repetition. Reading aloud was the main activity used by Sullivan, Fisher, and Marshall (1986). Upon successful reading, the visual stimulus was removed so that the utterance could be repeated without this cue. Peach (1987) wanted to improve sentence repetition by treating memory span. The patient started with a task of pointing to pictures in a sequence spoken by the clinician. Then, the patient was asked to repeat words in the order spoken. Repetition improved during the period of treatment.

Other investigators focused on reducing phonemic paraphasias. Boyle (1989) employed a procedure in which the patient was instructed to look at a word and think about how it sounds and then read the word aloud. In Italy, Cubelli and others

(1988) had clients confront phonemic-graphemic structure with a few metalinguistic tasks. In one task, the patient was shown a picture (e.g., table or *tavolo*) and cards containing each syllable of the word (e.g., TA, VO, LO). The patient was asked to arrange the syllables in correct order and then read the word aloud. In another task, the clinician displayed a picture (e.g., table) and a letter (e.g., E). The patient had to decide if the letter belongs to the word for the picture.

Later, Peach (1996) reported on a therapy for a patient who was initially diagnosed with Wernicke's aphasia and who then later took on some characteristics of conduction aphasia. The phonologically-based procedure was centered on an oral reading task. The clinician's responses to error included having the patient write the word. If this did not improve spoken response, a phonemic error was paired with the correct sound in the beginning of another word to read. Repetition was another option for restimulation. A multiple-baseline design showed generalization to an untreated baseline rather than a sequential treatment effect on the baselines.

ANOMIC OR MILD APHASIAS

In his argument regarding global aphasia, Marshall (1987) suggested that we have paid less attention to the communicative needs of persons with mild aphasia. He advocated that we "reapportion treatment time so as to spend more hours with mildly impaired clients" (p. 70). With respect to the syndrome of anomic aphasia, the main linguistic goal is to improve word-finding. Yet, good comprehension and circumlocutions frequently facilitate communicative conversation, so that functional goals may pertain mainly to the handicap caused by anomia. That is, language treatment may be motivated by social and vocational needs.

Linebaugh's (1983) *Lexical Focus* consisted of hierarchies of cueing for a convergent naming task and, for the mildest anomic aphasias, a divergent categorical word-fluency task. A hierarchy of difficulty for categories was based on "width" of exemplars in a category. That is, an easy category was *sports,* and a more challenging narrow category was *water sports.*

Studies of cueing have had apparently contradictory results for anomic aphasia (see Table 11.6). Comparison of phonemic and semantic cues seems to depend on when cues are administered in a naming treatment interaction. In prestimulation, phonemic cues were more powerful than semantic cues. For restimulation upon error, phonemic and semantic cues were about equally effective a small percentage of the time.

READING IMPAIRMENTS

Theory-driven treatments of reading are based on identifying an impaired component of the reading process (see Table 6.5). The process-model and clinical analysis are centered around reading aloud or, namely, the processes leading from seeing a word to articulating a spoken response. Training may be directed at repairing the impaired component or compensating with an available alternative route. Pragmatically, we are minimally interested in *comprehension* or, namely, the activation of semantic memory upon seeing a word. In the next two sections, we shall be examining cases caused by closed head injury as well as stroke.

Peripheral Dyslexias

Peripheral dyslexias are considered to be caused by visual sensory or attentional disorders, although they have been reported in cases of anomic aphasia (see Table 6.6). **Pure alexia** is characterized by very slow or letter-by-letter reading, signified in part by the word-length effect. Stimulation has consisted of speeded reading tasks in which one patient matched letters and named nonwords rapidly (Arguin and Bub, 1994), another patient read aloud rapidly presented words (Lott and Friedman, 1995), and a third patient named letters as fast as possible (Lott and Friedman, 1996). These subjects were shown mainly to have increased their reading speed in the treatment tasks.

Treatment of **neglect dyslexia** is tied to treatment of left neglect, which draws from experimental findings of an influence of cues on attending to the left hemispace. Fundamental stimulation tasks are very much like assessment devices, such as crossing out tasks and line bisection tasks (see Chapter 8). Myers (1999) recommended the following compensatory strategies:

- verbal reminders, such as "go left" whenever a patient reaches the end of a line of text
- visual cues, such as a colored line in the left margin of a text
- tactile cues, such as a velcro strip in the left margin
- *anchors,* which are letters or numbers in the left edges of a field that a patient is told to seek

In addition, environmental management includes placing important objects in the right hemispace and encouraging others to stand to the patient's right during conversation.

Pizzamiglio and others (1992) studied 13 cases of RH infarction and hemorrhage. Left neglect training included a visual scanning task in which a computer presented a digit in different locations of the screen and subjects named the digit when presented. During reading tasks a red flashing anchor was placed to the left of a page, and a subject was cued to look for the anchor before starting to read or copy. Clinicians also used verbal reminders such as "look carefully to your left." Based on a pre-post test design, patients improved on some tests of neglect but not on others. In an assessment of simulated real life situations, unreported results were "encouraging." The researchers concluded that treatment demonstrated "considerable effectiveness."

Dyslexias with Aphasia

Phonological dyslexia has been diagnosed in patients with Broca's, anomic, conduction, and transcortical sensory aphasias. Key symptoms are a word superiority effect along with good word repetition, with a particular problem in reading aloud unfamiliar letter strings. Because pronunciation of unfamiliar letter strings depends on grapheme-phoneme conversion rules (see Figure 6.3), it is thought that a so-called *orthographic-phonological conversion* (OPC) mechanism is impaired.

Kendall, McNeil, and Small (1998) tried to repair the OPC for WT, a 42-year-old who had suffered a stroke 17 years prior to the treatment study. At the time of the study, WT had a mild nonfluent aphasia with good reading comprehension. The treatment consisted of "systematic exposure" to two conversion rules over six weeks. The rules are as follows:

- *c-rule:* when *c* comes before *a, o,* or *u,* it is produced as /k/; otherwise, as /s/
- *g-rule:* when *g* comes at the end of words or just before *a,o,* or *u,* it is produced as /g/; otherwise, as /dz/

As with most stimulation therapies for aphasia, the rules were not taught explicitly. WT practiced reading aloud words and nonwords embodying one of the rules (e.g., *cylecaber, girandole*). The clinician presented phonetic and morphological cues as restimulation upon error. Progress in treatment generalized to pronunciation of words involving other conversion rules.

Kendall's study was presented mainly to address a theoretical-clinical question rather than a functional-clinical question. We might ponder the circumstances in which an aphasic person may want or need OPC treatment when functional reading comprehension is pretty good. When does someone want to be good at reading aloud unfamiliar words? One possibility is that OPC may be important for a meticulous speller who writes letters and uses a computer.

Surface dyslexia has been found in patients with Broca's, anomic, and Wernicke's aphasias. The reading disorder differs from phonological dyslexia in that the OPC is intact. The patient pronounces nonwords and function words better than content words. With surface dyslexia, there is a strong regularity effect, and regularization errors are common (see Table 6.4). The disorder is thought to occur primarily in the graphemic lexicon or in access to it.

Several treatments have been reported for cases of closed head injury, a few with aphasia and at least one without aphasia (Weekes and Coltheart, 1996). Behrmann and Byng (1992) wanted to improve "use of the lexical procedure (via semantics) to access word-specific orthographic representations which are critical for irregular words" (p. 339). That is, the treatment was to repair the presumed impaired component rather than compensate with the alternative OPC route. For EE, who was traumatically injured due to a fall from a ladder, the treatment appeared to entail reading aloud irregular words such as *bough.* A picture (e.g., a tree) was used to help EE remember pronunciation.

Deep dyslexia has been diagnosed mainly in patients with Broca's aphasia. These patients produce many semantic paralexias when reading aloud and have a strong word-superiority effect that may be related to reading content words better than function words. Ambivalent diagnosis has been one problem with deep dyslexia, in that a disorder has been identified with OPC impairment (like phonological dyslexia) or with lexical-semantic mapping.

de Partz (1986) studied a business executive who had progressed over three months after an initial diagnosis of Wernicke's aphasia (also, Bachy-Langedock and de Partz, 1989). In cognitive terms, her general goal was to repair the OPC process by using spared lexical knowledge as "a relay" between the written word and pronunciation. The treatment proceeded in three stages. First, the patient worked on associating a letter with a word and reading aloud single syllables. Then, he associated letter combinations with words. Finally, he practiced whole word reading that was focused on certain conversion rules much like Kendall's procedure for phonological dyslexia. de Partz reported that one stage was "laborious," and the whole program appeared to take several months.

Reading treatments are summarized in Table 13.6, but the relationship between diagnosis and treatment is not straightforward. Hillis (1993) noted that different approaches have been effective for one diagnosis, that a single approach has been effective for different diagnoses, and that a given treatment may be successful for some patients but not others with the same diagnosis. We may be tempted to add that the theoretical objectives are difficult to grasp, partly because their wording across dyslexias is too similar to make out the distinctions. While some interesting treatment activities materialized amidst theory-driven efforts, investigators are continuing to work on the reliability and intelligibility of this general approach to reading rehabilitation.

DISCOURSE AND TEXT

For aphasia, we may find ourselves dealing with discourse or text as a functional context for practicing word- and sentence-level skills. Conversational discourse was reviewed in the previous chapter for this purpose. Mildly aphasic patients may have needs at this level, especially for those who are returning to employment involving conversational and writing skills. In wanting to resume work as a lecturer, Martin Exeter started to focus on discourse-level skills. It is also a level of unique expressive difficulty for patients with closed head injury (CHI) or right hemisphere dysfunction (RHD).

Models for Discourse-Level Treatment

There are few precedents regarding rehabilitation at the discourse level. When embarking on a relatively new area of treatment, we turn to our knowledge of the behavior for ideas about targets of treatment. Methods can be drawn from experimental procedures and from traditional principles of language therapeutics. We may check in on what other professions are doing regarding education of people to deal with discourse and text.

Let us first consider the nature of the behavior to be treated. We can establish specific goals for improving microstructural cohesion and macrostructural thematic and organizational coherence (e.g., Chapman and Ulatowska, 1992). With respect to cohesion, it is logical to think that we could direct a patient's attention to the relationship

TABLE 13.6 Treatments aimed at reading impairments. A crucial process is the alternate route to reading aloud (see Figure 6.3), which is often called orthographic-phonological conversion (OPC).

DYSLEXIAS	CASE	LESION	CLINICAL DIAGNOSIS	TREATMENT	REFERENCE
Peripheral	DM	left occipital hemorrhage	pure alexia with letter-by-letter reading	two-stage speeded reading tasks	Arguin and Bub (1994)
		RH strokes	left neglect	spatial scanning and cued reading tasks	Pizzamiglio, et al. (1992)
Phonological	WT	left fronto-temporal stroke	mild nonfluent aphasia with an impaired OPC	word and nonword reading aloud organized by OPC rules	Kendall, et al. (1998)
Surface	BL	left temporo-occipital stroke	no aphasia but an impaired graphemic lexicon	reading aloud words containing various vowel groups	Friedman and Robinson (1991)
	JB	CHI left temporal	aphasia with an impaired graphemic lexicon	homophone decisions for a sentence-completion task	Scott and Byng (1989)
	EE	CHI	aphasia with an impaired graphemic lexicon	reading aloud irregular words using a semantic memory aid	Behrmann and Byng (1992)
Deep	LR	LH stroke	moderate nonfluent aphasia	"phonologic treatment" bigraph reading aloud	Friedmann & Lott (1996)
	SP	left parieto-temporal hemorrhage	Wernicke's aphasia with impaired OPC	reading aloud letters and syllables with word associations	de Partz (1986)

between pronouns and antecedents (if a patient has a problem with microstructure). With respect to story telling and comprehension, we could direct a patient's attention to elements of setting, an initiating event, episodes, and resolution (if a patient has a problem with macrostructure).

Once we determine that a patient needs assistance with a feature or features of discourse, we can set up tasks modeled after basic research. If a patient has difficulty relating pronouns to antecedents, then one task might be to have a patient read sentence pairs and choose possible antecedents to a pronoun in the second sentence (Chapter 7). We can chart a course based on principles of programmed stimulation. We can heighten awareness of main ideas and provide cues (e.g., underlining) to facilitate identifying them. Like asking questions about thematic roles in a sentence, we could ask targeted questions such as "What is the main idea?" "Who is the main character?" We could start with short stories of just three or four sentences and then gradually increase the length of stories to comprehend or produce.

Another source of ideas is to borrow from instruction for other purposes, as Penn, Jones, and Joffe (1997) did for their "hierarchical discourse therapy." The education literature contains numerous approaches for improving text-level reading

TABLE 13.7 Some therapies for primary cognitive impairments caused by closed head injury.

FUNCTION	TREATMENT	ROLE IN DISCOURSE	REFERENCE
attention	computer-based attention tasks	topic maintenance	Ruff, Mahaffey, Engel et al. (1994)
memory	elaborative semantic strategy for recognition memory of words	remembering recent discourse and episodes that could be input to the discourse production system	Goldstein, Levin, Boake et al. (1990)
executive system	practice in analysis of a task, selecting a strategy, monitoring the activity, and evaluating its outcome	telling a complete story, following macrostructural organization to a conclusion	Lawson and Rice (1989)

abilities. Direct instruction and cooperative learning were compared for helping elementary students identify main ideas of expository paragraphs (Stevens, Slavin, and Farnish, 1991). Lorch and Lorch (1995) trained college students to rely on organizational signals (e.g., headings, summaries) to recall information in expository texts. Children with learning disabilities were taught to monitor adventure stories for internal inconsistencies (Chan, Cole, and Barfett, 1987).

CHI and RHD

Because problems with discourse are caused by primary cognitive impairments, direct treatments of attention, perception, and memory should generalize to discourse comprehension and production. Conversely, work on discourse and text is one means of improving primary cognitive functions (Ylvisaker and Szekeres, 1986). In her book on RHD, Tompkins (1995) wrote two chapters on principles and approaches to rehabilitation. Because there are few precedents for treatment of this clinical population, most of her suggestions were borrowed from pragmatic treatments for aphasia and from cognitive and social skills training for CHI.

Table 13.7 cites examples of treatment studies for primary impairments caused by CHI. The table also suggests relationships between a cognitive impairment and discourse processing abilities. Let us consider briefly how discourse is integrated into treatment of attention, memory, and executive function.

Selective or focused attention may be emphasized in the middle phase of recovery at RLA Levels IV to VI (Table 9.5). Ylvisaker and Szekeres (1986) recommended "listening to high interest stories or newspaper articles for specific information, listening to reports of events and then relaying that information to another person" (p. 481). Like word-monitoring experiments, a patient is asked to listen for specific information such as main ideas or the theme of an article or story. To improve access to episodic memory, Ylvisaker and Szekeres (1986) suggested that patients work on "describing main events in life, significant people and places" and "describing simple sequential tasks (e.g., shaving) or scripts for more complex events (e.g., going to a restaurant)" (p. 481).

Organizational features of discourse can be applied to work on executive control. Ylvisaker and Holland (1985) noted that "we have long recognized the need for patients to employ consciously [a] self-governing or charioteer function to facilitate their recovery" (p. 243). They called this capacity **self-coaching.** Especially at RLA Levels VII and VIII, a patient may practice identifying the structure of scripts or stories and imposing organization on information. Stories can be presented with implausible or illogical sequences to be recognized (e.g., *the waiter brought the food, and then he took the order*). Using picture sequences as cues, a patient can practice arranging them in a logical order for routines and story, telling stories with the pictures present, recalling the stories with the pictures removed (e.g., Yorkston, Stanton, and Beukelman, 1981).

Aphasia

Research reviewed in Chapter 7 indicated that aphasic people retain a sense for the connective and structural features of discourse. Schemas are embedded in an intact semantic memory. Someone with agrammatism can tell a story with a beginning, middle, and an end. Thus, treatment may not have the specific goal of improving story structure. Yet, limitations of working memory capacity can turn discourse into a strenuous activity for aphasic individuals. Slowed processing can put stress on reading text. Word-finding and grammatical difficulties do the same to discourse production and text writing.

During his rehabilitation, Martin Exeter was receiving encouragement from colleagues in the Netherlands and Belgium. They had been keeping in touch over e-mail. His colleagues were familiar with specialists in aphasia who, in turn, were accustomed to integrating aphasic people into social situations. In Europe, conferences on rehabilitation commonly included professionals and aphasic people. Psycholinguists suggested to Martin that he give an updated version of his speech at a meeting of rehabilitation specialists, many of whom were interested in his specialty of cognitive processing.

At the first hint of resurrecting his speech, Martin refused to consider it seriously because he did not think he could do it. He had not thought much about teaching during the months of arduous work on basic linguistic skills. Although some of his self-imposed treatment involved typing simple letters and other things on his computer, these abilities did not immediately translate into a desire or an attempt to write an article or a lecture. A small paragraph would take hours, especially after editing for spelling errors, grammatical mistakes, and empty words. For e-mail, he would have to compose in his word-processor and then import the letter into his e-mail system. All of this effort was tiring. He could only do a little at a time.

Eventually Martin's friends suggested that he seek advice and further help from a speech-language pathologist who was teaching on his campus. Neither he nor his colleagues in the Psychology Department had known much about the Department of Communicative Disorders, which, with hindsight, seemed strange considering that both departments were teaching about cognition and language. Nevertheless, Martin made an appointment with the faculty member who was teaching the aphasia course, Dr. Norma Johnson.

Collegiality and a mutual distaste for pomp quickly put Martin and Norma on a first name basis. After talking with him for a few minutes, Norma recognized that his aphasia was a relatively mild form. She knew that he had retained his knowledge and his recall. He described the circumstances of his stroke and explained his specialty in psychology. He also spoke of frustration in following conversation that seemed too fast for him, especially in a social group when the topic turned to politics. He needed some advice on managing other people in conversations, but his main problem appeared to be a lack of confidence in his ability to convey messages.

Norma was careful. Initially she wanted to see what Martin could do with respect to his area of expertise. She asked him to define basic concepts about memory and describe some memory experiments. Because writing was time-consuming and probably embarrassing in front of her, she gave him a list of terms to define on his computer at home. Martin was surprised when she concluded later that giving the lecture in Belgium was a reasonable goal. He would have to be patient. Writing would always be slow. He may not be ready for this year's conference, but maybe next year. She thought to herself that giving the lecture would be therapeutic in the long run.

Norma gave Martin some assignments and met with him occasionally to assess his work. He practiced writing in steps from definitions to explanations to a structured argument. They talked about the organization of a good lecture. He wrote outlines at home and then showed them to Norma. She found that her main task was to prove to him that his writing was good enough, even though it took time. She pointed out moments in their conversations that sounded like a strong part of a speech. "Just say that in Brussels," she said. Meetings with Norma decreased in frequency. He did speak to her class about his experiences with aphasia. Nine months after their first meeting, he practiced presenting a formal lecture to her.

If she were reporting to an insurance company, Norma would have documented Martin's initial status as "mild aphasia" and "currently not working as a lecturer in psychology." The initial goal was to become a lecturer. Later, documentation of progress would have been that he gave a one-hour lecture to her class.

SUMMARY AND CONCLUSIONS

This final chapter presented therapeutic approaches and techniques that address many of the specific symptoms and syndromes of aphasia and related language disorders. We continue to follow the fundamental principle of stimulating processes. In some instances, psycholinguistics and related cognitive sciences are being applied so that treatments may be focused on more clearly defined processes. Many of the procedures are experimental and hopefully encourage an appreciation for the effort to improve rehabilitation through an understanding of language functions and an application of scientific methodologies. One omission so far is a treatment that is sensitive to automatic processing.

Meanwhile, Martin and Jackie were met at the airport in Brussels by one of his psycholinguistics colleagues, who drove them to what sounded like the "Marmalade Hotel." When they got there, it turned out to be a Ramada Hotel. Because their flight had been delayed in London, they had only a couple of hours to unpack and rest before a dinner in the city with other hosts and speakers. After dinner, he and Jackie returned to their room where he practiced reading the manuscript, like that night three long years before.

The next day their host took them to the conference location, which had a long lobby with a glass front and colorful mosaics on the opposite wall inside. In the enormous lecture hall everything was red. Every seat had headphones. Looking up, Martin saw glass booths where interpreters would work. He whispered to Jackie that it felt like the United Nations. Yet, it also felt like Norma Johnson's classroom. When he was introduced, he picked up his outline and left the manuscript at his seat. He walked to the podium with ease. He was ready to get started.

References

Adams, M. L., Reich, A. R., & Flowers, C. R. (1989). Verbal-fluency characteristics of normal and aphasic speakers. *Journal of Speech and Hearing Research,* 32, 871–879.

Ahlsén, E., Nespoulous, J-L., Dordain,, M., Stark, J., Jarema, G., Kadzielawa, D., Obler, L. K., & Fitzpatrick, P. M. (1996). Noun phrase production by agrammatic patients: A cross-linguistic approach. *Aphasiology,* 10, 543–559.

Ahola, K., Vilkki, J., & Servo, A. (1996). Frontal tests do not detect frontal infarctions after ruptured intracranial aneurysm. *Brain and Cognition,* 31, 1–16.

Alajouanine, T. (1948). Aphasia and artistic realization. *Brain,* 71, 229–241.

Alajouanine, T. (1956). Verbal realization in aphasia. *Brain,* 79, 1–28.

Albert, M. L. (1976). Short-term memory and aphasia. *Brain and Language,* 3, 28–33.

Albert, M. L., & Bear, D. (1974). Time to understand. A case study of word deafness with reference to the role of time in auditory comprehension. *Brain,* 97, 373–384.

Albert, M. L., & Obler, L. K. (1978). *The bilingual brain.* New York: Academic Press.

Albert, M. L., Sparks, R., & Helm, N. A. (1973). Melodic intonation therapy. *Archives of Neurology,* 29, 130–131.

Alexander, M. P. (1988). Variability in the syndrome of Broca's aphasia in a rehabilitation hospital: Implications for research strategies. *Aphasiology,* 2, 219–224.

Alexander, M. P., Naeser, M. A., & Palumbo, C. L., (1987). Correlations of subcortical CT lesion sites and aphasia profiles. *Brain,* 110, 961–991.

Alexander, M. P., Fischette, M. R., & Fischer, R. S. (1989). Crossed aphasias can be mirror image or anomalous: Case reports, review and hypothesis. *Brain,* 112, 953–973.

Altmann, G. T. M., Garnham, A., & Henstra, J-A. (1994). Effects of syntax in human sentence parsing: Evidence against a structure-based proposal mechanism. *Journal of Experimental Psychology: Learning, Memory, and Cognition,* 20, 209–216.

Andersen, G. (1997). Post-stroke depression and pathological crying: Clinical aspects and new pharmacological approaches. *Aphasiology,* 11, 651–664.

Anderson, D. W., & McLauren, R. L. (Eds.). (1980). Report on the national head and spinal cord injury survey conducted by NINCDS. *Journal of Neurosurgery,* Supplement, 1–43.

Anderson, J. R. (1983). *The architecture of cognition.* Cambridge, MA: Harvard University Press.

Anderson, J. R. (1990). *Cognitive psychology and its implications* (3rd ed.). New York: W. H. Freeman.

Anderson, S. W., Damasio, H., Jones, R. D., & Tranel, D. (1991). Wisconsin Card Sorting Test performance as a measure of frontal lobe damage. *Journal of Clinical and Experimental Neuropsychology,* 13, 909–922.

Ansell, B. J., & Flowers, C. R. (1982). Aphasic adults' use of heuristic and structural linguistic cues for sentence analysis. *Brain and Language,* 16, 61–72.

Appell, J., Kertesz, A., & Fisman, M. (1982). A study of language functioning in Alzheimer patients. *Brain and Language,* 17, 73–91.

Aram, D. M. (1991). Acquired aphasia in children. In M. T. Sarno (Ed.). *Acquired aphasia* (2nd Ed.). New York: Academic Press.

Aram, D. M., Morris, R., & Hall, N. E. (1993). Clinical and research congruence in identifying children with specific language impairment. *Journal of Speech and Hearing Research,* 36, 580–591.

Arena, R., & Gainotti, G. (1978). Constructional apraxia and visuoperceptive disabilities in relation to laterality of cerebral lesions. *Cortex,* 14, 463–473.

Arguin, M., & Bub, D. (1993). Modulation of the directional attention deficit in visual neglect by hemispatial factors. *Brain and Cognition,* 22, 148–160.

Arguin, M., & Bub, D. N. (1994). Pure alexia: Attempted rehabilitation and its implications for interpretation of the deficit. *Brain and Language,* 47, 233–268.

Arguin, M., & Bub, D. (1997). Lexical constraints on reading accuracy in neglect dyslexia. *Cognitive Neuropsychology,* 14, 765–800.

Armstrong, E. M. (1993). Aphasia rehabilitation: A sociolinguistic perspective. In A. L. Holland & M. M. Forbes (Eds.), *Aphasia treatment: World perspectives* (pp. 263–290). San Diego, CA: Singular.

Arnett, P. A., Rao, S. M., Hussain, M., Swanson, S. J., & Hammeke, T. A. (1996). Conduction aphasia in multiple sclerosis: A case report with MRI findings. *Neurology,* 47, 576–578.

Arrigoni, G., & DeRenzi, E. (1964). Constructional apraxia and hemispheric locus of lesion. *Cortex,* 1, 170–197.

Arvedson, J. C., McNeil, M. R., & West, T. L. (1985). Prediction of Revised Token Test overall, subtest, and linguistic unit scores by two shortened versions. In R. H. Brookshire (Ed.), *Clinical aphasiology* (Vol. 15) (pp. 57–63). Minneapolis: BRK.

Ashcraft, M. H. (1989). *Human memory and cognition.* Gleview. IL: Scott, Foresman.

Ashcraft, M. H. (1994). *Human memory and cognition* (2nd ed.). New York: HarperCollins.

Aten, J. L. (1986). Functional communication treatment. In R. Chapey (Ed.), *Language intervention strategies in adult aphasia* (2nd Ed.) (pp. 266–276). Baltimore: Williams & Wilkins.

Au, R., Albert, M. L., & Obler, L. K. (1988). The relation of aphasia to dementia. *Aphasiology,* 161–174.

Avent, J. R., Edwards, D. J., Franco, C. R., Lucero, C. J., & Pekowsky, J. I. (1995). A verbal and nonverbal treatment comparison study in aphasia. *Aphasiology,* 9, 295–303.

Bachy-Langedock, N., & de Partz, M-P. (1989). Coordination of two reorganization therapies in a deep dyslexic patient with oral naming disorders. In X. Seron & G. Deloche (Eds.), *Cognitive approaches in neuropsychological rehabilitation* (pp. 211–248). Hillsdale, NJ: Lawrence Erlbaum.

Baddeley, A. D. (1986). *Working memory.* London: Oxford University Press.

Badecker, W., & Caramazza, A. (1987). The analysis of morphological errors in a case of acquired dyslexia. *Brain and Language,* 32, 278–305.

Badecker, W., & Caramazza, A. (1991). Morphological composition in the lexical output system. *Cognitive Neuropsychology,* 8, 335–368.

Bakar, M., Kirshner, H. S., & Wertz, R. T. (1996). Crossed aphasia. Functional brain imaging with PET or SPECT. *Archives of Neurology,* 53, 1026–1032.

Baker, E., Blumstein, S. E., & Goodglass, H. (1981). Interaction between phonological and semantic factors in auditory comprehension. *Neuropsychologia,* 19, 1–15.

Bamber, L. (1980). A retrospective study of language recovery in adult aphasics. Thesis, Memphis State University.

Barlow, D. H., & Hersen, M. (1984). *Single case experimental designs: Strategies for studying behavior change* (2nd ed.). New York: Pergamon.

Barton, M. I. (1971). Recall of generic properties of words in aphasic patients. *Cortex,* 7, 73–82.

Barton, M. I., Maruszewski, M., & Urrea, D. (1969). Variation of stimulus context and its effect on word-finding ability in aphasics. *Cortex,* 5, 351–365.

Basili, A. G., Diggs, C. C., & Rao, P. (1980). Auditory comprehension of brain-damaged subjects under competitive listening conditions. *Brain and Language,* 9, 362–371.

Basso, A. (1978). Aphasia rehabilitation. In Y. Lebrun, & R. Hoops (Eds.), *The management of aphasia* (pp. 9–21). Amsterdam: Swets & Zeitlinger.

Basso, A. (1989). Spontaneous recovery and language rehabilitation. In X. Seron & G. Deloche (Eds.), *Cognitive approaches in neuropsychological rehabilitation* (pp. 17–37). Hillsdale, NJ: Lawrence Erlbaum.

Basso, A. (1992). Prognostic factors in aphasia. *Aphasiology,* 6, 337–348.

Basso, A., Capitani, E., & Vignolo, L. A. (1979). Influence of rehabilitation on language skills in aphasic patients: A controlled study. *Archives of Neurology,* 36, 190–196.

Basso, A., Capitani, E., & Moraschini, S. (1982). Sex differences in recovery from aphasia. *Cortex,* 18, 469–475.

Basso, A., Lecours, A. R., Moraschini, S., & Vanier, M. (1985). Anatomo-clinical correlations of aphasias as defined through computerized tomography: Exceptions. *Brain and Language,* 26, 201–229.

Basso, A., Razzano, C., Faglioni, P., & Zanobio, M. E. (1990). Confrontation naming, picture description and action naming in aphasic patients. *Aphasiology,* 4, 185–196.

Basso, A., Taborelli, A., & Vignolo, L. A. (1978). Dissociated disorders of speaking and writing in aphasia. *Journal of Neurology, Neurosurgery, and Psychiatry,* 41, 556–563.

Bastiaanse, R., Edwards, S., & Kiss, K. (1996). Fluent aphasia in three languages: Aspects of spontaneous speech. *Aphasiology,* 10, 561–575.

Bastiaanse, R., Bosje, M., & Franssen, M. (1996). Deficit-oriented treatment of word-finding problems: Another replication. *Aphasiology,* 10, 363–383.

Bates, E. A., Chen, S., Tzeng, O., Li, P., & Opie, M. (1991). The noun-verb problem in Chinese aphasia. *Brain and Language,* 41, 203–233.

Bates, E. A., Friederici, A. D., & Wulfeck, B. B. (1987a). Comprehension in aphasia: A cross-linguistic study. *Brain and Language,* 32, 19–67.

Bates, E. A., Friederici, A. D., & Wulfeck, B. B. (1987b). Grammatical morphology in aphasia: Evidence from three languages. *Cortex,* 23, 545–574.

Bates, E. A., Friederici, A. D., Wulfeck, B. B., & Juarez, L. A. (1988). On the preservation of word order in aphasia: Cross-linguistic evidence. *Brain and Language,* 33, 323–364.

Bates, E. A., Hamby, S., & Zurif, E. (1983). The effects of focal brain damage on pragmatic expression. *Canadian Journal of Psychology,* 37, 59–84.

Bates, E. A., & Wulfeck, B. (1989). Comparative aphasiology: A cross-linguistic approach to language breakdown. *Aphasiology,* 3, 111–142.

Bates, E. A., Wulfeck, B., & MacWhinney, B. (1991). Cross-linguistic research in aphasia: An overview. *Brain and Language,* 41, 123–148.

Bauer, R. M., & Rubens, A. B. (1985). Agnosia. In K. M. Heilman & E. Valenstein (Eds)., *Clinical neuropsychology* (2nd Ed.) (pp. 187–241). New York: Oxford University Press.

Baum, S. R. (1988). Syntactic processing in agrammatism: Evidence from lexical decision and grammaticality judgement tasks. *Aphasiology,* 2, 117–136.

Baum, S. R. (1989). On-line sensitivity to local and long-distance syntactic dependencies in Broca's aphasia. *Brain and Language,* 37, 327–338.

Baum, S. R. (1997). Phonological, semantic, and mediated priming in aphasia. *Brain and Language,* 60, 347–359.

Baum, S. R., Blumstein, S. E., Naeser, M. A., & Palumbo, C. L. (1990). Temporal dimensions of consonant and vowel production: An acoustic and CT scan analysis of aphasic speech. *Brain and Language,* 39, 33–56.

Baum, S. R., Daniloff, J., Daniloff, R., & Lewis, J. (1982). Sentence comprehension by Broca's aphasics: Effects on suprasegmental variables. *Brain and Language,* 17, 261–271.

Baum, S. R., & Pell, M. D. (1997). Production of affective and linguistic prosody by brain-damaged patients. *Aphasiology,* 11, 177–198.

Bayles, K. A., Boone, D. R., Tomoeda, C. K., Slauson, T. J., & Kaszniak, A. W. (1989). Differentiating Alzheimer's patients from the normal elderly and stroke patients with aphasia. *Journal of Speech and Hearing Disorders,* 54, 74–87.

Bayless, J. D., Varney, N. R., & Roberts, R. J. (1989). Tinker Toy Test performance and vocational outcome in patients with closed head injuries. *Journal of Clinical and Experimental Neuropsychology,* 11, 913–917.

Beatty, W. W., Salmon, D. P., Bernstein, N., & Butters, N. (1987). Remote memory in a patient with amnesia due to hypoxia. *Psychological Medicine,* 17, 657–665.

Beauchamp, T. L., & Childress, J. F. (1994). *Principles of biomedical ethics* (4th Ed.). New York: Oxford University Press.

Beeson, P. M., Holland, A. L., & Murray, L. L. (1997). Naming famous people: An examination of tip-of-the-tongue phenomena in aphasia and Alzheimer's disease. *Aphasiology,* 11, 323–336.

Behrens, S. J. (1988). The role of the right hemisphere in the production of linguistic stress. *Brain and Language,* 33, 104–127.

Behrens, S. J. (1989). Characterizing sentence intonation in a right hemisphere-damaged population. *Brain and Language,* 37, 181–200.

Behrmann, M., & Bub, D. (1992). Surface dyslexia and dysgraphia: Dual routes, single lexicon. *Cognitive Neuropsychology,* 9, 209–252.

Behrmann, M., & Byng, S. (1992). A cognitive approach to the neurorehabilitation of acquired language disorders. In D. I. Margolin (Ed.), *Cognitive neuropsychology in clinical practice* (pp. 327–350). New York: Oxford University Press.

Béland, R., Lecours, A. R., Giroux, F., & Bois, M. (1993). The MT-86 ß Aphasia Battery: A subset of normative data in relation to age and level of school education (Part II). *Aphasiology,* 7, 359–382.

Bellaire, K. J., Georges, J. B., & Thompson, C. K. (1991). Establishing functional communication board use for nonverbal aphasic subjects. In T. E. Prescott (Ed.), *Clinical aphasiology* (Vol. 19) (pp. 219–228). Austin, TX: Pro-Ed.

Benson, D. F. (1967). Fluency in aphasia: Correlation with radioactive scan localization. *Cortex,* 3, 373–394.

Benson, D. F. (1979a). *Aphasia, Alexia, and Agraphia.* New York: Churchill Livingstone.

Benson, D. F. (1979b). Aphasia rehabilitation. *Archives of Neurology,* 36, 187–189.

Benson, D. F. & Stuss, D. T. (1986). *The frontal lobes.* New York: Raven.

Benton, A. L. (1985). Visuoperceptual, visuospatial, and visuoconstructive disorders. In K. M. Heilman

& E. Valenstein (Eds). *Clinical neuropsychology* (Second Edition) (pp. 151–185). New York: Oxford University Press.

Benton, A. L., & Hamsher, K. (1978). *Multilingual aphasia examination.* Iowa City: Benton Laboratory of Neuropsychology.

Benton, A. L., Hamsher, K., Varney, N. R., & Spreen O. (1983). *Contributions to neuropsychological assessment: A clinical manual.* New York: Oxford University Press.

Berman, M., & Peelle, L. M. (1967). Self-generated cues: A method for aiding aphasic and apractic patients. *Journal of Speech and Hearing Disorders,* 32, 372–376.

Berndt, R. S. (1987). Symptom co-occurrence and dissociation in the interpretation of agrammatism. In M. Coltheart, G. Sartori, & R. Job (Eds.). *The cognitive neuropsychology of language* (pp. 221–233). London: Erlbaum.

Berndt, R. S., & Caramazza, A. (1980). A redefinition of the syndrome of Broca's aphasia: Implications for a nueropsychological model of language. *Applied Psycholinguists,* 1, 225–278.

Berndt, R. S., Haendiges, A. N., Mitchum, C. C., & Sandson, J. (1997). Verb retrieval in aphasia. 2. Relationship to sentence processing. *Brain and Language,* 56, 107–137.

Berndt, R. S., Haendiges, A. N., Mitchum, C. C., & Wayland, S. C. (1996). An investigation of nonlexical reading impairments. *Cognitive Neuropsychology,* 13, 763–802.

Berndt, R. S., Mitchum, C. C., Haendiges, A. N., & Sandson, J. (1997). Verb retrieval in aphasia. I. Characterizing single word impairments. *Brain and Language,* 56, 68–106.

Berndt, R. S., Mitchum, C. C., & Wayland, S. (1997). Patterns of sentence comprehension in aphasia: A consideration of three hypotheses. *Brain and Language,* 60, 197–221.

Berndt, R. S., Salasoo, A., Mitchum, C. C., & Blumstein, S. E. (1988). The role of intonation cues in aphasic patients' performance of the grammaticality judgment task. *Brain and Language,* 34, 65–97.

Bernstein-Ellis, E., Wertz, R. T., Dronkers, N. F., & Milton, S. B. (1985). PICA performance by traumatically brain injured and left hemisphere CVA patients. In R. H. Brookshire (Ed.), *Clinical aphasiology* (Vol. 15) (pp. 97–106). Minneapolis: BRK.

Best, W. (1996). When racquets are baskets but baskets are biscuits, where do the words come from? A single case study of formal paraphasic errors in aphasia. *Cognitive Neuropsychology,* 13, 443–480.

Beukelman, D. R., Yorkston, K. M., & Dowden, P. A. (1985). *Communication augmentation: A casebook of clinical management.* San Diego: College-Hill Press.

Bihrle, A. M., Brownell, H. H., Powelson, J. A., & Gardner, H. (1986). Comprehension of humorous and nonhumorous materials by left and right brain damaged patients. *Brain and Cognition,* 5, 399–411.

Binder, L. M. (1986). Persisting symptoms after mild head injury: A review of the post-concussive syndrome. *Journal of Clinical and Experimental Neuropsychology,* 8, 323–346.

Binder, L. M. (1993). Assessment of malingering after mild head trauma with the Portland Digit Recognition Test. *Journal of Clinical and Experimental Neuropsychology,* 15, 170–182.

Bisiach, E., Capitani, E., Luzzatti, C., & Perani, D. (1981). Brain and the conscious representation of outside reality. *Neuropsychologia,* 19, 543–551.

Bisiach, E., & Luzzatti, C. (1978). Unilateral neglect of representational space. *Cortex,* 14, 129–135.

Bisiach, E., Vallar, G., Perani, D., Papagno, C., & Berti, A. (1986). Unawareness of disease following lesions of the right hemisphere: Anosognosia for hemiplegia and anosognosia for hemianopia. *Neuropsychologia,* 24, 471–482.

Black, F. W., & Strub, R. L. (1978). Digit repetition performance in patients with focal brain damage. *Cortex,* 14, 12–21.

Black, S. E. (1996). Focal cortical atrophy syndromes. *Brain and Cognition,* 31, 188–229.

Blomert, L., Kean, M-L., Koster, C., & Schokker, J. (1994). Amsterdam-Nijmegen Everyday Language Test: Construction, reliability and validity. *Aphasiology,* 8, 381–407.

Blomert, L., Koster, C., van Mier, H., & Kean, M-L. (1987). Verbal communication abilities of aphasic patients: The everyday language test. *Aphasiology,* 1, 463–474.

Blonder, L. X., Burns, A. F., Bowers, D., Moore, R. W., & Heilman, K. M. (1993). Right hemisphere facial expressivity during natural conversation. *Brain and Cognition,* 21, 44–56.

Bloom, M., & Fischer, J. (1982). *Evaluating practice: Guidelines for the accountable professional.* Englewood Cliffs, NJ: Prentice-Hall.

Bloom, R. L., Borod, J. C., Obler, L. K., & Gerstman, L. J. (1992). Impact of emotional content on discourse production in patients with unilateral brain damage. *Brain and Language,* 42, 153–164.

Bloom, R. L., Borod, J. C., Obler, L. K., & Gerstman, L. J. (1993). Suppression and facilitation of pragmatic performance: Effects of emotional content on discourse following right and left brain damage. *Journal of Speech and Hearing Research,* 36, 1227–1235.

Bloom, R. L., Borod, J. C, Obler, L. K., Santschi-Haywood, C., & Pick, L. (1995). An examination of coherence and cohesion in aphasia (abstract). *Brain and Language,* 51, 206–209.

Blumstein, S. E. (1973). *A phonological investigation of aphasic speech.* The Hague, Netherlands: Mouton.

Blumstein, S. E., Baker, E., & Goodglass, H. (1977). Phonological factors in auditory comprehension in aphasia. *Neuropsychologia,* 15, 19–30.

Blumstein, S. E., Byma, G., Kurowski, K., Hourihan, J., Brown, T., & Hutchinson, A. (1998). On-line processing of filler-gap constructions in aphasia. *Brain and Language,* 61, 149–168.

Blumstein, S. E., Cooper, W. E., Goodglass, H., Statlender, S., & Gottleib, J. (1980). Production deficits in aphasia: A voice-onset time analysis. *Brain and Language,* 9, 153–170.

Blumstein, S. E., Cooper, W. E., Zurif, E. B., & Caramazza, A. (1977). The perception and production of voice-onset time in aphasia. *Neuropsychologia,* 15, 371–383.

Blumstein, S. E., & Goodglass, H. (1972). The perception of stress as a semantic cue in aphasia. *Journal of Speech and Hearing Research,* 15, 800–806.

Blumstein, S. E., Goodglass, H., Statlender, S., & Biber, C. (1983). Comprehension strategies determining reference in aphasia: A study of reflexivization. *Brain and Language,* 18, 115–127.

Blumstein, S. E., Katz, B., Goodglass, H., Shrier, R., & Dworetsky, B. (1985). The effects of slowed speech on auditory comprehension in aphasia. *Brain and Language,* 24, 246–265.

Blumstein, S. E., Milberg, W., Dworetzky, B., Rosen, A., & Gershberg, F. (1991). Syntactic priming effects in aphasia: An investigation of local syntactic dependencies. *Brain and Language,* 40, 393–421.

Blumstein, S. E., Milberg, W., & Shrier, R. (1982). Semantic processing in aphasia: Evidence from an auditory lexical decision task. *Brain and Language,* 17, 301–315.

Blumstein, S. E., Tartter, V. C., Nigro, G., & Statlender, S. (1984). Acoustic cues for the perception of place of articulation in aphasia. *Brain and Language,* 22, 128–149.

Boles, L. (1997). A comparison of naming errors in individuals with mild naming impairment following post-stroke aphasia, Alzheimer's disease, and traumatic brain injury. *Aphasiology,* 11, 1043–1056.

Boller, F. (1968). Latent aphasias: Right and left "nonaphasic" brain-damaged patients compared. *Cortex,* 4, 245–256.

Boller, F., & Dennis, M. (Eds.). (1979). *Auditory comprehension: Clinical and experimental studies with the Token Test.* New York: Academic Press.

Boller, F., Kim, Y., & Mack, J. L. (1977). Auditory comprehension in aphasia. In H. Whitaker & H. Whitaker (Eds.), *Studies in neurolinguistics* (Vol. 3) (pp. 1–63). New York: Academic Press.

Boller, F. & Vignolo, L. A. (1966). Latent sensory aphasia in hemisphere-damaged patients: An experimental study with the Token Test. *Brain,* 89, 815–8

Borkowski, J. G., Benton, A. L., & Spreen, O. (1967). Word fluency and brain damage. *Neuropsychologia,* 5, 135–140.

Bornstein, R. A. (1988a). Entry into clinical neuropsychology: Graduate, undergraduate, and beyond. *Clinical Neuropsychologist,* 2, 213–220.

Bornstein, R. A. (1988b). Guidelines for continuing education in clinical neuropsychology. *Clinical Neuropsychologist,* 2, 25–29.

Borod, J. C., Carper, J. M., & Naeser, M. (1990). Long-term language recovery in left-handed aphasic patients. *Aphasiology,* 4, 561–572.

Borod, J. C., Fitzpatrick, P. M., Helm-Estabrooks, N., & Goodglass, H. (1989). The relationship between limb apraxia and the spontaneous use of communicative gesture in aphasia. *Brain and Cognition,* 10, 121–131.

Borod, J. C., Goodglass, H., & Kaplan, E. (1980). Normative data on the Boston Diagnostic Aphasia Examination, Parietal Lobe Battery, and the Boston Naming Test. *Journal of Clinical Neuropsychology,* 2, 209–215.

Borod, J. C., Koff, E., Perlman-Lorch, M., & Nicholas, M. (1986). The expression and perception of facial emotion in brain-damaged patients. *Neuropsychologia,* 24, 169–180.

Botez, M. I., Botez, T., & Aube, M. (1980). Amusia: Clinical and computerized scanning (CT) correlations. *Neurology,* 30, 359.

Bottenberg, D., & Lemme, M. L. (1991). Effect of shared and unshared listener knowledge on narratives of normal and aphasic adults. In T. E. Prescott (Ed.), *Clinical aphasiology* (Vol. 19) (pp. 109–116). Austin, TX: Pro-Ed.

Bottenberg, D. E., Lemme, M. L., & Hedberg, N. L. (1987). Effect of story content on narrative discourse of aphasic adults. In R. H. Brookshire (Ed.), *Clinical aphasiology* (Vol. 17) (pp. 202–209). Minneapolis: BRK.

Boyle, M. (1989). Reducing phonemic paraphasias in the connected speech of a conduction aphasic subject. In T. E. Prescott (Ed.), *Clinical aphasiology* (Vol. 18) (pp. 379–393). Boston: College-Hill/Little, Brown.

Boyle, M. (1994). Aphasia treatment planning in acute rehabilitation settings. *Special Interest Division 2 Newsletter,* 4(3), 6–9.

Boyle, M., & Coelho, C. A. (1995). Application of semantic feature analysis as a treatment for aphasic dysnomia. *American Journal of Speech-Language Pathology,* 4(4), 94–98.

Boyle, M., Coelho, C. A., & Kimbarow, M. L. (1991). Word fluency tasks: A preliminary analysis of variability. *Aphasiology,* 5, 171–182.

Bradley, D.C., Garrett, M. F., & Zurif, E. B. (1980). Syntactic deficits in Broca's aphasia. In D. Caplan (Ed.), *Biological studies of mental processes* (pp. 269–286). Cambridge, MA: MIT Press.

Branchereau, L., & Nespoulous, J-L. (1989). Syntactic parsing and the availability of prepositions in agrammatic patients. *Aphasiology,* 3, 411–422.

Brauer, D., McNeil, M. R., Duffy, J. R., Keith, R. L., & Collins, M. J. (1989). The differentiation of normal from aphasic performance using PICA discriminant function scores. In T. E. Prescott (Ed.), *Clinical aphasiology* (Vol. 18) (pp. 117–129). Boston: College-Hill/Little Brown.

Brenneise-Sarshad, R., Nicholas, L. E., & Brookshire, R. H. (1991). Effects of apparent listener knowledge and picture stimuli on aphasic and non-brain-damaged speakers' narrative discourse. *Journal of Speech and Hearing Research,* 34, 168–176.

Broca, P. (1960). Remarks on the seat of the faculty of articulate language, followed by an observation of aphemia. In G. von Bonin (Trans.), *Some papers on the cerebral cortex.* Springfield, IL: Charles C. Thomas.

Broida, H. (1977). Language therapy effects in long term aphasia. *Archives of Physical Medicine and Rehabilitation,* 58, 248–253.

Broida, H. (1979). *Coping with stroke.* San Diego: Singular.

Brookshire, R. H. (1967). Speech pathology and the experimental analysis of behavior. *Journal of Speech and Hearing Disorders,* 32, 215–227.

Brookshire, R. H. (1972). Effects of task difficulty on naming by aphasic subjects. *Journal of Speech and Hearing Research,* 15, 551–558.

Brookshire, R. H. (1975). Recognition of auditory sequences by aphasic, right-hemisphere-damaged and non-brain-damaged subjects. *Journal of Communication Disorders,* 8, 51–59.

Brookshire, R. H. (1983). Subject description and generality of results in experiments with aphasic adults. *Journal of Speech and Hearing Disorders,* 48, 342–346.

Brookshire, R. H. (1994). Group studies of treatment for adults with aphasia: Efficacy, effectiveness, and believability. *Special Interest Division 2 Newsletter,* 4(4), 5–14.

Brookshire, R. H. (1997). *Introduction to neurogenic communication disorders* (5th ed.). St. Louis, MO: Mosby.

Brookshire, R. H., & Nicholas, L. E. (1978). Effects of clinician request and feedback behavior on responses of aphasic individuals in speech and language treatment sessions. In R. H. Brookshire (Ed.), *Clinical aphasiology conference proceedings* (pp. 40–48). Minneapolis: BRK.

Brookshire, R. H., & Nicholas, L. E. (1980). Verification of active and passive sentences by aphasic and nonaphasic subjects. *Journal of Speech and Hearing Disorders,* 43, 437–447.

Brookshire, R. H., & Nicholas, L. E. (1984). Consistency of effects of slow rate and pauses on aphasic listeners' comprehension of spoken sentences. *Journal of Speech and Hearing Research,* 27, 323–328.

Brookshire, R. H., & Nicholas, L. E. (1993). *The Discourse Comprehension Test.* Tucson, AZ: Communication Skill Builders.

Brookshire, R. H., & Nicholas, L. E. (1994). Speech sample size and test-retest stability of connected speech measures for adults with aphasia. *Journal of Speech and Hearing Research,* 37, 399–407.

Brookshire, R. H., Nicholas, L. S., Krueger, K. M., & Redmond, K. J. (1978). The clinical interaction analysis system: A system for observational recording of aphasia treatment. *Journal of Speech and Hearing Disorders,* 43, 437–447.

Brown, G., & Yule, G. (1983). *Discourse analysis.* Cambridge, UK: Cambridge University Press.

Brown, J. I., Bennett, J. M., & Hanna, G. (1981). *The Nelson-Denny reading test.* Chicago: Riverside.

Brown, J. R., & Schuell, H. M. (1950). A preliminary report of a diagnostic test for aphasia. *Journal of Speech and Hearing Disorders,* 15, 21–28.

Brownell, H. H. (1988). The neuropsychology of narrative comprehension. *Aphasiology,* 2, 247–250.

Brownell, H. H., Bihrle, A. M., & Michelow, D. (1986). Basic and subordinate level naming by agrammatic and fluent aphasic patients. *Brain and Language,* 28, 42–52.

Brownell, H. H., Michel, D., Powelson, J. A., & Gardner, H. (1983). Surprise but not coherence: Sensitivity to verbal humor in right hemisphere patients. *Brain and Language,* 18, 20–27.

Brownell, H. H., Potter, H. H., Bihrle, A. M., & Gardner, H. (1986). Inference deficits in right brain-damaged patients. *Brain and Language,* 27, 310–321.

Brownell, H. H., Potter, H. H., Michelow, D., & Gardner, H. (1984). Sensitivity to lexical denotation and connotation in brain-damaged patients: A double dissociation? *Brain and Language,* 22, 253–265.

Brownell, H. H., Simpson, T. L., Bihrle, A. M., Potter, H. H., & Gardner, H. (1990). Appreciation of metaphoric alternative word meanings by left and right brain-damaged patients. *Neuropsychologia,* 28, 375–383.

Bruce, C., & Howard, D. (1988). Why don't Broca's aphasics cue themselves? An investigation of phonemic cueing and tip of the tongue information. *Neuropsychologia,* 26, 253–264.

Bruce, V., & Young, A. W. (1986). Understanding face recognition. *British Journal of Psychology,* 77, 305–327.

Brumfitt, S. (1993). Losing your sense of self: What aphasia can do. *Aphasiology,* 7, 569–574.

Bruyer, R. (1991). Covert face recognition in prosopagnosia: A review. *Brain and Cognition,* 15, 223–235.

Bryan, K. L. (1988). Assessment of language disorders after right hemisphere damage. *British Journal of Disorders of Communication,* 23, 111–125.

Bryan, K. L. (1989). Language prosody and the right hemisphere. *Aphasiology,* 3(4), 285–300.

Bub, D. N., & Arguin, M. (1995). Visual word activation in pure alexia. *Brain and Language,* 49, 77–103.

Bub, D. N., Black, S., Howell, J., & Kertesz, A. (1987). Speech output processes and reading. In M. Coltheart, G. Sartori, & R. Job (Eds.), *The cognitive neuropsychology of language* (pp. 79–110). London: Lawrence Erlbaum.

Buck, R., & Duffy, R. J. (1980). Nonverbal communication of affect in brain-damaged patients. *Cortex,* 16, 351–362.

Buckingham, H. W. (1981). Where do neologisms come from? In J. W. Brown (Ed.), *Jargonaphasia* (pp. 39–62). New York: Academic Press.

Buckingham, H. W. (1986). The scan-copier mechanism and the positional level of language production: Evidence from phonemic paraphasia. *Cognitive Science,* 10, 195–217.

Buckingham, H. W. (1987). Phonemic paraphasias and psycholinguistic production models for neologistic jargon. *Aphasiology,* 1, 381–401.

Buckingham, H. W. (1989). Mechanisms underlying aphasic transformations. In A. Ardila & P. Ostrosky-Solis (Eds.). *Brain organization of language and cognitive processes* (pp. 123–145). New York: Plenum.

Buckingham, H. W., & Kertesz, A. (1976). *Neologistic jargon aphasia.* Amsterdam: Swets and Zeitlinger.

Buckingham, H. W., & Rekart, D. M. (1979). Semantic paraphasia. *Journal of Communication Disorders,* 12, 197–209.

Burgess, C., & Simpson, G. B. (1988). Cerebral hemispheric mechanisms in the retrieval of ambiguous word meanings. *Brain and Language,* 33, 86–103.

Burke, H. L., Yeo, R. A., Delaney, H. D., & Conner, L. (1993). CT scan cerebral hemispheric asymmetries: Predictors of recovery from aphasia. *Journal of Clinical and Experimental Neuropsychology,* 15, 191–204.

Burns, M. S., & Canter, G. J. (1977). Phonemic behavior in aphasic patients with posterior cerebral lesions. *Brain and Language,* 4, 492–507.

Burns, M. S., Halper, A. S., & Mogil, S. I. (1985). *Clinical management of right hemisphere dysfunction.* Rockville, MD: Aspen.

Busch, C. R. (1993). Functional outcome: Reimbursement issues. In M. L. Lemme (Ed.), *Clinical aphasiology* (Vol. 21) (pp. 73–85). Austin, TX: Pro-Ed.

Busch, C. R. (1994). How is a treatment plan for an aphasic patient reviewed in terms of Medicare policy and guidelines? *Special Interest Division 2 Newsletter,* 4(3), 14–17.

Busch, C. R., Brookshire, R. H., & Nicholas, L. E. (1988). Referential communication by aphasic and nonaphasic adults. *Journal of Speech and Hearing Disorders,* 53, 475–482.

Butfield, E., & Zangwill, O. L. (1946). Reeducation in aphasia: A review of 70 cases. *Journal of Neurology, Neurosurgery, and Psychiatry,* 9, 75–79.

Butler-Hinz, S., Caplan, D., & Waters, G. (1990). Characteristics of syntactic and semantic comprehension deficits following closed head injury versus left cerebrovascular accident. *Journal of Speech and Hearing Research,* 33, 269–280.

Butters, N., & Barton, M. (1970). Effect of parietal lobe damage on the performance of reversible operations in space. *Neuropsychologia,* 8, 205–214.

Butters, N., Barton, M., & Brody, B. A. (1970). Role of the right parietal lobe in the mediation of cross-modal associations and reversible operations in space. *Cortex,* 6, 174–190.

Byng, S. (1988). Sentence processing deficits: Theory and therapy. *Cognitive Neuropsychology,* 5, 629–676.

Byng, S. (1994). A theory of the deficit: A prerequisite for a theory of therapy? M. L. Lemme (Ed.), *Clinical aphasiology* (Vol. 22) (pp. 265–274). Austin, TX: Pro-Ed.

Byng, S., Kay, J., Edmundson, A., & Scott, C. (1990). Aphasia tests reconsidered. *Aphasiology,* 4, 67–92.

Byng, S., Nickels, L., & Black, M. (1994). Replicating therapy for mapping deficits in agrammatism: Remapping the deficit? *Aphasiology,* 8, 315–341.

Byng, S., & Black, M. (1989). Some aspects of sentence production in aphasia. *Aphasiology,* 3, 241–263.

Cairns, H. S. (1984). Research in language comprehension. In R. C. Naremore (Ed.), *Language science: Recent advances* (pp. 211–242). San Diego: College-Hill.

Calvin, W. H., & Ojemann, G. A. (1980). *Inside the brain.* New York: Mentor.

Campbell, K. (1970). *Body and mind.* Garden City, NY: Anchor Books.

Campbell, R., & Manning, L. (1996). Optic aphasia: A case with spared action naming and associated disorders. *Brain and Language,* 53, 183–221.

Campbell, T. F., & Dollaghan, C. A. (1990). Expressive language recovery in severely brain-injured children and adoloescents. *Journal of Speech and Hearing Disorders,* 55, 567–581.

Cancelliere, A. E. B., & Kertesz, A. (1990). Lesion localization in acquired deficits of emotional expression and comprehension. *Brain and Cognition,* 13, 133–148.

Cannito, M. P., Hough, M., Vogel, D., & Pierce, R. S. (1996). Contextual influences on auditory comprehension of reversible passive sentences in aphasia. *Aphasiology,* 10, 235–251.

Cannito, M. P., Jarecki, J. M., & Pierce, R. S. (1986). Effects of thematic structure on syntactic comprehension in aphasia. *Brain and Language,* 27, 38–49.

Cannito, M. P., Vogel, D., & Pierce, R. S. (1989). Sentence comprehension in context: Influence of prior visual stimulation? In T. E. Prescott (Ed)., *Clinical Aphasiology* (Vol. 18) (pp. 433–446). Boston: College-Hill/Little, Brown.

Canter, G. J. (1988). Apraxia of speech and phonemic paraphasia. *Aphasiology,* 2, 251–254.

Canter, G. J., Trost, J. E., Burns, M. S. (1985). Contrasting speech patterns in apraxia of speech and phonemic paraphasia. *Brain and Language,* 24, 204–222.

Caplan, D. (1983). A note on the "word-order problem" in agrammatism. *Brain and Language,* 20, 155–165.

Caplan, D. (1985). Syntactic and semantic structures in agrammatism. In M-L. Kean (Ed.). *Agrammatism* (pp. 125–151). Orlando, FL: Academic Press.

Caplan, D. (1987). *Neurolinguistics and linguistic aphasiology: An introduction.* Cambridge, UK: Cambridge University Press.

Caplan, D. (1988). On the role of group studies in neuropsychological and pathopsychological research. *Cognitive Neuropsychology,* 5, 535–548.

Caplan, D. (1991). Agrammatism is a theoretically coherent aphasic category. *Brain and Language,* 40, 274–281.

Caplan, D., Baker, C., & Dehaut, F. (1985). Syntactic determinants of sentence comprehension in aphasia. *Cognition,* 21, 117–175.

Caplan, D., & Evans, K. L. (1990). The effects of syntactic structure on discourse comprehension in patients with parsing impairments. *Brain and Language,* 39, 206–234.

Caplan, D., & Futter, C. (1986). Assignment of thematic roles to nouns in sentence comprehension by an agrammatic patient. *Brain and Language,* 27, 117–134.

Caplan, D., & Hildebrandt, N. (1988). Specific deficits in syntactic comprehension. *Aphasiology,* 2, 255–258.

Caplan, D., Matthei, E., & Gigley, H. (1981). Comprehension of gerundive constructions in Broca's aphasia. *Brain and Language,* 13, 145–160.

Caplan, D., & Waters, G. S. (1990). Short-term memory and language comprehension: A critical review of the neuropsychological literature. In G. Vallar & T. Shallice (Eds). *Neuropsychological impairments of short-term memory* (pp. 337–389). Cambridge University Press.

Caplan, D., & Waters, G. S. (1995). Aphasic disorders of syntactic comprehension and working memory capacity. *Cognitive Neuropsychology,* 12, 637–650.

Caplan, D., & Waters, G. S. (1996). Syntactic processing in sentence comprehension under dual-task conditions in aphasic patients. *Language and Cognitive Processes,* 11, 525–551.

Caplan, D., Waters, G. S., & Hildebrandt, N. (1997). Determinants of sentence comprehension in aphasic patients in sentence-picture matching tasks. *Journal of Speech, Language, and Hearing Research,* 40, 542–555.

Cappa, S. F. (1997). Subcortical aphasia: Still a useful concept? *Brain and Language,* 58, 424–426.

Cappa, S. F., Cavallotti, G., & Vignolo, L. (1981). Phonemic and lexical errors in fluent aphasia: Correlation with lesion site. *Neuropsychologia,* 19, 171–177.

Cappa, S. F., Papagno, C., & Vallar, G. (1990). Language and verbal memory after right hemispheric stroke: A clinical-CT scan study. *Neuropsychologia,* 28, 503–509.

Cappa, S. F., Perani, D., Grassi, F., Bressi, S., Alberoni, M., Franceschi, M., Bettinardi, V., Todde, S., & Fazio, F. (1997). A PET follow-up study of recovery after stroke in acute aphasics. *Brain and Language,* 56, 55–67.

Cappa, S. F., & Vignolo, L. A. (1988). Sex differences in the site of brain lesions underlying global aphasia. *Aphasiology,* 2, 259–264.

Caramazza, A. (1986). On drawing inferences about the structure of normal cognitive systems from the analysis of patterns of impaired performance: The case for single-patient studies. *Brain and Cognition,* 5, 41–66.

Caramazza, A. (1988). Some aspects of language processing revealed through the analysis of acquired aphasia: The lexical system. *Annual Review of Neuroscience,* 11, 395–421.

Caramazza, A. (1989). Cognitive neuropsychology and rehabilitation: An unfulfilled promise? In X. Seron & G. Deloche (Eds.), *Cognitive approaches in neuropsychological rehabilitation* (pp. 383–398). Hillsdale, NJ: Lawrence Erlbaum.

Caramazza, A. (1997). How many levels of processing are there in lexical access? *Cognitive Neuropsychology,* 14, 177–208.

Caramazza, A., & Badecker, W. (1991). Clinical syndromes are not God's gift to cognitive neuropsychology: A reply to a rebuttal to an answer to a response to the case against syndrome-based research. *Brain and Cognition,* 16, 211–227.

Caramazza, A., Basili, A., Koller, J. J., & Berndt, R. S. (1981). A investigation of repetition and language processing in a case of conduction aphasia. *Brain and Language,* 14, 235–271.

Caramazza, A. & Berndt, R. S. (1978). Semantic and syntactic processes in aphasia: A review of the literature. *Psychological Bulletin,* 85, 898–918.

Caramazza, A., & Berndt, R. D. (1985). A multicomponential deficit view of agrammatic Broca's aphasia. In M-L. Kean (Ed.). *Agrammatism* (pp. 27–63). Orlando, FL: Academic Press.

Caramazza, A., Gordon, J., Zurif, E. B., & DeLuca, D. (1976). Right hemisphere damage and verbal problem-solving behavior. *Brain and Language,* 3, 41–46.

Caramazza, A., & Hillis, A. E. (1989). The disruption of sentence production: Some dissociations. *Brain and Language,* 36, 625–650.

Caramazza, A., Hillis, A. E., Rapp, B. C., & Romani, C. (1990). The multiple semantics hypothesis: Multiple confusions? *Cognitive Neuropsychology,* 7, 161–190.

Caramazza, A., & Zurif, E. B. (1976). Dissociation of alogorithmic and heuristic processes in language comprehension: Evidence from aphasia. *Brain and Language,* 3, 572–582.

Carlesimo, G. A., Fadda, L., & Caltagirone, C. (1993). Basic mechanisms of constructional apraxia in unilateral brain-damaged patients: Role of visuoperceptual and executive disorders. *Journal of Clinical and Experimental Neuropsychology,* 15, 342–358.

Carlomagno, S. (1994). *Pragmatic approaches to aphasia therapy.* San Diego, CA: Singular.

Carlomagno, S., Losanno, N., Emanuelli, S., & Casadio, P. (1991). Expressive language recovery or improved communicative skills: Effects of P. A. C. E.

therapy on aphasics' referential communication and story retelling. *Aphasiology,* 5, 419–424.

Carlomagno, S., & Parlato, V. (1989). Writing rehabilitation in brain-damaged adult patients: A cognitive approach. In X. Seron, & G. Deloche (Eds.). *Cognitive approaches in neuropsychological rehabilitation* (pp. 175–210). London: Erlbaum.

Carney, R., & Temple, C. M. (1993). Prosopanomia? A possible category-specific anomia for faces. *Cognitive Neuropsychology,* 10, 185–195.

Carpenter, R. L., & Rutherford, D. R. (1973). Acoustic cue discrimination in adult aphasia. *Journal of Speech and Hearing Research,* 16, 534–544.

Carroll, D. W. (1999). *Psychology of language* (3rd ed.). Pacific Grove, CA: Brooks/Cole.

Cavalli, M., DeRenzi, E., Faglioni, P., & Vitale, A. (1981). Impairment of right brain-damaged patients on a linguistic cognitive task. *Cortex,* 17, 545–556.

Cermak, L. S., & Moreines, J. (1976). Verbal retention deficits in aphasic and amnesic patients. *Brain and Language,* 3, 16–27.

Cermak, L. S., & O'Conner, M. (1983). The anterograde and retrograde retrieval ability of a patient with amnesia due to encephalitis. *Neuropsychologia,* 213–234.

Chan, L. K. S., Cole, P. G., & Barfett, S. (1987). Comprehension monitoring: Detection and identification of text inconsistencies by LD and normal students. *Learning Disability Quarterly,* 10, 114–124.

Chang, F. R. (1980). Active memory processes in visual sentence comprehension: Clause effects and pronominal reference. *Memory and Cognition,* 8, 58–64.

Chapey, R., Rigrodsky, S., & Morrison, E. B. (1977). Aphasia: A divergent semantic interpretation. *Journal of Speech and Hearing Disorders,* 42, 287–295.

Chapman, S. B., & Ulatowska, H. K. (1989). Discourse in aphasia: Integration deficits in processing reference. *Brain and Language,* 36, 651–668.

Chapman, S. B., & Ulatowska, H. K. (1992). Methodology for discourse management in the treatment of aphasia. *Clinics in Communication Disorders,* 2, 64–81.

Chenery, H. J., Ingram, J. C. L., & Murdoch, B. E. (1990). Automatic and volitional semantic processing in aphasia. *Brain and Language,* 38, 215–232.

Chertkow, H., Bub, D., Deaudon, C., & Whitehead, V. (1997). On the status of object concepts in aphasia. *Brain and Language,* 58, 203–232.

Chiaromonte, L. (1996). Measuring functional outcomes in the subacute and long-term care patient using the Rehabilitation Outcome Measure (ROM) [On-line]. Available: geriatricspt.org/pubs/gerinotes/Sep 1996/measure.html

Chomsky, N. (1968). *Language and mind.* New York: Harcourt Brace Jovanovich.

Christiansen, J. A. (1995a). Coherence violations and propositional usage in the narratives of fluent aphasics. *Brain and Language,* 51, 291–317.

Christiansen, J. A. (1995b). Getting to the point: Relevance in story production and comprehension by aphasic patients (abstract). *Brain and Language,* 51, 201–204.

Chusid, J. G. (1979). *Correlative neuroanatomy and functional neurology* (17th Ed.). Los Altos, CA: Lange Medical Publications.

Cicone, M., Wapner, W., & Gardner, H. (1980). Sensitivity to emotional expressions and situations in organic patients. *Cortex,* 16, 145–158.

Clark, A. E., & Flowers, C. R. (1987). The effect of semantic redundancy on auditory comprehension in aphasia. In R. H. Brookshire (Ed.), *Clinical aphasiology* (Vol. 17) (pp. 174–179). Minneapolis: BRK.

Clark, C. M., & Ryan, L. (1993). Implications of statistical tests of variance and means. *Journal of Clinical and Experimental Neuropsychology,* 15, 619–622.

Code, C., & Rowley, D. (1987). Age and aphasia type: The interaction of sex, time since onset and handedness. *Aphasiology,* 1, 339–346.

Coelho, C. A. (1987). Sign acquisition and use following traumatic brain injury: A case report. *Archives of Physical Medicine and Rehabilitation,* 68, 229–231.

Coelho, C. A. (1990). Acquisition and generalization of simple manual sign grammars by aphasic subjects. *Journal of Communication Disorders,* 23, 383–400.

Coelho, C. A. (1991). Manual sign acquisition and use in two aphasic subjects. In T. E. Prescott (Ed.), *Clinical aphasiology* (Vol. 19) (pp. 209–218). Austin, TX: Pro-Ed.

Coelho, C. A. (1995). Discourse production deficits following traumatic brain injury: A critical review of the recent literature. *Aphasiology,* 9, 409–429.

Coelho, C. A., & Duffy, R. J. (1985). Communicative use of signs in aphasia: Is acquisition enough? In R. H. Brookshire (Ed.), *Clinical aphasiology* (Vol 15). (pp. 222–228). Minneapolis: BRK.

Coelho, C. A., & Duffy, R. J. (1987). The relationship of the acquisition of manual signs to severity of aphasia: A training study. *Brain and Language,* 31, 328–345.

Coelho, C. A., & Duffy, R. J. (1990). Sign acquisition in two aphasic subjects with limb apraxia. *Aphasiology,* 4, 1–8.

Coelho, C. A., Liles, B. Z., & Duffy, R. J. (1991). Discourse analyses with closed head injured adults: Evidence for differing patterns of deficits. *Archives of Physical Medicine and Rehabilitation,* 72, 465–468.

Coelho, C. A., Liles, B. Z., Duffy, R. J., & Clarkson, J. V. (1993). Conversational patterns of aphasic, closed-head-injured, and normal speakers. In M. L. Lemme (Ed.), *Clinical aphasiology* (Vol. 21) (pp. 183–192). Austin, TX: Pro-Ed.

Cohen, R., Kelter, S., & Woll, G. (1980). Analytical competence and language impairment in aphasia. *Brain and Language,* 10, 331–347.

Cohen, R., & Woll, G. (1981). Facets of analytical processing in aphasia: A picture ordering task. *Cortex,* 17, 557–570.

Collins, A. M., & Loftus, E. F. (1975). A spreading activation theory of semantic processing. *Psychological Review,* 82, 407–428.

Collins, M. J. (1986a). *Diagnosis and treatment of global aphasia.* San Diego: Singular.

Collins, M. J. (1986b). Treatment of a severely aphasic person. In R. C. Marshall (Ed.), *Case studies in aphasia rehabilitation: For clinicians by clinicians* (pp. 105–118). Austin, Tx: Pro-Ed.

Collins, M. J. (1997). Global aphasia. In L. L. LaPointe (Ed.), *Aphasia and related neurogenic disorders* (2nd ed.). New York: Thieme.

Collins, M. J., McNeil, M. R., Lentz, S., Shubitowski, Y., & Rosenbek, J. C. (1984). Word fluency and aphasia: Some linguistic and not-so-linguistic considerations. In R. H. Brookshire (Ed.), *Clinical aphasiology* conference proceedings (pp. 78–84). Minneapolis: BRK.

Coltheart, M. (1987). Functional architecture of the language-processing system. In M. Coltheart, G. Sartori, & R. Job (Eds.), *The cognitive neuropsychology of language* (pp. 1–25). London: Lawrence Erlbaum.

Coltheart, M., Sartori, G., & Job, R. (Eds.). (1987). *The cognitive neuropsychology of language.* London: Lawrence Erlbaum.

Conway, M. A., & Rubin, D.C. (1993). The structure of autobiographical memory. In A. E. Collins, S. E. Gathercole, M. A. Conway, & P. E. Morris (Eds.), *Theories of memory* (pp. 103–137). Hillsdale, NJ: Lawrence Erlbaum.

Cook, L, Smith, D. S., & Truman, G. (1994). Using Functional Independence Measure profiles as an index of outcome in the rehabilitation of brain-injured patients. *Archives of Physical Medicine and Rehabilitation,* 75, 390–393.

Cooper, P. R. (Ed.). (1982). *Head injury.* Baltimore: Williams & Wilkins.

Cooper, W. E., Soares, C., Nicol, J., Michelow, D., & Goloskie, S. (1984). Clausal intonation after unilateral brain damage. *Language and Speech,* 27, 17–24.

Coppens, P. (1991). Why are Wernicke's aphasia patients older than Broca's? A critical view of the hypotheses. *Aphasiology,* 5, 279–290.

Corballis, M. C. (1997). Mental rotation and the right hemisphere. *Brain and Language,* 57, 100–121.

Corina, D., Kritchevsky, M., & Bellugi, U. (1996). Visual language processing and unilateral neglect: Evidence from American Sign Language. *Cognitive Neuropsychology,* 13, 321–356.

Cornett, B. S. (1994). Service delivery issues in health care settings. In R. Lubinski & C. Frattali (Ed.), *Professional issues in speech-language pathology and audiology: A textbook* (pp. 188–200). San Diego, CA: Singular.

Coslett, H. B., & Saffran, E. M. (1989). Preserved object recognition and reading comprehension in optic aphasia. *Brain,* 112, 1091–1110.

Coughlan, A. K., & Warrington, E. K. (1978). Word comprehension and word comprehension and word retrieval in patients with localised cerebral lesions. *Brain,* 101, 163–185.

Craig, H. K., Hinckley, J. J., Winkelseth, M., Carry, L., Walley, J., Bardach, L., Higman, B., Hilfinger, P., Schall, C., & Sheimo, D. (1993). Quantifying connected speech samples of adults with chronic aphasia. *Aphasiology,* 7, 155–164.

Crary, M. A., Haak, N.J., & Malinsky, A. E. (1989). Preliminary psychometric evaluation of an acute aphasia screening protocol. *Aphasiology,* 3, 611–618.

Crary, M. A., & Kertesz, A. (1988). Evolving error profiles during aphasia syndrome remission. *Aphasiology,* 2, 67–78.

Crary, M. A., & Rothi, L. J. G. (1989). Predicting the Western Aphasia Battery aphasia quotient. *Journal of Speech and Hearing Disorders,* 54, 163–166.

Crary, M. A., Wertz, R. T., & Deal, J. L. (1992). Classifying aphasias: Cluster analysis of Western

Aphasia Battery and Boston Diagnostic Aphasia Examination results. *Aphasiology,* 6, 29–36.

Crerar, M. A., Ellis, A. W., & Dean, E. C. (1996). Remediation of sentence processing deficits in aphasia using a computer-based microworld. *Brain and Language,* 52, 229–274.

Cripe, L. I. (1987). The neuropsychological assessment and management of closed head injury: General guidelines. *Cognitive Rehabilitation,* 5, 18–22.

Critchley, M. (1960). Jacksonian ideas and the future, with special reference to aphasia. *British Medical Journal,* 6, 6–11.

Croot, K., Patterson, K., & Hodges, J. R. (1998). Single word production in nonfluent progressive aphasia. *Brain and Language,* 61, 226–273.

Crosson, M., Moberg, P. J., Boone, J. R., Rothi, L. G., & Raymer, A. (1997). Category-specific naming deficit for medical terms after dominant thalamic/capsular hemorrhage. *Brain and Language,* 60, 407–442.

Crowder, R. G., & Wagner, R. K. (1992). *The psychology of reading: An introduction* (2nd ed.). New York: Oxford University Press.

Crowe, S. F. (1992). Dissociation of two frontal lobe syndromes by a test of verbal fluency. *Journal of Clinical and Experimental Neuropsychology,* 14, 327–339.

Crystal, D., Fletcher, P., & Garman, M. (1976). *The grammatical analysis of language disability.* New York: Elsevier.

Cubelli, R., Foresti, A., & Consolini, T. (1988). Reeducation strategies in conduction aphasia. *Journal of Communication Disorders,* 21, 239–249.

Cubelli, R., Nichelli, P., Bonito, V., De Tanti, A., & Inzaghi, M. G. (1991). Different patterns of dissociation in unilateral spatial neglect. *Brain and Cognition,* 15, 139–159.

Cullum, C. M., & Bigler, E. D. (1986). Ventricle size, cortical atrophy and the relationship with neuropsychological status in closed-head injury: A quantitative analysis. *Journal of Clinical and Experimental Neuropsychology,* 8, 437–452.

Cummings, J. L., & Benson, D. (1983). *Dementia: A clinical approach.* Boston: Butterworths.

Curtiss, S., Jackson, C. A., Kempler, D., Hanson, W. R., & Metter, E. H. (1986). Length vs. structural complexity in sentence comprehension in aphasia. In R. H. Brookshire (Ed.). *Clinical aphasiology* (Vol. 16) (pp. 45–55). Minneapolis: BRW

Cutting, L. (1978). Study of anosognosia. *Journal of Neurology, Neurosurgery, and Psychiatry,* 41, 548–555.

Cyr-Stafford, C. (1993). The dynamics of speech therapy in aphasia. In D. Lafond, Y. Joanette, J. Ponzio, R. Degiovani, & M. T. Sarno (Eds.), *Living with aphasia: Psychosocial issues* (pp. 103–116). San Diego, CA: Singular.

Dahlberg, C. C., & Jaffe, J. (1977). *Stroke: A doctor's personal story of his recovery.* New York: Norton.

Damasio, A. R., Van Hoesen, G. W., & Hyman, B. T. (1990). Reflections on the selectivity of neuropathological changes in Alzheimer's disease. In M. F. Schwartz (Ed.), *Modular deficits in Alzheimer-type dementia* (pp. 83–100). Cambridge, MA: Bradford/MIT Press.

Damasio, H. D., & Damasio, A. R. (1980). The anatomical basis of conduction aphasia. *Brain,* 103, 337–350.

Daniloff, J. K., Fritelli, G., Buckingham, H. W., Hoffman, P. R., & Daniloff, R. G. (1986). Amer-Ind versus ASL: Recognition and imitation in aphasic subjects. *Brain and Language,* 28, 95–113.

Daniloff, J. K., Llyod, L., & Fristoe, M. (1983). Amer-Ind transparency. *Journal of Speech and Hearing Disorders,* 48, 103–110.

Daniloff, J. K., Noll, J. D., Fristoe, M., & Lloyd, L. L. (1982). Gesture recognition in patients with aphasia. *Journal of Speech and Hearing Disorders,* 47, 43–49.

Darley, F. L. (1982). *Aphasia.* Philadelphia: W. B. Saunders.

Darvesh, S., & Freedman, M. (1996). Subcortical dementia: A neurobehavioral approach. *Brain and Cognition* , 31, 230–249.

David, R., Enderby, P., & Bainton, D. (1982). Treatment of acquired aphasia: Speech therapists and volunteers compared. *Journal of Neurology, Neurosurgery and Psychiatry,* 45, 957–961.

Davidoff, J., & De Bleser, R. (1994). Impaired picture recognition with preserved object naming and reading. *Brain and Cognition,* 24, 1–23.

Davidoff, J., & De Bleser, R. (1993). Optic aphasia: A review of past studies and reappraisal. *Aphasiology,* 7, 135–154.

Davis, G. A. (1973). Linguistics and language therapy: The sentence construction board. *Journal of Speech and Hearing Disorders,* 38, 205–214.

Davis, G. A. (1986). Questions of efficacy in clinical aphasiology. In R. H. Brookshire (Ed.), *Clinical aphasiology* conference proceedings (pp. 154–162). Minneapolis: BRK.

Davis, G. A. (1989). The cognitive cloud and language disorders. *Aphasiology,* 3, 723–734.

Davis, G. A. (1993). *A survey of adult aphasia and related language disorders.* Boston: Allyn & Bacon.

Davis, G. A., & Holland, A. L. (1981). Age in understanding and treating aphasia. In D. S. Beasley & G. A. Davis (Eds.), *Aging: Communication processes and disorders* (pp. 207–228). New York: Grune & Stratton.

Davis, G. A., O'Neil-Pirozzi, T. M., & Coon, M. (1997). Referential cohesion and logical coherence of narration after right hemisphere stroke. *Brain and Language,* 56, 183–210.

Davis, G. A., & Wilcox, M. J. (1985). *Adult aphasia rehabilitation: Applied pragmatics.* San Diego: Singular.

Davolt, S. (1998). Providers adapt to new Medicare payment plan. *ASHA Leader,* 3(24), pp. 1, 4.

Deal, J. L., & Deal, L. A. (1978). Efficacy of aphasia rehabilitation: Preliminary results. In R. H. Brookshire (Ed.), *Clinical aphasiology* conference proceedings (pp. 66–77). Minneapolis: BRK.

Deal, J. L., Deal, L., Wertz, R. T., Kitselman, K., & Dwyer, C. (1979). Right hemisphere PICA percentiles: Some speculations about aphasia. In R. H. Brookshire (Ed.), *Clinical aphasiology* conference proceedings (pp. 30–37). Minneapolis: BRK.

Dekoskey, S., Heilman, K. M., Bowers, D., & Valenstein, E. (1980). Recognition and discrimination of emotional faces and pictures. *Brain and Language,* 9, 206–214.

Delis, D.C., Wapner, W., Gardner, H., & Moses, Jr., J. A. (1983). The contribution of the right hemisphere to the organization of paragraphs. *Cortex,* 19, 43–50.

Dell, G. S., & O'Seaghdha, P. G. (1992). Stages of lexical access in language production. *Cognition,* 42, 287–314.

Dell, G. S., Schwartz, M. F., Martin, N., Saffran, E. M., & Gagnon, D. A. (1997). Lexical access in aphasic and nonaphasic speakers. *Psychological Review,* 104, 801–838.

Deloche, G., Dordain, M, & Kremin, H. (1993). Rehabilitation of confrontation naming in aphasia: Relations between oral and written modalities. *Aphasiology,* 7, 201–216.

Deloche, G., Hannequin, D., Dordain, M., Perrier, D., Cardebat, D, Metz-Lutz, M-N., Pichard, B., Quint, S., & Kremin, H. (1997). Picture written naming: Performance parallels and divergencies between aphasic patients and normal subjects. *Aphasiology,* 11, 219–234.

Deloche, G., & Seron, X. (1981). Sentence understanding and knowledge of the world. Evidences from a sentence-picture matching task performed by aphasic patients. *Brain and Language,* 14, 57–69.

DeLuca, J. (1992). Cognitive dysfunction after aneurysm of the anterior communicating artery. *Journal of Clinical and Experimental Neuropsychology,* 14, 924–935.

Denes, G., Perazzolo, C., Piani, A., & Piccione, F. (1996). Intensive versus regular speech therapy in global aphasia: A controlled study. *Aphasiology,* 10, 385–394.

de Partz, M-P. (1986). Re-education of a deep dyslexic patient: Rationale of the methods and results. *Cognitive Neuropsychology,* 3, 149–177.

DeRenzi, E. (1979). A shortened version of the Token Test. In F. Boller & M. Dennis (Eds.), *Auditory comprehension: Clinical and experimental studies with the Token Test* (pp. 33–44). New York: Academic Press.

DeRenzi, E. (1986). Prosopagnosia in two patients with CT-scan evidence of damage confined to the right hemisphere. *Neuropsychologia,* 24, 385–389.

DeRenzi, E., & Faglioni, P. (1978). Normative data and screening power of a shortened version of the Token Test. *Cortex,* 14, 41–49.

DeRenzi, E., Faglioni, P., & Scotti, G. (1969). Impairment of memory for position following brain damage. *Cortex,* 5, 274–284.

DeRenzi, E., & Ferrari, C. (1978). The Reporter's Test: A sensitive test to detect expressive disturbances in aphasics. *Cortex,* 14, 279–293.

DeRenzi, E., Liotti, M., & Nichelli, P. (1987). Semantic amnesia with preservation of autobiographic memory: A case report. *Cortex,* 23, 575–597.

DeRenzi, E., & Lucchelli, F. (1988). Ideational apraxia. *Brain,* 111, 1173–1188.

DeRenzi, E., Motti, F., & Nichelli, P. (1980). Imitating gestures: A quantitative approach to ideomotor apraxia. *Archives of Neurology,* 37, 6–10.

DeRenzi, E., & Nichelli, P. (1975) Verbal and nonverbal short-term memory impairment following hemispheric damage. *Cortex,* 11, 341–354.

DeRenzi, E., Scotti, G., & Spinnler, H. (1969). Perceptual and associative disorders of visual recognition. *Neurology,* 19, 634–642.

DeRenzi, E., & Vignolo, L. A. (1962). The Token Test: A sensitive test to detect receptive disturbances in aphasics. *Brain,* 85, 665–678.

Devescovi, A., Bates, E., D'Amico, S., Hernandez, A., Marangolo, P., Pizzamiglio, L., & Razzano, C. (1997). An on-line study of grammaticality judgements in normal and aphasic speakers of Italian. *Aphasiology,* 11, 543–579.

Diggs, C. C., & Basili, A. G. (1987). Verbal expression of right cerebrovascular accident patients: Convergent and divergent language. *Brain and Language,* 30, 130–146.

DiSimoni, F., Keith, R. L., Holt, D. L., & Darley, F. L. (1975). Practicality of shortening the Porch Index of Communicative Ability. *Journal of Speech and Hearing Research,* 18, 491–497.

DiSimoni, F., Keith, R. L., & Darley, F. L. (1980). Prediction of PICA overall score by short versions of the test. *Journal of Speech and Hearing Research,* 23, 511–516.

Dobkin, B. (1995). The economic impact of stroke. *Neurology* (Supplement 1), 45, S6–S9.

Dosher, B. A., & Corbett, A. T. (1982). Instrument inferences and verbal schemata. *Memory & Cognition,* 10, 531–539.

Doyle, P. J., & Goldstein, H. (1985). Experimental analysis of acquisition and generalization of syntax in Broca's aphasia. In R. H. Brookshire (Ed.), *Clinical aphasiology* (Vol. 15) (pp. 205–213). Minneapolis: BRK.

Doyle, P. J., Goldstein, H., & Bourgeois, M. S. (1987). Experimental analysis of syntax training in Broca's aphasia: A generalization and social validation study. *Journal of Speech and Hearing Disorders,* 52, 143–155.

Doyle, P. J., Thompson, C. K., Oleyar, K., Wambaugh, J., & Jackson, A. (1994). The effects of setting variables on conversational discourse in normal and aphasic adults. In M. L. Lemme (Ed.), *Clinical aphasiology* (Vol. 22) (pp. 135–144). Austin, TX: Pro-Ed.

Doyle, P. J., Tsironas, D., Goda, A. J., & Kalinyak, M. (1996). The relationship between objective measures and listeners' judgments of the communicative informativeness of the connected discourse of adults with aphasia. *American Journal of Speech-Language Pathology,* 5(3), 53–60.

Dronkers, N. F., Redfern, B. B., & Ludy, C. A. (1995). Lesion localization in chronic Wernicke's aphasia (abstract). *Brain and Language,* 51, 62–65.

Duffy, J. R. (1994). Schuell's stimulation approach to rehabilitation. In R. Chapey (Ed.), *Language intervention strategies in adult aphasia* (3rd Ed) (pp. 146–178). Baltimore: Williams & Wilkins.

Duffy, J. R. (1995). *Motor speech disorders: Substrates, differential diagnosis, and management.* St. Louis, MO: Mosby.

Duffy, J. R., & Duffy, R. J. (1989). The limb apraxia test: An imitative measure of upper limb apraxia. In T. E. Prescott (Ed.), *Clinical aphasiology* (Vol. 18) (pp. 145–160). Boston: College-Hill/Little, Brown.

Duffy, J. R., Duffy, R. J., & Uryase, D. (1989). The limb apraxia test: Development of a short form. In T. E. Prescott (Ed.), *Clinical aphasiology* (Vol. 18) (pp. 616–172). Boston: College-Hill/Little, Brown.

Duffy, J. R., Keith, R. L., Shane, H., & Podraza, B. L. (1976). Performance of normal (non-brain-injured) adults on the Porch Index of Communicative Ability. In R. H. Brookshire (Ed.), *Clinical Aphasiology Conference Proceedings* (p. 32–42). Minneapolis: BRK.

Duffy, J. R., & Liles, B. Z. (1979). A translation of Finkelnberg's (1870) lecture on aphasia as "asymbolia" with commentary. *Journal of Speech and Hearing Disorders,* 44, 156–168.

Duffy, J. R., & Myers, P. S. (1991). Group comparisons across neurologic communication disorders: Some methodological issues. In T. E. Prescott (Ed.), *Clinical aphasiology* (Vol. 19) (pp. 1–14). Austin, TX: Pro-Ed.

Duffy, R. J., & Buck, R. (1979). A study of the relationship between propositional (pantomime) and subpropositional (facial expression) extraverbal behaviors in aphasics. *Folia Phoniatrica,* 31, 129–136.

Duffy, R. J., & Duffy, J. R. (1981). Three studies of deficits in pantomimic expression and pantomimic recognition in aphasia. *Journal of Speech and Hearing Research,* 24, 70–84.

Duffy, R. J., & Duffy, J. R. (1984). *Assessment of Nonverbal Communication.* Tigard, OR: C. C. Publications.

Duffy, R. J., Duffy, J. R., & Pearson, K. (1975). Pantomime recognition in aphasia. *Journal of Speech and Hearing Research,* 18, 115–132.

Duffy, R. J., Duffy, J. R., & Mercaitis, P. A. (1984). Comparison of the performance of a fluent and a nonfluent aphasic on a pantomimic referential task. *Brain and Language,* 21, 260–273.

Duffy, R. J., & Ulrich, S. R. (1976). A comparison of impairments in verbal comprehension, speech, reading, and writing in adult aphasics. *Journal of Speech and Hearing Disorders,* 41, 110–119.

Duffy, R. J., Watt, J. H., & Duffy, J. R. (1994). Testing causal theories of pantomimic deficits in aphasia using path analysis. *Aphasiology,* 8, 361–379.

Duncan, J. (1986). Disorganisation of behaviour after frontal lobe damage. *Cognitive Neuropsychology,* 3, 271–290.

Edelman, G. (1987). Global aphasia: The case for treatment. *Aphasiology,* 1, 75–80.

Edwards, S., Garman, M., & Kent, R. (1993). The grammatical characterization of aphasic language. *Aphasiology,* 7, 217–220.

Ehrlich, J. S. (1988). Selective characteristics of narrative discourse in head-injured and normal adults. *Journal of Communication Disorders,* 21, 1–9.

Eisenson, J. (1949). Prognostic factors related to language rehabilitation in aphasic patients. *Journal of Speech and Hearing Disorders,* 14, 262–264.

Eisenson, J. (1954). *Examining for aphasia.* New York: The Psychological Corporation.

Eisenson, J. (1962). Language and intellectual findings associated with right cerebral damage. *Language and Speech,* 5, 49–53.

Eisenson, J. (1984). *Adult aphasia* (Second Edition). Englewood Cliffs, NJ: Prentice-Hall.

Ellis, A. W., Flude, B. M., & Young, A. W. (1987). "Neglect dyslexia" and the early visual processing of letters in words and nonwords. *Cognitive Neuropsychology,* 4, 439–464.

Ellis, A. W., Kay, J., & Franklin, S. (1992). Anomia: Differentiating between semantic and phonological deficits. In D. I. Margolin (Ed.), *Cognitive neuropsychology in clinical practice* (pp. 207–228). New York: Oxford University Press.

Ellis, A. W., Miller, D., & Sin, G. (1983). Wernicke's aphasia and normal language processing: A case study in cognitive neuropsychology. *Cognition,* 15, 111–114.

Ellis, A. W., & Young, A. W. (1988). *Human cognitive neuropsychology.* London: Erlbaum.

Elman, R. J. (1994). Aphasia treatment planning in an outpatient medical rehabilitation center: Where do we go from here? *Special Interest Division 2 Newsletter,* 4(3), 9–13.

Emerick, L. L., & Hatten, J. T. (1979). *Diagnosis and evaluation in speech pathology* (2nd ed.). Englewood Cliffs, NJ: Prentice-Hall.

Emmorey, K. D. (1987). The neurological substrates for prosodic aspects of speech. *Brain and Language,* 30, 305–320.

Emmorey, K., Hickok, G., & Klima, E. S. (1996). Differences in mental rotation within linguistic and nonlinguistic domains: Evidence from an ASL signer with right hemisphere damage (abstract). *Brain and Language,* 51, 176–179.

Erickson, R. J., Goldinger, S. D., & LaPointe, L. L. (1996). Auditory vigilance in aphasic individuals: Detecting nonlinguistic stimuli with full or divided attention. *Brain and Cognition,* 30, 244–253.

Fabbro, F., Clarici, A., & Bava, A. (1996). Effects of left basal ganglia lesions on language production. *Perceptual and Motor Skills,* 82, 1291–1298.

Faglioni, P., Spinnler, H., & Vignolo, L. (1969). Contrasting behavior of right and left hemisphere-damaged patients on a discriminative and a semantic task of auditory recognition. *Cortex,* 5, 366–389.

Farah, M. J., Stowe, R. M., & Levinson, K. L. (1996). Phonological dyslexia: Loss of a reading-specific component of the cognitive architecture? *Cognitive Neuropsychology,* 13, 849–868.

Ferguson, A. (1994). The influence of aphasia, familiarity and activity on conversational repair. *Aphasiology,* 8, 143–157.

Ferguson, A. (1998). Conversational turn-taking and repair in fluent aphasia. *Aphasiology,* 12, 1007–1031.

Ferreira, F., & Clifton, Jr., C. (1986). The independence of syntactic processing. *Journal of Memory and Language,* 25, 348–368.

Ferreira, F., & Henderson, J. M. (1990). The use of verb information in syntactic parsing: Evidence from eye movements and word-by-word self-paced reading. *Journal of Experimental Psychology: Learning, Memory, and Cognition,* 16, 555–568.

Ferro, J. M. (1992). The influence of infarct location on recovery from global aphasia. *Aphasiology,* 6, 415–430.

Ferro, J. M., & Kertesz, A. (1987). Comparative classification of aphasic disorders. *Journal of Clinical and Experimental Neuropsychology,* 9, 365–375.

Ferro, J. M., Santos, M. E., Castro-Caldas, A., & Mariano, G. (1980). Gesture recognition in aphasia. *Journal of Clinical Neuropsychology,* 2, 277–292.

Feyereisen, P. (1991). Communicative behaviour in aphasia. *Aphasiology,* 5, 323–334.

Feyereisen, P., Barter, D., Goosens, M., & Clarebaut, N. (1988). Gestures and speech referential communication by aphasic subjects: Channel use and efficiency. *Aphasiology,* 2, 21–32.

Feyereisen, P., & Seron, X. (1982). Nonverbal communication and aphasia: A review. I. Comprehension. *Brain and Language,* 16, 191–212.

Fillenbaum, S., Jones, L. V., & Wepman, J. M. (1961). Some linguistic features of speech from aphasic patients. *Language and Speech,* 4, 91–108.

Fink, R. B., Martin, N., Schwartz, M. F., Saffran, E. M., & Myers, J. L. (1993). Facilitation of verb retrieval skills in aphasia: A comparison of two approaches. In M. L. Lemme (Ed.), *Clinical aphasiology* (Vol. 21) (pp. 263–275). Austin, Tx: Pro-Ed.

Fink, R. B., Schwartz, M. F., & Myers, J. L. (1997). Effects of multilevel training on verb retrieval: Is more always better? (abstract). *Brain and Language,* 60, 41–44.

Fink, R. B., Schwartz, M. F., Rochon, E., Myers, J. L., Socolof, G. S., & Bluestone, R. (1995). Syntax stimulation revisited: An analysis of generalization of treatment effects. *American Journal of Speech-Language Pathology,* 4(4), 99–104.

Fisher, C. M. (1982). Disorientation for place. *Archives of Neurology,* 39, 33–36.

Fishman, S. (1988). *A bomb in the brain.* New York: Avon.

Fitch-West, J. (1983). Heightening visual imagery: A new approach to aphasia therapy. In E. Perecman (Ed.), *Cognitive processing in the right hemisphere* (pp. 215–228). New York: Academic Press.

Fitch-West, J., & Sands, E. S. (1987). *Bedside Evaluation Screening Test.* Rockville, MD: Aspen.

Flanagan, O. J. (1984). *The science of the mind.* Cambridge, MA: Bradford/MIT Press.

Fletcher, C. R., & Bloom, C. P. (1988). Causal reasoning in the comprehension of simple narrative texts. *Journal of Memory and Language,* 27, 235–244.

Flowers, C. R., & Wyse, M. (1985). Assessing gestural intelligibility of normal and aphasic subjects. In R. H. Brookshire (Ed.), *Clinical aphasiology* (Vol. 15) (pp. 64–71). Minneapolis: BRK.

Flude, B. M., Ellis, A. W., & Kay, J. (1989). Face processing and name retrieval in an anomic aphasic: Names are stored separately from semantic information about familiar people. *Brain and Cognition,* 11, 60–72.

Fodor, J. A. (1983). *The modularity of mind.* Cambridge, MA: Bradford/MIT Press.

Foldi, N. S. (1987). Appreciation of pragmatic interpretations of indirect commands: Comparison of right and left hemisphere brain-damaged patients. *Brain and Language,* 31, 88–108.

Folstein, M. F., Folstein, S. E., & McHugh, P. R. (1975). Mini-mental state. *Journal of Psychiatric Research,* 12, 189–198.

Forster, K. I., & Chambers, S. M. (1973). Lexical access and naming time. *Journal of Verbal Learning and Verbal Behavior,* 12, 627–635.

Fortinski, R. H., Granger, C. V., & Selzer, G. B. (1981). The use of functional assessment in understanding home care needs. *Medical Care,* 19, 489–497.

Foss, D. J., & Hakes, D. T. (1978). *Psycholinguistics: An introduction to the psychology of language.* Englewood Cliffs, NJ: Prentice-Hall.

Franklin, S. (1989). Dissociations in auditory word comprehension: Evidence from nine fluent aphasic patients. *Aphasiology,* 6, 63–84.

Franklin, S., Howard, D., & Patterson, K. (1994). Abstract word meaning deafness. *Cognitive Neuropsychology,* 11, 1–34.

Franklin, S., Howard, D., & Patterson, K. (1995). Abstract word anomia. *Cognitive Neuropsychology,* 12, 549–566.

Frattali, C. M. (1992). Functional assessment of communication: Mergin public policy with clinical views. *Aphasiology,* 6, 63–84.

Frattali, C. M. (1994). Quality improvement. In R. Lubinski & C. Frattali (Ed.), *Professional issues in speech-language pathology and audiology: A textbook* (pp. 246–259). San Diego, CA: Singular.

Frattali, C. M., & Lynch, C. (1989). Functional assessment: Current issues and future challenges. *Asha,* 31, 70–74.

Frattali, C. M., Thompson, C. M., Holland, A. L., Wohl, C. B., & Ferketic, M. M. (1995). The FACS of life: ASHA FACS—A functional outcome measure for adults. *Asha,* 37(4), 40–46.

Frazier, L., & Friederici, A. (1991). On deriving the properties of agrammatic comprehension. *Brain and Language,* 40, 51–66.

Frazier, L., & Rayner, K. (1982). Making and correcting errors during sentence comprehension: Eye movements in the analysis of structurally ambiguous sentences. *Cognitive Psychology,* 14, 178–210.

Friederici, A. D. (1982). Syntactic and semantic processes in aphasic deficits: The availability of prepositions. *Brain and Language,* 15, 249–258.

Friederici, A. D. (1983). Aphasics' perception of words in sentential context: Some real-time processing evidence. *Neuropsychologia,* 21, 351–358.

Friederici, A. D. (1985). Levels of processing and vocabulary types: Evidence from on-line comprehension in normals and agrammatics. *Cognition,* 19, 133–166.

Friederici, A. D. (1988). Agrammatic comprehension: Picture of a computational mismatch. *Aphasiology,* 2, 279–284.

Friederici, A. D., & Frazier, L. (1992). Thematic analysis in agrammatic comprehension: Syntactic structures and task demands. *Brain and Language,* 42, 1–29.

Friederici, A. D., Schonle, P. W., & Garrett, M. F. (1982). Syntactically and semantically based computations: Processing of prepositions in agrammatism. *Cortex,* 18, 525–534.

Friederici, A. D., Wessels, J. M. I., Emmorey, K., & Bellugi, U. (1992). Sensitivity to inflectional morphology in aphasia: A real-time processing perspective. *Brain and Language,* 43, 747–763.

Friedman, R. B. (1996). Phonological text alexia: Poor pseudoword reading plus difficulty reading functors and affixes in text. *Cognitive Neuropsychology,* 13, 869–886.

Friedman, R. B., Beeman, M., Lott, S. N., Link, K., Grafman, J., & Robinson, S. (1993). Modality-specific phonological alexia. *Cognitive Neuropsychology,* 10, 549–568.

Friedman, R. B., & Lott, S. N. (1996). Phonologic treatment for deep dyslexia using bigraphs instead of graphemes (abstract). *Brain and Language,* 55, 116–119.

Friedman, R. B., & Robinson, S. R. (1991). Whole-word training therapy in a stable surface alexic patient: It works. *Aphasiology,* 5, 521–528.

Friedrich, F. J., Glenn, C. G., & Marin, O. S. M. (1984). Interruption of phonological coding in conduction aphasia. *Brain and Language,* 22, 266–291.

Friedrich, F. J., Martin, R., & Kemper, S. J. (1985). Consequences of a phonological coding deficit on sentence processing. *Cognitive Neuropsychology,* 2, 385–412.

Fukkink, R. (1996). The internal validity of aphasiological single-subject studies. *Aphasiology,* 10, 741–754.

Funnell, E., & Allport, A. (1989). Symbolically speaking: Communicating with Blissymbols in aphasia. *Aphasiology,* 3, 279–300.

Funnell, E., & Sheridan, J. (1992). Categories of knowledge? Unfamiliar aspects of living and nonliving things. *Cognitive Neuropsychology,* 9, 135–154.

Gaddie, A., Naeser, M. A., Palumbo, C. L., & Stiassny-Eder, D. (1989). Recovery of auditory comprehension after one year: A computed tomography scan study. In T. E. Prescott (Ed.), *Clinical aphasiology* (Vol. 18) (pp. 463–478). Boston: College-Hill/Little, Brown.

Gagnon, D. A., & Schwartz, M. F. (1997). Serial position effects in aphasics' neologisms (abstract). *Brain and Language,* 60, 87–89.

Gainotti, G. (1972). Emotional behavior and hemispheric side of lesion. *Cortex,* 8, 41–55.

Gainotti, G. (1976). The relationship between semantic impairment in comprehension and naming in aphasic patients. *British Journal of Disorders of Communication,* 11, 57–61.

Gainotti, G., Caltagirone, C., & Ibba, A. (1975). Semantic and phonemic aspects of auditory language comprehension in aphasia. *Linguistics,* 154/5, 15–29.

Gainotti, G., Caltagirone, C., & Miceli, G. (1983). Selective impairment of semantic-lexical discrimination in right-brain-damaged patients. In E. Perecman (Ed.). *Cognitive processing in the right hemisphere* (pp. 149–167). New York: Academic Press.

Gainotti, G., Caltagirone, C., Miceli, G., & Masullo, C. (1981). Selective semantic-lexical impairment of language comprehension in right brain-damaged patients. *Brain and Language,* 13, 201–211.

Gainotti, G., Carlomagno, S., Craca, A., & Silveri, M. C. (1986). Disorders of classificatory activity in aphasia. *Brain and Language,* 28, 181–195.

Gainotti, G., & Lemmo, M. A. (1976). Comprehension of symbolic gestures in aphasia. *Brain and Language,* 3, 451–460.

Gainotti, G., & Tiacci, C. (1970). Patterns of drawing disability in right and left hemispheric patients. *Neuropsychologia,* 8, 379–384.

Gallaher, A. J. (1979). Temporal reliability of aphasic performance on the Token Test. *Brain and Language,* 7, 34–41.

Gallaher, A. J., & Canter, G. J. (1982). Reading and listening comprehension in Broca's aphasia: Lexical versus syntactical errors. *Brain and Language,* 17, 183–192.

Gandour, J., & Dardarananda, R. (1982). Voice onset time in aphasia: Thai. I. Perception. *Brain and Language*, 17, 24–33.

Gandour, J., & Dardarananda, R. (1983). Identification of tonal contrasts in Thai aphasic patients. *Brain and Language,* 18, 98–114.

Gandour, J., Marshall, R. C., Kim, S. Y., & Neuburger, S. (1991). On the nature of conduction aphasia: A longitudinal case study. *Aphasiology,* 5, 291–306.

Gandour, J., Petty, S. H., & Dardarananda, R. (1988). Perception and production of tone in aphasia. *Brain and Language,* 35, 201–240.

Gansler, D. A., Covall, S., McGrath, N., & Oscar-Berman, M. (1996). Measures of prefrontal dysfunction after closed head injury. *Brain and Cognition,* 30, 194–204.

Gardner, H. (1974). *The Shattered Mind.* New York: Vintage Books.

Gardner, H. (1982). Missing the point: Language and the right hemisphere. In H. Gardner, *Art, mind, and brain: A cognitive approach to creativity* (pp. 309–317). New York: Basic Books.

Gardner, H. (1983). *Frames of mind: The theory of multiple intelligences.* New York: Basic Books.

Gardner, H., Brownell, H. H., Wapner, W., & Michelow, D. (1983). Missing the point: The role of the right hemisphere in the processing of complex linguistic materials. In E. Perecman (Ed.). (1983). *Cognitive processing in the right hemisphere* (pp. 169–191). New York: Academic Press.

Gardner, H., & Denes, G. (1973). Connotative judgements by aphasic patients on a pictorial adaptation of the semantic differential. *Cortex,* 9, 183–196.

Gardner, H., Denes, G., & Weintraub, S. (1975). Comprehending a word: The influence of speed and redundancy on auditory comprehension in aphasia. *Cortex,* 11, 155–162.

Gardner, H., Denes, G., & Zurif, E. B. (1975). Critical reading at the sentence level in aphasics. *Cortex,* 11, 60–72.

Gardner, H., Ling, P. K., Flamm, L., & Silverman, J. (1975). Comprehension and appreciation of humorous material following brain damage. *Brain,* 98, 399–412.

Gardner, H., Zurif, E. B., Berry, T., & Baker, E. (1976). Visual communication in aphasia. *Neuropsychologia,* 14, 275–292.

Garnham, A. (1985). *Psycholinguistics: Central topics.* London: Methuen.

Garrett, M. F. (1984). The organization of processing structure for language production: Applications to aphasic speech. In D. Caplan, A. R., Lecours, & A. Smith (Eds.), *Biological perspectives on language* (pp. 172–193). Cambridge, MA: MIT Press.

Gates, W. H. (1978). *Gates-MacGinitie reading tests.* Chicago: Riverside.

Germani, M. J., & Pierce, R. S. (1995). Semantic attribute knowledge in adults with right and left hemisphere damage. *Aphasiology,* 9, 1–21.

Gernsbacher, M. A. (Ed.). (1994). *Handbook of psycholinguistics.* San Diego, CA: Academic Press.

Gerratt, B., & Jones, D. (1987). Aphasic performance on a lexical decision task: Multiple meanings and word frequency. *Brain and Language,* 30, 106–115.

Geschwind, N. (1965). Disconnexion syndromes in animals and man. *Brain,* 88, 237–294, 585–644.

Geschwind, N. (1967). The varieties of naming errors. *Cortex,* 3, 96–112.

Glass, A. V., Gazzaniga, M. S., & Premack, D. (1973). Artificial language training in global aphasia. *Neuropsychologia,* 11, 95–103.

Glassman, R. B. (1978). The logic of the lesion experiment and its role in the neural sciences. In S. Finger (Ed.), *Recovery from brain damage: Research and theory.* New York: Plenum Press.

Gleason, J. B., Goodglass, H., Green, E., Ackerman, N., & Hyde, M. R. (1975). The retrieval of syntax in Broca's aphasia. *Brain and Language,* 2, 451–471.

Gleason, J. B., Goodglass, H., Obler, L., Green, E., Hyde, M. R., & Weintraub, S. (1980). Narrative strategies of aphasic and normal-speaking subjects. *Journal of Speech and Hearing Research,* 23, 370–382.

Glindemann, R., & Springer, L. (1995). An assessment of PACE therapy. In C. Code & D. J. Müller (Eds.), *The treatment of aphasia: From theory to practice* (pp. 90–107). San Diego, CA: Singular.

Glindemann, R., Willmes, K., Huber, W., & Springer, L. (1991). The efficacy of modeling in PACE-therapy. *Aphasiology,* 5, 425–430.

Glosser, G., & Deser, T. (1991). Patterns of discourse production among neurological patients with fluent language disorders. *Brain and Language,* 40, 67–88.

Glosser, G., & Goodglass, H. (1991). Idiosyncratic word associations following right hemisphere damage. *Journal of Clinical and Experimental Neuropsychology,* 13, 703–710.

Glosser, G., Wiener, M., & Kaplan, E. (1986). Communicative gestures in aphasia. *Brain and Language,* 27, 345–359.

Glosser, G., Wiener, M., & Kaplan, E. (1988). Variations in aphasic language behaviors. *Journal of Speech and Hearing Disorders,* 53, 115–124.

Gobble, E. M., Dunson, L., Szekeres, S. F., & Cornwall, J. (1987). Avocational programming for the severely impaired head injured individual. In M. Ylvisaker & E. M. Gobble (Eds.), *Community reentry for head injured adults* (pp. 349–380). Boston: College-Hill/Little, Brown.

Godefroy, O., & Rousseaux, M. (1996). Divided and focused attention in patients with lesion of the prefrontal cortex. *Brain and Cognition,* 30, 155–174.

Godfrey, C. M., & Douglass, E. (1959). The recovery process in aphasia. *Canadian Medical Association Journal,* 80, 618–624.

Godfrey, H. P. D., Partridge, F. M., Knight, R. G., & Bishara, S. (1993). Course of insight disorder and emotional dysfunction following closed-head injury: A controlled cross-sectional follow-up study. *Journal of Clinical and Experimental Neuropsychology,* 15, 503–515.

Goldberg, E. (1990). Associative agnosias and the functions of the left hemisphere. *Journal of Clinical and Experimental Neuropsychology,* 12, 467–484.

Golden, C. J., Hemmeke, T. A., & Purisch, A. D. (1980). *The Luria-Nebraska Neuropsychological Battery.* Los Angeles: Western Psychological Services.

Goldenberg, G., & Artner, C. (1991). Visual imagery and knowledge about the visual appearance of objects in patients with posterior cerebral artery lesions. *Brain and Cognition,* 15, 160–186.

Goldenberg, G., & Spatt, J. (1994). Influence of size and site of cerebral lesions on spontaneous recovery of aphasia and on success of language therapy. *Brain and Language,* 47, 684–698.

Goldstein, F. C., Levin, H. S., Boake, C., & Lohrey, J. H. (1990). Facilitation of memory performance through induced semantic processing in survivors of severe closed-head injury. *Journal of Clinical and Experimental Neuropsychology,* 12, 286–300.

Goldstein, K. (1942). *Aftereffects of brain injuries in war.* New York: Grune & Stratton.

Goldstein, K. (1948). *Language and language disturbances.* New York: Grune & Stratton.

Golper, L. A. C. (1992). *Sourcebook for medical speech pathology.* San Diego, CA: Singular.

Goodenough, C., Zurif, E. B., Weintraub, S., & Von Stockert, T. (1977). Aphasics' attention to grammatical morphemes. *Language and Speech,* 20, 11–19.

Goodglass, H. (1989). Commentary: Cognitive psychology and clinical aphasiology. *Aphasiology,* 4, 93–97.

Goodglass, H., Barton, M. I., & Kaplan, E. F. (1968). Sensory modality and object-naming in aphasics. *Journal of Speech and Hearing Research,* 11, 488–496.

Goodglass, H., Blumstein, S. E., Gleason, J. B., Hyde, M. R., Green, E., & Statlender, S. (1979). The effect of syntactic encoding on sentence comprehension in aphasia. *Brain and Language,* 7, 201–209.

Goodglass, H., Fodor, I. G., & Schulhoff, C. (1967). Prosodic factors in grammar—evidence from aphasia. *Journal of Speech and Hearing Research,* 10, 5–20.

Goodglass, H., Hyde, M. R., Blumstein, S. (1969). Frequency, picturability and availability of nouns in aphasia. *Cortex,* 5, 104–119.

Goodglass, H., & Kaplan, E. (1979). Assessment of cognitive deficit in the brain-injured patient. In M. S. Gazzaniga (Ed.), *Handbook of behavioral neurobiology* (Vol. 2). New York: Plenum.

Goodglass, H., & Kaplan, E. (1983). *The assessment of aphasia and related disorders* (Second Edition). Philadelphia: Lea & Febiger.

Goodglass, H., Kaplan, E., Weintraub, S., & Ackerman, N. (1976). The "tip-of-the-tongue" phenomenon in aphasia. *Cortex,* 12, 145–153.

Goodglass, H., Klein, B., Carey, P. W., & Jones, K. J. (1966). Specific semantic word categories in aphasia. *Cortex,* 2, 74–89.

Goodglass, H., & Mayer, J. (1958). Agrammatism in aphasia. *Journal of Speech and Hearing Disorders,* 23, 99–111.

Goodglass, H., & Menn, L. (1985). Is agrammatism a unitary phenomenon? In M-L. Kean (Ed.), *Agrammatism* (pp. 1–26). Orlando, FL: Academic Press.

Goodglass, H., Quadfasel, F. A., & Timberlake, W. H. (1964). Phrase length and the type and severity of aphasia. *Cortex,* 1, 133–153.

Goodglass, H., & Stuss, D. T. (1979). Naming to picture versus description in three aphasic subgroups. *Cortex,* 15, 199–211.

Goodglass, H., Wingfield, A., & Ward, S. E. (1997). Judgments of concept similarity by normal and aphasic subjects: Relation to naming and comprehension. *Brain and Language,* 56, 138–158.

Gordon, B., & Caramazza, A. (1983). Closed- and open-class lexical access in agrammatic and fluent aphasics. *Brain and Language,* 19, 335–345.

Gordon, J. K., & Baum, S. R. (1994). Rhyme priming in aphasia: The role of phonology in lexical access. *Brain and Language,* 47, 661–683.

Gow, D. W., & Caplan, D. (1996). An examination of impaired acoustic-phonetic processing in aphasia. *Brain and Language,* 52, 386–407.

Graf, P., & Schacter, D. (1985). Implicit and explicit memory for new associations in normal and amnesic subjects. *Journal of Experimental Psychology: Learning, Memory and Cognition,* 11, 501–518.

Graham, K. S., Lambon Ralph, M. A., & Hodges, J. R. (1997). Determining the impact of autobiographical experience on "meaning": New insights from investigating sports-related vocabulary and knowledge in two cases with semantic dementia. *Cognitive Neuropsychology,* 14, 801–838.

Granger, C. V., Cotter, A. C., Hamilton, B. B., & Fiedler, R. C. (1993). Functional assessment scales: A study of persons after stroke. *Archives of Physical Medicine and Rehabilitation,* 74, 133–138.

Gray, K. F., & Cummings, J. L. (1994). Neuroimaging in dementia. In A. Kertesz (Ed.), *Localization and neuroimaging in neuropsychology* (pp. 621–651). San Diego, CA: Academic Press.

Greitemann, G., & Wolf, E. (1991). Making dynamic use of different modes of expression: The efficacy of the PACE-approach. Paper presented to the Academy of Aphasia, Rome.

Grice, L. P. (1975). Logic and conversation. In P. Cole & J. L. Morgan (Ed.), *Syntax and semantics: Speech acts* (Vol. 3) (pp. 41–58). New York: Academic Press.

Griffiths, K. M., Cook, M. L., & Newcombe, R. L. G. (1988). Cube copying after cerebral damage. *Journal of Clinical and Experimental Neuropsychology,* 10, 800–812.

Grober, E., Perecman, E., Kellar, L., & Brown, J. (1980). Lexical knowledge in anterior and posterior aphasics. *Brain and Language,* 10, 318–330.

Grodzinsky, Y. (1984). The syntactic characterization of agrammatism. *Cognition,* 16, 99–120.

Grodzinsky, Y. (1986). Language deficits and the theory of syntax. *Brain and Language,* 27, 135–159.

Grodzinsky, Y. (1989). Agrammatic comprehension of relative clauses. *Brain and Language,* 37, 480–499.

Grodzinsky, Y. (1991). There is an entity called agrammatic aphasia. *Brain and Language,* 41, 555–564.

Grodzinsky, Y., Swinney, D., & Zurif, E. (1985). Agrammatism: Structural deficits and antecedent processing disruptions. In M-L. Kean (Ed.). *Agrammatism* (pp. 65–81). Orlando, FL: Academic Press.

Groher, M. (1977). Language and memory disorders following closed head trauma. *Journal of Speech and Hearing Research,* 20, 212–223.

Grosjean, F. (1982). *Life with two languages: An introduction to bilingualism.* Cambridge, MA: Harvard University Press.

Grosjean, F. (1985). Polyglot aphasics and language mixing: A comment on Perecman (1984). *Brain and Language,* 26, 349–355.

Grosjean, F. (1989). Neurolinguists, beware! The bilingual is not two monolinguals in one person. *Brain and Language,* 36, 3–15.

Grossman, M. (1981). A bird is a bird is a bird: Making reference within and without superordinate categories. *Brain and Language,* 12, 313–331.

Grossman, M. (1988). Drawing deficits in brain-damaged patients' freehand pictures. *Brain and Cognition,* 8, 189–205.

Grossman, M., Carey, S., Zurif, E., & Diller, L. (1986). Proper and common nouns: Form class judgments in Broca's aphasia. *Brain and Language,* 28, 114–125.

Grossman, M., & Haberman, S. (1982). Aphasics' selective deficits in appreciating grammatical agreements. *Brain and Language,* 16, 109–120.

Grossman, M., & Wilson, M. (1987). Stimulus categorization by brain-damaged patients. *Brain and Cognition,* 6, 55–71.

Gruen, A. K., Frankle, B. C., & Schwartz, R. (1990). Word fluency generation skills of head-injured patients in an acute trauma ceneter. *Journal of Communication Disorders,* 23, 163–170.

Haaland, K. Y., & Flaherty, D. (1984). The different types of limb apraxia errors made by patients with left vs. right hemisphere damage. *Brain and Cognition,* 3, 370–384.

Haarmann, H. J., & Kolk, H. H. J. (1991). Syntactic priming in Broca's aphasics: Evidence for slow activation. *Aphasiology,* 5, 247–264.

Haarmann, H. J., & Kolk, H. H. J. (1994). On-line sensitivity to subject-verb agreement violations in Broca's aphasics: The role of syntactic complexity and time. *Brain and Language,* 46, 493–516.

Haarmann, H. J., Just, M. A., & Carpenter, P. A. (1997). Aphasic sentence comprehension as a resource deficit: A computational approach. *Brain and Language, 59*, 76–120.

Haberlandt, K. (1994). *Cognitive psychology.* Boston: Allyn and Bacon.

Haberlandt, K. F., & Graesser, A. C. (1990). Integration and buffering of new information. In A. C. Graesser & G. H. Bower (Eds.), *Inferences and text comprehension* (pp. 71–88). San Diego: Academic Press.

Hadar, U., Wenkert-Olenik, D., Krauss, R., & Soroker, N. (1998). Gesture and processing of speech: Neuropsychological evidence. *Brain and Language,* 62, 107–126.

Haendiges, A. N., Berndt, R. S., & Mitchum, C. C. (1996). Assessing the elements contributing to a "mapping" deficit: A targeted treatment study. *Brain and Language,* 52, 276–302.

Hageman, C. F., & Folkestad, A. (1986). Performance of aphasic listeners on an expanded Revised Token Test subtest presented verbally and nonverbally. In R. H. Brookshire (Ed.), *Clinical aphasiology* (Vol. 16) (pp. 227–233). Minneapolis: BRK.

Hageman, C. F., & Lewis, D. L. (1983). The effects of intrastimulus pause on the quality of auditory comprehension in aphasia. In R. H. Brookshire (Ed.), *Clinical aphasiology conference proceedings* (pp. 177–185). Minneapolis, MN: BRK.

Hageman, C. F., McNeil, M., Rucci-Zimmer, S., & Cariski, D. (1982). The reliability of patterns of auditory processing deficits: Evidence from the Revised Token Test. In R. H. Brookshire (Ed.), *Clinical aphasiology* conference proceedings (pp. 230–234). Minneapolis: BRK.

Hagen, C. (1973). Communication abilities in hemiplegia: Effect of speech therapy. Archives of Physical Medicine and Rehabilitation, 54, 454–463.

Hagen, C. (1981). Language disorders secondary to closed head injury: Diagnosis and treatment. *Topics in Language Disorders,* 1, 73–87.

Hagiwara, H., & Caplan, D. (1990). Syntactic comprehension in Japanese aphasics: Effects of category and thematic role order. *Brain and Language,* 38, 159–170.H-L

Hagoort, P. (1989). Processing of lexical ambiguities: A comment on Milberg, Blumstein, and Dworetzky (1987). *Brain and Language,* 36, 335–348.

Hagoort, P. (1993). Impairments of lexical-semantic processing in aphasia: Evidence from the processing of lexical ambiguities. *Brain and Language,* 45, 189–232.

Hagoort, P. (1997). Semantic priming in Broca's aphasics at a short SOA: No support for an automatic access deficit. *Brain and Language,* 56, 287–300.

Hagoort, P., Brown, C., & Swaab, T. (1995). Semantic deficits in right hemisphere patients (abstract). *Brain and Language,* 51, 161–163.

Halligan, P. W., & Marshall, J. C. (1994). Toward a principled explanation of unilateral neglect. *Cognitive Neuropsychology,* 11, 167–206.

Halstead, W. C., & Wepman, J. M. (1949). The Halstead-Wepman aphasia screening test. *Journal of Speech and Hearing Disorders,* 14, 9–15.

Hamilton, B. B., Laughlin, J. A., Granger, C. V., & Kayton, R. M. (1991). Interrater agreement of the seven-level Functional Independence Measure (FIM) (abstract). *Archives of Physical Medicine and Rehabilitation,* 72, 790.

Handel, S. (1989). *Listening: An introduction to the perception of auditory events.* Cambridge, MA: Bradford/MIT Press.

Hanlon, R. E., Brown, J. W., & Gerstman, L. J. (1990). Enhancement of naming in nonfluent aphasia through gesture. *Brain and Language,* 38, 298–314.

Hanna, G., Schell, L. M., & Schriener, R. (1977). *The Nelson reading skills test.* Chicago: Riverside.

Hannay, H. J., & Levin, H. S. (1989). Visual continous recognition memory in normal and closed head-injured adolescents. *Journal of Clinical and Experimental Neuropsychology,* 11, 444–460.

Hanson, W. R., & Cicciarelli, A. W. (1978). The time, amount, and pattern of language improvement in adult aphasics. *British Journal of Disorders of Communication,* 13, 59–63.

Hanson, W. R., Metter, E. J., & Riege, W. H. (1989). The course of chronic aphasia. *Aphasiology,* 3, 19–30.

Haravon, A., Obler, L. K., & Sarno, M. T. (1994). A method for microanalysis of discourse in brain-damaged patients. In R. L. Bloom, L. K. Obler, S. De Santi, & J. S. Ehrlich (Eds.), *Discourse analysis and applications: Studies in adult clinical populations* (pp. 47–80). Hillsdale, NJ: Lawrence Erlbaum.

Hartje, W., Kerschensteiner, M., Poeck, K., & Orgass, B. (1973). A cross-validation study on the Token Test. *Neuropsychologia,* 11, 119–121.

Hartley, L. L., & Levin, H. S. (1990). Linguistic deficits after closed head injury: A current appraisal. *Aphasiology,* 4, 353–370.

Harvey, M., Milner, A. D., & Roberts, R. C. (1995). An investigation of hemispatial neglect using the Landmark Task. *Brain and Cognition,* 27, 59–78.

Hathaway, S. R., & McKinley, J. C. (1951). *The Minnesota Multiphasic Personality Inventory Manual* (Revised). New York: Psychological Corporation.

Haut, M. W., Petros, T. V., Frank, R. G., & Haut, J. S. (1991). Speed of processing within semantic memory following severe closed head injury. *Brain and Cognition,* 17, 31–41.

Haynes, W. O., & Oratio, A. R. (1978). A study of clients' perceptions of therapeutic effectiveness. *Journal of Speech and Hearing Disorders,* 43, 21–33.

Head, H. (1920). Aphasia and kindred disorders of speech. *Brain,* 43, 87–165.

Heeschen, C. (1980). Strategies of decoding actor-object relations by aphasic patients. *Cortex,* 16, 5–19.

Heeschen, C., & Kolk, H. (1988). Agrammatism and paragrammatism. *Aphasiology,* 2, 299–302.

Heilman, K. M., & Bowers, D. (1995). Reply to Warrington-Rudge comment on "Apperceptive visual agnosia: A case study." *Brain and Cognition,* 28, 178–179.

Heilman, K. M., Bowers, D., Speedie, L., & Coslett, H. B. (1984). Comprehension of affective and non-affective prosody. *Neurology,* 34, 917–921.

Heilman, K. M., Rothi, L., Campanella, D., & Wolfson, S. (1979). Wernicke's and global aphasia without alexia. *Archives of Neurology,* 36, 129–133.

Heilman, K. M., Safran, A., & Geschwind, N. (1971). Closed head trauma and aphasia. *Journal of Neurology, Neurosurgery, and Psychiatry,* 34, 265–269.

Heilman, K. M., & Scholes, R. J. (1976). The nature of comprehension errors in Broca's, conduction and Wernicke's aphasics. *Cortex,* 12, 258–265.

Heilman, K. M., Schwartz, H. D., & Watson, R. T. (1978). Hypoarousal in patients with the neglect syndrome and emotional indifference. *Neurology,* 28, 229–232.

Heilman, K. M., & Valenstein, E. (1985). *Clinical neuropsychology* (Second Edition). New York: Oxford University Press.

Heilman, K. M., Watson, R. T., & Valenstein, E. (1985). Neglect and related disorders. In K. M. Heilman & E. Valenstein (Eds.), *Clinical neuropsychology* (2nd ed.) (pp. 243–293). New York: Oxford University Press.

Helm, N. A., & Barresi, B. (1980). Voluntary conrol of involuntary utterances: A treatment approach for severe aphasia. In R. H. Brookshire (Ed.), *Clinical aphasiology conference proceedings* (pp. 308–315). Minneapolis: BRK.

Helm-Estabrooks, N. (1981). *Helm Elicited Language Program for Syntax Stimulation (HELPSS).* Chicago: Riverside.

Helm-Estabrooks, N. (1983). Exploiting the right hemisphere for language rehabilitation: Melodic intonation therapy. In E. Perecman (Ed.), *Cognitive processing in the right hemisphere* (pp. 229–240). New York: Academic Press.

Helm-Estabrooks, N. (1991). *Test of Oral and Limb Apraxia (TOLA).* Chicago: Riverside.

Helm-Estabrooks, N., & Albert, M. L. (1991). *A manual of aphasia therapy.* Chicago: Riverside

Helm-Estabrooks, N., Fitzpatrick, P. M., & Barresi, B. N. (1981). Response of an agrammatic patient to a syntax stimulation program for aphasia. *Journal of Speech Hearing Disorders,* 46, 422–427.

Helm-Estabrooks, N., Fitzpatrick, P. M., & Barresi, B. N. (1982). Visual action therapy for global aphasia. *Journal of Speech and Hearing Disorders,* 47, 385–389.

Helm-Estabrooks, N., & Hotz, G. (1990). *Brief Test of Head Injury (BTHI).* Chicago: Riverside.

Helm-Estabrooks, N., Nicholas, M., & Morgan, A. R. (1989). *Melodic Intonation Theapy (MIT).* Chicago: Riverside.

Helm-Estabrooks, N., & Ramsberger, G. (1986). Treatment of agrammatism in long-term Broca's aphasia. *British Journal of Disorders of Communication,* 21, 39–45.

Helm-Estabrooks, N., Ramsberger, G., Morgan, A. R., & Nicholas, M. (1989). *Boston Assessment of Severe Aphasia (BASA).* Chicago: Riverside

Henderson, L. W., Frank, E. M., Pigatt, T., Abramson, R. K., & Houston, M. (1998). Race, gender, and educational level effects on Boston Naming Test scores. *Aphasiology,* 12, 901–911.

Henley, S., Pettit, S., Todd-Pokropek, A., & Tupper, A. (1985). Who goes home? Predictive factors in stroke recovery. *Journal of Neurology, Neurosurgery, and Psychiatry,* 48, 1–6.

Herrmann, M. (1997). Studying psychosocial problems in aphasia: Some conceptual and methodological considerations. *Aphasiology,* 11, 717–725.

Herrmann, M., Johannsen-Horbach, H., & Wallesch, C-W. (1993a). Empathy and aphasia rehabilitation—are there contradictory requirements of treatment and psychological support? *Aphasiology,* 7, 575–579.

Herrmann, M., Johannsen-Horbach, H., & Wallesch, C-W. (1993b). The psychosocial aspects of aphasia. In D. Lafond, Y. Joanette, J. Ponzio, R. Degiovani, & M. T. Sarno (Eds.), *Living with aphasia: Psychosocial issues* (pp. 187–206). San Diego, CA: Singular.

Herrmann, M., Koch, U., Johannsen-Horbach, H., & Wallesch, C-W. (1989). Communicative skills in chronic and severe nonfluent aphasia. *Brain and Language,* 37, 339–352.

Herrmann, M., & Wallesch, C. W. (1989). Psychosocial changes and psychosocial adjustment with chronic and severe nonfluent aphasia. *Aphasiology,* 3, 513–526.

Herrmann, M., & Wallesch, C. W. (1990). Expectations of psychosocial adjustment in aphasia: A MAUT study with the Code-Muller Scale of Psychosocial Adjustment, *Aphasiology,* 4, 527–538.

Hersh, D. (1998). Beyond the 'plateau': Disharge dilemmas in chronic aphasia. *Aphasiology,* 12, 207–218.

Hickok, G., Say, K., Bellugi, U., & Klima, E. S. (1996). The basis of hemispheric asymmetries for language and spatial cognition: Clues from focal brain damage in two deaf native signers. *Aphasiology,* 10, 577–591.

Hier, D. B., & Kaplan, J. (1980). Verbal comprehension deficits after right hemisphere damage. *Applied Psycholinguistics,* 1, 279–294.

Hillis, A. E. (1993). The role of models of language processing in rehabilitation of language impairments. *Aphasiology,* 7, 5–26.

Hillis, A. E., & Caramazza, A. (1989). The graphemic buffer and attentional mechanisms. *Brain and Language,* 36, 208–235.

Hillis, A. E., & Caramazza, A. (1992). The reading process and its disorders. In D. I. Margolin (Ed.), *Cognitive neuropsychology in clinical practice* (pp. 229–261). New York: Oxford University Press.

Hillis, A. E., & Caramazza, A. (1995a). Converging evidence for the interaction of semantic and sublexical phonological information in accessing lexical representations for spoken output. *Cognitive Neuropsychology,* 12, 187–227.

Hillis, A. E., & Caramazza, A. (1995b). Spatially specific deficits in processing graphemic representations in reading and writing. *Brain and Language,* 48, 263–308.

Hillis, A. E., Rapp, B. C., Romani, C., & Caramazza, A. (1990). Selective impairment of semantics in lexical processing. *Cognitive Neuropsychology,* 7, 191–244.

Hodges, J. R., & McCarthy, R. A. (1993). Autobiographical amnesia resulting from bilateral paramedian thalamic infarction. *Brain,* 116, 921–940.

Hodges, J. R., Patterson, K., & Tyler, L. K. (1994). Loss of semantic memory: Implications for the modularity of mind. *Cognitive Neuropsychology,* 11, 505–542.

Hoen, B., Thelander, M., & Worsley, J. (1997). Improvement in psychological well-being of people with aphasia and their families: Evaluation of a community-based programme. *Aphasiology,* 11, 681–691.

Hofstede, B. T. M., & Kolk, H. H. J. (1994). The effects of task variation on the production of grammatical morphology in Broca's aphasia: A multiple case study. *Brain and Language,* 46, 278–328.

Holland, A. L. (1970). Case studies in aphasia rehabilitation using programmed instruction. *Journal of Speech and Hearing Disorders,* 35, 377–390.

Holland, A. L. (1975). Aphasics as communicators: A model and its implications. Paper presented to the American Speech and Hearing Association, November, Washington, D.C.

Holland, A. L. (1977). Some practical considerations in aphasia rehabilitation. In M. Sullivan & M. S. Kommers (Eds.), *Rationale for adult aphasia therapy* (pp. 167–180). University of Nebraska Medical Center.

Holland, A. L. (1980a). *Communicative abilities in daily living.* Baltimore: University Park Press.

Holland, A. L. (1980b). The usefulness of treatment for aphasia: A serendipitous study. In R. H. Brookshire (Ed.), *Clinical aphasiology conference proceedings* (pp. 240–247). Minneapolis: BRK.

Holland, A. L. (1982). When is aphasia aphasia? The problem of closed head injury. In R. H. Brookshire (Ed.), *Clinical aphasiology conference proceedings* (pp. 345–349). Minneapolis: BRK.

Holland, A. L. (1991). Pragmatic aspects of intervention in aphasia. *Journal of Neurolinguistics,* 6, 197–211.

Holland, A. L. (1994). Cognitive neuropsychological theory and treatment for aphasia: Exploring the strengths and limitations. M. L. Lemme (Ed.), *Clinical aphasiology* (Vol. 22) (pp. 275–282). Austin, TX: Pro-Ed.

Holland, A. L. (1995). Patient inputs to increasing understanding of communicative drawing. *Aphasiology,* 9, 57–59.

Holland, A. L. (1998). Why can't clinicians talk to aphasic adults? Comments on supported conversation for adults with aphasia: Methods and resources for training conversational partners. *Aphasiology,* 12, 844–846.

Holland, A. L., & Beeson, P. M. (1993). Finding a new sense of self: What the clinician can do to help. *Aphasiology,* 7, 581–584.

Holland, A. L., & Forbes, M. M. (1993). *Aphasia treatment: World perspectives.* San Diego, CA: Singular.

Holland, A. L., Fromm, D. S., DeRuyter, F., & Stein, M. (1996). Treatment efficacy: Aphasia. *Journal of Speech and Hearing Research,* 39, S27-S36.

Holland, A. L., Greenhouse, J., Fromm, D., & Swindell, C. S. (1989). Predictors of language restitution following stroke: A multivariate analysis. *Journal of Speech and Hearing Research,* 32, 232–238.

Holland, A. L., & Harris, A. (1968). Aphasia rehabilitation using programmed instruction: An intensive case history. In H. N. Sloane & B. D. Macaulay (Eds.), *Operant procedures in remedial speech and language training* (pp. 197–218). New York: Houghton Mifflin.

Holland, A. L., & Sonderman, J. C. (1974). Effects of a program based on the Token Test for teaching comprehension skills to aphasics. *Journal of Speech and Hearing Research,* 17, 589–598.

Holland, A. L., Swindell, C. S., & Forbes, M. M. (1985). The evolution of initial global aphasia: Implications for prognosis. In R. H. Brookshire (Ed.), *Clinical aphasiology* (Vol. 15) (pp. 169–175). Minneapolis: BRK.

Holtzapple, P., Pohlman, K., LaPointe, L. L., & Graham, L. F. (1989). Does SPICA and PICA? In T. E. Prescott (Ed.), *Clinical aphasiology* (Vol. 18). (pp. 131–144). Boston: College-Hill/ Little, Brown.

Hom, J., & Reitan, R. M. (1990). Generalized cognitive function after stroke. *Journal of Clinical and Experimental Neuropsychology,* 12, 644–654.

Hopper, T., & Holland, A. L. (1998). Situation-specific training for adults with aphasia: An example. *Aphasiology,* 12, 933–944.

Horner, J., Dawson, D., Heyman, A., & Fish, A. M. (1992). The usefulness of the Western Aphasia Battery for differential diagnosis of Alzheimer dementia and focal stroke syndromes: Preliminary evidence. *Brain and Language,* 42, 77–88.

Hough, M. S. (1990). Narrative comprehension in adults with right and left hemisphere brain-damage: Theme organization. *Brain and Language,* 38, 253–277.

Howard, D., Patterson, K., Franklin, S., Orchard-Lisle, V., & Morton, J. (1985a). The facilitation of picture naming in aphasia. *Cognitive Neuropsychology,* 2, 49–80.

Howard, D., Patterson, K., Franklin, S., Orchard-Lisle, V., & Morton, J. (1985b). Treatment of word retrieval deficits in aphasia. *Brain,* 108, 817–829.

Howes, D. H. (1964). Application of the word-frequency concept for aphasia. In A. V. S. de Reuck & M. O'Conner (Eds.), *Disorders of the language.* London: Churchill.

Huber, M. (1946). Linguistic problems of brain-injured servicemen. *Journal of Speech and Hearing Disorders,* 11, 143–147.

Huber, W., & Gleber, J. (1982). Linguistic and nonlinguistic processing of narratives in aphasia. *Brain and Language,* 16, 1–18.

Huber, W., Poeck, K., & Willmes, K. (1984). The Aachen Aphasia Test. In F. C. Rose (Ed.), *Progress in aphasiology* (pp. 291–303). New York: Raven Press.

Hubert, M. D., & Degiovani, R. (1993). Associations for persons with aphasia. In D. Lafond, Y. Joanette, J. Ponzio, R. Degiovani, & M. T. Sarno (Eds.), *Living with aphasia: Psychosocial issues* (pp. 279–310). San Diego, CA: Singular.

Huff, F. J., Collins, C., Corkin, S., & Rosen, J. T. (1986). Equivalent forms of the Boston Naming Test. *Journal of Clinical and Experimental Neuropsychology,* 8, 556–562.

Humphreys, G. W., & Riddoch, M. J. (1987). *To see but not to see: A case study of visual agnosia.* London: Erlbaum.

Humphreys, G. W., & Riddoch, M. J. (1988). On the case for multiple semantic systems: A reply to Shallice. *Cognitive Neuropsychology,* 5, 143–150.

Illes, J., Metter, E. J., Dennings, R., Jackson, C., Kempler, D., & Hanson, W. R. (1989). Spontaneous language production in mild aphasia: Relationship to left prefrontal glucose hypometabolism. *Aphasiology,* 3, 527–537.

Itoh, M., Sasanuma, S., Hirose, H., Yoshioka, H., & Sawashima, M. (1983). Velar movements during speech in two Wernicke aphasic patients. *Brain and Language,* 19, 283–292.

Itoh, M., Sasanuma, S., Tatsumi, I. F., Murakami, S., Fukusako, Y., & Suzuki, T. (1982). Voice onset time characteristics in apraxia of speech. *Brain and Language,* 17, 193–210.

Jackson, S. T., & Tompkins, C. A. (1989). Clinical utility of a semantic categorization task. In T. E. Prescott (Ed.), *Clinical aphasiology* (Vol. 18) (pp. 369–378). Boston: College-Hill/Little, Brown.

Jenkins, J. J., & Schuell, H. M. (1964). Further work on language deficit in aphasia. *Psychological Review,* 71, 87–93.

Jennett, B., & Teasdale, G. (1981). *Management of head injuries.* Philadelphia: F. A. Davis.

Joanette, Y., & Goulet, P. (1986). Criterion-specific reduction of verbal fluency in right-brain-damaged right-handers. *Neuropsychologia,* 24, 875–879.

Joanette, Y., Goulet, P., & Le Dorze, G. (1988). Impaired word naming in right-brain-damaged right-handers: Error types and time-course analyses. *Brain and Language,* 34, 54–64.

Joanette, Y., Goulet, P., Ska, B., & Nespoulous, J-L. (1986). Informative content of narrative discourse in right-brain-damaged right-handers. *Brain and Language,* 29, 81–105.

Joanette, Y., Lecours, A. R., Lepage, Y., & Lamoureux, M. (1983). Language in right-handers with right-hemisphere lesions: A preliminary study including anatomical, genetic and social factors. *Brain and Language,* 20, 217–248.

Johannsen-Horback, H., Cegla, B., Mager, U., Schempp, B., & Wallesch, C. W. (1985). Treatment of chronic global aphasia with a non-verbal communication system. *Brain and Language,* 24, 74–82.

Johnson, G. (1991). *In the palaces of memory: How we build the worlds inside our heads.* New York: Knopf.

Johnson-Laird, P. N. (1983). *Mental models.* Cambridge, UK: Cambridge University Press.

Jonkers, R., & Bastiaanse, R. (1997). Verb retrieval in isolation and sentence context in Broca's aphasics: The effect of transivity (abstract). *Brain and Language,* 60, 33–36.

Junque, C., Vendrell, P., Vendrell-Brucet, J. M., & Tobena, A., (1989). Differential recovery in naming in bilingual aphasics. *Brain and Language,* 36, 16–22.

Just, M. A., Carpenter, P. A., & Keller, T. A. (1996). The capacity theory of comprehension: New frontiers of evidence and arguments. *Psychological Review,* 103, 773–780.

Just, M. A., Davis, G. A., Carpenter, P. A. (1977). A comparison of aphasic and normal adults in a sentence-verification task. *Cortex,* 13, 402–423.

Kaczmarek, B. L. J. (1984). Neurolinguistic analysis of verbal utterances in patients with focal lesions of frontal lobes. *Brain and Language,* 21, 52–58.

Kagan, A. (1998). Supported conversation for adults with aphasia: Methods and resources for training conversation partners. *Aphasiology,* 12, 816–830.

Kagan, A., & Gailey, G. F. (1993). Functional is not enough: Training conversation partners for aphasic adults. In A. L. Holland & M. M. Forbes (Eds.), *Aphasia treatment: World perspectives* (pp. 199–225). San Diego, CA: Singular.

Kahn, H. J., Joanette, Y., Ska, B., & Goulet, P. (1990). Discourse analysis in neuropsychology: Comment on Chapman and Ulatowska. *Brain and Language,* 38, 454–461.

Kaplan, E. (1988). The process approach to neuropsychological assessment. *Aphasiology,* 2, 309–312.

Kaplan, E., Goodglass, H., & Weintraub, (1983). *The Boston Naming Test.* Philadelphia: Lea & Febiger.

Kaplan, J. A., Brownell, H. H., Jacobs, J. R., & Gardner, H. (1990). The effects of right hemisphere damage on the pragmatic interpretation of conversational remarks. *Brain and Language,* 38, 315–333.

Kapur, N. (1994). Remembering Norman Schwarzkopf: Evidence for two distinct long-term fact learning mechanisms. *Cognitive Neuropsychology,* 11, 661–670.

Karbe, H, Thiel, A., Weber-Luxenburger, G., Herholz, K., Kessler, J., & Heiss, W-D. (1998). Brain plasticity in poststroke aphasia: What is the contribution of the right hemisphere? *Brain and Language,* 64, 215–230.

Kashiwagi, T., Kashiwagi, A., Kunimoi, Y., Yamadori, A., Tanabe, H. & Okuda, J. (1994). Preserved capacity to copy drawings in severe aphasics with little premorbid experience. *Aphasiology,* 8, 427–442.

Katz, R. C. (1995). Aphasia treatment and computer technology. In C. Code & D. J. Müller (Eds.), *The treatment of aphasia: From theory to practice* (pp. 253–285). San Diego, CA: Singular.

Katz, R. C., & Wertz, R. T. (1992). Computerized hierarchical reading treatment in aphasia. *Aphasiology,* 6, 165–178.

Katz, W. F. (1988). An investigation of lexical ambiguity in Broca's aphasics using an auditory lexical priming technique. *Neuropsychologia,* 26, 747–752.

Katzman, R., Brown, T., Fuld, P., Peck, A., Schechter, R., & Schimmel, H. (1983). Validation of a short orientation-memory-concentration test of cognitive impairment. *American Journal of Psychiatry,* 14, 734–739.

Kay, J., & Ellis, A. W. (1987). A cognitive neuropsychological case study of anomia: Implications for psychological models of word retrieval. *Brain,* 110, 613–629.

Kay, J., Lesser, R., & Coltheart, M. (1992). *PALPA: Psycholinguistic Assessments of Language Processing in Aphasia.* Hove, UK: Lawrence Erlbaum.

Kay, J., Lesser, R., & Coltheart, M. (1996a). Psycholinguistic assessments of language processing in aphasia (PALPA): An introduction. *Aphasiology,* 10, 159–180.

Kay, J., Lesser, R., & Coltheart, M. (1996b). PALPA: The proof of the pudding is in the eating. *Aphasiology,* 10, 202–215.

Kay, J., & Patterson, K. E. (1985). Routes to meaning in surface dyslexia. In K. E. Patterson, J. C. Marshall, & M. Coltheart (Eds.), *Surface dyslexia: Neuropsychological and cognitive studies of phonological reading* (pp. 79–104). London: Lawrence Erlbaum.

Kazdin (1982). *Single-case research designs: Methods for clinical and applied settings.* New York: Oxford University Press.

Kearns, K. P. (1985). Response elaboration training for patient initiated utterances. In R. H. Brookshire (ed.), *Clinical Aphasiology* (Vol. 15) (pp. 196–204). Minneapolis: BRK.

Kearns, K. P. (1986a). Flexibility of single-subject experimental designs. Part II: Design selection and arrangement of experimental phases. *Journal of Speech and Hearing Disorders,* 51, 204–214.

Kearns, K. P. (1986b). Systematic programming of verbal elaboration skills in chronic Broca's aphasia. In R. C. Marshall (Ed.), *Case studies in aphasia rehabilitation: For clinicians by clinicians* (pp. 225–244). Austin, Tx: Pro- Ed.

Kearns, K. P. (1994). Group therapy for aphasia: Theoretical and practical considerations. In R. Chapey (Ed.), *Language intervention strategies in adult aphasia* (3rd Ed.) (pp. 304–321). Baltimore: Williams & Wilkins.

Kearns, K. P., & Salmon, S. J. (1984). An experimental analysis of auxiliary and copula verb generalization in aphasia. *Journal of Speech and Hearing Disorders,* 49, 152–163.

Kearns, K. P., & Simmons, N. N. (1983). A practical procedure for the grammatical analysis of aphasic language impairments: The LARSP. In R. H. Brookshire (Ed.), *Clinical aphasiology conference proceedings* (pp. 4–14). Minneapolis: BRK.

Kearns, K. P., & Yedor, K. (1991). An alternating treatments comparison of loose training and a convergent treatment strategy. In T. E. Prescott (Ed.), *Clinical aphasiology* (Vol. 20) (pp. 223–238). Austin, Tx: Pro-Ed.

Keefe, K. A. (1995). Applying basic neuroscience to aphasia therapy: What the animals are telling us. *American Journal of Speech-Language Pathology,* 4(4), 88–93.

Keenan, J. S., & Brassell, E. G. (1975). *Aphasia Language Performance Scales.* Murfreesboro, TN: Pinnacle Press.

Kendall, D. L., McNeil, M. R., & Small, S. L. (1998). Rule-based treatment for acquired phonological dyslexia. *Aphasiology,* 12, 587–600.

Kenin, M., & Swisher, L. P. (1972). A study of pattern of recovery in aphasia. *Cortex,* 8, 56–68.

Kennedy, M., & Murdoch, B. E. (1991). Patterns of speech and language recovery following left striatocapsular haemorrhage. *Aphasiology,* 5, 489–510.

Kennedy, M., & Murdoch, B. E. (1994). Thalamic aphasia and striato-capsular aphasia as independent aphasic syndromes. *Aphasiology,* 8, 303–313.

Kerschensteiner, M., Poeck, K., & Brunner, E. (1972). The fluency-nonfluency dimension in the classification of aphasic speech. *Cortex,* 8, 233–247.

Kertesz, A. (1979). *Aphasia and associated disorders: Taxonomy, localization, and recovery.* New York: Grune & Stratton.

Kertesz, A. (1981). The anatomy of jargon. In J. W. Brown (Ed.), *Jargonaphasia* (pp. 63–112). New York: Academic Press.

Kertesz, A. (1982). *Western Aphasia Battery.* New York: Grune & Stratton.

Kertesz, A. (1990). What should be the core of aphasia tests? (The authors promise but fail to deliver). *Aphasiology,* 4, 97–102.

Kertesz, A. (1994). Frontal lesions and function. In A. Kertesz (Ed.), *Localization and neuroimaging in neuropsychology* (pp. 567–598). San Diego, CA: Academic Press.

Kertesz, A., Benson, D. F., (1970). Neologistic jargon—a clinicopatholgical study. *Cortex,* 6, 362–386.

Kertesz, A., Ferro, J. M., & Shewan, C. M. (1984). Apraxia and aphasia: The functional-anatomical basis for their dissociation. *Neurology,* 34, 40–47.

Kertesz, A., Harlock, W., & Coates, R. (1979). Computer topographic localiztion, lesion size and prognosis in aphasia. *Brain and Language,* 8, 34–50.

Kertesz, A., Lau, W. K., & Polk, M. (1993). The structural determinants of recovery in Wernicke's aphasia. *Brain and Language,* 44, 153–165.

Kertesz, A., Lesk, D., & McCabe, P. (1977). Isotope localization of infarcts in aphasia. *Archives of Neurology,* 34, 590–601.

Kertesz, A., & McCabe, P. (1975). Intelligence and aphasia: Performance of aphasics on Raven's Coloured Progressive Matrices (RCPM). *Brain and Language,* 2, 387–395.

Kertesz, A., & McCabe, P. (1977). Recovery patterns and prognosis in aphasia. *Brain,* 100, 1–18.

Kertesz, A., & Munoz, D. G. (1997). Primary progressive aphasia. *Clinical Neuroscience,* 4, 95–102.

Kertesz, A., & Phipps, J. B. (1977). Numerical taxonomy of aphasia. *Brain and Language,* 4, 1–10.

Kertesz, A., & Poole, E. (1974). The aphasia quotient: The taxonomic approach to measurement of aphasic disability. *Canadian Journal of Neurological Sciences,* 1, 7–16.

Kiernan, R. J., Mueller, J., Langston, J. W., & Van Dyke, C. (1987). The neurobehavioral cognitive status examination: A brief but differentiated approach to cognitive assessment. *Annals of Internal Medicine,* 107, 481–485.

Kimbarow, M. L., Vangel, Jr., S. J., Lichtenberg, P. A. (1996). The influence of demographic variables on normal elderly subjects' performance on the Boston Naming Test. In M. L. Lemme (Ed.), *Clinical aphasiology* (Vol. 24) (pp. 135–144). Austin, TX: Pro-Ed.

Kimmel, D.C. (1974). *Adulthood and aging.* New York: John Wiley.

Kintsch, W. (1994). The psychology of discourse processing. In M. A. Gernsbacher (Ed.), *Handbook of psycholinguistics* (pp. 721–740). San Diego, CA: Academic Press.

Kirk, A., & Kertesz, A. (1994). Cortical and subcortical aphasias compared. *Aphasiology,* 8, 65–82.

Kirshner, H. S., Casey, P. F., Henson, J., & Heinrich, J. J. (1989). Behavioural features and lesion localization in Wernicke's aphasia. *Aphasiology,* 3, 169–176.

Kirshner, H. S., Webb, W. G., & Duncan, G. W. (1981). Word deafness in Wernicke's aphasia. *Journal of Neurology, Neurosurgery, and Psychiatry,* 45, 197–201.

Klein, D., Behrmann, M., & Doctor, E. (1994). The evolution of deep dyslexia: Evidence for the spontaneous recovery of the semantic reading route. *Cognitive Neuropsychology,* 11, 579–611.

Klima, E. S., Bellugi, U., & Poizner, H. (1988). Grammar and space in sign aphasiology. *Aphasiology,* 2, 319–328.

Knopman, D. S., Selnes, O. A., Niccum, N., & Rubens, A. B. (1984). Recovery of naming in aphasia: Relationship to fluency, comprehension and CT findings. *Neurology,* 34, 1461–1471.

Koemeda-Lutz, M., Cohen, R., Meier, E. (1987). Organization of and access to semantic memory in aphasia. *Brain and Language,* 30, 321–337.

Kohlmeyer, K. (1976). Aphasia due to focal disorders of cerebral circulation: Some aspects of localization and of spontaneous recovery. In Y. Lebrun & R. Hoops (Eds.), *Recovery in aphasics* (pp. 79–95). Amsterdam: Swets & Zeitlinger.

Kohn, S. E., & Friedman, R. B. (1986). Word-meaning deafness: A phonological-semantic dissociation. *Cognitive Neuropsychology,* 3, 291–308.

Kohn, S. E., & Goodglass, H. (1985). Picture-naming in aphasia. *Brain and Language,* 24, 266–283.

Kohn, S. E., & Smith, K. L. (1990). Between-word speech errors in conduction aphasia. *Cognitive Neuropsychology,* 7, 133–156.

Kohn, S. E., & Smith, K. L. (1995). Serial effects of phonemic planning during word production. *Aphasiology,* 9, 209–222.

Kolk, H. H. J., & Blomert, L. (1985). On the Bradley hypothesis concerning agrammatism: The nonword-interference effect. *Brain and Language,* 26, 94–105.

Kolk, H. H. J., & Friederici, A. D. (1985). Strategy and impairment in sentence understanding by Broca's and Wernicke's aphasics. *Cortex,* 21, 47–67.

Kolk, H. H. J., & Heeschen, C. (1990). Adaptation symptoms and impairment symptoms in Broca's aphasia. *Aphasiology,* 4, 221–232.

Kolk, H. H. J., & Heeschen, C. (1992). Agrammatism, paragrammatism and the management of language. *Language and Cognitive Processes,* 7, 89–130.

Kolk, H. H. J., & van Grunsven, M. M. (1985). Agrammatism as a variable phenomenon. *Cognitive Neuropsychology,* 2, 347–384.

Koul, R. K., & Lloyd, L. L. (1998). Comparison of graphic symbol learning in individuals with aphasia and right hemisphere brain damage. *Brain and Language,* 62, 398–421.

Koyama, Y., Ishiai, S., Seki, K., & Nakayama, T. (1997). Distinct processes in line bisection according to severity of left unilateral spatial neglect. *Brain and Cognition,* 35, 271–281.

Kraat, A. W. (1990). Augmentative and alternative communication: Does it have a future in aphasia rehabilitation? *Aphasiology,* 312–338.

Kudo, T. (1984). The effect of semantic plausibility on sentence comprehension in aphasia. *Brain and Language,* 21, 208–218.

Labourel, D., & Martin, M-M. (1993). The person with aphasia and the family. In D. Lafond, Y. Joanette, J. Ponzio, R. Degiovani, & M. T. Sarno (Eds.), *Living with aphasia: Psychosocial issues* (pp. 151–172). San Diego, CA: Singular.

Laine, M., & Niemi, J. (1997). Reading morphemes. *Aphasiology,* 11, 913–926.

Laine, M., & Martin, N. (1996). Lexical retrieval deficit in picture naming: Implications for word production models. *Brain and Language,* 53, 283–314.

Lambier, J. D., & Bradley, D. (1991). The effects of physical similarity on pantomime recognition in aphasia. *Aphasiology,* 5, 23–37.

LaPointe, L. L. (1985). Aphasia therapy: Some principles and strategies for treatment. In D. F. Johns (Ed.), *Clinical management of neurogenic communicative disorders* (pp. 179–241). Boston: Little, Brown.

LaPointe, L. L., & Erickson, R. J. (1991). Auditory vigilance during divided task attention in aphasic individuals. *Aphasiology,* 5, 511–520.

LaPointe, L. L., & Horner, J. (1998). *Reading Comprehension Battery for Aphasia* (Rev. Ed.) Austin, TX: Pro-Ed.

Lapointe, S. G. (1985). A theory of verb form use in the speech of agrammatic aphasics. *Brain and Language,* 24, 100–155.

Lasky, E. Z., Weidner, W. E., & Johnson, J. P. (1976). Influence of linguistic complexity, rate of presentation, and interphrase pause time on auditory-verbal comprehension of adult aphasic patients. *Brain and Language,* 3, 386–395.

Laurence, S., & Stein, D. G. (1978). Recovery after brain damage and the concept of localization of function. In S. Finger (Ed.), *Recovery from brain damage: Research and theory* (pp. 369–407). New York: Plenum Press.

Lawson, M. J., & Rice, D. N. (1989). Effects of training in use of executive strategies on a verbal memory problem resulting from closed head injury. *Journal of Clinical and Experimental Neuropsychology,* 11, 842–854.

Layman, S., & Greene, E. (1988). The effect of stroke on object recognition. *Brain and Cognition,* 7, 87–114.

Lecours, A. R., & Nespoulous, J-L. (1988). The phonetic-phonemic dichotomy in aphasiology. *Aphasiology,* 2, 329–336.

Lecours, A. R., & Vanier-Clement, M. (1976). Schizophasia and jargonaphasia. *Brain and Language,* 3, 516–565.

Le Dorze, G., Boulay, N., Gaudreau, J., & Brassard, C. (1994). The contrasting effects of a semantic versus a formal-semantic technique for the facilitation of naming in a case of anomia. *Aphasiology,* 8, 127–141.

Le Dorze, G., & Brassard, C. (1995). A description of the consequences of aphasia on aphasic persons and their relatives and friends, based on the WHO model of chronic diseases. *Aphasiology,* 9, 239–255.

Le Dorze, G., Croteau, C., & Joanette, Y. (1993). Perspectives on aphasia intervention in French-speaking Canada. In A. L. Holland & M. M. Forbes (Eds.), *Aphasia treatment: World perspectives* (pp. 87–114). San Diego, CA: Singular.

Le Dorze, G., & Nespoulous, J-L. (1989). Anomia in moderate aphasia: Problems in accessing the lexical representation. *Brain and Language,* 37, 381–400.

LeDoux, J. D., & Hirst, W. (Eds). (1986). *Mind and brain: Dialogues in cognitive neuroscience.* Cmabridge, UK: Cambridge University Press.

Le May, A., David, R., & Thomas, A. P. (1988). The use of spontaneous gesture by aphasic patients. *Aphasiology,* 2, 137–146.

Lendrem, W., & Lincoln, N. B. (1985). Spntaneous recovery of language in patients with aphasia between 4 and 34 weeks after stroke. *Journal of Neurology, Neurosurgery, and Psychiatry,* 48, 743–748.

Leonard, C. L., & Baum, S. R. (1997). The influence of phonological and orthographic information on auditory lexical access in brain-damaged patients: A preliminary investigation. *Aphasiology,* 11, 1031–1041.

Lesgold, A. M., Roth, S. F., & Curtis, M. E. (1979). Foregrounding effects in discourse comprehension. *Journal of Verbal Learning and Verbal Behavior,* 18, 291–308.

Lesser, R. (1974). Verbal comprehension in aphasia: An English version of three Italian tests. *Cortex,* 10, 247–263.

Lesser, R. (1976). Verbal and non-verbal components of the Token Test. *Neuropsychologia,* 14, 79–85.

Lesser, R. (1995). Making psycholinguistic assessments accessible. In C. Code & D. J. Müller

(Eds.), *The treatment of aphasia: From theory to practice* (pp. 164–172). San Diego, CA: Singular.

Letourneau, P. Y. (1993). The psychological effects of aphasia. In D. Lafond, Y. Joanette, J. Ponzio, R. Degiovani, & M. T. Sarno (Eds.), *Living with aphasia: Psychosocial issues* (pp. 65–86). San Diego, CA: Singular.

Levelt, W. J. M. (1989). *Speaking: From intention to articulation.* Cambridge, MA: MIT Press.

Levin, H. S. (1981). Aphasia in closed head injury. In M. T. Sarno (Ed.), *Acquired aphasia* (pp. 427–463). New York: Academic Press.

Levin, H. S., Benton, A. L., & Grossman, R. G. (1982). *Neurobehavioral consequences of closed head injury.* New York: Oxford University Press.

Levin, H. S., Goldstein, F. C., High, W. M., & Williams, D. (1988). Automatic and effortful processing after severe closed head injury. *Brain and Cognition,* 7, 283–297.

Levin, H. S., Grossman, R. G., & Kelly, P. J. (1976). Aphasic disorders in patients with closed head injury. *Journal of Neurology, Neurosurgery, and Psychiatry,* 39, 1062–1070.

Levin, H. S., Grossman, R. G., Sarwar, M., & Meyers, C. A. (1981). Linguistic recovery after closed head injury. *Brain and Language,* 12, 360–374.

Levin, H. S., O'Donnell, V. M., & Grossman, R. G. (1979). The Galveston orientation and amnesia test: A practical scale to assess cognition after head injury. *Journal of Nervous and Mental Disease,* 167, 675–684.

Levine, D. N., & Sweet, E. (1983). Localization of lesions in Broca's aphasia. In A. Kertesz (Ed.), *Localization in neuropsychology* (pp. 185–208). New York: Academic Press.

Levinson, S. C. (1983). *Pragmatics.* Cambridge, UK: Cambridge University Press.

Lezak, M. D. (1979). Recovery of memory and learning functions following traumatic brain injury. *Cortex,* 15, 63–72.

Lezak, M. D. (1982). The problem of assessing executive functions. *International Journal of Psychology,* 17, 281–297.

Lezak, M. D. (1983). *Neuropsychological assessment* (2nd Ed.). New York: Oxford University Press.

Lezak, M. D., & O'Brien, K. P. (1988). Longitudinal study of emotional, social, and physical changes after traumatic brain injury. *Journal of Learning Disability,* 21, 456–465.

Li, E. C., Kitselman, K., Dusatko, D., & Spinelli, C. (1988). The efficacy of PACE in the remediation of naming deficits. *Journal of Communication Disorders,* 21, 491–503.

Li, E. C., & Williams, S. E. (1989). The efficacy of two types of cues in aphasic patients. *Aphasiology,* 3, 619–626.

Li, E. C., & Williams, S. E. (1990). The effects of grammatic class and cue type on cueing responsiveness in aphasia. *Brain and Language,* 38, 48–60.

Liles, B. Z., & Brookshire, R. H. (1975). The effects of pause time on auditory comprehension of aphasic subjects. *Journal of Communication Disorders, 8,* 221–236.

Liles, B. Z., Coelho, C. A., Duffy, R. J., & Zalagens, M. R. (1989). Effects of elicitation procedures on the narratives of normal and closed head-injured adults. *Journal of Speech and Hearing Disorders,* 54, 356–366.

Lincoln, N. B., & Ells, P. (1980). A shortened version of the PICA. *British Journal of Disorders of Communication,* 15, 183–187.

Lincoln, N. B., & McGuirk, E. (1987). Letter to the editor. *Aphasiology,* 1, 442–443.

Lincoln, N. B., McGuirk, E., Mully, G. P., Lendrem, W., Jones, A. C., & Mitchell, J. R. A. (1984). The effectiveness of speech therapy for aphasic stroke patients: A randomized controlled trial. *Lancet,* 1, 1197–1200.

Linebarger, M. C. (1990). Neuropsychology of sentence parsing. In A. Caramazza (Ed.), *Cognitive neuropsychology and neurolinguistics: Advances in models of cognitive function and impairment* (pp. 55–122). Hillsdale, NJ: Lawrence Erlbaum.

Linebarger, M., Schwartz, M. F., & Saffran, E. M. (1983). Sensitivity to grammatical structure in so-called agrammatic aphasics. *Cognition,* 13, 361–392.

Linebaugh, C. W. (1983). Treatment of anomic aphasia. In W. H. Perkins (Ed.), *Language handicaps in adults* (pp. 35–44). New York: Thieme-Stratton.

Linebaugh, C. W., Margulies, C. P., & Mackisack-Morin, E. L. (1984). The effectiveness of comprehension-enhancing strategies employed by spouses of aphasic patients. In R. H. Brookshire (Ed.), *Clinical aphasiology conference proceedings* (pp. 188–197). Minneapolis: BRK.

Linebaugh, C. W., & Young-Charles, H. Y. (1978). The counseling needs of the families of aphasic patients. In R. H. Brookshire (Ed.), *Clinical aphasiology conference proceedings* (pp. 304–313). Minneapolis: BRK.

Lohman, T., Ziggas, D., & Pierce, R. S. (1989). Word fluency performance on common categories by subjects with closed head injuries. *Aphasiology,* 3, 685–694.

Lomas, J., & Kertesz, A. (1978). Patterns of spontaneous recovery in aphasic groups: A study of adult stroke patients. *Brain and Language,* 5, 388–401.

Lomas, J., Pickard, L., Bester, S., Elbard, H., Finlayson, A., & Zoghaib, C. (1989). The Communicative Effectiveness Index: Development and psychometric evaluation of a functional communication measure for adult aphasia. *Journal of Speech and Hearing Disorders,* 54, 113–124.

Lorch, R. F., & Lorch, E. P. (1995). Effects of organizational signals on text-processing strategies. *Journal of Educational Psychology,* 87, 537–544.

Lott, S. N., & Friedman, R. B. (1996). A speeded letter-by-letter reading treatment for pure alexia (abstract). *Brain and Language,* 55, 20–22.

Love, R. J., & Webb, W. J. (1977). The efficacy of cueing techniques in Broca's aphasia. *Journal of Speech and Hearing Disorders,* 42, 170–178.

Loverso, F. L., & Milione, J. (1992). Training and generalization of expressive syntax in nonfluent aphasia. *Clinics in Communication Disorders,* 2, 43–53.

Loverso, F. L., Prescott, T. E., & Selinger, M. (1988). Cueing verbs: A treatment strategy for aphasic adults. *Journal of Rehabilitation Research,* 25, 47–60.

Loverso, F. L., Prescott, T. E., & Selinger, M. (1992). Microcomputer treatment applications in aphasiology. *Aphasiology* , 6, 155–164.

Loverso, F. L., Prescott, T. E., Selinger, M., & Riley, L. (1989). Comparison of two modes of aphasia treatment: Clinician and computer-clinician assisted. In T. E. Prescott (Ed.), *Clinical aphasiology* (Vol. 18) (pp. 297–320). Boston: College-Hill/Little, Brown.

Loverso, F. L., Selinger, M., & Prescott, T. E. (1979). Application of verbing strategies to aphasia treatment. In R. H. Brookshire (Ed.), *Clinical aphasiology conference proceedings* (pp. 229–238). Minneapolis: BRK.

Lowell, S., Beeson, P. M., & Holland, A. L. (1995). The efficacy of a semantic cueing procedure on naming performance of adults with aphasia. *American Journal of Speech-Language Pathology,* 4(4), 109–114.

Lubinski, R. (1981). Environmental language intervention. In R. Chapey (Ed.), *Language intervention strategies in adult aphasia* (1st ed.) (pp. 223–248). Baltimore: Williams & Wilkins.

Lubinski, R. (1988). A model for intervention: Communication skills, effectiveness, and opportunity. In B. B. Shadden (Ed.), *Communication behavior and aging: A sourcebook for clinicians* (pp. 295–308). Baltimore: Williams & Wilkins.

Lubinski, R., Duchan, J., & Weitzner-Lin, B. (1980). Analysis of breakdowns and repairs in aphasic adult communication. In R. H. Brookshire (Ed.), *Clinical aphasiology conference proceedings* (pp. 111–116). Minneapolis: BRK.

Lukatela, G., Frost, S. J., & Turvey, M. T. (1998). Phonological priming by masked nonword primes in the lexical decision task. *Journal of Memory and Language,* 39, 666–683.

Luria, A. R. (1966). *Higher cortical functions in man.* New York: Basic Books.

Luria, A. R. (1970a). The functional organization of the brain. *Scientific American,* 222(3), 66–78.

Luria, A. R.(1970b). *Traumatic aphasia.* The Hague, Netherlands: Mouton.

Luzzatti, C., Willmes, K., Taricco, M., Colombo, C., & Chiesa, G. (1989). Language disturbances after severe head injury: do neurological or other associated cognitive disorders influence type, severity and evolution of the verbal impairment? A preliminary report. *Aphasiology,* 3, 643–654.

Lyon, J. G. (1989). Communicative partners: Their value in reestablishing communication with aphasic adults. In T. E. Prescott (Ed). *Clinical aphasiology* (Vol. 18) (pp. 11–17). Austin, TX: Pro-Ed.

Lyon, J. G. (1992). Communication use and participation in life for adults with aphasia in natural settings: The scope of the problem. *American Journal of Speech-Language Pathology,* 1(3), 7–14.

Lyon, J. G. (1995). Communicative drawing: An augmentative mode of interaction. *Aphasiology,* 9, 84–94.

Lyon, J. G., Cariski, D., Keisler, L., Rosenbek, J., Levine, R., Kumpula, J., Ryff, C., Coyne, S., & Blanc, M. (1997). Communication partners: Enhancing participation in life and communication for adults with aphasia in natural settings. *Aphasiology,* 11, 693–708.

Lyon, J. G., & Helm-Estabrooks, N. (1987). Drawing: Its communicative significance for expressively restricted aphasic adults. *Topics in Language Disorders,* 8, 61–71.

Lyon, J. G., & Sims, E. (1989). Drawing: Its use as a communicative aid with aphasic and normal adults. In T. E. Prescott (Ed.), *Clinical aphasiology* (Vol. 18) (pp. 339–355). Boston: College-Hill/Little, Brown.

MacDonald, M. C., Pearlmutter, N.J., & Seidenberg, M. S. (1994). The lexical nature of syntactic ambiguity resolution. *Psychological Review,* 101, 676–703.

Mack, J. L., & Boller, F. (1979). Components of auditory comprehension: Analysis of errors in a revised Token Test. In F. Boller & M. Dennis (Eds.), *Auditory comprehension: Clinical and experimental studies with the Token Test* (pp. 45–70). New York: Academic Press.

MacWhinney, B., & Osman-Sagi, J. (1991). Inflectional marking in Hungarian aphasics. *Brain and Language,* 41, 165–183.

MacWhinney, B., Osman-Sagi, J., & Slobin, D. I. (1991). Sentence comprehension in aphasia in two clear case-marking languages. *Brain and Language,* 41, 234–249.

Maher, L. M., Chatterjee, A., Rothi, L. J. G., & Heilman, K. M. (1995). Agrammatic sentence production: The use of a temporal-spatial strategy. *Brain and Language,* 49, 105–124.

Mahoney, F. I., & Barthel, D. (1965). Functional evaluation: The Barthel Index. *Maryland Medical Journal,* 14, 56–61.

Mandler, J. M. (1987). On the psychological reality of story structure. *Discourse Processes,* 10, 1–29.

Margolin, D. I. (1992). Probing the multiple facets of human intelligence: The cognitive neuropsychologist as clinician. In D. I. Margolin (Ed.), *Cognitive neuropsychology in clinical practice* (pp. 18–40). New York: Oxford University Press.

Mariner, W. K. (1994). Outcomes assessment in health care reform: Promise and limitations. *American Journal of Law & Medicine,* 20, 36–57.

Marks, M. M., Taylor, M., & Rusk, H. A. (1957). Rehabilitation of the aphasic patient: A survey of three years' experience in a rehabilitation setting. *Neurology,* 7, 837–843.

Marr, D. (1982). *Vision: A computational investigation into the human representation and processing of visual information.* San Francisco: W. H. Freeman.

Marsh, N. V., & Knight, R. G. (1991). Behavioral assessment of social competence following severe head injury. *Journal of Clinical and Experimental Neuropsychology,* 13, 729–740.

Marshall, J., Pound, C., White-Thomson, M., & Pring, T. (1990). The use of picture/word matching tasks to assist word retrieval in aphasic patients. *Aphasiology,* 4, 167–184.

Marshall, J., Pring, T., & Chiat, S. (1993). Sentence processing therapy: Working at the level of the event. *Aphasiology,* 7, 177–199.

Marshall, J., Pring, T., & Chiat, S. (1998). Verb retrieval and sentence production in aphasia. *Brain and Language,* 63, 159–183.

Marshall, J., Robson, J., Pring, T., & Chiat, S. (1998). Why does monitoring fail in jargon aphasia? Comprehension, judgment, and therapy evidence. *Brain and Language,* 63, 79–107.

Marshall, J. C., & Halligan, P. W. (1989). Does the midsagittal plane play any privileged role in "left" neglect? *Cognitive Neuropsychology,* 6, 403–422.

Marshall, R. C. (1976). Word retrieval behavior of aphasic adults. *Journal of Speech and Hearing Disorders,* 41, 444–451.

Marshall, R. C. (1987). Reapportioning time for aphasia rehabilitation: A point of view. *Aphasiology,* 1, 59–74.

Marshall, R. C., Freed, D. B., & Phillips, D. S. (1997). Communicative efficiency in severe aphasia. *Aphasiology,* 11, 373–384.

Marshall, R. C., & Tompkins, C. A. (1982). Verbal self-correction behaviors of fluent and nonfluent aphasic subjects. *Brain and Language,* 15, 292–306.

Marshall, R. C., Wertz, R. T., Weiss, D. G., Aten, J. L., Brookshire, R. H., Garcia-Bunuel, L., Holland, A. L., Kurtzke, J. F., LaPointe, L. L., Milianti, F. J., Brannegan, R., Greenbaum, H., Vogel, D., Carter, J., Barnes, N. S., & Goodman, R. (1989). Home treatment for aphasic patients by trained nonprofessionals. *Journal of Speech and Hearing Disorders,* 54, 462–470.

Martin, R. C. (1987). Articulatory and phonological deficits in short-term memory and their relation to syntactic processing. *Brain and Language,* 32, 159–192.

Martin, R. C. (1995). Working memory doesn't work: A critique of Miyake et al.'s capacity theory of aphasic comprehension deficits. *Cognitive Neuropsychology,* 12, 623–636.

Martin, R. C., & Blossom-Stach, C. (1986). Evidence of syntactic deficits in a fluent aphasic. *Brain and Language,* 28, 196–234.

Martin, R. C., & Feher, E. (1990). The consequences of reduced memory span for the comprehension of semantic versus syntactic information. *Brain and Language,* 38, 1–20.

Mauthe, R. W., Haaf, D.C., Hayn, P., & Krall, J. M. (1996). Predicting discharge destination of stroke patients using a mathematical model based on six items from the Functional Independence Measure. *Archives of Physical Medicine and Rehabilitation,* 77, 10–13.

Mazzocchi, F., & Vignolo, L. A. (1978). Computer assisted tomography in neuropsychological research: A simple procedure for lesion mapping. *Cortex,* 14, 136–144.

Mazzocchi, F., & Vignolo, L. A. (1979). Localization of lesions in aphasia: Clinical-CT scan correlations in stroke patients. *Cortex,* 15, 627–654.

Mazzoni, M., Vista, M., Pardossi, L., Avila, L., Bianchi, F., & Moretti, P. (1992). Spontaneous evolution of aphasia after ischaemic stroke. *Aphasiology,* 6, 387–396.

McCarthy, R. A., & Warrington, E. K. (1985). Category-specificity in an agrammatic patient: The relative impairment of verb retrieval and comprehension. *Neuropsychologia,* 23, 709–727.

McCarthy, R. A., & Warrington, E. K. (1986). Visual associative agnosia: A clinico-anatomical study of a single case. *Journal of Neurology, Neurosurgery, and Psychiatry,* 49, 1233–1240.

McCarthy, R. A., & Warrington, E. K. (1990). *Cognitive neuropsychology: A clinical introduction.* San Diego, CA: Academic Press.

McCleary, C. (1988). The semantic organization and classification of fourteen words by aphasic patients. *Brain and Language,* 34, 183–202.

McCleary, C., & Hirst, W. (1986). Semantic classification in aphasia: A study of basic, superordinate, and function relations. *Brain and Language,* 27, 199–209.

McCrae, K., Jared, D., & Seidenberg, M. S. (1990). On the roles of frequency and lexical access in word naming. *Journal of Memory and Language,* 29, 43–65.

McDermott, F. B., Horner, J., & DeLong, E. R. (1996). Evolution of acute aphasia as measured by the Western Aphasia Battery. In M. L. Lemme (Ed.), *Clinical aphasiology* (Vol. 24) (pp. 159–172). Austin, TX: Pro-Ed.

McDonald, S. (1993). Viewing the brain sideways? Frontal versus right hemisphere explanations of non-aphasic language disorders. *Aphasiology,* 7, 535–549.

McDonald, S., & Pearce, S. (1998). Requests that overcome listener reluctance: Impairment associated with executive dysfunction in brain injury. *Brain and Language,* 61, 88–104.

McDonald, S., Tate, R. L., & Rigby, J. (1994). Error types in ideomotor apraxia: A qualitative analysis. *Brain and Cognition,* 25, 250–270.

McDonald, S., & van Sommers, P. (1993). Pragmatic language skills after closed head injury: Ability to negotiate requests. *Cognitive Neuropsychology,* 10, 297–315.

McDonald, S., & Wales, R. (1986). An investigation of the ability to process inferences in language following right hemisphere brain damage. *Brain and Language,* 29, 68–80.

McGlinchey-Berroth, R., Milberg, W. P., Verfaellie, M., Alexander, M., & Kilduff, P. T. (1993). Semantic processing in the neglected visual field: Evidence from a lexical decision task. *Cognitive Neuropsychology,* 10, 79–108.

McGlynn, S. M., & Schacter, D. L. (1989). Unawareness of deficits in neuropsychological syndromes. *Journal of Clinical and Experimental Neuropsychology,* 11, 143–205.

McIntosh, K. W., Ramsberger, G., & Prescott, T. E. (1996). Relationships between and among language impairment, communication disability and quality of life outcome assessments in aphasic patients (abstract). *Brain and Language,* 55, 23–26.

McKhann, G., Drachman, D., Folstein, M., Katzman, R., Price, D., & Stadlin, E. M. (1984). Clinical diagnosis of Alzheimer's disease: Report of the NINCDS-ADRDA work group under the auspices of the Department of Health and Human Services Task Force on Alzheimer's disease. *Neurology,* 34, 939–944.

McNeil, M. R., & Hageman, C. F. (1979). Auditory processing deficits in aphasia evidenced on the Revised Token Test: Incidence and prediction of across subtest and across item within subtest patterns. In R. H. Brookshire (Ed.), *Clinical aphasiology conference proceedings* (pp. 47–69). Minneapolis: BRK.

McNeil, M. R., & Kimelman, M. D. Z. (1986). Toward an integrative information-processing structure of auditory comprehension and processing in adult aphasia. *Seminars in Speech and Language,* 7, 123–146.

McNeil, M. R., Odell, K., & Tseng, C-H. (1991). Toward the integration of resource allocation into a general theory of aphasia. In T. E. Prescott (Ed.), *Clinical aphasiology* (Vol. 20) (pp. 21–40). Austin, TX: Pro-Ed.

McNeil, M. R., & Prescott, T. E. (1978). Revised Token Test. Baltimore, MD: University Park Press.

McReynolds, L. V., & Kearns, K. P. (1983). *Single-subject experimental designs in communicative disorders.* Baltimore: University Park Press.

McReynolds, L. V., & Thompson, C. K. (1986). Flexibility of single-subject experimental designs. Part I: Review of the basics of single-subject designs. *Journal of Speech and Hearing Disorders,* 51, 194–203.

Mehler, J., Morton, J., & Jusczyk, P. W. (1984). On reducing language to biology. *Cognitive Neuropsychology,* 1, 83–116.

Meikle, M., Wechsler, E., Tupper, A., Benenson, M., Butler, J., Mulhall, D., & Stern, G. (1979). Comparative trial of volunteer and professional treatments of dysphasia after stroke. *British Medical Journal,* 2, 87–89.

Mendez, M. F., & Benson, D. F. (1985). Atypical conduction aphasia: A disconnection syndrome. *Archives of Neurology,* 42, 886–891.

Menn, L., & Obler, L. K. (1990). Cross-language data and theories of agrammatism. In L. Menn & L. K. Obler (Eds.), *Agrammatic aphasia: A cross-linguistic narrative sourcebook* (pp. 1369–1389). Philadelphia: John Benjamins.

Menn, L., Reilly, K. F., Hayashi, M., Kamio, A., Fujita, I., & Sasanuma, S. (1998). The interaction of preserved pragmatics and impaired syntax in Japanese and English aphasic speech. *Brain and Language,* 61, 183–225.

Mentis, M. & Prutting, C. A. (1987). Cohesion in the discourse of normal and head-injured adults. *Journal of Speech and Hearing Research,* 30, 88–98.

Mesulam, M. M. (1982). Slowly progressive aphasia without generalized dementia. *Annals of Neurology,* 11, 592–598.

Metter, E. J. (1985). Feature: Letter. *Asha,* 27, 43.

Metter, E. J. (1986). Medical aspects of stroke rehabilitation. In R. Chapey (Ed.), *Language intervention strategies in adult aphasia* (2nd ed.) (pp. 141–159). Baltimore: Williams & Wilkins.

Metter, E. J. (1987). Neuroanatomy and physiology of aphasia: Evidence from positron emission tomography. *Aphasiology,* 1, 3–33.

Metter, E. J., & Hanson, W. R. (1994). Use of positron emission tomography to study aphasia. In A. Kertesz (Ed.), *Localization and neuroimaging in neuropsychology* (pp. 123–149). San Diego, CA: Academic Press.

Miceli, G., Amitrano, A., Capasso, R., & Caramazza, A. (1996). The treatment of anomia resulting from output lexical damage: Analysis of two cases. *Brain and Language,* 52, 150–174.

Miceli, G., Gainotti, G., Caltagirone, C., & Masulo, C. (1980). Some aspects of phonological impairment in aphasia. *Brain and Language,* 11, 159–170.

Miceli, G., Mazzucchi, A., Menn, L., & Goodglass, H. (1983). Contrasting cases of Italian agrammatic aphasia without comprehension disorder. *Brain and Language,* 19, 65–97.

Miceli, G., Silveri, M. C., Nocentini, U., & Caramazza, A. (1988). Patterns of dissociation in comprehension and production of nouns and verbs. *Aphasiology,* 2, 351–358.

Miceli, G., Silveri, M. C., Romani, C., & Caramazza, A. (1989). Variation in the pattern of omissions and substitutions of grammatical morphemes in the spontaneous speech of so-called agrammatic patients. *Brain and Language,* 36, 447–492.

Miceli, G., Silveri, M. C., Villa, G., & Caramazza, A. (1984). On the basis for the agrammatic's difficulty in producing main verbs. *Cortex,* 20, 207–220.

Milberg, W., & Blumstein, S. (1981). Lexical decision and aphasia: Evidence for semantic processing. *Brain and Language,* 14, 371–385.

Milberg, W., & Blumstein, S. (1989). Reaction time methodology and the aphasic patient: A reply to Hagoort. *Brain and Language,* 36, 349–353.

Milberg, W., Blumstein, S. E., & Dworetzky, B. (1987). Processing of lexical ambiguities in aphasia. *Brain and Language,* 31, 151–170.

Miller, R., & Groher, M. (1990). *Medical speech pathology.* Rockville, MD: Aspen.

Milner, B., Corkin, S., & Teuber, H-L. (1968). Further analysis of the hippocampal amnesic syndrome: 14-year follow-up of H. M. *Neuropsychologia,* 6, 215–234.

Milton, S. B., Wertz, R. T., Katz, R. C., & Prutting, C. A. (1981). Stimulus saliency in the sorting behavior of aphasic adults. In R. H. Brookshire (Ed.),

Clinical aphasiology conference proceedings (pp. 46–54). Minneapolis: BRK.

Mitchell, D.C., & Corley, M. M. B. (1994). Immediate biases in parsing: Discourse effects or experimental artifacts? *Journal of Experimental Psychology: Learning, Memory, and Cognition,* 20, 217–222.

Mitchum, C. C., Haendiges, A. N., & Berndt, R. S. (1993). Model-guided treatment to improve written sentence production: A case study. *Aphasiology,* 7, 71–109.

Mitchum, C. C., Haendiges, A. N., & Berndt, R. S. (1995). Treatment of thematic mapping in sentence comprehension: Implications for normal processing. *Cognitive Neuropsychology,* 12, 503–547.

Mitchum, C. C., Ritgert, B., Sandson, J., & Berndt, R. S. (1990). The use of response analysis in confrontation naming. *Aphasiology,* 4, 261–279.

Miyake, A., Carpenter, P. A., & Just, M. A. (1994). A capacity approach to syntactic comprehension disorders: Making normal adults perform like aphasic patients. *Cognitive Neuropsychology,* 11, 671–717.

Miyake, A., Carpenter, P. A., & Just, M. A. (1995). Reduced resources and specific impairments in normal and aphasic sentence comprehension. *Cognitive Neuropsychology,* 12, 651–679.

Mogil, S., Bloom, D., Gray, L., & Lefkowitz, N. (1978). A unique method for the follow-up of aphasic patients. In R. H. Brookshire (Ed.), *Clinical aphasiology* conference proceedings (pp. 314–317). Minneapolis: BRK.

Mohr, J., Pessin, M., Finkelstein, S., Funkenstein, H., Duncan, G., & Davis, K. (1978). Broca's aphasia: pathologic and clinical. *Neurology,* 28, 311–324.

Mohr, J. P., Weiss, G., Caveness, W. F., Dillon, J. D., Kistler, J. P., Meirowsky, A. M., & Rish, B. L. (1980). Language and motor deficits following penetrating head injury in Vietnam. *Neurology,* 30, 1273–1279.

Moir, A., & Jessel, D. (1991). *Brain sex: The real difference between men and women.* New York: Laurel.

Monoi, H., Fukusako, Y., Itoh, M., & Sasanuma, S. (1983). Speech sound errors in patients with conduction and Broca's aphasia. *Brain and Language,* 20, 175–194.

Moore, B. D., & Papanicolaou, A. C. (1992). Dichotic listening in aphasics: Response to Niccum and Speaks. *Journal of Clinical and Experimental Neuropsychology,* 14, 641–645.

Moore, W. H. (1989). Language recovery in aphasia: A right hemisphere perspective. *Aphasiology,* 3, 101–110.

Morgan, A. L. R., & Helm-Estabrooks, N. (1987). Back to the drawing board: A treatment program for nonverbal aphasic patients. In R. H. Brookshire (Ed.), *Clinical aphasiology* (Vol. 17) (pp. 64–72). Minneapolis: BRK.

Morley, G. K., Lundgren, S., & Haxby, J. (1979). Comparison and clinical applicability of auditory comprehension scores on the Behavioral Neurology Deficit Examination, Boston Diagnostic Aphasia Examination, Porch Index of Communicative Ability and Token Test. *Journal of Clinical Neuropsychology,* 1, 249–258.

Morrow, L. Ratcliff, G., & Johnston, S. (1985). Externalising spatial knowledge in patients with right hemisphere lesions. *Cognitive Neuropsychology,* 2, 265–274.

Morrow, L., Vrtunski, P. B., Kim, Y., & Boller, F. (1981). Arousal responses to emotional stimuli and laterality of lesion. *Neuropsychologia,* 19, 65–71.

Morse, H. N. (1968). Aberrational man—tour de force of legal psychiatry. *Journal of Forensic Science,* 13, 1–32, 177–222.

Morton, J. (1985). The problem with amnesia: The problem with human memory. *Cognitive Neuropsychology,* 2, 281–290.

Morton, N., & Morris, R. G. (1995). Image transformation dissociated from visuospatial working memory. *Cognitive Neuropsychology,* 12, 767–791.

Mowrer, D. E. (1982). *Methods of modifying speech behaviors: Learning theory in speech pathology* (Second Edition). Prospect Heights, IL: Waveland Press.

Murdoch, B. E. (1988). Computerized tomographic scanning: Its contributions to the understanding of the neuroanatomical basis of aphasia. *Aphasiology,* 2, 437–462.

Murdoch, B. E., Afford, R. J., Ling, A. R., & Ganguley, B. (1986). Acute computerized tomographic scans: Their value in the localiztion of lesions and as prognostic indicators in aphasia. *Journal of Communication Disorders,* 19, 311–345.

Murdoch, B. E., Kennedy, M., McCallum, W., & Siddle, K. J. (1991). Persistent aphasia following a purely subcortical lesion: A magnetic resonance imaging study. *Aphasiology,* 5, 183–196.

Murray, L. L., Holland, A. L., & Beeson, P. M. (1995). The dissociation of attention and language skills in mild aphasia (abstract). *Brain and Language,* 51, 56–59.

Murray, L. L., Holland, A. L., & Beeson, P. M. (1997). Accuracy monitoring and task demand evaluation in aphasia. *Aphasiology,* 11, 401–414.

Murray, L. L., Holland, A. L., & Beeson, P. M. (1998). Spoken language of individuals with mild fluent aphasia under focused and divided-attention conditions. *Journal of Speech Language and Hearing Research,* 41, 213–227.

Myers, P. S. (1979). Profiles of communication deficits in patients with right cerebral hemisphere damage. In R. H. Brookshire (Ed.), *Clinical aphasiology conference proceedings* (pp. 38–46). Minneapolis: BRK.

Myers, P. S. (1986). Right hemisphere communication impairment. In R. Chapey (Ed.), *Language intervention strategies in adult aphasia* (2nd Ed.) (pp. 444–461). Baltimore: Williams & Wilkins.

Myers, P. S. (1999). *Right hemisphere damage.* San Diego, CA: Singular.

Myers, P. S., & Brookshire, R. H. (1994). The effects of visual and inferential complexity on the picture descriptions of non-brain-damaged and right-hemisphere-damaged adults. In M. L. Lemme (Ed.), *Clinical aphasiology* (Vol. 22) (pp. 25–34). Austin, TX: Pro-Ed.

Myers, P. S., & Linebaugh, C. W. (1984). The use of context-dependent pictures in aphasia rehabilitation. In R. H. Brookshire (Ed.), *Clinical aphasiology conference proceedings* (pp. 145–158). Minneapolis: BRK.

Myers, P. S., Linebaugh, C. W., & Mackisack-Morin, L. (1985). Extracting implicit meaning: Right versus left hemisphere damage. In R. H. Brookshire (Ed.), *Clinical aphasiology* (Vol. 15). (pp. 72–82). Minneapolis: BRK.

Myers, P. S., & Mackisack, E. L. (1986). Defining single versus dual definition idioms: The performance of right hemisphere and non-brain-damaged adults. In R. H. Brookshire (Ed.), *Clinical aphasiology* (Vol. 16) (pp. 267–274). Minneapolis: BRK.

Nadeau, S. E., & Crosson, B. (1997). Subcortical aphasia. *Brain and Language,* 58, 355–402.

Naeser, M. A. (1988). Some effects of subcortical white matter lesions on language behavior in aphasia. *Aphasiology,* 2, 363–368.

Naeser, M. A. (1994). Neuroimaging and recovery of auditory comprehension and spontaneous speech in aphasia with some implications for treatment of severe aphasia. In A. Kertesz (Ed.), *Localization and neuroimaging in neuropsychology* (pp. 245–296). San Diego, CA: Academic Press.

Naeser, M. A., Alexander, M. P., Helm-Estabrooks, N., Levine, H. L., Laughlin, S. A., Geschwind, N. (1982). Aphasia with predominantly subcortical lesion sites: description of three capsular/putaminal aphasia syndromes. *Archives of Neurology,* 28, 545–551.

Naeser, M. A., & Hayward, R. W. (1978). Lesion localization in aphasia with cranial computed tomography and the Boston Diagnostic Aphasia Exam. *Neurology,* 28, 545–551.

Naeser, M. A., Hayward, R. W., Laughlin, S. A., & Zatz, L. M. (1981). Quanitative CT scan studies in aphasia. I. Infarct size and CT numbers. *Brain and Language,* 12, 140–164.

Naeser, M. A., Palumbo, C. L., Prete, M. N., Fitzpatrick, P. M., Mimura, M., Samaraweera, R., & Albert, M. L. (1998). Visible changes in lesion borders on CT scan after five years poststroke, and long-term recovery in aphasia. *Brain and Language,* 62, 1–28.

Nagata, K., Yunoki, K., Kabe, S., Suzuki, A., & Araki, G. (1986). Regional cerebral blood flow correlates of aphasia outcome in cerebral haemorrhage and cerebral infarction. *Stroke,* 17, 417–423.

Nass, R., deCoudres Peterson, H., & Koch, D. (1989). Differential effects of congenital left and right brain injury on intelligence. *Brain and Cognition,* 9, 258–266.

Neely, J. H. (1976). Semantic priming and retrieval from lexical memory: Evidence for facilitatory and inhibitory processes. *Memory & Cognition,* 13, 140–144.

Neils, J., Baris, J. M., Carter, C., Dell'aira, A. L., Nordloh, S. J., Weiler, E., & Weisiger, B. (1995). Effects of age, education, and living environment on Boston Naming Test performance. *Journal of Speech and Hearing Research,* 38, 1143–1149.

Neppe, V., Chen, A., Davis, J. T, et al. (1992). The application of Screening Cerebral Assessment of Neppe (BROCAS SCAN) to a neuropsychiatric population. *Journal of Neuropsychiatry and Clinical Neuroscience,* 4, 85–94.

Nespoulous, J., Dordain, M., Perron, C., Ska, B., Bub, D., Caplan, D., Mehler, J., & Lecours, A. R. (1988). Agrammatism in sentence production without comprehension deficits: Reduced availability of syntactic structures and/or of grammatical morphemes? A case study. *Brain and Language,* 33, 273–295.

Newcombe, F. (1969). *Missile wounds to the brain: A study of psychological deficits.* Oxford: Clarendon Press.

Newcombe, F., Oldfield, R. C., Ratcliff, G. G., & Wingfield, A. (1971). Recognition and naming of object-drawings by men with focal brain wounds. *Journal of Neurology, Neurosurgery, and Psychiatry,* 34, 329–340.

Newhoff, M. N., & Davis, G. A. (1978). A spouse intervention program: Planning, implementation and problems of evaluation. In. R. H. Brookshire (Ed.), *Clinical aphasiology conference proceedings* (pp. 318–326). Minneapolis: BRK.

Niccum, N., & Speaks, C. (1991). Interpretation of outcome of dichotic listening tests following stroke. *Journal of Clinical and Experimental Neuropsychology,* 13, 614–628.

Nichelli, P., Rinaldi, M., & Cubelli, R. (1989). Selective spatial attention and length representation in normal subjects and in patients with unilateral spatial neglect. *Brain and Cognition,* 9, 57–70.

Nichelli, P., Venneri, A., Pentore, R., & Cubelli, R. (1993). Horizontal and vertical neglect dyslexia. *Brain and Language,* 44, 264–283.

Nickels, L. (1995). Getting it right? Using aphasic naming errors to evaluate theoretical models of spoken word production. *Language and Cognitive Processes,* 10, 13–45.

Nickels, L., & Best, W. (1996). Therapy for naming deficits (part II): Specifics, surprises and suggestions. *Aphasiology,* 10, 109–136.

Nicholas, L. E., & Brookshire, R. H. (1979). An analysis of how clinicians respond to unacceptable patients responses in aphasia treatment sessions. In R. H. Brookshire (Ed.), *Clinical aphasiology conference proceedings* (pp. 131–138). Minneapolis: BRK.

Nicholas, L. E., & Brookshire, R. H. (1986). Consistency of the effects of rate of speech on brain-damaged adults' comprehension of narrative discourse. *Journal of Speech and Hearing Research,* 29, 462–470.

Nicholas, L. E., & Brookshire, R. H. (1987). Error analysis and passage dependency of test items from a standardized test of multiple-sentence reading comprehension for aphasic and non-brain-damaged adults. *Journal of Speech and Hearing Disorders,* 52, 358–366.

Nicholas, L. E., & Brookshire, R. H. (1993). A system for quantifying the informativeness and efficiency of the connected speech of adults with aphasia. *Journal of Speech and Hearing Research,* 36, 338–350.

Nicholas, L. E., & Brookshire, R. H. (1995a). Comprehension of spoken narrative discourse by adults with aphasia, right-hemisphere brain damage, or traumatic brain injury. *American Journal of Speech-Language Pathology,* 4(3), 69–81.

Nicholas, L. E., & Brookshire, R. H. (1995b). Presence, completeness, and accuracy of main concepts in the connected speech of non-brain-damaged adults and adults with aphasia. *Journal of Speech and Hearing Research,* 38, 145–156.

Nicholas, L. E., Brookshire, R. H., MacLennan, D. L., Schumacher, J. G., & Porrazzo, S. A. (1989). Revised administration and scoring procedures for the Boston Naming Test and norms for non-brain-damaged adults. *Aphasiology,* 3, 569–580.

Nicholas, L. E., MacLennan, D. L., & Brookshire, R. H. (1986). Validity of multiple-sentence reading comprehension tests for aphasic adults. *Journal of Speech and Hearing Disorders,* 51, 82–87.

Nicholas, M., Obler, L. K., Albert, M. L., & Helm-Estabrooks, N. (1985). Empty speech in Alzheimer's disease and fluent aphasia. *Journal of Speech and Hearing Research,* 28, 405–410.

Nicol, J. L., Jakubowicz, & Goldblum, M-C. (1996). Sensitivity to grammatical marking in English-speaking and French-speaking non-fluent aphasics. *Aphasiology,* 10, 593–622.

Niemi, J., & Laine, M. (1989). The English language bias in neurolinguistics: New languages give new perspectives. *Aphasiology,* 3, 155–160.

Nolan, K. A., & Caramazza, A. (1982). Modality-independent impairments in word processing in a deep dyslexic patient. *Brain and Language,* 16, 237–266.

Nolan, K. A., & Caramazza, A. (1983). An analysis of writing in a case of deep dyslexia. *Brain and Language,* 20, 305–328.

Noll, J. D., & Randolf, S. R. (1978). Auditory semantic, syntactic, and retention errors made by aphasic subjects on the Token Test. *Journal of Communication Disorders,* 11, 543–553.

Obler, L. K., & Albert, M. L. (1977). Influence of aging on recovery from aphasia in polyglots. *Brain and Language,* 4, 460–463.

Obler, L. K., & Albert, M. L. (1981). Language in the elderly aphasic and the dementing patient. In M. T. Sarno (Ed.), *Acquired aphasia* (pp. 385–398). New York: Academic Press.

Obler, L. K., Goral, M., & Albert, M. L. (1995). Variability in aphasia research: Aphasia subject selection in group studies. *Brain and Language,* 48, 341–350.

Oczkowski, W. J., & Barreca, S. (1993). The Functional Independence Measure: Its use to identify rehabilitation needs in stroke survivors. *Archives of Physical Medicine and Rehabilitation,* 74, 1291–1294.

Oleyar, K. S., Doyle, P. J., Keefe, K., & Goldstein, H. (1991). The effects of a time-delay procedure on comprehension of verb-noun commands in severe aphasia. In T. E. Prescott (Ed.), *Clinical aphasiology* (Vol. 20) (pp. 271–284). Austin, Tx: Pro-Ed.

Orgass, B., & Poeck, K. (1966). Clinical validation of a new test for aphasia: An experimental study of the Token Test. *Cortex,* 2, 222–243.

Orgass, B., & Poeck, K. (1969). Assessment of aphasia by psychometric methods. *Cortex,* 5, 317–330.

Ostrin, R. K., & Schwartz, M. F. (1986). Reconstructing from a degraded trace: A study of sentence repetition in agrammatism. *Brain and Language,* 28, 328–345.

Ostrin, R. K., & Tyler, L. K. (1993). Automatic access to lexical semantics in aphasia: Evidence from semantic and associative priming. *Brain and Language,* 45, 147–159.

Paivio, A., & Begg, I. (1981). *Psychology of language.* Englewood Cliffs, NJ: Prentice-Hall.

Paradis, M. (1977). Bilingualism and aphasia. In H. Whitaker & H. A. Whitaker (Eds.), *Studies in neurolinguistics* (Vol. 3) (pp. 65–122). New York: Academic Press.

Paradis, M., (1987). *The assessment of bilingual aphasia.* Hillsdale, NJ: Lawrence Erlbaum.

Paradis, M. (1990). Language lateralization in bilinguals: Enough already! *Brain and Language,* 39, 576–586.

Paradis, M., Goldblum, M-C., & Abidi, R. (1982). Alternate antagonism with paradoxical translation behavior in two bilingual aphasic patients. *Brain and Language,* 15, 55–69.

Paradis, M., & Goldblum, M-C. (1989). Selective crossed aphasia in a trilingual aphasic patient followed by reciprocal antagonism. *Brain and Language,* 36, 62–75.

Parasuraman, R., Mutter, S. A., & Molloy, R. (1991). Sustained attention following mild closed head injury. *Journal of Clinical and Experimental Neuropsychology,* 13, 789–811.

Parisi, D., & Pizzamiglio, L. (1971). Syntactic comprehension in aphasia. *Cortex,* 6, 204–215.

Parkin, A. J., Yeomans, J., & Bindschaedler, C. (1994). Further characterization of the executive memory impairment following frontal lobe lesions. *Brain and Cognition,* 26, 23–42.

Parr, S. (1992). Everyday reading and writing practices of normal adults: Implications for aphasia assessment. *Aphasiology,* 6, 273–283.

Parr, S. (1994). Coping with aphasia: Conversations with 20 aphasic people. *Aphasiology,* 8, 457–466.

Parr, S. (1996). Everyday literacy in aphasia: Radical approaches to functional assessment and therapy. *Aphasiology,* 10, 469–479.

Parry, F. M., Young, A. W., Saul, J. S. M., & Moss, A. (1991). Dissociable face processing impairments after brain injury. *Journal of Clinical and Experimental Neuropsychology,* 13, 545–558.

Parsons, C. L. (1987a). Call me irresponsible, but don't try to mislead me. *Aphasiology,* 1, 443–444.

Parsons, C. L. (1987b). Is there support for assumptions underlying 'Reapportioning time for aphasia rehabilitation: A point of view'? *Aphasiology,* 1, 81–86.

Parsons, C. L., Lambier, J. D., & Miller, A. (1988). Phonological processes and phonemic paraphasias. *Aphasiology,* 2, 45–54.

Pashek, G. V., & Holland, A. L. (1988). Evolution of aphasia in the first year post-stroke. *Cortex,* 24, 411–423.

Patronas, N.J., Deveikis, J. P., & Schellinger, D. (1987). The use of computed tomography in studying the brain. In H. G. Mueller & V. C. Geoffrey (Eds.), *Communication disorders in aging: Assessment and management* (pp. 107–134). Washington, DC: Gallaudet University Press.

Patterson, K. E. (1978). Phonemic dyslexia: Errors of meaning and the meaning of errors. *Quarterly Journal of Experimental Psychology,* 30, 587–608.

Patterson, K. E. (1979). What is right with "deep" dyslexic patients? *Brain and Language,* 8, 111–129.

Patterson, K. E., & Wilson, B. (1990). A ROSE is a ROSE or a NOSE: A deficit in initial letter identification. *Cognitive Neuropsychology,* 7, 447–478.

Patterson, K. W., Purell, C., & Morton, J. (1983). The facilitation of word retrieval in aphasia. In C. Code & D. J. Muller (Eds.), *Aphasia therapy* (pp. 76–87). London: Edward Arnold.

Patterson, M. B., & Mack, J. L. (1985). Neuropsychological analysis of a case of reduplicative paramnesia. *Journal of Clinical and Experimental Neuropsychology,* 7, 111–121.

Peach, R. K. (1987). A short-term memory treatment approach to the repetition deficit in conduction aphasia. In R. H. Brookshire (Ed.), *Clinical aphasiology* (Vol. 17) (pp. 35–45). Minneapolis: BRK.

Peach, R. K. (1996). Treatment for aphasic phonological output planning deficits. In M. L. Lemme (Ed.), *Clinical aphasiology* (Vol. 24) (pp. 109–120). Austin, TX: Pro-Ed.

Peach, R. K., Canter, G. J., & Gallaher, A. J. (1988). Comprehension of sentence structure in anomic and conduction aphasia. *Brain and Language,* 35, 119–137.

Peach, R. K., & Rubin, S. S. (1994) Treatment of global aphasia. In R. Chapey (Ed.), *Language intervention strategies in adult aphasia* (3rd Ed) (pp. 429–445). Baltimore: Williams & Wilkins.

Peach, R. K., Rubin, S. S., & Newhoff, M. (1994). A topographic event-related potential analysis of the attention deficit for auditory processing in aphasia. In M. L. Lemme (Ed.), *Clinical aphasiology* (Vol. 22) (pp. 81–96). Austin, TX: Pro-Ed.

Pease, D. M., & Goodglass, H. (1978). The effects of cuing on picture naming in aphasia. *Cortex,* 14, 178–189.

Pell, M. D., & Baum, S. R. (1997). Unilateral brain damage, prosodic comprehension deficits, and the acoustic cues to prosody. *Brain and Language,* 57, 195–214.

Pendleton, M. G., Heaton, R. K., Lehman, R. A. W., & Hulihan, D. (1982). Diagnostic utility of the Thurstone Word Fluency Test in neuropsychological evaluations. *Journal of Clinical Neuropsychology,* 4, 307–318.

Pendley, A., & Ramsberger, G. (1996). Self-awareness in patients with right hemisphere damage. In M. L. Lemme (Ed.), *Clinical aphasiology* (Vol. 24) (pp. 243–253). Austin, TX: Pro-Ed.

Penfield, W., & Perot, P. (1963). The brain's record of visual and auditory experience: A final summary and discussion. *Brain,* 86, 595–696.

Penn, C., Jones, D., & Joffe, V. (1997). Hierarchical discourse therapy: A method for the mild patient. *Aphasiology,* 11, 601–613.

Peper, M., & Irle, E. (1997). The decoding of emotional concepts in patients with focal cerebral lesions. *Brain and Cognition,* 34, 360–387.

Perecman, E. (1984). Spontaneous translation and language mixing in a polyglot aphasic. *Brain and Language,* 23, 43–63.

Peretz, I. (1993). Auditory atonalia for melodies. *Cognitive Neuropsychology,* 10, 21–56.

Peterson, L. N., & Kirshner, H. S. (1981). Gestural impairment and gestural ability in aphasia: A review. *Brain and Language,* 14, 333–348.

Petocz, A., & Oliphant, G. (1988). Closed-class words as first syllables do interfere with lexical decisions for nonwords: Implications for theories of agrammatism. *Brain and Language,* 34, 127–146.

Phillips, P. P., & Halpin, G. (1978). Language impaiment evaluation in aphasic patients. *Archives of Physical Medicine and Rehabilitation,* 59, 327–329.

Pickersgill, M. J., & Lincoln, N. B. (1983). Prognostic indicators and the pattern of recovery of communication in aphasic stroke patients. *Journal of Neurology, Neurosurgery, and Psychiatry,* 46, 130–139.

Pierce, R. S. (1988). Influence of prior and subsequent context on comprehension in aphasia. *Aphasiology,* 2, 577–582.

Pierce, R. S., & Beekman, L. A. (1985). Effects of linguistic and extralinguistic context on semantic and syntactic processing in aphasia. *Journal of Speech and Hearing Research,* 28, 250–254.

Pierce, R. S., Jarecki, J., & Cannito, M. (1990). Single word comprehension in aphasia: Influence of array size, picture relatedness and situational context. *Aphasiology,* 4, 155–166.

Pierce, R. S., & Wagner, C. M. (1985). The role of context in facilitating syntactic decoding in aphasia. *Journal of Communication Disorders,* 18, 203–219.

Pimental, P. A., & Kingsbury, N. A. (1989). *Mini inventory of right brain injury.* Austin, TX: Pro-Ed.

Pizzamiglio, L., Antonucci, G., Judica, A., Montenero, P., Razzano, C., & Zoccolotti, P. (1992). Cognitive rehabilitation of the hemineglect disorder in chronic patients with unilateral right-brain damage. *Journal of Clinical and Experimental Neuropsychology,* 14, 901–923.

Pizzamiglio, L., & Appicciafuoco, A. (1971). Semantic comprehension in aphasia. *Journal of Communication Disorders,* 3, 280–288.

Pizzamiglio, L., Mammucari, A., & Razzano, C. (1985). Evidence for sex differences in brain organization in recovery in aphasia. *Brain and Language,* 25, 213–223.

Plourde, G., Joanette, Y., Fontaine, F. S., Laplante, L., & Renaseau-Leclerc, C. (1993). The severity of visual hemineglect follows a bimodal frequency distribution. *Brain and Cognition,* 21, 131–139.

Poeck, K., Huber, W., & Willmes, K. (1989). Outcome of intensive language treatment in aphasia. *Journal of Speech and Hearing Disorders,* 54, 471–478.

Poeck, K., & Hartje, W. (1979). Performance of aphasic patients in visual versus auditory presentation of the Token Test: Demonstration of a supramodal deficit. In F. Boller & M. Dennis (Eds.), *Auditory comprehension: Clinical and experimental studies with the Token Test* (pp. 107–116). New York: Academic Press.

Poeck, K., & Pietron, H. (1981). The influence of stretched speech presentation on Token Test performance of aphasic and right brain damaged patients. *Neuropsychologia,* 19, 133–136.

Poizner, H., Klima, E. S., & Bellugi, U. (1987). *What the hands reveal about the brain.* Cambridge, MA: MIT Press.

Ponsford, J., & Kinsella, G. (1992). Attentional deficits following closed-head injury. *Journal of Clinical and Experimental Neuropsychology,* 14, 822–838.

Ponzio, J., & Degiovani, R. (1993). Typical behavior of persons with aphasia and their families. In D. Lafond, Y. Joanette, J. Ponzio, R. Degiovani, & M. T. Sarno (Eds.), *Living with aphasia: Psychosocial issues* (pp. 117–128). San Diego, CA: Singular.

Porch, B. E. (1967). *Porch Index of Communicative Ability, Volume I: Theory and development.* Palo Alto, CA: Consulting Psychologists Press.

Porch, B. E. (1971). *Porch Index of Communicative Ability, Volume II: Administration, scoring, and interpretation* (Second Edition). Palo Alto, CA: Consulting Psychologists Press.

Porch, B. E. (1981). *Porch Index of Communicative Ability, Volume II: Administration, scoring, and interpretation* (Third Edition). Palo Alto, CA: Consulting Psychologists Press.

Porch, B. E. (1986). Therapy subsequent to the Porch Index of Communicative Ability (PICA). In R. Chapey (Ed.), *Language intervention strategies in adult aphasia* (2nd ed.) (pp. 295–303). Baltimore: Williams & Wilkins.

Porch, B. E., Collins, M., Wertz, R. T., & Friden, T. P. (1980). Statistical prediction of change in aphasia. *Journal of Speech and Hearing Research,* 23, 312–321.

Porch, B. E., & Palmer, P. M. (1986). Right hemisphere PICA percentiles revised. In R. H. Brookshire (Ed.), *Clinical aphasiology* (Vol 16) (pp. 275–280). Minneapolis: BRK.

Porch, B. E., & Porec, J. P. (1977). Medical-legal application of PICA results. In R. H. Brookshire (Ed.), *Clinical aphasiology* conference proceedings (pp. 302–309). Minneapolis: BRK.

Porec, J. P., & Porch, B. E. (1977). The behavorial charactoristics of "simulated" aphasia. In R. H. Brookshire (Ed.), *Clinical aphasiology* conference proceedings (pp. 297–301). Minneapolis: BRK.

Porter, J. L., & Dabul, B. (1977). The application of transactional analysis to therapy with wives of adult aphasic patients. *Asha,* 19, 244–248.

Posner, M. I., Walker, J. A., Friedrich, F. J., & Rafal, R. D. (1984). Effects of parietal lobe injury on covert orienting of visual attention. *Journal of Neuroscience,* 4, 1863–1874.

Posner, M. I., Walker, J. A., Friedrich, F. J., & Rafal, R. D. (1987). How do the parietal lobes direct covert attention. *Neuropsychologia,* 25, 135–146.

Prather, P. A., Love, T., Finkel, L., & Zurif, E. B. (1994). Effects of slowed processing on lexical activation: Automaticity without encapsulation (abstract). *Brain and Language,* 47, 326–329.

Prescott, T. E., Gruber, J. L., Olson, M., & Fuller, K. C. (1987). Hanoi revisited. In R. H. Brookshire (Ed.), *Clinical aphasiology* (Vol. 17) (pp. 249–259). Minneapolis: BRK.

Prescott, T. E., Loverso, F. L., & Selinger, M. (1984). Differences between normal and left brain damaged (aphasic) subjects in a nonverbal problem solving task. In R. H. Brookshire (Ed.), *Clinical aphasiology conference proceedings* (pp. 235–240). Minneapolis: BRK.

Prescott, T. E., Selinger, M., & Loverso, F. L. (1982). An analysis of learning, generalization, and maintenance of verbs by an aphasic patient. In R. H. Brookshire (Ed.), *Clinical aphasiology conference proceedings* (pp. 178–182). Minneapolis: BRK.

Price, C. J., & Humphreys, G. W. (1992). Letter by letter reading? Functional deficits and compensatory strategies. *Cognitive Neuropsychology,* 9, 427–457.

Price, C. J., & Humphreys, G. W. (1993). Attentional dyslexia: The effects of co-occurring deficits? *Cognitive Neuropsychology,* 10, 569–592.

Prigatano, G. P. (1987). Recovery and cognitive retraining after craniocerebral trauma. *Journal of Learning Disabilities,* 20, 603–613.

Pring, T., Hamilton, A., Harwood, A., & Macbride, L. (1993). Generalization of naming after picture/word matching tasks: Only items appearing in therapy benefit. *Aphasiology,* 7, 383–394.

Prins, R. S., Snow, C. E., & Wagenaar, E.(1978). Recovery from aphasia: Spontaneous speech versus language comprehension. *Brain and Language,* 6, 192–211.

Prior, M., Kinsella, G., & Giese, J. (1990). Assessment of musical processing in brain-damaged patients: Implications for laterality of music. *Journal of Clinical and Experimental Neuropsychology,* 12, 301–312.

Prutting, C. A., & Kirchner, D. M. (1987). A clinical appraisal of the pragmatic aspects of language. *Journal of Speech and Hearing Disorders,* 52, 105–119.

Purdy, M. H., Belanger, S., & Liles, B. Z. (1993). Right-hemisphere-damaged subjects' ability to use context in inferencing. In M. L. Lemme (Ed.), *Clinical aphasiology* (Vol. 21) (pp. 135–143). Austin, TX: Pro-Ed.

Purdy, M. H., Duffy, R. J., & Coelho, C. A. (1994). An investigation of the communicative use of trained symbols following multimodality training. In M. L. Lemme (Ed.), *Clinical aphasiology* (Vol. 22) (pp. 345–356). Austin, TX: Pro-Ed.

Quinteros, B., Williams, D. R. R., White, C. A. M., & Pickering, M. (1984). The costs of using trained and supervised volunteers as part of a speech therapy service for dysphasic patients. *British Journal of Disorders of Communication,* 19, 205–212.

Rao, P. R. (1995). Drawing conclusions on the efficacy of 'drawing' as a treatment for persons with severe aphasia. *Aphasiology,* 9, 59–62.

Rapp, B. C., Hillis, A. E., & Caramazza, A. (1993). The role of representations in cognitive theory: More on multiple semantics and the agnosias. *Cognitive Neuropsychology,* 10, 235–250.

Ratcliff, G. (1979). Spatial thought, mental rotation, and the right hemisphere. *Neuropsychologia,* 17, 49–53.

Raven, J. C. (1962). *Coloured Progressive Matrices Sets, A, Ab, B.* London: H. K. Lewis.

Raymer, A. M., Maher, L. M., Foundas, A. L., Heilman, K. M., & Rothi, L. J. G. (1997). The significance of body part as tool errors in limb apraxia. *Brain and Cognition,* 34, 287–292.

Raymer, A. M., Moberg, P., Crosson, B., Nadeau, S., & Rothi, L. J. (1997). Lexical-semantic deficits in two patients with dominant thalamic infarction. *Neuropsychologia,* 35, 211–219.

Raymer, A. M., Thompson, C. K., Jacobs, B., & Le Grand, H. R. (1993). Phonological treatment of naming deficits in aphasia: Model-based generalization analysis. *Aphasiology,* 7, 27–53.

Rayner, K., & Pollatsek, A. (1989). *The psychology of reading.* Englewood Cliffs, NJ: Prentice-Hall.

Read, D. E. (1981). Solving deductive reasoning problems after unilateral temporal lobectomy. *Brain and Language,* 12, 116–127.

Reitan, R. M., & Wolfson, D. (1985). *The Halstead-Reitan Neuropsychological Test Battery: Theory and clinical interpretation.* Tucson, AZ: Neuropsychology Press.

Rice, B., Paull, A., & Muller, D. J. (1987). An evaluation of a social support group for spouses of aphasic partners. *Aphasiology,* 1, 247–256.

Riddoch, M. J. (1990). Loss of visual imagery: A generation deficit. *Cognitive Neuropsychology,* 7, 249–274.

Riddoch, M. J., & Humphreys, G. W. (1987). Visual object processing in optic aphasia: A case of semantic access agnosia. *Cognitive Neuropsychology,* 4, 131–185.

Riddoch, M. J., Humphreys, G. W., Cleton, P., & Ferry, P. (1990). Interaction of attentional and lexical processes in neglect dyslexia. *Cognitive Neuropsychology,* 7, 479–518.

Riddoch, M. J., Humphreys, G. W., Coltheart, M., & Funnell, E. (1988). Semantic systems or system? Neuropsychological evidence re-examined. *Cognitive Neuropsychology,* 5, 3–26.

Riedel, K., & Studdert-Kennedy, M. (1985). Extending formant transitions may not improve aphasics' perception of stop consonant place of articulation. *Brain and Language,* 24, 223–232.

Riege, W. H., Metter, E. J., & Hanson, W. R. (1980). Verbal and nonverbal recognition memory in aphasic and nonaphasic stroke patients. *Brain and Language,* 10, 60–70.

Rimel, R. W., & Jane, J. A. (1983). Characteristics of the head-injured patient. In M. Rosenthal, E. R. Griffith, M. R. Bond, & J. D. Miller (Eds.), *Rehabilitation of the head injured adult* (pp. 9–22). Philadelphia: F. A. Davis.

Rinnert, C., & Whitaker, H. A. (1973). Semantic confusions by aphasic patients. *Cortex,* 9, 56–81.

Rispens, J., Bastiaanse, R., van Zonneveld, R., Jarema, G., & Edwards, S. (1997). Negation in agrammatism: A crosslinguistic comparison (abstract). *Brain and Language,* 60, 75–78.

Rivers, D. L., & Love, R. J. (1980). Language performance on visual processing tasks in right hemisphere lesion cases. *Brain and Language,* 10, 348–366.

Roach, A., Schwartz, M. F., Martin, N., Grewal, R. S., & Brecher, A. (1996). The Philadelphia Naming Test: Scoring and rationale. In M. L. Lemme (Ed.), *Clinical aphasiology* (Vol. 24) (pp. 121–134). Austin, TX: Pro-Ed..

Roberts, J. A., & Wertz, R. T. (1989). Comparison of spontaneous and elicited oral-expressive language in aphasia. In T. E. Prescott (Ed)., *Clinical aphasiology* (Vol. 18) (pp. 479–488). Boston: College-Hill/Little, Brown.

Robey, R. R. (1998). A meta-analysis of clinical outcomes in the treatment of aphasia. *Journal of Speech, Language, and Hearing Research,* 41, 172–187.

Robey, R. R., & Dalebout, S. D. (1998). A tutorial on conducting meta-analyses of clinical outcome research. *Journal of Speech Language and Hearing Research,* 41, 1227–1241.

Robey, R. R., Schultz, M. C., Crawford, A. B., & Sinner, C. A. (1999). Single-subject clinical-outcome research: Designs, data, effect sizes, and analyses. *Aphasiology,* 13, 445–473.

Robin, D. A., & Schienberg, S. (1990). Subcortical lesions and aphasia. *Journal of Speech and Hearing Disorders,* 55, 90–100.

Robinson, R. G., Kubos, K. L., Starr, L. B., Rao, K., & Price, T. R. (1984). Mood disorders in stroke patients: Importance of location of lesion. *Brain,* 107, 81–93.

Rogers, C. R. (1951). *Client-centered therapy.* Boston: Houghton Mifflin.

Rogers, C. R. (1961). *On becoming a person.* Boston: Houghton Mifflin.

Rolak, L. A. (Ed.). (1993). *Neurology secrets.* Philadelphia: Hanley & Belfus.

Rollin, W. J. (1987). *The psychology of communication disorders in individuals and their families.* Englewood Cliffs, NJ: Prentice-Hall.

Roman, M., Brownell, H. H., Potter, H. H., Seibold, M. S., & Gardner, H. (1987). Script knowledge in right hemisphere-damaged and in normal elderly adults. *Brain and Language,* 31, 151–170.

Romani, C. (1994). The role of phonological short-term memory in syntactic parsing: A case study. *Language and Cognitive Processes,* 9, 29–67.

Rosch, E. (1975). Cognitive representations of semantic categories. *Journal of Experimental Psychology: General,* 104, 192–233.

Rose, S. (1989). *The conscious brain* (Revised Edition). New York Paragon.

Rosenbek, J. C. (1982). When is aphasia aphasia? In R. H. Brookshire (Ed.), *Clinical aphasiology conference proceedings* (pp. 360–366). Minneapolis: BRK.

Rosenbek, J. C., LaPointe, L. L., & Wertz, R. T. (1989). *Aphasia: A clinical approach.* San Diego: Singular.

Rosenberg, B., Zurif, E., Brownell, H., Garrett, M., & Bradley, D. (1985). Grammatical class effects in relation to normal and aphasic sentence processing. *Brain and Language,* 26, 287–303.

Ross, E. D. (1981). The aprosodias: Functional-anatomic organization of the affective components of language in the right hemisphere. *Archives of Neurology,* 38, 561–569.

Ross, E. D., & Mesulam, M. (1979). Dominant language functions of the right hemisphere? Prosody and emotional gesturing. *Archives of Neurology,* 36, 144–148.

Ross, G. W., Cummings, J. L., & Benson, D. F. (1990). Speech and language alterations in dementia syndromes: Characteristics and treatment. *Aphasiology,* 4, 339–352.

Rothi, L. J. G., Mack, L., Verfaellie, M., Brown, P., & Heilman, K. M. (1988). Ideomotor apraxia: Error pattern analysis. *Aphasiology,* 2, 381–388.

Rubens, A. B. (1977a). The role of changes within the central nervous system during recovery from aphasia. In M. Sullivan & M. S. Kommers (Eds.), *Rationale for adult aphasia therapy* (pp. 28–43). University of Nebraska Medical Center.

Rubens, A. B. (1977b). What neurologists expect of clinical aphasiologists. In R. H. Brookshire (Ed.), *Clinical aphasiology conference proceedings* (pp. 1–4). Minneapolis: BRK.

Ruff, R., Mahaffey, R., Engel, J., Farrow, C., Cox, D., & Karzmark, P. (1994). Efficacy study of THINKable in the attention and memory training of traumatically head-injured patients. *Brain Injury,* 8, 3–14.

Russell, W. R., & Espir, M. L. E. (1961). *Traumatic aphasia.* London: Oxford University Press.

Ryalls, J. H. (1986). What constitutes a primary disturbance of speech prosody? A reply to Shapiro and Danly. *Brain and Language,* 29, 183–187.

Ryalls, J. H., & Behrens, S. J. (1988). An overview of changes in fundamental frequency associated with cortical insult. *Aphasiology,* 2, 107–116.

Ryff, C. D. (1989). Happiness is everything, or is it? Explorations on the meaning of psychological well-being. *Journal of Personality and Social Psychology,* 57, 1069–1081.

Sacks, O. (1985). *The man who mistook his wife for a hat and other clinical tales.* New York: Summit.

Saffran, E. M., & Marin, O. S. M. (1975). Immediate memory for word lists and sentences in a patient with deficient auditory-verbal short-term memory. *Brain and Language,* 2, 420–433.

Saffran, E. M., & Schwartz, M. F. (1988). "Agrammatic" comprehension it's not: Alternatives and implications. *Aphasiology,* 2, 389–394.

Saffran, E. M., Schwartz, M. F., & Linebarger, M. C. (1998). Semantic influences on thematic role assignment: Evidence from normals and aphasics. *Brain and Language,* 62, 255–297.

Saffran, E. M., Schwartz, M. F., & Marin, O. S. M. (1980). The word order problem in agrammatism. II. Production. *Brain and Language,* 10, 263–280.

Salvatore, A. P. (1985). Experimental analysis of acquisition and generalization of syntax in Broca's aphasia. In R. H. Brookshire (Ed.), *Clinical aphasiology* (Vol. 15) (pp. 214–221). Minneapolis: BRK.

Salvatore, A. P., Trunzo, M. J., Holtzapple, P., & Graham, L. (1983). Investigation of the sentence hierarchy of the Helm Elicited Language Program for Syntax Stimulation. In R. H. Brookshire (Ed.), *Clinical aphasiology conference proceedings* (pp. 73–84). Minneapolis: BRK.

Samples, J. M., & Lane, V. W. (1980). Language gains in global aphasia over a three-year period: Case study. *Journal of Communication Disorders,* 13, 49–57.

Samuels, J. A., & Benson, D. F. (1979). Some aspects of language comprehension in anterior aphasia. *Brain and Language,* 8, 275–286.

Sanders, S. B. (1986). Maximum recovery: By what definition? In R. C. Marshall (Ed.), *Case studies in aphasia rehabilitation: For clinicians by clinicians* (pp. 89–104). Austin, Tx: Pro-Ed.

Sanders, S. B. & Davis, G. A. (1978). A comparison of the Porch Index of Communicative Ability and the Western Aphasia Battery. In R. H. Brookshire (Ed.), *Clinical aphasiology conference proceedings* (pp. 117–126). Minneapolis: BRK.

Sanders, S. B., Davis, G. A., & Wells, R. (1981). Influence of the preposition in language comprehension subtests of the PICA. In R. H. Brookshire (Ed.), *Clinical aphasiology conference proceedings* (pp. 115–119). Minneapolis: BRK.

Sanders, S. B., Hamby, E. I., & Nelson, M. (1984). *You are not alone: Organizing your local stroke club.* Nashville, Tennessee Affiliate of the American Heart Association.

Sands, E., Sarno, M. T., & Shankweiler, D. (1969). Long-term assessment of language function in aphasia due to stroke. *Archives of Physical Medicine and Rehabilitation,* 50, 202–207.

Sarno, J. E., Sarno, M. T., & Levita, E. (1971). Evaluating language improvement after completed stroke. *Archives of Physical Medicine and Rehabilitation,* 52, 73–78.

Sarno, M. T. (1969). *The functional communication profile manual of directions.* Rehabilitation Monograph 42, New York University Medical Center.

Sarno, M. T. (1980). The nature of verbal impairment after closed head injury. *Journal of Nervous and Mental Disease,* 168, 685–692.

Sarno, M. T. (1981). Recovery and rehabilitation in aphasia. In M. T. Sarno (Ed.), *Acquired aphasia* (pp. 485–529). New York: Academic Press.

Sarno, M. T. (1993). Aphasia rehabilitation: Psychosocial and ethical considerations. *Aphasiology,* 7, 321–334.

Sarno, M. T., Buonaguro, A., & Levita, E. (1987). Aphasia in closed head injury and stroke. *Aphasiology,* 1, 331–338.

Sarno, M. T., & Levita, E. (1971). Natural course of recovery in severe aphasia. *Archives of Physical Medicine and Rehabilitation,* 52, 175–178.

Sarno, M. T., & Levita, E. (1979). Recovery in treated aphasia during the first year post-stroke. *Stroke,* 10, 663–670.

Sarno, M. T., & Levita, E. (1981). Some observations on the nature of recovery in global aphasia after stroke. *Brain and Language,* 13, 1–12.

Sarno, M. T., Silverman, M., & Sands, E. (1970). Speech therapy and language recovery in severe aphasia. *Journal of Speech and Hearing Research,* 13, 607–623.

Sartori, G., Job, R., Miozzo, M., Zago, S., & Marchiori, G. (1993). Category-specific form-knowledge deficit in a patient with herpes simplex virus encephalitis. *Journal of Clinical and Experimental Neuropsychology,* 15, 280–299.

Schacter, D. L. (1987). Implicit memory: History and current status. *Journal of Experimental Psychology: Learning, Memory, and Cognition,* 13, 501–518.

Schacter, D. L. (1996). *Searching for memory: The brain, the mind, and the past.* New York: BasicBooks.

Schacter, D. L., & Graf, P. (1986). Preserved learning in amnesic patients: Perspectives from research on direct priming. *Journal of Clinical and Experimental Neuropsychology,* 8, 727–743.

Schacter, D. L., Harbluk, J. L., & McLachlan, D. R. (1984). Retrieval without recollection: An experimental analysis of source amnesia. *Journal of Verbal Learning and Verbal Behavior,* 23, 593–611.

Scheinberg, S., & Holland, A. (1980). Conversational turn-taking in Wernicke's aphasia. In R. Brookshire (Ed.), *Clinical aphasiology conference proceedings* (pp. 106–110). Minneapolis: BRK.

Scherer, N.J., & Olswang, L. B. (1989). Using structured discourse as a language intervention technique with autistic children. *Journal of Speech and Hearing Disorders,* 54, 383–394.

Scherzer, E. (1992). Functional assessment: A clinical perspective. *Aphasiology,* 6, 101–104.

Schlanger, B. B., Schlanger, P., & Gerstman, L. J. (1976). The perception of emotionally toned sentences by right hemisphere-damaged and aphasic subjects. *Brain and Language,* 3, 396–403.

Schlanger, P. H., & Schlanger, B. B. (1970). Adapting role playing activities with aphasic patients. *Journal of Speech and Hearing Disorders,* 35, 229–235.

Schmitter-Edgecombe, M. E., Marks, W., Fahy, J. F., & Long, C. J. (1992). Effects of severe closed-head injury on three stages of information processing. *Journal of Clinical and Experimental Neuropsychology,* 14, 717–737.

Schnitzer, M. L. (1978). Toward a neurolinguistic theory of language. *Brain and Language,* 6, 342–361.

Schonle, P. W. (1988). Compound noun stimulation: An intensive treatment approach for severe aphasia. *Aphasiology,* 2, 401–404.

Schriefers, H., Meyer, A. S., & Levelt, W. J. M. (1990). Exploring the time course of lexical access in language production: Picture-word interference studies. *Journal of Memory and Language,* 29, 86–102.

Schuell, H. M. (1957). A short examination for aphasia. *Neurology,* 7, 625–634.

Schuell, H. M. (1966). A re-evaluation of the short examination for aphasia. *Journal of Speech and Hearing Disorders,* 31, 137–147.

Schuell, H. M. (1969). Aphasia in adults. In Human communication and its disorders—an overview. Bethesda, MD: U.S. Department of Health, Education, and Welfare.

Schuell, H. M. (1973). *Differential diagnosis of aphasia with the Minnesota test* (2nd ed., revised by Sefer, J. W.). Minneapolis: University of Minnesota Press.

Schuell, H. M., & Jenkins, J. J. (1959). The nature of language deficit in aphasia. *Psychological Review,* 66, 45–67.

Schuell, H. M., & Jenkins, J. J. (1961). Reduction of vocabulary in aphasia. *Brain,* 84, 243–261.

Schuell, H. M., Jenkins, J. J., & Jimenez-Pabon, E. (1964). *Aphasia in adults.* New York: Harper and Row.

Schuell, H. M., Jenkins, J. J., & Landis, L. (1961). Relationships between auditory comprehension and word frequency in aphasia. *Journal of Speech and Hearing Research,* 4, 30–36.

Schwartz-Cowley, R., & Stepanik, M. J. (1989). Communication disorders and treatment in the acute trauma center setting. *Topics in language disorders,* 9, 1–14.

Schwartz, M. F. (1987). Patterns of speech production deficit within and across aphasia syndromes: Application of a psycholinguistic model. In M. Coltheart, G. Sartori, & R. Job (Eds.). *The cognitive neuropsychology of language* (pp. 163–199). London: Erlbaum.

Schwartz, M. F., Linebarger, M. C., & Saffran, E. M. (1985). The status of the syntactic deficit theory of agrammatism. In M-L. Kean (Ed.), *Agrammatism* (pp. 83–124). Orlando, FL: Academic Press.

Schwartz, M. F., Linebarger, M. C., Saffran, E. M., & Pate, D. S. (1987). Syntactic transparency and sentence interpretation in aphasia. *Language and Cognitive Processes,* 2, 85–114.

Schwartz, M. F. Saffran, E. M., Fink, R., Myers, J., & Martin, N. (1994). Mapping therapy: A treatment programme for agrammatism. *Aphasiology,* 8, 19–54.

Schwartz, M. F., Saffran, E. M., & Marin, O. S. M. (1980). The word order problem in agrammatism. I. Comprehension. *Brain and Language,* 10, 249–262.

Schweich, M., & Bruyer, R. (1993). Heterogeneity in the cognitive manifestations of prosopagnosia:

The study of a group of single cases. *Cognitive Neuropsychology,* 10, 529–548.

Schweinberger, S. R. (1995). Personal name recognition and associative priming in patients with unilateral brain damage. *Brain and Cognition,* 29, 23–35.

Schweinberger, S. R., Buse, C., Freeman, Jr., R. B., Schonle, P. W., & Sommer, W. (1992). Memory search for faces and digits in patients with unilateral brain lesions. *Journal of Clinical and Experimental Neuropsychology,* 14, 839–856.

Scott, C., & Byng, S. (1989). Computer assisted remediation of homophone comprehension disorder in surface dyslexia. *Aphasiology,* 3, 301–320.

Searle, J. R. (1969). *Speech acts.* London: Cambridge University Press.

Searle, J. R. (Ed.). (1979). *Expression and meaning.* Cambridge, UK: Cambridge University Press.

Seidenberg, M. S. (1988). Cognitive neuropsychology and language: The state of the art. *Cognitive Neuropsychology,* 5, 403–426.

Seidenberg, M. S., Tanenhaus, M. K., Leiman, J. M., & Bienkowski, M. (1982). Automatic access of the meanings of ambiguous words in context: Some limitations of knowledge-based processing. *Cognitive Psychology,* 14, 489–537.

Sekuler, E. B., & Behrmann, M. (1996). Perceptual cues in pure alexia. *Cognitive Neuropsychology,* 13, 941–974.

Selinger, M., Walker, K. A., Prescott, T. E., & Davis, R. E. (1993). A possible explanation of problem-solving deficits based on resource allocation. *Aphasiology,* 7, 165–176.

Senelick, R. C., Rossi, P. W., & Dougherty, K. (1994). *Living with stroke: A guide for families.* Chicago: Contemporary Books.

Seron, X., & Deloche, G. (1981). Processing of locatives "in," "on," and "under" by aphasic patients: An analysis of the regression hypothesis. *Brain and Language,* 14, 70–80.

Seron, X., & Deloche, G. (Eds.). (1989). *Cognitive approaches in neuropsychological rehabilitation.* Hillsdale, NJ: Lawrence Erlbaum.

Seron, X., Deloche, G., Moulard, G., & Rouselle, M. (1980). A computer-based therapy for the treatment of aphasic subjects with writing disorders. *Journal of Speech and Hearing Disorders,* 45, 45–58.

Seron, X., & de Partz, M-P. (1993). The re-education of aphasics: Between theory and practice. In A. L. Holland & M. M. Forbes (Eds.), *Aphasia treatment: World perspectives* (pp. 131–144). San Diego, CA: Singular.

Seron, X., Van Der Kaa, M., Remitz, A., & Van Der Linden, M. (1979). Pantomime interpretation and aphasia. *Neuropsychologia,* 17, 661–668.

Seron, X., Van Der Kaa, M., Van Der Linden, M., Remitz, A., & Feyereisen, P. (1982). Decoding paralinguistic signals: Effect of semantic and prosodic cues on aphasics' comprehension. *Journal of Communication Disorders,* 15, 223–231.

Shallice, T. (1987). Impairments of semantic processing: Multiple dissociations. In M. Coltheart, G. Sartori, & R. Job (Eds.). *The cognitive neuropsychology of language* (pp. 111–127). London: Erlbaum.

Shallice, T. (1988a). *From neuropsychology to mental structure.* Cambridge, UK: Cambridge University Press.

Shallice, T. (1988b). Specialisation within the semantic system. *Cognitive Neuropsychology,* 5, 133–142.

Shallice, T. (1993). Multiple semantics: Whose confusions? *Cognitive Neuropsychology,* 10, 252–262.

Shallice, T., & Warrington, E. K. (1977). Auditory-verbal short-term memory impairment and spontaneous speech. *Brain and Language,* 4, 479–491.

Shankweiler, D., Crain, S., Gorrell, P., & Tuller, B. (1989). Reception of language in Broca's aphasia. *Language and Cognitive Processes,* 4, 1–34.

Shankweiler, D., & Harris, K. S. (1966). An experimental approach to the problem of articulation in aphasia. *Cortex,* 2, 277–292.

Shapiro, B. E., & Danly, M. (1985). The role of the right hemisphere in the control of speech prosody in propositional and affective contexts. *Brain and Language,* 25, 19–36.

Shapiro, B. E., Grossman, M., & Gardner, H. (1981). Selective musical processing deficits in brain damaged populations. *Neuropsychologia,* 19, 161–169.

Shapiro, L. P. (1997). Tutorial: An introduction to syntax. *Journal of Speech and Hearing Research,* 40, 254–272.

Shapiro, L. P., Gordon, B., Hack, N., & Killackey, J. (1993). Verb-argument structure processing in complex sentences in Broca's and Wernicke's aphasia. *Brain and Language,* 45, 423–447.

Shapiro, L. P., & Levine, B. A. (1990). Verb processing during sentence comprehension in aphasia. *Brain and Language,* 38, 21–47.

Shattuck-Hufnagel, S. (1979). Speech errors as evidence for a serial ordering mechanism in speech production. In W. E. Cooper & E. C. T. Walker

(Eds.), *Sentence processing: Psycholinguistic studies presented to Merrill Garrett* (pp. 295–342). Hillsdale, NJ: Erlbaum.

Sheehan, V. M. (1946). Rehabilitation of aphasics in an army hospital. *Journal of Speech and Hearing Disorders,* 11, 149–157.

Shelton, J. R., Martin, R. C., & Yaffee, L. S. (1992). Investigating a verbal short-term memory deficit and its consequences for language processing. In D. I. Margolin (Ed.), *Cognitive neuropsychology in clinical practice* (pp. 131–167). New York: Oxford University Press.

Shelton, J. R., Weinrich, M., McCall, D., & Cox, D. M. (1996). Differentiating globally aphasic patients: Data from in-depth language assessments and production training using C-VIC. *Aphasiology,* 10, 319–342.

Shepard, R. N., & Metzler, J. (1971). Mental rotation of three-dimensional objects. *Science,* 171, 701–703.

Sherer, M., Parsons, O. A., Nixon, S. J., & Adams, R. L. (1991). Clinical validity of the Speech-Sounds Perception Test and the Seashore Rhythm Test. *Journal of Clinical and Experimental Neuropsychology,* 13, 741–751.

Sheridan, J., & Humphreys, G. W. (1993). A verbal-semantic category-specific recognition impairment. *Cognitive Neuropsychology,* 10, 143–184.

Sherman, J. C., & Schweickert, J. (1989). Syntactic and semantic contributions to sentence comprehension in agrammatism. *Brain and Language,* 37, 419–439.

Shewan, C. M. (1976). Error patterns in auditory comprehension of adult aphasics. *Cortex,* 12, 325–336.

Shewan, C. M. (1979). *Auditory Comprehension Test for Sentences.* Chicago: Biolinguistics Clinical Institutes.

Shewan, C. M. (1982). To hear is not to understand: Auditory processing deficits and factors influencing performance in aphasic individuals. In N.J. Lass (Ed.), *Speech and language: Advances in basic research and practice* (Vol. 7) (pp. 1–70). New York: Academic Press.

Shewan, C. M. (1988). The Shewan Spontaneous Language Analysis (SSLA) system for aphasic adults: Description, reliability, and validity. *Journal of Communication Disorders,* 21, 103–138.

Shewan, C. M., & Bandur, D. L. (1986). *Treatment of aphasia: A language-oriented approach.* San Diego: Singular.

Shewan, C. M., & Canter, G. J. (1971). Effects of Vocabulary, syntax, and sentence legnth on auditory comprehension in aphasic patients. *Cortex,* 7, 209–226.

Shewan, C. M. & Kertesz, A. (1980). Reliability and validity charactoristics of the Western Aphasia Battery (WAB). *Journal of Speech and Hearing Disorders,* 45, 308–324.

Shewan, C. M., & Kertesz, A. (1984). Effects of speech and language treatment on recovery from aphasia. *Brain and Language,* 23, 272–299.

Shimberg, E. F. (1990). *Strokes: What families should know.* New York: Ballantine.

Shum, D. H. K., McFarland, K. A., Bain, J. D., & Humphreys, M. S. (1990). Effects of closed-head injury on attentional processes: An information-processing stage analysis. *Journal of Clinical and Experimental Neuropsychology,* 12, 247–264.

Sidtis, J. J., & Volpe, B. T. (1988). Selective loss of complex-pitch or speech discrimination after unilateral lesion. *Brain and Language,* 34, 235–245.

Sies, L. F. (Eds.). (1974). *Aphasia theory and therapy: Selected lectures and papers of Hildred Schuell.* Baltimore: University Park Press.

Silberman, E. K., & Weingartner, H. (1986). Hemispheric lateralization of functions related to emotion. *Brain and Cognition,* 5, 322–354.

Silverman, F. H. (1989). *Communication for the speechless* (Second Edition). Englewood Cliffs, NJ: Prentice-Hall.

Simmons, N. N. (1989). A trip down Easy Street. In T. E. Prescott (Ed). *Clinical aphasiology* (Vol. 18) (pp. 19–30). Austin, TX: Pro-Ed.

Simmons-Mackie, N. N., & Damico, J. S. (1996). The contribution of discourse markers to communicative competence in aphasia. *American Journal of Speech-Language Pathology,* 5, 37–43.

Simmons-Mackie, N. N., & Damico, J. S. (1997). Reformulating the definition of compensatory strategies in aphasia. *Aphasiology,* 11, 761–781.

Simpson, G. B., & Burgess, C. (1985). Activation and selection processes in the recognition of ambiguous words. *Journal of Experimental Psychology: Human Perception and Performance,* 11, 28–39.

Skelly, M. (1975). Aphasic patients talk back. *American Journal of Nursing,* 75, 1140–1142.

Skelly, M. (1979). *Amer-Ind gestural code based on universal American Indian hand talk.* New York: Elsevier.

Skilbeck, C. E., Wade, D. T., Hewer, R. L., & Wood, V. A. (1983). Recovery after stroke. *Journal of Neurology, Neurosurgery, and Psychiatry,* 46, 5–8.

Smith, A. (1971). Objective indices of severity of chronic aphasia in stroke patients. *Journal of Speech and Hearing Disorders,* 36, 167–207.

Smith, F. (1982). *Understanding reading: A psycholinguistic analysis of reading and learning to read* (Third Edition). New York: Holt, Rinehart and Winston.

Smith, L. (1987). Nonverbal competency in aphasic stroke patients' conversation. *Aphasiology,* 1, 127–139.

Smith, S. D., & Bates, E. (1987). Accessibility of case and gender contrasts for agent-object assignment in Broca's aphasics and fluent anomics. *Brain and Language,* 30, 8–32.

Smith, S. D., & Mimica, I. (1984). Agrammatism in a case-inflected language: Comprehension of agent-object relations. *Brain and Language,* 21, 274–290.

Snow, P., Douglas, J., & Ponsford, J. (1995). Discourse assessment following traumatic brain injury: A pilot study examining some demographic and methodological issues. *Aphasiology,* 9, 365–380.

Snow, P., Douglas, J., & Ponsford, J. (1997). Procedural discourse following traumatic brain injury. *Aphasiology,* 11, 947–968.

Snowden, J. S., Griffiths, H. L., & Neary, D. (1996). Semantic-episodic memory interactions in semantic dementia: Implications for retrograde memory function. *Cognitive Neuropsychology,* 13, 1101–1138.

Solin, D. (1989). The systematic misrepresentation of bilingual-crossed aphasia data and its consequences. *Brain and Language,* 36, 92–116.

Solso, R. L. (1988). *Cognitive psychology* (2nd ed.). Boston: Allyn & Bacon.

Solso, R. L. (1991). *Cognitive psychology* (3rd ed.). Boston: Allyn & Bacon.

Sparks, R. W. (1978). Parastandardized examination guidelines for adult aphasia. *British Journal of Disorders of Communication,* 13, 135–146.

Sparks, R. W., Helm, N. A., & Albert, M. L. (1974). Aphasia rehabilitation resulting from melodic intonation therapy. *Cortex,* 10, 303–316.

Sparks, R. W., & Holland, A. L. (1976). Method: Melodic intonation therapy for aphasia. *Journal of Speech and Hearing Disorders,* 41, 287–297.

Spellacy, F. J., & Spreen, O. (1969). A short form of the Token Test. *Cortex,* 5, 390–397.

Sperber, D., & Wilson, D. (1986). *Relevance: Communication and cognition.* Cambridge, MA: Harvard University Press.

Spinnler, H., & Vignolo, L. (1966). Impaired recognition of meaningful sounds in aphasia. *Cortex,* 2, 337–348.

Spreen, O., & Benton, A. L. (1977). *Neurosensory center comprehensive examination for aphasia* (NCCEA) (Revised). Victoria, British Columbia: Neuropsychology Laboratory, University of Victoria.

Springer, L., Glindemann, R., Huber, W., & Willmes K. (1991). How efficacious is PACE-therapy when "Language Systematic Training" is incorporated? *Aphasiology,* 5, 391–399.

Springer, S. P. & Deutsch, G. (1998). *Left brain, right brain* (5th ed.). New York: W. H. Freeman.

Squire, L. R. (1987). *Memory and brain.* New York: Oxford University Press.

Stambrook, M., Moore, A. D., Peters, L. C., Zubek, E., McBeath, S., & Friesen, I. C. (1991). Head injury and spinal cord injury: Differential effects on psychosocial functioning. *Journal of Clinical and Experimental Neuropsychology,* 13, 521–530.

Stanton, K., Yorkston, K. M., Kenyon, V. T., & Beukelman, D. R. (1981). Language utilization in teaching reading to left neglect patients. In R. H. Brookshire (Ed.), *Clinical aphasiology conference proceedings* (pp. 262–271). Minneapolis: BRK.

Starkstein, S. E., & Robinson, R. G. (1988). Aphasia and depression. *Aphasiology,* 2, 1–20.

State University of New York at Buffalo (1990). *Guide for use of the uniform data set for medical rehabilitation* . Buffalo, NY: Research Foundation.

Stein, N. L., & Glenn, C. G. (1979). An analysis of story comprehension in elementary school children. In R. O. Freedle (Ed.), *New directions in discourse processes* (pp. 53–120). Norwood, NJ: Ablex.

Stemmer, B., Giroux, F., & Joanette, Y. (1994). Production and evaluation of requests by right hemisphere brain-damaged individuals. *Brain and Language,* 47, 1–31.

Stern, B. H. (1995). The neuropsychologist in a mild traumatic brain injury case: How to conduct the direct examination. *Trial,* June, 66–73.

Sternberg, S. (1975). Memory scanning: New findings and current controversies. In D. Deutsch & J. A. Deutsch (Eds.), *Short-term memory.* New York: Academic Press.

Stevens, R. J., Slavin, R. E., & Farnish, A. M. (1991). The effects of cooperative learning and direct instruction in reading comprehension strategies on main idea identification. *Journal of Educational Psychology,* 83, 8–16.

Stimley, M. A., & Noll, J. D. (1991). The effects of semantic and phonemic prestimulation cues on picture naming in aphasia. *Brain and Language,* 41, 496–509.

Stimley, M. A., & Noll, J. D. (1994). The effects of communication partner familiarity on the verbal abilities of aphasic adults. *Aphasiology,* 8, 173–180.

Strand, E. A. (1995). Ethical issues related to progressive disease. *Special Interest Division 2 Newsletter,* 5(3), 3–8.

Strohner, H., Cohen, R., Kelter, S., & Woll, G. (1978). "Semantic" and "acoustic" errors of aphasic and schizophrenic patients in a sound-picture matching task. *Cortex,* 14, 391–403.

Stubbs, M. (1983). *Discourse analysis: The sociolinguistic analysis of natural language.* Chicago, IL: University of Chicago Press.

Stuss, D. T., & Levine, B. (1996). The dementias: Nosological and clinical factors related to diagnosis. *Brain and Cognition,* 31, 99–113.

Sullivan, M. P., & Brookshire, R. H. (1989). Can generalization differentiate whether learning or facilitation of a process occurred? In T. E. Prescott (Ed.), *Clinical aphasiology* (Vol. 18) (pp. 247–256). Boston: College-Hill/Little, Brown.

Sullivan, M. P., Fisher, B., & Marshall, R. C. (1986). Treating the repetition deficit in conduction aphasia. In R. H. Brookshire (Ed.), *Clinical aphasiology* (Vol. 16) (pp. 172–180). Minneapolis: BRK.

Sundet, K. (1986). Sex differences in cognitive impairment following unilateral brain damage. *Journal of Clinical and Experimental Neuropsychology,* 8, 51–61.

Sunderland, A., Harris, J. E., & Baddeley, A. D. (1983). Do laboratory tests predict everyday memory? A neuropsychological study. *Journal of Verbal Learning and Verbal Behavior,* 22, 341–357.

Swindell, C. S., Boller, F., & Holland, A. L. (1988). Expressive language characteristics in probable Alzheimer's disease. *Aphasiology,* 2, 411–416.

Swindell, C. S., Holland, A. L., & Fromm, D. (1984). Classification of aphasia: WAB type versus clinical impression. In R. H. Brookshire (Ed.), *Clinical aphasiology conference proceedings* (pp. 48–54). Minneapolis: BRK.

Swindell, C. S., Holland, A. L., Fromm, D., & Greenhouse, J. B. (1988). Characteristics of recovery of drawing ability in left and right brain-damaged subjects. *Brain and Cognition,* 7, 16–30.

Swinney, D. A. (1979). Lexical access during sentence comprehension: (Re)consideration of context effects. *Journal of Verbal Learning and Verbal Behavior,* 20, 645–660.

Swinney, D. A., & Zurif, E. (1995). Syntactic processing in aphasia. *Brain and Language,* 50, 225–239.

Swinney, D. A., Zurif, E., & Cutler, A. (1980). Effects of sentential stress and word class upon comprehension in Broca's aphasics. *Brain and Language,* 10, 132–144.

Swinney, D. A., Zurif, E., & Nicol, J. (1989). The effects of focal brain damage on sentence processing: An examination of the neurological organization of a mental module. *Journal of Cognitive Neuroscience,* 1, 25–37.

Swisher, L., & Hirsh, I. J. (1972). Brain damage and the ordering of two temporally successive stimuli. *Neuropsychologia,* 10, 137–152.

Swisher, L. P., & Sarno, M. T. (1969). Token Test scores of three matched patient groups: Left brain-damaged with aphasia; right brain-damaged without aphasia, non-brain damaged. *Cortex,* 5, 264–273.

Taft, M. (1990). Lexical processing of functionally constrained words. *Journal of Memory and Language,* 29, 245–257.

Tainturier, M-J. & Caramazza, A. (1996). The status of double letters in graphemic representations. *Journal of Memory and Language,* 35, 53–73.

Tanner, D. C., & Gerstenberger, D. L. (1988). The grief response in neuropathologies of speech and language. *Aphasiology,* 2, 79–84.

Tanridag, O., Kirshner, H. S., & Casey, P. F. (1987). Memory functions in aphasic and non-aphasic stroke patients. *Aphasiology,* 1, 201–214.

Taylor, M. L. (1965). A measurement of functional communication in aphasia. *Archives of Physical Medicine and Rehabilitation,* 46, 101–107.

Taylor, M. L., & Marks, M. M. (1959). *Aphasia rehabilitation manual and therapy kit.* New York: McGraw-Hill.

Terman, L. M., & Merrill, M. A. (1937). *Measureing intelligence.* Boston: Houghton Mifflin.

Tesak, J., & Niemi, J. (1997). Telegraphese and agrammatism: A cross-linguistic study. *Aphasiology,* 11, 145–155.

Thompson, C. K. (1989). Generalization research in aphasia: A review of the literature. In T. E. Prescott

(Ed). *Clinical aphasiology* (Vol. 18) (pp. 195–222). Austin, TX: Pro-Ed.

Thompson, C. K., and Byrne, M. E. (1984). Across setting generalization of social conventions in aphasia: An experimental analysis of "loose training." In R. H. Brookshire (ed.), *Clinical aphasiology conference proceedings* (pp. 132–144). Minneapolis: BRK.

Thompson, C. K., & Kearns, K. P. (1981). An experimental analysis of acquisition, generalization, and maintenance of naming behavior in a patient with anomia. In R. H. Brookshire (Ed.), *Clinical aphasiology conference proceedings* (pp. 35–45. Minneapolis: BRK.

Thompson, C. K., Lange, K. L., Schneider, S. L., & Shapiro, L. P. (1997). Agrammatic and non-brain-damaged subjects' verb and verb argument structure production. *Aphasiology,* 11, 473–490.

Thompson, C. K., & McReynolds, L. V. (1986). Wh-interrogative production in agrammatic aphasia: An experimental analysis of auditory-visual stimulation and direct-production treatment. *Journal of Speech and Hearing Research,* 29, 193–206.

Thompson, C. K., & Shapiro, L. P. (1994). A linguistic-specific approach to treatment of sentence production deficits in aphasia. In M. L. Lemme (Ed.), *Clinical aphasiology* (Vol. 22) (pp. 307–324). Austin, Tx: Pro-Ed.

Thompson, C. K., Shapiro, L. P., Ballard, K. J., Jacobs, B. J., Schneider, S. L., & Tait, M. E. (1997). Training and generalized production of wh- and NP-movement structures in agrammatic aphasia. *Journal of Speech, Language, and Hearing Research,* 40, 228–244.

Thompson, C. K., Shapiro, L. P., Tait, M. E., Jacobs, B. J., & Schneider, S. L. (1996). Training Wh-question production in agrammatic aphasia: Analysis of argument and adjunct movement. *Brain and Language,* 52, 175–228.

Thompson, C. K., Shapiro, L. P., Tait, M. E., Jacobs, B. J., Schneider, S. L., & Ballard, K. J. (1995). A system for the linguistic analysis of agrammatic language production (abstract). *Brain and Language,* 51, 124–129.

Thompson, J., & Enderby, P. (1979). Is all of your Schuell really necessary? *British Journal of Disorders of Communication,* 14, 195–201.

Thomson, A. M., Taylor, R., Fraser, D., & Whittle, I. R. (1997). Stereotactic biopsy of nonpolar tumors in the dominant hemisphere: a prospective study of effects on language functions. *Journal of Neurosurgery,* 86, 923–926.

Thorndyke, P. W. (1977). Cognitive structures in comprehension and memory of narrative discourse. *Cognitive Psychology,* 9, 77–110.

Togher, L., Hand, L., & Code, C. (1997). Measuring service encounters with the traumatic brain injury population. *Aphasiology,* 11, 491–504.

Tompkins, C. A. (1990). Knowledge and strategies for processing lexical metaphor after right or left hemisphere brain damage. *Journal of Speech and Hearing Research,* 33, 307–316.

Tompkins, C. A. (1995). *Right hemisphere communication disorders: Theory and management.* San Diego, CA: Singular.

Tompkins, C. A., Bloise, C. G. R., Timko, M. L., & Baumgaertner, A. (1994). Working memory and inference revision in brain-damaged and normally aging adults. *Journal of Speech and Hearing Research,* 37, 896–912.

Tompkins, C. A., Boada, R., & McGarry, K. (1992). The access and processing of familiar idioms by brain-damaged and normally aging adults. *Journal of Speech and Hearing Research,* 35, 626–637.

Tompkins, C. A., & Flowers, C. R. (1987). Contextual mood priming following left and right hemisphere damage. *Brain and Cognition,* 6, 361–376.

Tompkins, C. A., Holland, A. L., Ratcliff, G., Costello, A., Leahy, L. F., & Cowell, V. (1990). Predicting cognitive recovery from closed head-injury in children and adolescents. *Brain and Cognition,* 13, 86–97.

Tompkins, C. A., Jackson, S. T., & Schulz, R. (1990). On prognostic research in adult neurologic disorders. *Journal of Speech and Hearing Research,* 33, 398–401.

Tonkovich, J. D., & Loverso, F. (1982). A training matrix approach for gestural acquisition by the agrammatic patient. In R. H. Brookshire (Ed.), *Clinical aphasiology conference proceedings* (pp. 283–288). Minneapolis: BRK.

Toolan, M. J. (1988). *Narrative: A critical linguistic introduction.* London: Routledge.

Trahan, D. E., Larrabee, G. J., & Quintana, J. W. (1990). Visual recognition memory in normal adults and patients with unilateral vascular lesions. *Journal of Clinical and Experimental Neuropsychology,* 12, 857–872.

Trexler, L. E., & Zappala, G. (1988). Neuropathological determinants of acquired attention disorders in traumatic brain injury. *Brain and Cognition,* 8, 291–302.

Trueblood, W., & Schmidt, M. (1993). Malingering and other validity considerations in the neuropsychological evaluation of mild head injury. *Journal of Clinical and Experimental Neuropsychology,* 15, 578–590.

Trupe, E. H. (1984). Reliability of rating spontaneous speech in the Western Aphasia Battery: Implications for classification. In R. H. Brookshire (Ed.), *Clinical aphasiology conference proceedings* (pp. 55–69). Minneapolis: BRK.

Trupe, E. H., & Hillis, A. (1985). Paucity vs. verbosity: Another analysis of right hemisphere communication deficits. In R. H. Brookshire (Ed.) *Clinical Aphasiology* (Vol. 15) (pp. 83–96). Minneapolis: BRK.

Tseng, C-H., McNeil, M. R., & Milenkovic, P. (1993). An investigation of attention allocation deficits in aphasia. *Brain and Language,* 45, 276–296.

Tucker, D. M., Watson, R. T., & Heilman, K. M. (1977). Discrimination and evocation of affectively intoned speech in patients with right parietal disease. *Neurology,* 27, 947–950.

Tulving, E. (1972). Episodic and semantic memory. In E. Tulving & W. Donaldson (Eds.), *Organization of memory* (pp. 382–403). New York: Academic Press.

Tulving, E., Schacter, D. L., McLachlan, D. R., & Moscovitch, M. (1988). Priming of semantic autobiographical knowledge: A case study of retrograde amnesia. *Brain and Cognition,* 8, 3–20.

Tyler, L. K. (1985). Real-time comprehension processes in agrammatism: A case study. *Brain and Language,* 26, 259–275.

Tyler, L. K. (1987). Spoken language comprehension in aphasia: A real-time processing perspective. In M. Coltheart, G. Sartori, & R. Job (Eds.), *The cognitive neuropsychology of language* (pp. 145–162). London: Erlbaum.

Tyler, L. K. (1988). Spoken language comprehension in a fluent aphasic patient. *Cognitive Neuropsychology,* 5, 375–400.

Tyler, L. K. (1989). Syntactic deficits and the construction of local phrases in spoken language comprehension. *Cognitive Neuropsychology,* 6, 333–355.

Tyler, L. K., & Cobb, H. (1987). Processing bound grammatical morphemes in context: The case of an aphasic patient. *Language and Cognitive Processes,* 2, 245–262.

Tyler, L. K., & Moss, H. E. (1997). Imageability and category-specificity. *Cognitive Neuropsychology,* 14, 293–318.

Tyler, L. K., Ostrin, R. K., Cooke, M., & Moss, E. (1995). Automatic access of lexical information in Broca's aphasics: Against the automaticity hypothesis. *Brain and Language,* 48, 131–162.

Udell, R., Sullivan, R. A., & Schlanger, P. H. (1980). Legal competency of aphasic patients: Role of speech-language pathologists. *Archives of Physical Medicine and Rehabilitation,* 61, 374–375.

Ulatowska, H. K., Allard, L., Reyes, B. A., Ford, J., & Chapman, S. (1992). Conversational discourse in aphasia. *Aphasiology,* 6, 325–330.

Ulatowska, H. K., Cannito, M. P., Hayashi, M. M., & Fleming, S. G. (1985). Language abilities in the elderly. In H. K. Ulatowska (Ed.), *The aging brain: Communication in the elderly* (pp. 125–140). San Diego: Singular.

Ulatowska, H. K., Doyel, A. W., Stern, R. F., & Haynes, S. M. (1983). Production of procedural discourse in aphasia. *Brain and Language,* 18, 315–341.

Ulatowska, H. K., Freedman-Stern, R., Doyel, A. W., Macaluso-Haynes, S., & North, A. J. (1983). Production of narrative discourse in aphasia. *Brain and Language,* 19, 317–334.

Ulatowska, H. K., Macaluso-Haynes, S., & Mendel-Richardson, S. (1976). The assessment of communicative competence in aphasia. In R. H. Brookshire (Ed.), *Clinical aphasiology* conference proceedings (pp. 22–31). Minneapolis: BRK.

Uryase, D., Duffy, R. J., & Liles, B. Z. (1990). Analysis and description of narrative discourse in right-hemisphere-damaged adults: A comparison to neurologically normal and left-hemisphere-damaged aphasic adults. In T. E. Prescott (Ed.), *Clinical aphasiology* (Vol. 19). Austin, TX: Pro-Ed.

Uzell, B. P., Dolinskas, C. A., Wiser, R. F., & Langfitt, T. W. (1987). Influence of lesions detected by computed tomography on outcome and neuropsychological recovery after severe head injury. *Neurosurgery,* 20, 396–402.

Vakil, E., Blachstein, H., & Hoofien, D. (1991). Automatic temporal order judgment: The effect of intentionality of retrieval on closed-head-injured patients. *Journal of Clinical and Experimental Neuropsychology,* 13, 291–298.

Valdois, S., Joanette, Y., & Nespoulous, J-L. (1989). Intrinsic organization of sequences of phonemic approximations: A preliminary study. *Aphasiology,* 3, 55–74.

Vallar, G., & Baddeley, A. D. (1984). Fractionation of working memory: Neuropsychological evidence for a phonological short-term store. *Journal of Verbal Learning and Verbal Behavior,* 23, 151–161.

Vallar, G., & Baddeley, A. D. (1987). Phonological short-term store and sentence processing. *Cognitive Neuropsychology,* 4, 417–438.

Vallar, G., Perani, D., Cappa, S. F., Messa, C., Lenzi, G. L., & Fazio, F. (1988). Recovery from aphasia and neglect after subcortical stroke: Neuropsychological and cerebral perfusion study. *Journal of Neurology, Neurosurgery, and Psychiatry,* 51, 1269–1276.

Van Allen, M. W., Benton, A. L., & Gordon, M. C. (1966). Temporal discrimination in brain-damaged patients. *Neuropsychologia,* 4, 159–167.

Van Demark, A. A., Lemmer, E. C., & Drake, M. L. (1982). Measurement of reading comprehension in aphasia with the RCBA. *Journal of Speech and Hearing Disorders,* 47, 288–291.

Van der Linden, M., Coyette, F., & Seron, X. (1992). Selective impairment of the "central executive" component of working memory: A single case study. *Cognitive Neuropsychology,* 9, 301–326.

Van der Linden, M., Brédart, S., Depoorter, N., & Coyette, F. (1996). Semantic memory and amnesia: A case study. *Cognitive Neuropsychology,* 13, 391–414.

van Dijk, T. A., & Kintsch, W. (1983). *Strategies of discourse comprehension.* New York: Academic Press.

Van Eeckhout, P. (1993). Aphasia and artistic creation. In D. Lafond, Y. Joanette, J. Ponzio, R. Degiovani, & M. T. Sarno (Eds.), *Living with aphasia: Psychosocial issues* (pp. 87–102). San Diego, CA: Singular.

Van Lancker, D. R., & Kempler, D. (1987). Comprehension of familiar phrases by left- but not by right-hemisphere damaged patients. *Brain and Language,* 32, 265–277.

Van Lancker, D. R., Kreiman, J., & Cummings, J. (1989). Voice perception deficits: Neuroanatomical correlates of phonagnosia. *Journal of Clinical and Experimental Neuropsychology,* 11, 665–674.

Varney, N. R. (1980). Sound recognition in relation to aural language comprehension in aphasia. *Journal of Neurology, Neurosurgery, and Psychiatry,* 43, 71–75.

Varney, N. R. (1982). Pantomime recognition defect in aphasia: Implications for the concept of asymbolia. *Brain and Language,* 15, 32–39.

Varney, N. R. (1984). Phonemic imperception in aphasia. *Brain and Language,* 21, 85–94.

Varney, N. R., & Benton, A. L. (1978). *Pantomime Recognition Test.* Iowa City: Benton Laboratory of Neuropsychology.

Varney, N. R., & Benton, A. L. (1982). Qualitative aspects of pantomime recognition defect in aphasia. *Brain and Cognition,* 1, 132–139.

Verfaellie, M., Bowers, D., & Heilman, K. M. (1988). Hemispheric asymmetries in mediating inattention, but not selective attention. *Neuropsychologia,* 26, 521–532.

Vignolo, L. A. (1964). Evolution of aphasia and language rehabilitation: A retrospective exploratory study. *Cortex,* 1, 344–367.

Vignolo, L. A., Boccardi, E., & Caverni, L. (1986). Unexpected CT-scan findings in global aphasia. *Cortex,* 22, 55–69.

Visch-Brink, E. G., van Harskamp, F., Van Amerongen, N. M., Wielaert, S. M., & van de Sandt-Koenderman, M. E. (1993). *A multidisciplinary approach to aphasia therapy.* In A. L. Holland & M. M. Forbes (Eds.), Aphasia treatment: World perspectives (pp. 227–262). San Diego, CA: Singular.

Vogel, D., & Costello, R. M. (1986). Bilingual aphasic adults: Measures of word retrieval. In R. H. Brookshire (Ed.). *Clinical aphasiology* (Vol. 16) (pp. 80–86). Minneapolis: BRK.

Wade, D. T., Hewer, R. L., David, R. M., & Enderby, P. M. (1986). Aphasia after stroke: Natural history and associated deficits. *Journal of Neurology, Neurosurgery, and Psychiatry,* 49, 11–16.

Wahrborg, P. (1989). Aphasia and family therapy. *Aphasiology,* 3, 479–482.

Wahrborg, P. (1991). *Assessment and management of emotional reactions to brain damage and aphasia.* San Diego: Singular.

Wahrborg, P., & Borenstein, P. (1990). The aphasic person and his/her family: What about the future? *Aphasiology,* 4, 371–380.

Walker-Batson, D., Barton, M. M., Wendt, J. S., & Reynolds, S. (1987). Symbolic and affective non-verbal deficits in left- and right-hemisphere injured adults. *Aphasiology,* 1, 257–262.

Wallace, G. L., & Canter, G. J. (1985). Effects of personally relevant language materials on the performance of severely aphasic individuals. *Journal of Speech and Hearing Disorders,* 50, 385–390.

Wallander, J. L., Conger, A. J., & Conger, J. C. (1985). Development and evaluation of a behaviorally referenced rating system for heterosocial skills. *Behavioral Assessment,* 7, 137–153.

Wallesch, C-W., Bak, T., & Schulte-Mönting, J. (1992). Acute aphasia—patterns and prognosis. *Aphasiology,* 6, 373–385.

Wallesch, C-W., Henriksen, L., Kornhuber, H-H., & Paulson, O. B. (1985). Observations on regional cerebral blood flow in cortical and subcortical structures during language production in normal man. *Brain and Language,* 25, 224–233.

Wallesch, C-W., Johannsen-Horbach, H., Bartels, C., & Herrmann, M. (1997). Mechanisms of and misconceptions about subcortical aphasia. *Brain and Language,* 58, 403–409.

Wallesch, C-W., Kornhuber, H. H., Brunner, R. J., Kunz, T., Hollerbach, B., & Suger, G. (1983). Lesions of the basal ganglia, thalamus, and deep white matter: Differential effects on language functions. *Brain and Language,* 20, 286–304.

Wang, L., & Goodglass, H. (1992). Pantomime, praxis, and aphasia. *Brain and Language,* 42, 402–418.

Wapner, W., Hamby, S., & Gardner, H. (1981). The role of the right hemisphere in the apprehension of complex linguistic materials. *Brain and Language,* 14, 15–33.

Warrington, E. K. (1975). The selective impairment of semantic memory. *Quarterly Journal of Experimental Psychology,* 27, 635–657.

Warrington, E. K. (1991). Right neglect dyslexia: A single case study. *Cognitive Neuropsychology,* 8, 193–212.

Warrington, E. K., & James, M. (1986). Visual object recognition in patients with right hemisphere lesions: Axes or features. *Perception,* 15, 355–366.

Warrington, E. K., & McCarthy, R. (1983). Category-specific access dysphasia. *Brain,* 106, 859–878.

Warrington, E. K., & McCarthy, R. (1987). Categories of knowledge: Further fractionations and an attempted integration. *Brain,* 110, 1273–1296.

Warrington, E. K., & Rudge, P. (1995). A comment on apperceptive agnosia. *Brain and Cognition,* 28, 173–177.

Warrington, E. K., & Sanders, H. I. (1971). The fate of old memories. *Quarterly Journal of Experimental Psychology,* 23, 432–444.

Warrington, E. K., & Shallice, T. (1969). The selective impairment of auditory verbal short-term memory. *Brain,* 92, 885–896.

Warrington, E. K., & Shallice, T. (1984). Category-specific semantic impairments. *Brain,* 107, 829–854.

Warrington, E. K., & Taylor, A. M. (1978). Two categorical stages of object recognition. *Perception,* 7, 695–705.

Wasserstein, J., Zappulla, R., Rosen, J., Gerstman, L., & Rock, D. (1987). In search of closure: Subjective contour illusions, gestalt completion tests, and implications. *Brain and Cognition,* 6, 1–14.

Waters, G. S., & Caplan, D. (1996). The capacity theory of sentence comprehension: Critique of Just and Carpenter (1992). *Psychological Review,* 103, 761–772.

Waters, G. S., Caplan, D., & Hildebrandt, N. (1991). On the structure of verbal short-term memory and its functional role in sentence comprehension: Evidence from neuropsychology. *Cognitive Neuropsychology,* 8, 81–126.

Watt, S., Jokel, R., & Behrmann, M. (1997). Surface dyslexia in nonfluent progressive aphasia. *Brain and Language,* 56, 211–233.

Webb, D-M. (1991). Increasing carryover and independent use of compensatory strategies in brain injured patients. *Cognitive Rehabilitation,* 9(3), 28–35.

Webb, W. G., & Love, R. J. (1983). Reading problems in chronic aphasia. *Journal of Speech and Hearing Disorders,* 48, 164–171.

Webster, E. J., & Newhoff, M. (1981). Intervention with families of communicatively impaired adults. In D. S. Beasley & G. A. Davis (Eds.), *Aging: Communication processes and disorders* (pp. 229–240). New York: Grune & Stratton.

Webster, J. S., Cottam, G., Gouvier, W. D., Blanton, P., Beissel, G. F., & Wofford, J. (1988). Wheelchair obstable course performance in right cerebral vascular accident victims. *Journal of Clinical and Experimental Neuropsychology,* 11, 295–310.

Webster, J. S., Godlewski, M. C., Hanley, G. L., & Sowa, M. V. (1992). A scoring method for logical memory that is sensitive to right-hemisphere dysfunction. *Journal of Clinical and Experimental Neuropsychology,* 14, 222–238.

Wechsler, D. (1945). A standardized memory scale for clinical use. *Journal of Psychology,* 19, 87–95.

Wechsler, D. (1955). *Wechsler Adult Intelligence Scale.* New York: Psychological Corporation.

Wechsler, D. (1981). *Wechsler Adult Intelligence Scale—Revised.* New York: Psychological Corporation.

Weddell, R. A. (1989) Recognition memory for emotional facial expressions in patients with focal cerebral lesions. *Brain and Cognition,* 11, 1–17.

Weekes, B., & Coltheart, M. (1996). Surface dyslexia and surface dysgraphia: Treatment studies and their theoretical implications. *Cognitive Neuropsychology,* 13, 277–315.

Weidner, W. E., & Lasky, E. Z. (1976). The interaction of rate and complexity of stimulus on the performance of adult aphasic subjects. *Brain and Language,* 3, 34–40.

Weinrich, M., McCall, D., Weber, C., Thomas, K., & Thornburg, L. (1995). Training on an iconic communication system for severe aphasia can improve natural language production. *Aphasiology,* 9, 343–364.

Weinrich, M., Shelton., J. R., Cox, D. M., & McCall, D. (1997). Remediating production of tense morphology improves verb retrieval in chronic aphasia. *Brain and Language,* 58, 23–45.

Weintraub, S., Mesulam, M., & Kramer, L. (1981). Disturbances in prosody: A right-hemisphere contribution to language. *Archives of Neurology,* 38, 742–744.

Weisenburg, T. H.,& McBride, K. E. (1935). *Aphasia.* New York: Commonwealth Fund.

Weiss, H. D. (1982). Neoplasms. In M. A. Samuels (Ed.), *Manual of Neurologic Therapeutics with Essentials of Diagnosiss* (Second Edition). Boston: Little, Brown.

Wepman, J. M. (1951). *Recovery from aphasia.* New York: Ronald Press.

Wepman, J. M. (1968). Aphasia therapy: Some "relative" comments and some purely personal prejudices. In J. W. Black & E. G. Jancosek (Eds.), *Proceedings of the conference on language retraining for aphasics* (pp. 95–107). Columbus, OH: Ohio State University.

Wepman, J. M. (1972). Aphasia therapy: A new look. *Journal of Speech and Hearing Disorders,* 37, 203–214.

Wepman, J. M., & Jones, L. V. (1961). *Studies in aphasia: An approach to testing.* Chicago: Education-Industry Service.

Wepman, J. M., Jones, L. V., Bock, R. D., & Van Pelt, D. (1960). Studies in aphasia: Background and theoretical formulations. *Journal of Speech and Hearing Disorders,* 25, 323–332.

Wepman, J. M., & Van Pelt, D. (1955). A theory of cerebral language disorders based on therapy. *Folia Phoniatrica,* 7, 223–235.

Wernicke, C. (1977). The aphasia symptom complex: A psychological study on an anatomic basis. In G. H. Eggert (Trans.), *Wernicke's works on aphasia: A sourcebook and review.* The Hague, Netherlands: Mouton.

Wertz, R. T. (1983). Classifying the aphasias: Commodious or chimerical? In R. H. Brookshire (Ed.), *Clinical aphasiology conference proceedings* (pp. 296–303). Minneapolis: BRK.

Wertz, R. T. (1985). Neuropathologies of speech and language: An introduction to patient management. In D. F. Johns (Ed.), *Clinical management of neurogenic communicative disorders* (Second Edition) (pp. 1–96). Boston: Little, Brown.

Wertz, R. T., Auther, L. L., & Ross, K. B. (1997). Aphasia in African-Americans and Caucasians: Severity, improvement, and rate of improvement. *Aphasiology,* 11, 533–542.

Wertz, R. T., Collins, M. J., Weiss, D. G., Kurtzke, J. F., Friden, T., Brookshire, R. H., Pierce, J., Holzapple, P., Hubbard, D. J., Porch, B. E., West, J. A., Davis, L., Matovich, V., Morley, G. K., & Resurreccion, E. (1981). Veterans Administration cooperative study on aphasia: A comparison of individual and group treatment. *Journal of Speech and Hearing Research,* 24, 580–594.

Wertz, R. T., Deal, J. L., Holland, A. L., Kurtzke, J. F., & Weiss, D. G. (1986). Comments on an uncontrolled aphasia no treatment trial. *Asha,* 28, 31.

Wertz, R. T., Deal, J. L., & Robinson, A. J. (1984). Classifying the aphasias: A comparison of the Boston Diagnostic Aphasia Examination and the Western Aphasia Battery. In R. H. Brookshire (Ed.), *Clinical aphasiology conference proceedings* (pp. 40–47). Minneapolis: BRK.

Wertz, R. T., Deal, L. M., & Deal, J. L. (1980). Prognosis in aphasia: Investigation of the High-Overall Predition (HOAP) method and the Short-Direct or HOAP-Slope method to predict change in PICA performance. In R. H. Brookshire (Ed.), *Clinical aphasiology conference proceedings* (pp. 164–173). Minneapolis: BRK.

Wertz, R. T., & Dronkers, N. F. (1994). PICA performance following left or right hemisphere brain damage: Influence of side and severity. M. L. Lemme (Ed.), *Clinical aphasiology* (Vol. 22) (pp. 157–164).

Wertz, R. T., Dronkers, N. F., & Shubitowski, Y. (1986). Discriminant function analysis of performance by normals and left hemisphere, right hemisphere, and bilaterally brain damaged patients on a word fluency measure. In R. H. Brookshire (Ed.),

Clinical aphasiology (Vol. 16) (pp. 257–266). Minneapolis: BRK.

Wertz, R. T., Kitselman, K. P., & Deal, L. A. (1981). Classifying the aphasias: Methods, prognostic implications, and efficacy of treatment. Miniseminar at the American Speech-Language-Hearing Association Convention, Los Angeles, November.

Wertz, R. T., Weiss, D. G., Aten, J. L., Brookshire, R. H., Garcia-Bunuel, L., Holland, A. L., Kurtzke, J. F., LaPointe, L. L., Milianti, F. J., Brannegan, R., Greenbaum, H., Marshall, R. C., Vogel, D., Carter, J., Barnes, N. S., & Goodman, R. (1986). Comparison of clinic, home, and deferred language treatment for aphasia: A Veterans Administration cooperative study. *Archives of Neurology,* 43, 653–658.

West, J. A. (1973). Auditory comprehension in aphasic adults: Improvement through training. *Archives of Physical Medicine and Rehabilitation,* 54, 78–86.

Westbury, C., & Bub, D. (1997). Primary progressive aphasia: A review of 112 cases. *Brain and Language,* 60, 381–406.

Weylman, S. T., Brownell, H. H., Roman, M., & Gardner, H. (1989). Appreciation of indirect requests by left- and right-brain-damaged patients: The effects of verbal context and conventionality of wording. *Brain and Language,* 36, 580–591.

Whitaker, H. A., & Noll, J. D. (1972). Some linguistic parameters of the Token Test. *Neuropsychologia,* 10, 395–404.

Whiteley, A. M., & Warrington, E. M. (1977). Prosopagnosia: A clinical, psychological and anatomical study of three patients. *Journal of Neurology, Neurosurgery, and Psychiatry,* 40, 395–403.

Whiteley, A. M., & Warrington, E. K. (1978). Selective impairment of topographical memory: A single case study. *Journal of Neurology, Neurosurgery, and Psychiatry,* 41, 575–578.

Wiig, E. H., & Secord, W. A. (1994). Language disabilities in school-age children and youth. In G. H. Shames, E. H. Wiig, & W. A. Secord (Eds.). *Human communication disorders: An introduction* (4th ed.) (pp. 212–247). New York: Merrill.

Wilcox, M. J., Davis, G. A., & Leonard, L. L. (1978). Aphasics' comprehension of contextually conveyed meaning. *Brain and Language,* 6, 362–377.

Williams, S. E., & Canter, G. J. (1982). The influence of situational context on naming performance in aphasic syndromes. *Brain and Language,* 17, 92–106.

Williams, S. E., & Canter, G. J. (1987). Action-naming performance in four syndromes of aphasia. *Brain and Language,* 32, 124–136.

Williams, S. E., & Seaver, E. J. (1986). A comparison of speech sound durations in three syndromes of aphasia. *Brain and Language,* 29, 171–182.

Willmes, K. (1990). Statistical methods for a single-case study approach to aphasia therapy research. *Aphasiology,* 4, 415–436.

Willmes, K. (1995). Aphasia therapy research: Some psychometric considerations and statistical methods for the single-case study approach. In C. Code & D. J. Müller (Eds.), *The treatment of aphasia: From theory to practice* (pp. 286–308). San Diego, CA: Singular.

Willmes, K. Poeck, K., Weniger, D., & Huber, W. (1983). Facet theory applied to the construction and validation of the Aachen Aphasia Test. *Brain and Language,* 18, 259–276.

Wingfield, A., & Wayland, S. C. (1988). Object-naming in aphasia: Word-initial phonology and response activation. *Aphasiology,* 2, 423–426.

Winner, E., & Gardner, H. (1977). Comprehension of metaphor in brain damaged patients. *Brain,* 100, 717–729.

Winograd, E., & Killinger, W. A. (1983). Relating age at encoding in early childhood to adult recall: Development of flashbulb memories. *Journal of Experimental Psychology: General,* 112, 413–422.

Wulf, H. H. (1979). *My world alone.* Detroit: Wayne State University Press.

Wulfeck, B. B. (1988). Grammaticality judgments and sentence comprehension in agrammatic aphasia. *Journal of Speech and Hearing Research,* 31, 72–80.

Wulfeck, B., Bates, E., & Capasso, R. (1991). A cross-linguistic study of grammaticality judgments in Broca's aphasia. *Brain and Language,* 41, 311–336.

Yasuda, K., & Ono, Y. (1998). Comprehension of famous personal and geographical names in global aphasic subjects. *Brain and Language,* 61, 274–287.

Yedor, K. E., Conlon, C. P., & Kearns, K. P. (1993). Measurements predictive of generalization of response elaboration training. In M. L. Lemme (Ed.), *Clinical aphasiology* (Vol. 21) (pp. 213–223). Austin, Tx: Pro-Ed.

Yiu, E. M-L., & Worrall, L. E. (1996). Sentence production ability of a bilingual Cantonese/

English agrammatic speaker. *Aphasiology,* 10, 505–522.

Ylvisaker, M., & Holland, A. L. (1985). Coaching, self-coaching, and rehabilitation of head injury. In D. F. Johns (Ed.), *Clinical managagement of neurogenic communicative disorders* (2nd ed. (pp. 243–257). Boston: Little, Brown.

Ylvisaker, M., & Szekeres, S. F. (1986). Management of the patient with closed head injury. In R. Chapey (Ed.), *Language intervention strategies in adult aphasia* (2nd ed.) (pp. 474–490). Baltimore: Williams & Wilkins.

Yorkston, K. M., & Beukelman, D. R. (1980). An analysis of connected speech samples of aphasic and normal speakers. *Journal of Speech and Hearing Disorders,* 45, 27–36.

Yorkston, K. M., Marshall, R. C., & Butler, M. (1977). Imposed delay of response: Effects on aphasics' auditory comprehension of visually and nonvisually cued material. *Perceptual and Motor Skills,* 44, 647–655.

Yorkston,, K. M., Stanton, K. M., & Beukelman, D. R. (1981). Language-based compensatory training for closed-head-injured patients. In R. H. Brookshire (Ed.), *Clinical aphasiology conference proceedings* (pp. 293–300). Minneapolis: BRK.

Young, A. W., & De Haan, E. H. F. (1988). Boundaries of covert recognition in prosopagnosia. *Cognitive Neuropsychology,* 5, 317–336.

Young, A. W., Newcombe, F., & Ellis, A. W. (1991). Different impairments contribute to neglect dyslexia. *Cognitive Neuropsychology,* 8, 177–192.

Young, J. Z. (1986). What's in a brain? In C. Coen (Ed.), *Functions of the brain* (pp. 1–10). Oxford, UK: Clarendon.

Zangwill, O. (1946). Intelligence in aphasia. In A. De Reuck & M. O'Conner (Eds.), *Disorders of language* (pp. 261–274). London: Churchill.

Zatorre, R. J. (1989). On the representation of multiple languages in the brain: Old problems and new directions. *Brain and Language,* 36, 127–147.

Zingeser, L. B., & Berndt, R. S. (1988). Grammatical class and context effects in a case of pure anomia: Implications for models of lexical processing. *Cognitive Neuropsychology,* 5, 473–516.

Zingeser, L. B., & Berndt, R. S. (1990). Retrieval of nouns and verbs in agrammatism and anomia. *Brain and Language,* 39, 14–32.

Zoccolotti, P., Scabini, D., & Violani, C. (1982). Electrodermal responses in patients with unilateral brain damage. *Journal of Clinical Neuropsychology,* 4, 143–150.

Zraick, R. I., & Boone, D. R. (1991). Spouse attitudes toward the person with aphasia. *Journal of Speech and Hearing Research,* 34, 123–128.

Zurif, E. B., Caramazza, A., Myerson, R., & Galvin, J. (1974). Semantic feature representations for normal and aphasic language. *Brain and Language,* 1, 167–188.

Zurif, E. B., Gardner, H., & Brownell, H. H. (1989). The case against the case against group studies. *Brain and Cognition,* 10, 237–255.

Zurif, E. B., Swinney, D., Prather, P., Soloman, J., & Bushell, C. (1993). An on-line analysis of syntactic processing in Broca's and Wernicke's aphasia. *Brain and Language,* 45, 448–464.

Author Index

Subject Index